George Davey-Smith, best wishes from Hugh

MONICA
Monograph and Multimedia Sourcebook

World's largest study of heart disease, stroke, risk factors, and population trends 1979–2002

Edited by Hugh Tunstall-Pedoe

Prepared by Hugh Tunstall-Pedoe (Dundee), Kari Kuulasmaa (Helsinki), Hanna Tolonen (Helsinki), Moira Davidson (Dundee), Shanthi Mendis (Geneva)

with 64 other contributors

for

The WHO MONICA Project

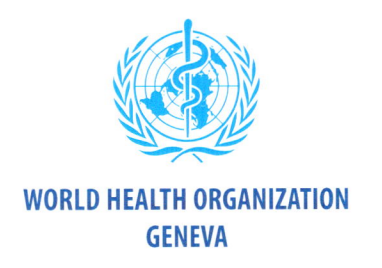

WORLD HEALTH ORGANIZATION
GENEVA

WHO Library Cataloguing-in-Publication Data

MONICA monograph and multimedia sourcebook / edited by Hugh Tunstall-
    Pedoe ; prepared by Hugh Tunstall-Pedoe . . . [et al.] with 64 other contributors
    for the WHO MONICA Project.

With accompanying CD-ROM.

1.Cardiovascular diseases—epidemiology   2.Coronary disease—epidemiology
3.Cerebrovascular accident—epidemiology   4.Program development
5.Epidemiologic methods   6.Multicenter studies   7.Resource guides
I.Tunstall-Pedoe, Hugh.   II.WHO MONICA Project.

ISBN 92 4 156223 4   (NLM classification: WG 16)

© Copyright World Health Organization (WHO) and the WHO MONICA Project Investigators 2003

All rights reserved. Extracts of the document may be reviewed, reproduced or translated for research or private study but not for sale or for use for commercial purposes. Any use of information in this Monograph should be accompanied by citation of the Editor, the section author(s) where relevant, and WHO MONICA Project. Any use of the document other than for educational or other non-commercial purposes, requires explicit, prior authorization in writing. Applications and enquiries should be directed in the first instance to the Office of Cardiovascular Diseases, World Health Organization, 1211 Geneva 27, Switzerland who will consult the relevant MONICA Investigators as appropriate.

The designations employed and the presentation of the information in this Monograph do not imply the expression of any opinion whatsoever on the part of WHO, or the WHO MONICA Project Investigators, concerning the legal status of any country, territory, city or area or of its authorities, or concerning the delimitation of its frontiers or boundaries.

The mention of specific companies or of certain manufacturers' products does not imply that they are endorsed or recommended by the WHO or WHO MONICA Project Investigators in preference to others of a similar nature that are not mentioned. Errors and omissions excepted, the names of proprietary products are identified by initial capital letters. The views expressed are those of the authors concerned and/or of the editor, and not necessarily those of the World Health Organization.

Note that this copyright notice applies to the printed text, graphics and other illustrations of this Monograph. The CD-ROMs which come with it are covered by their own copyright notice.

Designed in New Zealand • Typeset in Hong Kong • Printed in Singapore

Contents

Acknowledgements	ix
Contributors	x
Welcome to the Monograph from Minneapolis *Russell Luepker*	xii
Congratulations! *Dag Thelle*	xiii
MONICA and the World Health Organization *Derek Yach*	xiv
MONICA: the European Contribution *Philippe Busquin*	xv
Editor's Introduction *Hugh Tunstall-Pedoe*	xvi
Glossary, Abbreviations and Nicknames *Hugh Tunstall-Pedoe*	xviii

Background, Development and Organization of MONICA — 1

1	Background to the WHO MONICA Project *Hugh Tunstall-Pedoe*	1
2	MONICA Hypotheses and Study Design *Hugh Tunstall-Pedoe*	3
3	Organization Chart of the WHO MONICA Project *Hugh Tunstall-Pedoe*	6
4	Council of Principal Investigators (CPI) and MONICA Congresses and Symposia *Marco Ferrario, Hugh Tunstall-Pedoe*	7
5	MONICA Steering Committee (MSC) *Stephen Fortmann, Hugh Tunstall-Pedoe*	9
6	MONICA Management Centre (MMC) *Hugh Tunstall-Pedoe, Shanthi Mendis*	11
7	MONICA Data Centre (MDC) *Kari Kuulasmaa*	13
8	MONICA Quality Control Centres (MQCs) *Hugh Tunstall-Pedoe*	15
9	MONICA Reference Centres (MRCs) *Hugh Tunstall-Pedoe*	18
10	Recruitment of Populations *Jaakko Tuomilehto, Zbyněk Píša, Hugh Tunstall-Pedoe*	20
11	Communications in MONICA *Hugh Tunstall-Pedoe*	22
12	Quality Assurance *Dale Williams, Kari Kuulasmaa*	25
13	Ethics and Confidentiality *Alun Evans, Hugh Tunstall-Pedoe*	26
14	MONICA and the Prevention of Cardiovascular Disease *Pekka Puska*	28
15	Reminiscences of MONICA's Rapporteur *Hugh Tunstall-Pedoe*	30

Administrative Data — 35

16	Routine Mortality Data *Annette Dobson*	35
17	Demographic Data *Vladislav Moltchanov*	36
18	Health Services *Michael Hobbs*	37
19	Other Documents Used in MONICA *Hugh Tunstall-Pedoe*	38

Coronary-Event Registration and Coronary Care — 41

20	Registration of Coronary Events, Hot and Cold Pursuit *Hugh Tunstall-Pedoe*	41
21	Coronary-Event Registration Record Form *Hugh Tunstall-Pedoe*	43
22	Minnesota Coding of the Electrocardiogram (ECG) *Hugh Tunstall-Pedoe*	44
23	Diagnosing Myocardial Infarction and Coronary Death *Hugh Tunstall-Pedoe*	46
24	Acute Coronary Care *Diego Vanuzzo*	48
25	Treatment Scores *Hugh Tunstall-Pedoe*	50

Stroke Registration — 53

26	Registration of Stroke Events *Kjell Asplund*	53
27	Diagnosis of Stroke *Kjell Asplund*	54

Population Surveys — 57

28	Sampling *Kari Kuulasmaa*	57
29	Recruitment and Response Rates *Andrzej Pająk, Hermann Wolf*	58
30	Questionnaire Design and Contents *Hanna Tolonen, Kari Kuulasmaa*	59
31	Smoking *Alun Evans, Hugh Tunstall-Pedoe*	61

32	Blood Pressure	*Hans-Werner Hense*	62
33	Cholesterol	*Marco Ferrario*	64
34	Height, Weight and Waist Circumference	*Susana Sans*	66
35	Risk-Factor Scores	*Hanna Tolonen*	68

Data Handling, Quality Assessment and Publication 71

36	Data Transfer, Checking and Management	*Esa Ruokokoski, Markku Mähönen*	71
37	Event Rates, Case Fatality and Trends	*Hugh Tunstall-Pedoe*	72
38	Population Prevalence and Trends	*Hanna Tolonen*	74
39	Age Standardization	*Hanna Tolonen*	75
40	Statistical Analysis—relating changes in risk factors and treatments to changes in event rates	*Annette Dobson*	77
41	Preparation of Manuscripts and Presentations	*Kjell Asplund*	78
42	Making Graphics for MONICA	*Hanna Tolonen*	80

MONICA Optional Studies 83

43	Optional Studies—Beyond the Core	*Hugh Tunstall-Pedoe*	83
44	MONICA Optional Study on Nutrition	*Daan Kromhout*	85
45	MONICA Optional Study on Antioxidant Vitamins and Polyunsaturated Fatty Acids (PUFA)	*Hugh Tunstall-Pedoe*	85
46	MONICA Optional Psychosocial Substudy (MOPSY)	*Aushra Shatchkute*	86
47	MONICA Optional Study of Physical Activity (MOSPA)	*Deborah Jones*	87
48	MONICA Optional Study on Drugs	*Eberhard Greiser, Katrin Janhsen*	88
49	MONICA Optional Study on Haemostatic Risk Factors	*John Yarnell, Evelyn McCrum, Alun Evans*	89

MONICA Populations 91

50	Introduction to Population Pages	*Hugh Tunstall-Pedoe*	91
51	Australia-Newcastle (AUS-NEW, AN)	*Annette Dobson*	93
52	Australia-Perth (AUS-PER, AP)	*Michael Hobbs, Konrad Jamrozik*	94
53	Belgium-Ghent/Charleroi (BEL-GCH, BE)	*Guy De Backer, Stefaan De Henauw, Marcel Kornitzer*	95
54	Canada-Halifax (CAN-HAL, CA)	*Hermann Wolf, Ronald Gregor, Iqbal Bata*	96
55	China-Beijing (CHN-BEI, CN)	*Zhaosu Wu*	97
56	Czech Republic (CZE-CZE, CZ)	*Zdenka Škodová, Zbyněk Píša*	98
57	Denmark-Glostrup (DEN-GLO, DN)	*Marianne Schroll*	99
58	Finland (FIN-FIN, FI)	*Jaakko Tuomilehto*	100
59	France-Country Coordinating Centre	*Pierre Ducimetière, Annie Bingham*	102
60	France-Lille (FRA-LIL, FL)	*Philippe Amouyel*	103
61	France-Strasbourg (FRA-STR, FS)	*Dominique Arveiler*	104
62	France-Toulouse (FRA-TOU, FT)	*Jean Ferrières*	105
63	Germany-Augsburg (GER-AUG, GA)	*Ulrich Keil*	106
64	Germany-Bremen (GER-BRE, GB)	*Eberhard Greiser, Katrin Janhsen*	107
65	Germany-East Germany (GER-EGE, GE)	*Lothar Heinemann*	108
66	Iceland (ICE-ICE, IC)	*Nikulás Sigfússon*	109
67	Italy-Country Coordinating Centre	*Simona Giampaoli*	110
68	Italy-Brianza (ITA-BRI, IT)	*Marco Ferrario, Giancarlo Cesana*	111
69	Italy-Friuli (ITA-FRI, IF)	*Diego Vanuzzo, Lorenza Pilotto*	112
70	Lithuania-Kaunas (LTU-KAU, LT)	*Juozas Bluzhas, Stase Domarkiene*	113
71	New Zealand-Auckland (NEZ-AUC, NZ)	*Alistair Stewart*	114
72	Poland-Tarnobrzeg Voivodship (POL-TAR, PT)	*Andrzej Pająk, Roman Topór-Mądry*	115
73	Poland-Warsaw (POL-WAR, PW)	*Stefan Rywik*	116
74	Russia-Moscow (RUS-MOS, RM)	*Vladislav Moltchanov, Hugh Tunstall-Pedoe, Svetlana Shalnova*	117
75	Russia-Novosibirsk (RUS-NOV, RN)	*Sofia Malyutina, Yuri Nikitin*	118
76	Spain-Catalonia (SPA-CAT, SP)	*Susana Sans, Ignacio Balaguer-Vintró*	119
77	Sweden-Gothenburg (SWE-GOT, SG)	*Lars Wilhelmsen*	120
78	Sweden-Northern Sweden (SWE-NSW, SN)	*Kjell Asplund*	121
79	Switzerland (SWI-SWI, SW)	*Vincent Wietlisbach*	122
80	United Kingdom-Belfast (UNK-BEL, UB)	*Alun Evans*	123
81	United Kingdom-Glasgow (UNK-GLA, UG)	*Hugh Tunstall-Pedoe, Caroline Morrison*	124
82	United States-Stanford (USA-STA, US)	*Stephen Fortmann*	125
83	Yugoslavia-Novi Sad (YUG-NOS, YU)	*Milutin Planojevic, Djordje Jakovljevic*	126
84	Former MONICA Populations	*Kari Kuulasmaa, Hugh Tunstall-Pedoe*	127

MONICA Publications | 129

85	MONICA Publications list	129
86	Abstracts of MONICA Publications	131
87	MONICA Publications on the World Wide Web	146
88	MONICA Memo (list only: for text see CD-ROMs)	148

MONICA Graphics | 157

89	MONICA Graphics *Hugh Tunstall-Pedoe, Hanna Tolonen* (See below for listing)	157

Appendix | 239

Index | 241

CD-ROMs | 244

Introduction to CD-ROMs *Kari Kuulasmaa* 244
CD-ROMs, in back cover, contain own contents and authorship credits

List of MONICA Graphics

Populations, data collection and official mortality | 158

G1	Populations outside Europe used in testing the MONICA hypotheses	159
G2	European populations used in testing the MONICA hypotheses	159
G3	Death rates from various causes: first three years of coronary-event registration	161
G4	Death rates from various causes: final three years of coronary-event registration	161
G5	Ranking of populations by proportion of all deaths from cardiovascular causes: first three years of coronary-event registration	163
G6	Populations by proportion of all deaths from cardiovascular causes: final three years of coronary-event registration	163
G7	Populations using different methods of identifying non-fatal cases for coronary-event registration	165
G8	Years of coronary-event registration in different populations	165
G9	Years of stroke registration in different populations	167
G10	Timing of risk factor surveys in different populations	167
G11	Periods used for testing the MONICA coronary-care (treatment or second) hypothesis	169

Coronary events: incidence, case fatality and mortality rates | 170

G12	Coronary-event rates: first three years of registration	171
G13	Coronary-event rates: final three years of registration	171
G14	Coronary-event rates by calendar year of registration	173
G15	Average annual change in coronary-event rates	173
G16	Case fatality for coronary events: first three years of registration	175
G17	Case fatality for coronary events: final three years of registration	175
G18	Average annual change in case fatality	177
G19	Populations ranked by ten-year average MONICA coronary heart disease (CHD) mortality rates showing official unvalidated rates	177
G20	Populations ranked by average annual change in MONICA CHD mortality rates, showing unvalidated (from routine mortality reporting) trend equivalents	179
G21	Change in coronary end points, by population, against coronary-event quality score	179
G22	Average annual change in MONICA coronary heart disease (CHD) mortality rates	181
G23	Changes in MONICA coronary heart disease (CHD) mortality rates divided between changes in coronary-event rates and changes in case fatality	181
G24	Spot maps of changes in coronary end points in men	183
G25	Spot maps of changes in coronary end points in women	183

Strokes: incidence, case fatality and mortality rates | 184

G26	Overall stroke rates: first three years and final three years of registration	185
G27	Overall stroke rates by calendar year of registration	185

G28	Stroke case fatality: first three and final three years of registration	187
G29	Average annual change in stroke-event rates and in case fatality	187
G30	Stroke mortality rates: first three years and final three years of registration	189
G31	Changes in stroke mortality rates divided between changes in stroke-event rates and changes in case fatality	189
G32	Spot maps of changes in stroke end points in men	191
G33	Spot maps of changes in stroke end points in women	191
G34	Change in stroke end points, by population, against stroke-event quality scores	193
G35	Event rates and case fatality: subarachnoid haemorrhage	193

Risk factors: daily cigarette smoking — 194

G36	Prevalence of daily cigarette smokers in the initial risk-factor survey	195
G37	Prevalence of daily cigarette smokers in the final risk-factor survey	195
G38	Ten-year change in prevalence of daily cigarettes smokers	197
G39	Spot maps of population changes in prevalence of daily cigarette smoking	197

Risk factors: systolic blood pressure — 198

G40	Average systolic blood pressure in the initial risk-factor survey	199
G41	Average systolic blood pressure in the final risk-factor survey	199
G42	Ten-year change in average systolic blood pressure	201
G43	Spot maps of population changes in average systolic blood pressure	201

Risk factors: total blood cholesterol — 202

G44	Average blood cholesterol concentration in the initial risk-factor survey	203
G45	Average blood cholesterol concentration in the final risk-factor survey	203
G46	Ten-year change in average blood cholesterol concentration	205
G47	Spot maps of population changes in average blood cholesterol concentration	205

Risk factors: obesity, body mass index — 206

G48	Average body mass index (BMI) in the initial risk-factor survey	207
G49	Average body mass index (BMI) in the final risk-factor survey	207
G50	Ten-year change in average body mass index (BMI)	209
G51	Spot maps of population changes in average body mass index (BMI)	209

Risk factors: risk-factor score — 210

G52	Average coronary risk-factor score in the initial risk-factor survey	211
G53	Average coronary risk-factor score in the final risk-factor survey	211
G54	Ten-year change in average coronary risk-factor score	213
G55	Spot maps of population changes in average coronary risk-factor score	213

Risk factors: risk-factor quality scores — 214

G56	Scatter plots by population of change in risk factors against their quality scores	215

Eight evidence-based treatments in coronary care — 216

G57	Change in beta blocker use before myocardial infarction	217
G58	Change in beta blocker use during myocardial infarction	217
G59	Change in antiplatelet (aspirin) use before myocardial infarction	219
G60	Change in antiplatelet (aspirin) use during myocardial infarction	219
G61	Change in angiotensin converting enzyme (ACE) inhibitor use before myocardial infarction	221
G62	Change in angiotensin converting enzyme (ACE) inhibitor use during myocardial infarction	221
G63	Change in coronary artery revascularization (bypass graft or angioplasty) before myocardial infarction	223
G64	Change in thrombolytic drug use during myocardial infarction	223
G65	Change in Equivalent Treatment Score	225
G66	Populations ranked by change in Equivalent Treatment Score	225
G67	Scatter plot of change in Equivalent Treatment Score against the acute coronary care quality score	227
G68	Spot maps of population changes in Equivalent Treatment Score	227

Hypotheses: coronary disease and coronary risk factors — 228

G69	First MONICA hypothesis: change in coronary-event rates against change in coronary risk-factor score, full registration period	229
G70	First MONICA hypothesis: change in coronary-event rates against change in coronary risk-factor score, lagged registration period	229

G71	First MONICA hypothesis: change in coronary-event rates against change in individual coronary risk factors, full coronary-event registration period	231
G72	First MONICA hypothesis: change in coronary-event rates against change in individual coronary risk factors, lagged coronary-event registration period	231

Hypotheses: stroke and stroke risk factors   232

G73	First MONICA stroke hypothesis: change in stroke-event rates against change in stroke risk-factor score, full stroke-event registration period	233
G74	First MONICA stroke hypothesis: change in stroke-event rates against change in stroke risk-factor score, lagged stroke-event registration period	233
G75	Change in stroke-event rates against change in individual stroke risk factors, full stroke-event registration period	235
G76	Change in stroke-event rates against change in individual stroke risk factors, lagged stroke-event registration period	235

Hypotheses: coronary care   236

G77a	Second MONICA hypothesis: change in case fatality against change in Equivalent Treatment Score	237
G77b	Second MONICA hypothesis: change in coronary-event rates against change in Equivalent Treatment Score	237
G77c	Second MONICA hypothesis: change in MONICA coronary heart disease (CHD) mortality rates against change in Equivalent Treatment Score	237

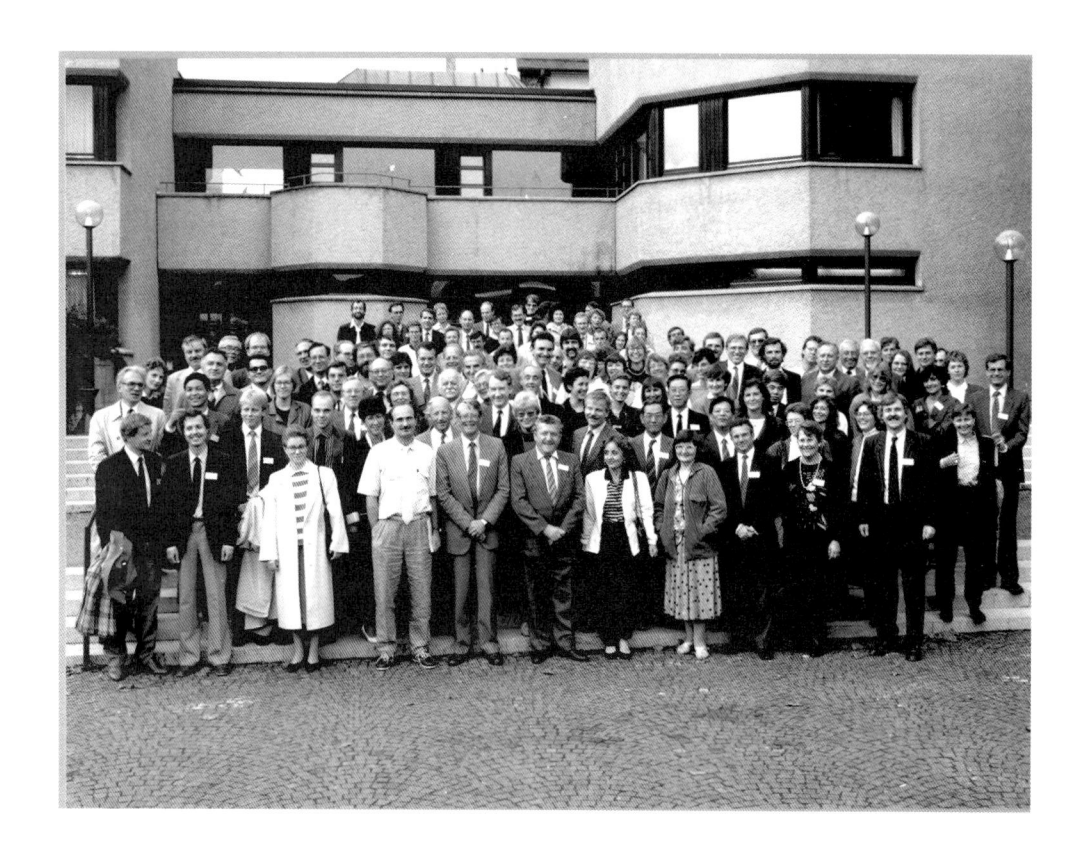

Acknowledgements

The MONICA Centres were funded predominantly by regional and national governments, research councils, and research charities. The World Health Organization (WHO) was responsible for coordination. It was assisted in the organization of congresses and workshops by local staff and fund raising efforts. WHO also supported the MONICA Data Centre (MDC) in Helsinki. In addition, generous long-term support for the MDC was provided by the National Public Health Institute of Finland (KTL), as well as through repeated contributions made to WHO by the National Heart, Lung, and Blood Institute, National Institutes of Health, Bethesda, Maryland, USA. These supported the MDC and the Quality Control Centre for Event Registration in Dundee. The completion of the MONICA Project was made possible by a generous Concerted Action Grant from the European Commission under its BIOMED programme: BMH4-96-1693: MONICA:Multinational MONItoring of trends and determinants in CArdiovascular disease. Subsequently, archiving of MONICA data and substantial funding for the production of this Monograph were provided by a Shared Cost Grant from the BIOMED 2 Third Call from the European Commission, Contract BMH4-CT98-3183: the MORGAM Project: MONica Risk, Genetics, Archiving and Monograph. Recurrent grants to support data analysis and the preparation of publications were also gratefully received from ASTRA Hässle AB, Sweden, Hoechst AG, Germany, Hoffmann-La Roche Ltd, Switzerland, the Institut de Recherches Internationales Servier (IRIS), France, and Merck & Co. Inc., Whitehouse Station, NJ, USA. Preparation of this Monograph was supported by all these grants. Final production costs were financed by the BIOMED 2 grant from the European Commission, by the World Health Organization, and by specific grants from the British Heart Foundation (funding production costs of the Monograph CD-ROMs) the Swedish Heart and Chest Foundation, AstraZeneca , the Becel Institute from Unilever, Boehringer-Ingelheim, GlaxoSmithKline, Merck and Co. Inc., Whitehouse Station, NJ, USA and Pfizer Inc.

Abstracts of MONICA publications are reproduced with the permission of their journal publishers. Many photographs were provided by MONICA investigators and other colleagues. Thanks are due to Caroline Morrison in Glasgow and Alun Evans in Belfast for photographs of MONICA activities, and to the MONICA Data Centre for photographs taken at MONICA Principal Investigator meetings in the 1980s. The Editor recorded several photographs for the Monograph and downloaded others from the internet. WHO Headquarters, pages xx and 9 courtesy Pierre Virot/WHO; and Stanford, page 125 courtesy Stanford News Service.

The *MONICA Monograph and Multimedia Sourcebook* has been written and produced by the MONICA collaboration without any personal payments.

The World Health Organization and the WHO MONICA Project acknowledge the outstanding contribution to this project of Hugh Tunstall-Pedoe of the Cardiovascular Epidemiology Unit, Institute of Cardiovascular Research, University of Dundee, Scotland, in masterminding, leading and managing it from its inception, and as editor, principal author and fund-raiser; also that of Kari Kuulasmaa and Hanna Tolonen and their colleagues in the former MONICA Data Centre, now the International CVD Epidemiology Unit of the National Public Health Institute in Helsinki, Finland.

Contributors

Origins of contributors are not stated if they are implicit in their contributions

Amouyel, Philippe	*Editorial Advisory Group.* #60 France-Lille
Arveiler, Dominique	#61 France-Strasbourg
Asplund, Kjell	*Editorial Advisory Group.* #26 Registration of Stroke Events, #27 Diagnosis of Stroke, #41 Preparation of Manuscripts and Presentations, #78 Sweden-Northern Sweden
Balaguer-Vintró, Ignacio	#76 Spain-Catalonia
Bata, Iqbal	#54 Canada-Halifax
Beaglehole, Robert	*Editorial Advisory Group. Auckland, New Zealand and Geneva, Switzerland*
Bingham, Annie	#59 France-Country Coordinating Centre
Bluzhas, Juozas	#70 Lithuania-Kaunas
Busquin, Philippe	MONICA: the European Contribution
Cesana, Giancarlo	#68 Italy-Brianza
De Backer, Guy	#53 Belgium-Ghent/Charleroi
De Henauw, Stefaan	#53 Belgium-Ghent/Charleroi
Davidson, Moira	*Prepared by Group. Dundee, Scotland, UK*
Dobson, Annette	*Editorial Advisory Group.* #16 Routine Mortality Data, #40 Statistical Analysis, #51 Australia-Newcastle
Domarkiene, Stase	#70 Lithuania-Kaunas
Ducimetière, Pierre	#59 France-Country Coordinating Centre
Evans, Alun	*Editorial Advisory Group.* #13 Ethics and Confidentiality, #31 Smoking, #49 MONICA Optional Study on Haemostatic Risk Factors, #80 United Kingdom-Belfast
Ferrario, Marco	*Editorial Advisory Group.* #4 Council of Principal Investigators (CPI) and MONICA Congresses and Symposia, #33 Cholesterol, #68 Italy-Brianza
Ferrières, Jean	#62 France-Toulouse
Fortmann, Stephen	*Editorial Advisory Group.* #5 MONICA Steering Committee (MSC), #82 USA-Stanford
Giampaoli, Simona	#67 Italy-Country Coordinating Centre
Gregor, Ronald	#54 Canada-Halifax
Greiser, Eberhard	#48 MONICA Optional Study on Drugs, #64 Germany-Bremen
Gutzwiller, Felix	*Editorial Advisory Group. Zurich, Switzerland*
Heinemann, Lothar	#65 Germany-East Germany
Hense, Hans-Werner	#32 Blood Pressure. *Münster, Germany*
Hobbs, Michael	*Editorial Advisory Group.* #18 Health Services, #52 Australia-Perth
Jakovljevic, Djordje	#83 Yugoslavia-Novi Sad
Janhsen, Katrin	#48 MONICA Optional Study on Drugs, #64 Germany-Bremen
Jones, Deborah	#47 MONICA Optional Study on Physical Activity (MOSPA).
Keil, Ulrich	*Editorial Advisory Group.* #63 Germany-Augsburg
Kornitzer, Marcel	#53 Belgium-Ghent/Charleroi
Kromhout, Daan	#44 MONICA Optional Study on Nutrition
Kuulasmaa, Kari	*Prepared by Group.* #7 MONICA Data Centre (MDC), #12 Quality Assurance, #28 Sampling, #30 Questionnaire Design and Contents, #84 Former MONICA Populations, #92 Introduction to CD-ROMs
Luepker, Russell	Welcome to the Monograph from Minneapolis
McCrum, Evelyn	#49 MONICA Optional Studies on Haemostatic Risk Factors
Mähönen, Markku	#36 Data Transfer, Checking and Management. *Helsinki, Finland*
Malyutina, Sofia	#75 Russia-Novosibirsk
Mendis, Shanthi	*Prepared by Group.* #6 MONICA Management Centre (MMC)
Moltchanov, Vladislav	#17 Demographic Data, #74 Russia-Moscow. *Helsinki, Finland*
Morrison, Caroline	#81 United Kingdom-Glasgow

Nikitin, Yuri	#75 Russia-Novosibirsk
Pająk, Andrzej	*Editorial Advisory Group.* #29 Recruitment and Response Rates, #72 Poland-Tarnobrzeg Voivodship
Pilotto, Lorenza	#69 Italy-Friuli
Planojevic, Milutin	#83 Yugoslavia-Novi Sad
Píša, Zbyněk	#10 Recruitment of Populations, #56 Czech Republic
Puska, Pekka	#14 MONICA and the Prevention of Cardiovascular Disease
Rywik, Stefan	*Editorial Advisory Group.* #73 Poland-Warsaw
Ruokokoski, Esa	#36 Data Transfer, Checking and Management. *Helsinki, Finland*
Sans, Susana	*Editorial Advisory Group.* #34 Height, Weight and Waist Circumference, #76 Spain-Catalonia
Schroll, Marianne	#57 Denmark-Glostrup
Shalnova, Svetlana	#74 Russia-Moscow
Shatchkute, Aushra	*Editorial Advisory Group.* #46 MONICA Optional Psychosocial Substudy (MOPSY)
Sigfússon, Nikulás	#66 Iceland
Škodová, Zdenka	#56 Czech Republic
Stewart, Alistair	#71 New Zealand-Auckland
Thelle, Dag	Congratulations! *Gothenburg, Sweden*
Tolonen, Hanna	*Prepared by Group.* #30 Questionnaire Design and Content, #35 Risk-Factor Scores, #38 Population Prevalence and Trends, #39 Age Standardization, #42 Making Graphics for MONICA, #89 MONICA Graphics. *Helsinki, Finland*
Topór-Mądry, Roman	#72 Poland-Tarnobrzeg Voivodship
Tunstall-Pedoe, Hugh	*Monograph Editor. Prepared by Group.* Editor's Introduction, Glossary, Abbreviations and Nicknames, #1 Background to the WHO MONICA Project, #2 MONICA Hypotheses and Study Design, #3 Organization Chart of the WHO MONICA Project, #4 Council of Principal Investigators (CPI) and MONICA Congresses and Symposia, #5 MONICA Steering Committee (MSC), #6 MONICA Management Centre (MMC), #8 MONICA Quality Control Centres (MQCs), #9 MONICA Reference Centres (MRCs), #10 Recruitment of Populations, #11 Communications in MONICA, #13 Ethics and Confidentiality, #15 Reminiscences of MONICA's Rapporteur, #19 Other Documents Used in MONICA, #20 Registration of Coronary Events, Hot and Cold Pursuit, #21 Coronary-Event Registration Record Form, #22 Minnesota Coding of the Electrocardiogram (ECG), #23 Diagnosing Myocardial Infarction and Coronary Death, #25 Treatment Scores, #31 Smoking, #37 Event Rates, Case Fatality and Trends, #43 Optional Studies—Beyond the Core, #45 MONICA Optional Study on Antioxidant Vitamins and Polyunsaturated Fatty Acids (PUFA), #50 Introduction to Population Pages, #74 Russia-Moscow, #81 United Kingdom-Glasgow, #84 Former MONICA Populations, #89 MONICA Graphics, (as well as all unattributed sections, helped by Kari Kuulasmaa and Hanna Tolonen).
Tuomilehto, Jaakko	#10 Recruitment of Populations, #58 Finland
Vanuzzo, Diego	#24 Acute Coronary Care, #69 Italy-Friuli
Wietlisbach, Vincent	#79 Switzerland
Wilhelmsen, Lars	#77 Sweden-Gothenburg
Williams, Dale	#12 Quality Assurance
Wolf, Hermann	#29 Recruitment and Response Rates, #54 Canada-Halifax
Yach, Derek	MONICA and the World Health Organization
Yarnell, John	#49 MONICA Optional Study on Haemostatic Risk Factors.
Zhaosu, Wu	#55 China-Beijing

Welcome to the Monograph from Minneapolis

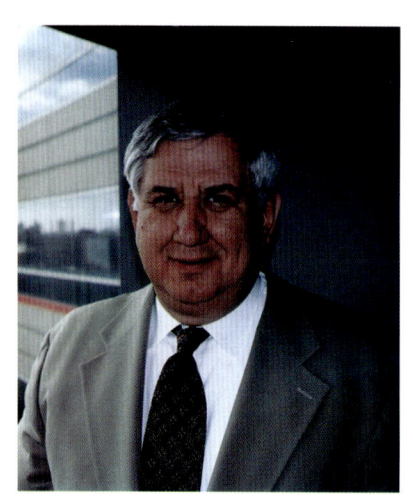

Russell Luepker

*For references see later introductory sections, particularly **#1 Background to the WHO MONICA Project.***

Cardiovascular epidemiology is a fairly recent discipline. Until 1975, it concentrated on identifying and substantiating the role played by classic risk factors in determining individual risk, as done, for example in the Framingham study, and also how they related to population disease rates, as, for example in the Seven Countries Study. Standardized methods of measurement were developed both in Minneapolis and elsewhere and formalized with the publication, in 1968 by the World Health Organization, of *Cardiovascular Survey Methods*, now entering its third edition.

In the mid-1970s there came the realization that mortality from coronary heart disease was falling in the United States. The seminal *Conference on the Decline in Coronary Heart Disease Mortality* was organized in Bethesda, USA in 1978. Its sponsor, the National Heart Lung and Blood Institute in Washington began to fund studies of cardiovascular disease trends in whole communities, such as the Minnesota Heart Survey—which ran concurrently with the planning and launch of the WHO MONICA Project—and later the ARIC study.

Despite consultation with and input of American expertise in the planning of MONICA, the major monitoring initiatives in the USA that began before or at the same time as MONICA were not completely compatible. This left only one US centre, Stanford, as a full MONICA participant providing data. American investigators, centrally funded and closely linked with one another, envied the great heterogeneity of the populations involved in the WHO MONICA Project. They did not, however, envy the consequent problems for standardization and data quality that MONICA struggled successfully to overcome. MONICA is a landmark study in our understanding of and efforts to control cardiovascular disease.

Having chaired the session of the European Congress of Cardiology in Vienna in 1998 at which many MONICA graphics were first displayed, I am delighted to now see them in print. On behalf of its American friends, I welcome the MONICA Monograph.

Russell Luepker
Division of Epidemiology, School of Public Health
University of Minnesota, Minneapolis USA

Congratulations!

The WHO MONICA Project was set up to explore trends in cardiovascular disease in different populations. These eventually encompassed 38 populations in 21 countries on four continents, but the biggest contributor was Europe. Never intended as a study of national disease trends, the Project nevertheless stimulated friendly international rivalry. When the closing date for entry was fixed for 1985 some of us realized that our own countries could never be represented. We were doomed to spend the next 15 years or so on the outside looking in—a regret shared, for example by Austrian, Dutch, English, Greek, Portuguese, and Republic of Ireland colleagues as well as by myself, a Norwegian.

During the 1980s and 1990s we watched your collaborative struggle to make the MONICA Project a success. Recently we have been stimulated and fascinated by the study results. Now you are sharing all aspects of the study with us in this Monograph and Multimedia Sourcebook. Apart from its scientific contribution, MONICA has ignited vivid interest around the world, disseminating both the concepts and the disciplined practice of cardiovascular epidemiology. The Monograph will further spread this learning and teaching process on the interface of cardiology and public health.

On behalf of all those on the outside involved in the epidemiology and prevention of cardiovascular disease, I would like to send my congratulations and best wishes to the MONICA family on this momentous publication. I encourage both insiders and outsiders to make maximum use of this amazing resource.

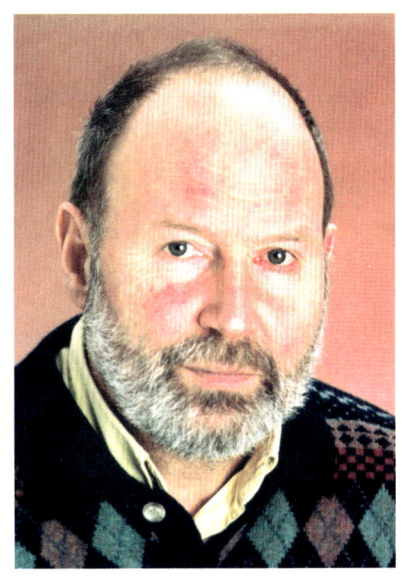

Dag Thelle
Cardiovascular Epidemiology and Prevention
Sahlgrenska University Hospital, Gothenburg, Sweden

MONICA and the World Health Organization

With the end of the Second World War, and the consequent foundation of the World HealthOrganization (WHO) in 1948, improved nutrition, education, immunization, quarantine, insecticides, antibiotics and other biomedical products helped to reduce the rates of many diseases caused by deficiency, bacteria and parasites. In many old and new industrializing countries however, life expectancy failed to improve proportionately, because of a rise in deaths from heart disease. Through the International Classification of Diseases, and the international format for death certificates, WHO helped to standardize recording and international comparison of death rates. Successive World Health Statistics Annuals reported striking differences in cardiovascular death rates between countries, but they also showed alarming increases in cardiovascular mortality in a large proportion of those countries that were able to provide such data.

In the 1960s and 1970s the European Regional Office of WHO convened expert groups to plan collaborative studies of cardiovascular disease and risk factors. It fostered the international standardization of definitions, for example of myocardial infarction, and the measurement of morbidity as in the European Myocardial Infarction Registers, as well as encouraging prevention.

At the end of the 1970s, intense interest in population trends in cardiovascular disease precipitated an initiative from the then Cardiovascular Diseases Unit at WHO Headquarters in Geneva. This encouraged those investigators intending to measure disease and risk-factor trends in their own populations to come together, to standardize their definitions and their measurements, and to combine their findings. This initiative led to the WHO MONICA Project.

MONICA was a huge undertaking—impossible without the pivotal role of WHO, but also the support of other organizations. This support included funding of participating centres by governments and charities, support for the MONICA Data Centre by the National Public Health Institute in Helsinki, Finland (KTL), and important supplementary funding for quality control, coordination and data analysis from the National Institutes of Health in Washington, and later from the European Commission and others, and now for publication of this Monograph.

MONICA combined the old with the new. It emphasized standardized measurement of mortality, morbidity, risk factors and medical care. In addition, it combined these potentially routine activities with the publication of quality control results on the Internet, the testing of hypotheses, and the publication of study results in prestigious scientific journals. These hypotheses could not have been tested within one population alone nor without WHO.

In this Monograph MONICA provides unique data on cardiovascular risk factors, mortality, morbidity and medical care from its numerous populations. It's release will bring added value to WHO's endeavour to place 'risks to health' on the global health agenda through the 2002 *World Health Report*. The WHR 2002 provides new estimates of the impact of current risk levels on present and projected mortality and morbidity. It highlights the urgent need to address core risk factors common to major noncommunicable diseases including cardiovascular disease. Further the new global estimates reiterate the need to take action on tobacco use, physical inactivity, overweight and lack of fruit and vegetables, as well as their intermediate manifestations; elevated cholesterol, blood pressure and blood sugar. The challenge is substantive and demands complex multisectoral approaches including upstream policy interventions, cost-effective health promotion and practice of clinical prevention.

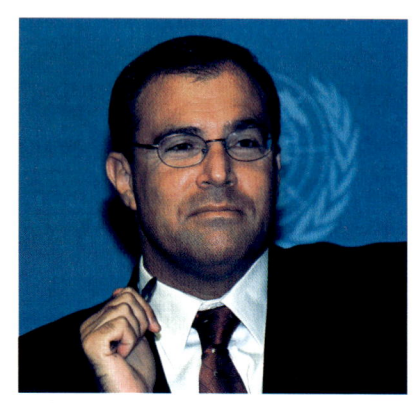

Derek Yach
Executive Director, Noncommunicable Diseases and Mental Health Cluster
World Health Organization, Geneva, Switzerland

MONICA: the European Contribution

The World Health Organization MONICA Project is an international study of cardiovascular disease that was initiated 23 years ago. It covers 38 populations in 21 countries and on four continents. The importance to the Project of contributions from Asia, Australasia, and North America should not be overlooked, however, the largest contribution in terms of numbers of populations and countries has come from the continent of Europe; from members of the European Union, its candidate members, and other countries in Europe which are closely linked to it and to each other. It was this predominance of European centres that enabled MONICA participants, when funding was scarce during its later years, to bid successfully to the European Commission for two different grants for funds to facilitate research coordination, data analysis and publications. The second of these grants substantially contributed towards funding preparation, editorial work and production of this Monograph.

Although many in Europe see themselves increasingly as European, Member States nonetheless encompass a great diversity of populations with large disparities in lifestyle and disease rates. These are well demonstrated in the following pages. MONICA and the World Health Organization have pioneered the standardized collection of disease, lifestyle and risk-factor data. This experience is now feeding back into the drafting of European guidelines for standard data sets for disease and risk-factor monitoring.

The publication of this Monograph is a major milestone for the World Health Organization and the MONICA investigators. Those involved should be proud of their achievement. That pride will be shared by the organizations and individuals who—in their different ways—helped bring this enterprise to its completion.

Philippe Busquin
European Commissioner for Research, Brussels, Belgium

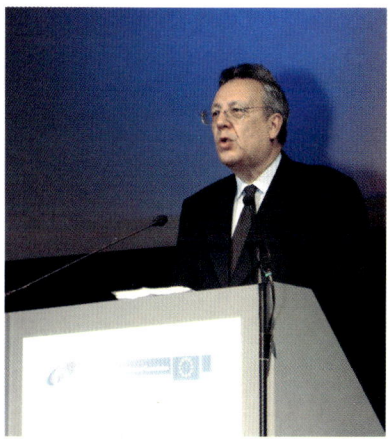

Philippe Busquin

Editor's Introduction

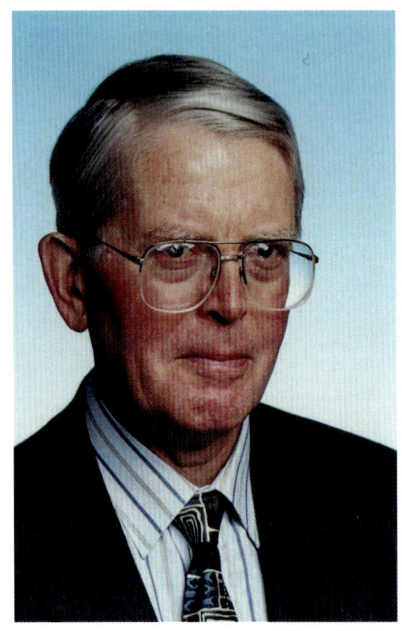

Hugh Tunstall-Pedoe

This Monograph marks the completion of the WHO MONICA Project. Extending to four continents over 23 years, MONICA is the largest and longest research project ever undertaken on heart disease and stroke. We are now sharing with a world readership the excitement and achievement of all that was put into MONICA—and what we and others have gained from it.

International collaboration is not easy, particularly with modern pressures on individual performance and rapid results. The 'MONICA family' has collaborated since 1979. In that time world systems and alliances changed, crises came and went, wars were fought, heads of state appeared and disappeared, but the 21 nationalities and 38 research groups in MONICA moved forward together.

MONICA evolved through different phases:
- development of the original concept and research plan
- standardization of methods, recruitment and training
- quality assurance in parallel with data collection
- publication of cross-sectional data
- maintaining and re-evaluating methods, training and quality assurance
- data processing and data analysis
- publication of quality assessments
- publication of main longitudinal results
- evaluation of the project and dissemination of findings.

This publication, from the final phase, brings everything together in a 'Monograph and Multimedia Sourcebook', to be used at the level of sophistication that the reader wants. It contains:

- explanations of what the study is about
- descriptions of the participating populations, the local study teams and their work
- abstracts of MONICA collaborative publications, with full references
- 79 graphics of the key MONICA results, with explanatory notes
- finally two CD-ROMs containing:
    a. The MONICA Manual
    b. MONICA Quality assessment reports
    c. methodological appendices to published papers
    d. MONICA Data Books incorporating tables of most of the variables
    e. a 20% sub-set of the MONICA Database for exploration
    f. slide shows covering each of the main MONICA topics
    g. copies of MONICA Memos.

This book can also be used as a textbook on epidemiology for students of medicine, nursing, social sciences and public health. Through its Data Books, it is a source of material for student exercises. The 20% sample Database is a challenge for those interested in data analysis.

The Monograph has been designed for a readership ranging from the general public to journalists and politicians, to medical administrators, medical students, the medical and para-medical professions and different medical specialities. The Monograph should be of interest to anyone interested in cardiac

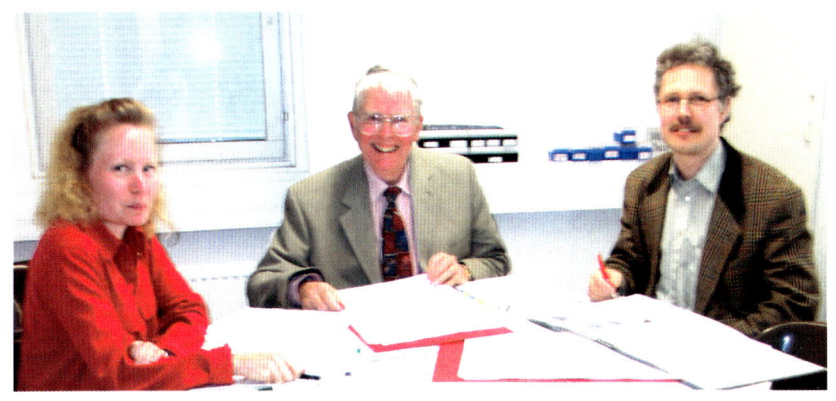

Hanna Tolonen (Helsinki), Hugh Tunstall-Pedoe (Dundee) and Kari Kuulasmaa (Helsinki) planning the Monograph in Helsinki, February 2001

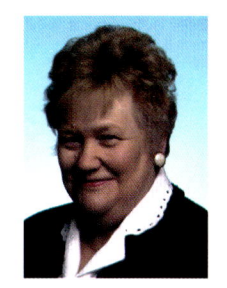

Moira Davidson (Dundee)

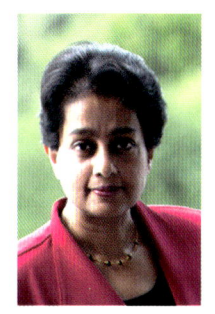

Shanthi Mendis (Geneva)

disease and stroke, in public health and epidemiology, and the wider issues of primary and secondary prevention, lifestyle, risk factors and health policy.

Whether you wish to browse through the graphics, assimilating information from them and the notes, or to read the book systematically, we hope you will share our excitement in the size and scope of this exercise. See how, by sharing our objectives and standardizing our methods, we have been able to draw conclusions for the public good from the variety of experiences of our different populations. The Monograph illustrates the value of international collaboration in understanding and controlling chronic diseases and their causes, and in the dissemination of sound scientific methods. The success of the Monograph will be judged by how much it stimulates health workers and administrators in different countries to think like epidemiologists—on a world scale—and to collaborate in tackling other similar challenges to world health.

Hugh Tunstall-Pedoe
Editor, MONICA Monograph and Multimedia Sourcebook

Glossary, Abbreviations and Nicknames

age standardization, age standardized, age adjusted
rates and outcomes vary with age. Comparison of groups with differing age structure can be misleading unless differences are adjusted for. See #39

AMI/MI
acute myocardial infarction. Heart muscle (myocardium) dies when the coronary artery feeding it is blocked. May be fatal but coronary deaths are not all infarct cases. See #23

attack rate
used in MONICA for 'incidence' of fatal plus non-fatal event rates. See #37

BMI
body mass index. Indicator of obesity: weight in kilograms divided by square of height in metres. See #34

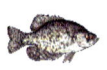

CARPFISH
nickname of manuscript group working on the MONICA Second (coronary care) Hypothesis and materials it produced. 'Coronary Artery Revascularization Procedures For Improving Survival from Heart attack'. Still found in some MONICA Web directories.

CAD
coronary artery disease. See CHD

case fatality
proportion of cases of the disease that are fatal within a specified time from onset; in MONICA 28 days, unless otherwise stated. Fatality percent = 100 − survival percent. Do not confuse fatality with mortality. See #37

CHD
coronary heart disease, also known as ischaemic heart disease (IHD). Caused by narrowing or obstruction of the coronary arteries by atheromatous (fatty) deposits and thrombosis, and resulting impairment of the blood supply to the myocardium or heart muscle.

cholesterol
also total, blood, serum or plasma cholesterol. Measured concentration of cholesterol in serum or plasma without regard to the accompanying lipoprotein, as millimoles per litre (mmol/l). Milligrams per decilitre is also used. 5 mmol/l = 192 mg/dl. One of three major, classic risk factors. See #33

CI, 95%CI
confidence interval. Wide interval means poor precision. 95% is the probability that the CI includes the value that is being estimated.

cold pursuit
registration of events from hospital discharge records, usually weeks or months after the event, extracting data from written material. Opposite of hot pursuit. See #20

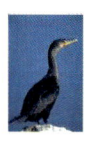

CORMORANT
nickname for first MONICA final-results paper and accompanying material. Derived from 'CORonary MORtality And Nonfatal Trends'. Found on MONICA Website directories.

coronary death
not all coronary deaths are from myocardial infarction so classification is complex. Can be sudden, but this is not a specific criterion in MONICA. See #23

coronary event
coronary heart attack, such as acute myocardial infarction or coronary death. MONICA excluded chronic angina pectoris and heart failure. See #23

CVD
cardiovascular diseases—diseases of the heart and blood vessels.

EARWIG
nickname of manuscript group and materials for the First (risk factor) MONICA Hypothesis, derived from 'EventuAl Results WorkIng Group". Found in MONICA Website directories.

event rate
rates compare disease in populations by standardizing denominator and time period, such as rate per 100 000 per year. Calculation involves time and denominator, not just numbers of events. See #37

HDL-cholesterol
high density lipoprotein cholesterol—a fifth to one third of the total cholesterol found in blood, serum or plasma—can be distinguished by its density and other physical and biological characteristics. It has been found to be a marker for reduced coronary risk in that high levels are protective, so its behaviour is paradoxical compared with total cholesterol. See cholesterol. See #33

hot pursuit
registration of events through hospital admissions. Allows interview of patients when information is incomplete. Daily surveillance of acute services is necessary and expensive. See cold pursuit. See #20

hypotheses, MONICA main hypotheses
MONICA enunciated two main coronary hypotheses: the First on coronary risk factors, the Second on coronary care. See #2. Stroke hypotheses came later, involving fewer centres and fewer events.

ICD, ICD-8, ICD-9, ICD-CM
International Classification of Diseases, published by World Health Organization, and used worldwide to code diseases and causes of death. The 8th edition 1965 was used by some Scandinavian MCCs, 9th edition 1977 by most MCCs, 10th edition not in use during MONICA. Clinical Modification (CM)—complex system used in some MCCs for hospital episodes.

Manual
MONICA 'bible', *WHO MONICA Project MONICA Manual*, contains the protocol and manual of operations for the study.

Originally in hard copy, then on the website, now on CD-ROM.

MCC
MONICA Collaborating Centre.

MDC
MONICA Data Centre, National Public Health Institute (KTL), Helsinki, Finland. See #7.

MMC
MONICA Management Centre at World Health Organization Headquarters in Geneva, Switzerland. See #6.

mmHg
millimetres of mercury, traditional unit for measuring blood pressure. The official international unit, although not in general use, is kilopascals. In conversion 100 mmHg is equal to 13.3 kPa.

mmol/l
millimoles per litre (mmol/l), standard (SI) units, replaced milligrams per decilitre (mg/dl) for reporting laboratory results in many countries. For cholesterol (not for other analytes) 10 mmol/l = 387 mg/dl.

MONICA
MONICA Project: 'MONItoring of trends and determinants in CArdiovascular disease'. WHO MONICA Project is international, MONICA a local label.

Monograph CD-ROM(s)
Compact Disk(s) accompanying this Monograph contains the MONICA Manual, Quality Assessment reports, Data Books, unpublished appendices to manuscripts, a 20% random sample of most of the MONICA Database, slide shows and other items.

MRC
MONICA Reference Centre, coordinating MONICA Optional Study in a specific area. See #9

MQC
MONICA Quality Control Centre. See #8

MSC
MONICA Steering Committee. See #5

mortality or mortality rate
see event rate. Applies to a defined population, or a sex and age group within it, and is usually disease specific. Differs in meaning from fatality or fatality rate. See #37

official mortality, routine mortality
MONICA centres obtained routine death certificate data from the statistical offices serving their populations. Official mortality rates in MONICA were statistics based on this routine certification. See #16

prevention
in epidemiological terms, anything which reduces disease rates in the population. In cardiovascular epidemiology and cardiology, primary prevention means interfering with the disease process before it causes illness or symptoms while secondary prevention is delaying or preventing progress of the disease once it is apparent. Other classifications are used elsewhere in public health.

primary prevention
see prevention.

quality assessment, quality assurance, quality control
all involved in attempting to produce a standardized set of data for analysis—where any deficiencies are known and quantified. See #12

Rapporteur
World Health Organization title of person responsible for drafting reports on meetings.

registration, register
procedures involved in identifying disease events, obtaining relevant clinical information, coding, classifying and listing them. (A register is primarily a list.) See #20

risk factor
personal characteristic associated with increased risk of a disease. Classic risk factors, smoking, blood pressure and cholesterol are considered causal for cardiovascular disease; obesity measured as body mass index (BMI) is more controversial.

RU
Reporting Units are geographical sub-units of population which can be detected in all data records in MONICA. Some populations had a number of different suburbs or towns as Reporting Units, others had one RU for a whole city.

RUA
combinations (Aggregates) of Reporting Units used in MONICA analyses.

secondary prevention
see prevention.

SBP
Systolic blood pressure, the upper of the two readings taken routinely in blood pressure measurement. A classic coronary risk factor, as is diastolic blood pressure, which features in the survey Data Book, but not in this Monograph.

SI
Système International. International convention for standardizing units of measurement.

stroke
cerebrovascular disease, the acute illness precipitated by local derangement of the blood supply to the brain, either by obstruction to the artery concerned (ischaemic stroke) or rupture and bleeding into the brain (haemorrhagic stroke), or into the membrane around it (subarachnoid haemorrhage).

sudden death
see coronary death.

total cholesterol
see cholesterol.

WHO
World Health Organization.

WWW
World Wide Web. MONICA Web publications in the public domain are found at http://www.ktl.fi/publications/monica/. An internal password-protected website exists at http://www.ktl.fi/monica/internal/ for the use of MONICA Investigators. Data in the public domain are replicated on the Monograph CD-ROMs enclosed with this publication.

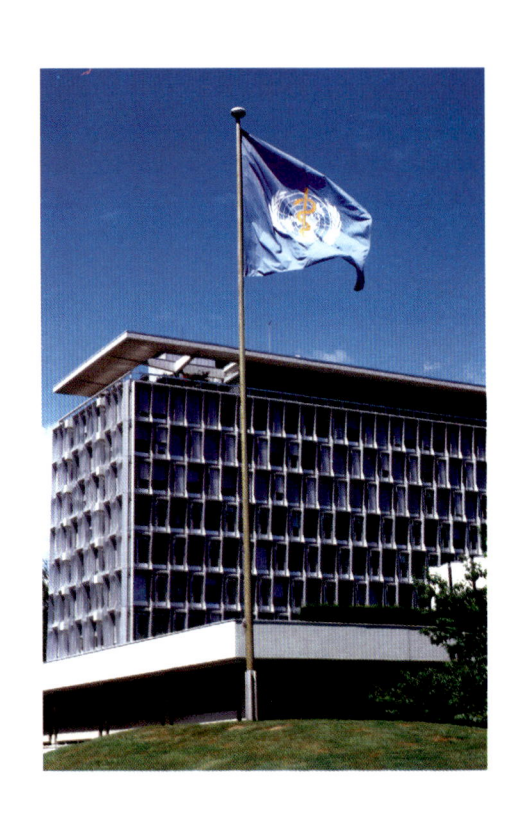

Background, Development and Organization of MONICA

#1 Background to the WHO MONICA Project

The post-war epidemic
Peace and prosperity and the control of infections through antibiotics and vaccination all promised longer life expectancy after the Second World War. However, this promise was not fulfilled in many countries, particularly in men. A new form of heart disease, going under different names—degenerative, arteriosclerotic, atheromatous, ischaemic, or coronary heart disease—but basically one condition, was rapidly increasing. The most economically advanced and industrialized countries seemed at greatest risk. Large increases in such mortality had begun in many different countries, some as early as the 1920s, but in others only a decade or two later. These countries, led by the United States of America, initiated studies to identify the causes of this disease, previously labelled as *degenerative* and, by implication, a manifestation, and therefore inevitable consequence, of increasing age.

MONICA is built on:
- Framingham
- Seven Countries
- Cardiovascular Survey Methods
- European Myocardial Infarction Registers

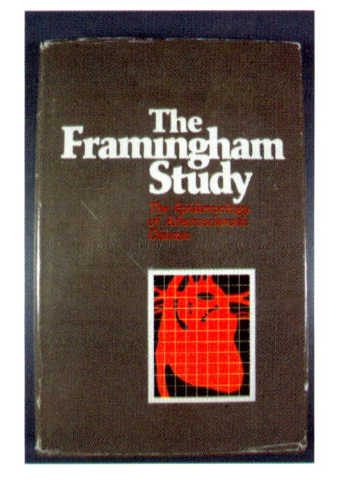

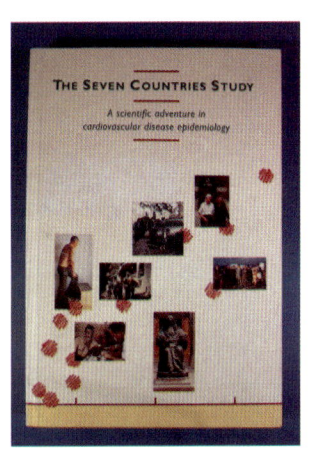

Framingham
The Framingham Study, the best-known study, and a model for many others, was launched in the early 1950s (*1*). Several thousand men and women in Framingham, Massachusetts, were examined for certain personal factors, suspected, and subsequently shown through many years of follow-up, to be powerful and consistent indicators of increased risk of coronary heart disease. The concept of *risk factors* was born. The most consistent and powerful of these in explaining coronary risk, the classic risk factors, were cigarette smoking, blood pressure and blood (serum or plasma, also known as total) cholesterol. Others were less common (diabetes mellitus), less consistent (obesity and exercise) or less readily measured (diet, alcohol and psychosocial factors).

Seven Countries
Soon after the initiation of the Framingham Study came an international collaboration led from Minneapolis in the United States, the *Seven Countries Study* (*2*). It sought to explain the large variation in death rates from coronary heart disease in different countries. Study populations, some occupational, some residential, in seven countries extended over the full range of mortality rates, from Finland (high) to the United States of America, the Netherlands, Italy, Yugoslavia, and Greece to Japan (low). This study found the classic Framingham risk factors to be of differing importance in determining variation in coronary risk between whole populations in different countries. Obesity and physical exercise accounted for little, as did cigarette smoking. Blood pressure was of some significance, but the dominant role went to cholesterol. The average blood cholesterol concentration varied significantly across populations. It correlated with the amount and type of fat in the diet and correlated strongly with population coronary disease rates.

Cardiovascular Survey Methods and ten-day seminars

For cross-population comparability, studies in cardiovascular epidemiology needed standardized methods of ascertainment and people who knew how to use them. By the 1960s the former were sufficiently developed for the World Health Organization to publish a manual prepared by Henry Blackburn from Minneapolis and the *Seven Countries Study* and Geoffrey Rose from the London School of Hygiene and the British Whitehall Study (*3*), the now classic *Cardiovascular Survey Methods* (*4*). Through the Research Committee and the Council on Epidemiology of what was then the International Society and Federation of Cardiology, an international faculty of teachers initiated annual ten-day teaching seminars. The first took place in Makarska in Yugoslavia in 1968 (*5*). They continue to this day. They introduced the concepts of cardiovascular epidemiology and of conducting field surveys to likely candidates, often trainees in cardiology. The seminars produced a cadre of young initiates, and a network of contacts for international collaboration.

Coronary care and the European Myocardial Infarction Registers

During the 1950s and early 1960s ambulatory treatment of angina pectoris, the chronic symptom of coronary heart disease, consisted of pain relief with a limited range of nitrate drugs. For myocardial infarction (coronary thrombosis), an acute medical emergency, treatment was morphine, anticoagulants and extended bed-rest. Management was then revolutionized by the electronic monitoring of patients with myocardial infarction in coronary care units (*6*), with potential resuscitation from cardiac arrest by electric defibrillation and mouth-to-mouth respiration. New drugs were being introduced. Claims that cardiac mortality was being halved in such units fitted strangely with rising population mortality rates. This led to an initiative by the European Regional Office of the World Health Organization in the late 1960s to establish *Myocardial Infarction Community Registers* (*7*) in which the incidence and outcome of acute coronary events would be studied on a whole-population basis. Both hospitalized myocardial infarction, and out of hospital coronary deaths would be studied together to assess the known and potential impact of coronary care. The registers established standardized techniques for heart attack registration not previously incorporated in *Cardiovascular Survey Methods*. They also confirmed that the great majority of coronary deaths were occurring in the community, outside hospital, and largely inaccessible to hospital-based acute coronary care.

The American decline and the Bethesda Conference

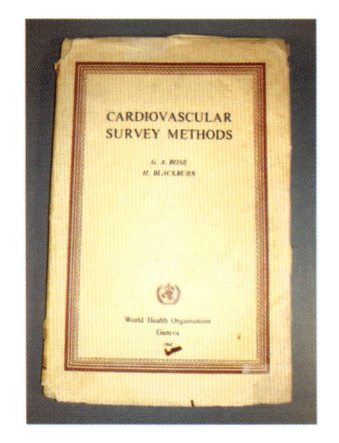

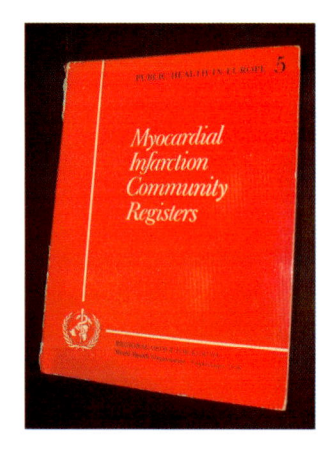

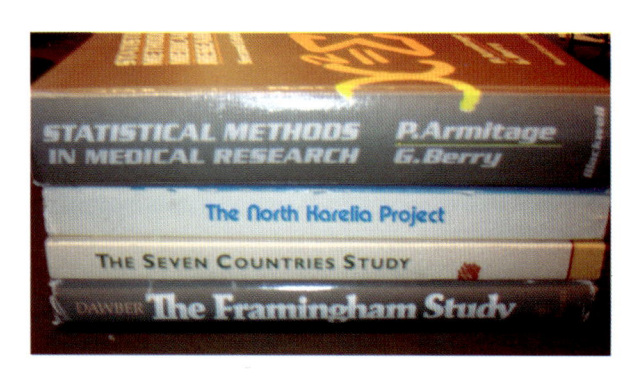

Concealed from immediate recognition by the instability of intermittent winter influenza epidemics, mortality rates from coronary heart disease in the United States of America began to decline in the early 1960s. Similar trends appeared in other New World countries such as Australia and Canada, while coronary disease mortality was still rising or stable elsewhere. The decline in mortality in the United States caused considerable excitement. It was analysed at a seminal conference organized by the US National Heart Lung and Blood Institute at Bethesda in Maryland, USA in 1978 (*8*). At this conference Píša, of the World Health Organization in Geneva, with Epstein (later also important in MONICA) showed comparative data on trends in cardiovascular mortality after the Second World War for a number of different countries (*8*), work that Píša later extended with Uemura (*9*). The Bethesda conference demonstrated that the American decline was probably genuine, but inadequately explained. Despite thirty years of cardiovascular research, information on risk factors, morbidity and mortality was incompletely integrated. There had been variation and inconsistency in the definitions and populations studied. What was needed was long-term monitoring of mortality, morbidity and risk factors in the same defined populations experiencing different trends in mortality, to establish the underlying patterns and associations. This was the background to the WHO MONICA Project, first proposed after the Bethesda conference in 1979, and undertaken across four continents in the 1980s and 1990s, in parallel with similar studies that took place in the United States of America (*10–13*).

References

1. Dawber TR. *The Framingham Study. The Epidemiology of Atherosclerotic Disease*, Cambridge, Mass., Harvard University Press, 1980.
2. Keys A. *Seven Countries: A Multivariate Analysis of Death and Coronary Heart Disease*, Cambridge, Mass., and London, England, Harvard University Press, 1980.
3. Reid DD, Hamilton PJS, McCartney P, Rose G, Jarrett RJ, Keen H. Smoking and other risk factors for coronary heart disease in British civil servants. *Lancet*, 1976, 2:979–984. PMID: 62262.
4. Rose G, Blackburn H. *Cardiovascular Survey Methods*, Geneva, World Health Organization, 1968 (Monograph Series No. 56).
5. Blackburn H. *If it isn't fun*, Minneapolis, 2001, ISBN 1-887268-03-0.
6. Day HW. Acute coronary care—a five-year report. *American Journal of Cardiology*, 1968, 21:252–257. PMID: 5635664.
7. World Health Organization Regional Office for Europe. *Myocardial infarction community registers*, Copenhagen, 1976 (Public Health in Europe 5).
8. Havlik RJ, Feinleib M, eds. *Proceedings of the Conference on the Decline in Coronary Heart Disease Mortality, October 24–25, 1978*, Washington, DC: National Heart, Lung and Blood Institute, 1979, NIH publication No.79–1610, DHES.
9. Uemura K, Píša Z. Recent trends in cardiovascular disease mortality in 27 industrialized countries. *World Health Statistics Quarterly*, 1985, 38:142–162. PMID: 4036160.
10. Gillum RF, Hannan PJ, Prineas RJ, Jacobs DR Jr, Gomez-Marin O, Luepker RV, Baxter J, Kottke TE, Blackburn H. Coronary heart disease mortality trends in Minnesota 1960–1980: the Minnesota Heart Survey. *American Journal of Public Health*, 1984, 74:360–362. PMID: 6703165.
11. The ARIC Investigators. The Atherosclerosis Risk in Communities (ARIC) Study: design and objectives. *American Journal of Epidemiology*, 1989, 129:687–702. PMID: 2646917.
12. McGovern PG, Pankow JS, Shahar E, Doliszny KM, Folsom AR, Blackburn H, Luepker RV. Recent trends in acute coronary heart disease—mortality, morbidity, medical care and risk factors. The Minnesota Heart Survey Investigators. *New England Journal of Medicine*, 1996, 334:884–890. PMID: 8669676.
13. Rosamond WD, Folsom AR, Chambless LE, Wang CH, ARIC Investigators. Coronary heart disease trends in four United States communities. The Atherosclerosis Risk in Communities (ARIC) study 1987–1996. *International Journal of Epidemiology*, 2001, Suppl 1:S17–S22. PMID: 11759846.

Hugh Tunstall-Pedoe

#2 MONICA Hypotheses and Study Design

Introduction

The following aims, objectives and hypotheses of the MONICA Project are taken from the original protocol of the early 1980s. The protocol has undergone subsequent minor revisions. Numbered notes and commentary are provided as explanations for the current reader.

- multinational monitoring of cardiovascular disease, risk factors and medical care
- seeking answers beyond any single country
- largest such study ever undertaken

Name

Multinational Monitoring of Trends and Determinants in Cardiovascular Disease. Hence the MONICA Project (*1*).

Objectives

To measure the trends in cardiovascular mortality and coronary heart disease and stroke morbidity and to assess the extent to which these trends are related to changes in known risk factors, daily living habits, health care, or major socioeconomic features measured at the same time in defined communities in different countries (*2*).

Hypotheses

Changes in cardiovascular mortality might be related to a change in disease incidence (3), or a change in case fatality, or both. A change in incidence could be related to change in any of the known factors such as cigarette smoking, blood pressure, blood cholesterol, diet, weight and exercise (4), or other unrecorded factors. A change in case fatality could be related to changes in medical care, or in the natural history of the disease.

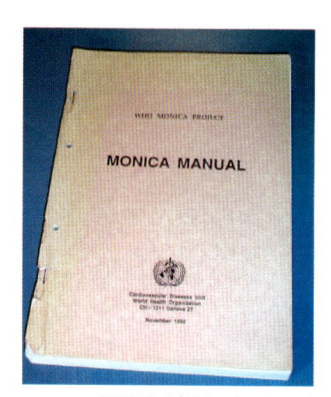

The MONICA study will involve measurement of:

a. incidence rates (3)
b. case fatality
c. risk-factor levels (4)
d. medical care (5).

These can be used to test six possible associations:

a. risk factors versus incidence
b. medical care versus case fatality
c. incidence versus case fatality
d. medical care versus incidence
e. risk factors versus case fatality
f. medical care versus risk factors.

MONICA's 'bible'—the Manual

Although the six associations can be tested within the MONICA Project for both coronary heart disease and stroke, a small number of main null hypotheses have been formulated:

Main (coronary) null hypothesis

For the population Reporting Units there is no relationship between:

- 10-year trends in the major CVD risk factors of serum cholesterol, blood pressure and cigarette consumption, (4) and
- 10-year trends in incidence rates (fatal plus non-fatal attack rates) (3) of coronary heart disease.

Second main (coronary) null hypothesis

For the population Reporting Units there is no relationship between:

- 10-year trends in case fatality rate (percentage of attacks that are fatal within 28 days), and
- 10-year trends in acute coronary care (5).

(Stroke hypotheses)

An analogous first hypothesis was subsequently formulated for stroke (replacing coronary heart disease with stroke, but otherwise identical), whereas a second main null hypothesis related trends in stroke and coronary-event rates (6). (For the population Reporting Units there is no difference in 10-year trends in event rates between stroke and coronary events.)

Contemporary notes for this Monograph

1. The name MONICA was an abbreviation of 'monitoring cardiovascular disease'. It was suggested by Dr Tom Strasser who attended one of the early planning meetings in Geneva as a member of the WHO staff.
2. The ambitious sweeping objective owed much to the original MONICA Chairman, Dr Fred Epstein. It was followed in the protocol by a caution from the Rapporteur. 'Collaborating Centres may wish to cover all these areas, but the basic protocol covers key items only, leaving the rest as local options'. There were components of the objective for which there were

then (and arguably still are) no standard cross-cultural methods of measurement.

3. The term 'incidence' is used loosely in ordinary medical parlance whereas in epidemiology it means the rate at which disease occurs in those previously free of the disease. In registering coronary heart disease it could be defined in several different ways. It was not possible in many MONICA populations to distinguish new from recurrent coronary events especially where these occurred as sudden deaths outside hospital. Likewise we only had information on the total population denominator, not how much of it was disease-free. MONICA in reality therefore used attack rates for incidence—that is the event rate for new and recurrent attacks combined. Angina pectoris was not included in incidence, which was confined to the major acute coronary events of myocardial infarction and coronary death. First event rates were calculated for those populations where reasonable data were available, but the denominator was the whole population, including those surviving previous non-fatal events.

4. In retrospect it is interesting to note the minor inconsistencies in the development of the protocol. It was revised a number of times. This applies to the key risk factors. When challenged by Dr Jeremiah Stamler at one of the early meetings in Geneva, to formulate null hypotheses in advance, we specified cigarette smoking, blood pressure and cholesterol, leaving out obesity, exercise and diet which had been mentioned previously. Obesity was subsequently brought back in the risk-factor score that was eventually used, although it made a very minor contribution, particularly in women, because of the small size of the coefficients that it attracted. Blood pressure became the systolic blood pressure. (See #35 *Risk-Factor Scores*.)

5. The hypotheses were formulated before MONICA had a clear statement of how and when medical care was to be recorded. This explains inconsistent use of the terms 'medical care', and 'acute coronary care' and 'medical care in the attack' used in different documents. Information on coronary care was recorded in relation to coronary events, including medication before the onset and at hospital discharge. This was specified by good fortune, as the impending importance of secondary prevention of recurrent attacks was not fully appreciated at the time. It was decided to record administrative information on medical care as a separate data item fairly late in MONICA. Although collected retrospectively, it was not incorporated into the hypothesis-testing analyses. (See #18 *Health Services*.)

6. Stroke hypotheses were formulated considerably later than those for coronary events. Stroke care was not a core data item. The status of stroke registration itself was officially 'core' but in practice 'optional'. This was because centres could not be excluded from MONICA for refusing to study stroke, but centres that could do it needed to be able to inform their funding bodies that stroke was a core element of the study. It was recognized that without extending the age-range above 65, numbers of strokes being registered would make it unlikely that trends could be estimated with confidence, unless they were large.

Study design

The basic design of the MONICA Project first involved the designation of defined populations. Within each population, certain annual routine administrative data were required. These included demographic information on numbers by age and sex and official or routine data on numbers of deaths from different causes. MONICA investigators were then responsible for undertaking registration of all coronary events within defined age groups (25–64) in both sexes over a period of ten years. Population risk-factor surveys were to be conducted at least at the beginning and the end of this period, and optionally in the middle. Coronary care was also to be monitored at least at the beginning and at the end, so that both of these data components were discontinuous. Centres were strongly encouraged to register strokes in the same populations at the same time as the acute coronary events.

Reference
MONICA Web Publications are also accessible on the Monograph CD-ROM
WHO MONICA Project. MONICA Manual. (1998–1999). Available from URL: http://www.ktl.fi/publications/monica/manual/index.htm, URN:*NBN:fi-fe19981146*. MONICA Web Publication 1. (The older version of the Manual is archived on the CD-ROM.)

Hugh Tunstall-Pedoe

#3 Organization Chart of the WHO MONICA Project

The policy-making and management structure of the WHO MONICA Project is made up of the following components:

- Council of Principal Investigators—*CPI* (see #4)
- Principal Investigators—*PIs*
- MONICA Steering Committee—*MSC* (see #5)
- MONICA Management Centre—*MMC* (see #6)
- MONICA Data Centre—*MDC* (see #7)
- MONICA Quality Control Centres—*MQCs* (see #8)
- MONICA Collaborating Centres—*MCCs* (see #50–#84)
- MONICA Reference Centres—*MRCs* (see #9 and #43–#49)

Hugh Tunstall-Pedoe

WHO MONICA PROJECT: Organizational Chart

```
                    COUNCIL OF
              PRINCIPAL INVESTIGATORS
                 (MONICA Parliament)
                          |
  MONICA MANAGEMENT       |         MONICA DATA CENTRE
       CENTRE         MONICA         National Public Health
  Cardiovascular Diseases  STEERING COMMITTEE     Institute,
   Programme, WHO,                         Helsinki
      Geneva
                          |
                    Publications
                    Coordinator
                          |
              QUALITY CONTROL CENTRES(a)
                          |
              MONICA COLLABORATING CENTRES
                          |
                 REFERENCE CENTRES OF
                 OPTIONAL STUDIES(b)
```

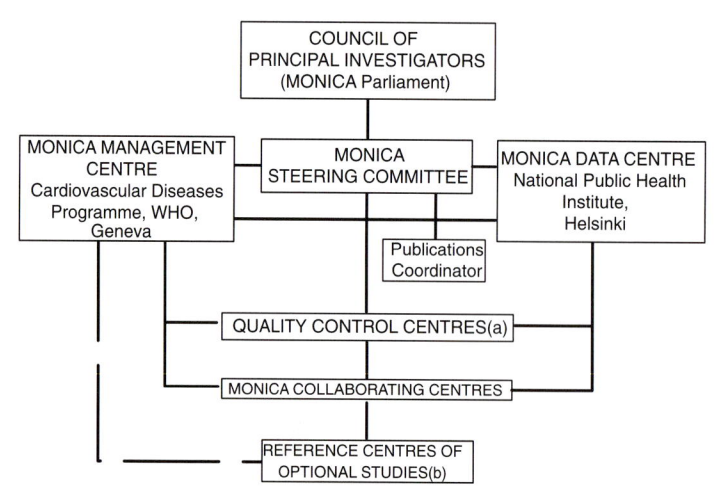

a) Quality Control Centres:
   Lipids (Prague)
   ECG (Budapest)
   Event Registration (Dundee)
   Health Services (Perth)

b) Reference Centres:
   Psychosocial (WHO, Copenhagen)
   Nutrition (Bilthoven)
   Vitamins (Bern)
   Physical activity (Atlanta)
   Drugs (Bremen)
   Haemostatic factors (Belfast)

#4 Council of Principal Investigators (CPI) and MONICA Congresses and Symposia

Early meetings

Five preliminary meetings, involving a total of 61 different people were held between 1979 and 1981 to initiate what became the WHO MONICA Project. These meetings were held 17–19 September and 17–19 December 1979 in Geneva, 27–28 June 1980 in Paris, 13–14 April and 12–15 October 1981 in Geneva. (See #1 *Background to the WHO MONICA Project* and #15 *Reminiscences of MONICA's Rapporteur.*) These meetings led to the publication and distribution in October 1982 of the document *Proposal for the Multinational Monitoring of Trends and Determinants in Cardiovascular Disease and Protocol* (*1*).

- Council of Principal Investigators was MONICA's parliament
- frequency of meetings limited by the cost
- quality control, administration
- networking on problems and optional studies
- election of new members of MONICA Steering Committee
- scientific congresses and symposia were separate

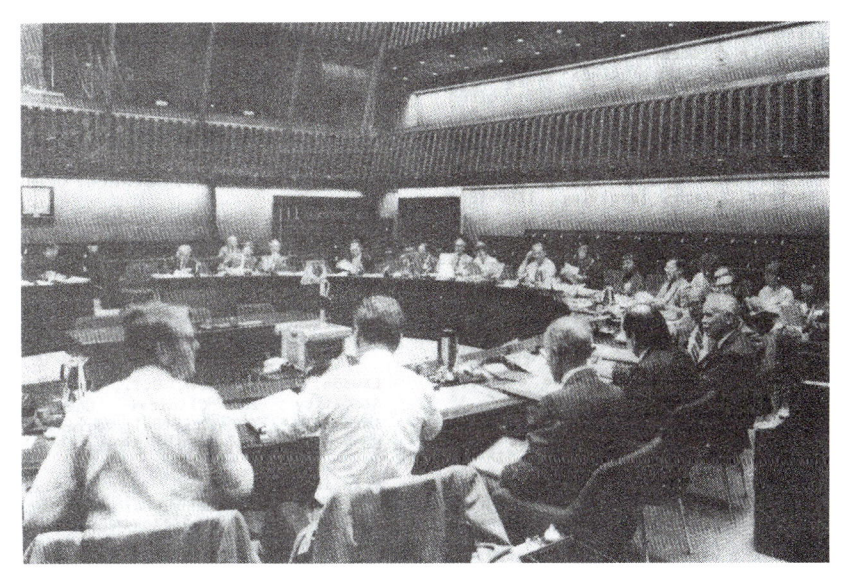

First numbered CPI: CPI-1

This (*1*) was the working document for the first numbered Council of Principal Investigators meeting (CPI) that took place in Geneva from 30 November to 3 December 1982. It was this meeting which began to give MONICA its structure for the next two decades by setting up the MONICA Steering Committee and initiating MONICA Memos and work on the *Manual of Operations* (*2*). This and subsequent Councils of Principal Investigators (CPI) were the MONICA Parliament, the highest policy and decision-making body of the WHO MONICA Project. They were composed of the designated Principal Investigators (PIs), who were the responsible scientific officer(s) of each MONICA Collaborating Centre (MCC), and MONICA country coordinators, if any; ex-officio staff including heads of the MONICA Management Centre (MMC), MONICA Data Centre (MDC), MONICA Quality Control Centres (MQCs) and MONICA Reference Centres (MRCs), Principal Investigators from Associate MONICA Centres, team members from MONICA Centres; consultants and support staff. For the full constitution see the MONICA Manual (*3*).

Council of Principal Investigators Meeting, Geneva, 1982 showing (l to r) Hugh Tunstall-Pedoe, Zbyněk Píša, Fred Epstein, Vadim Zaitsev and Martti Karvonen (photo scanned from MONICA Newsletter of April 1983)

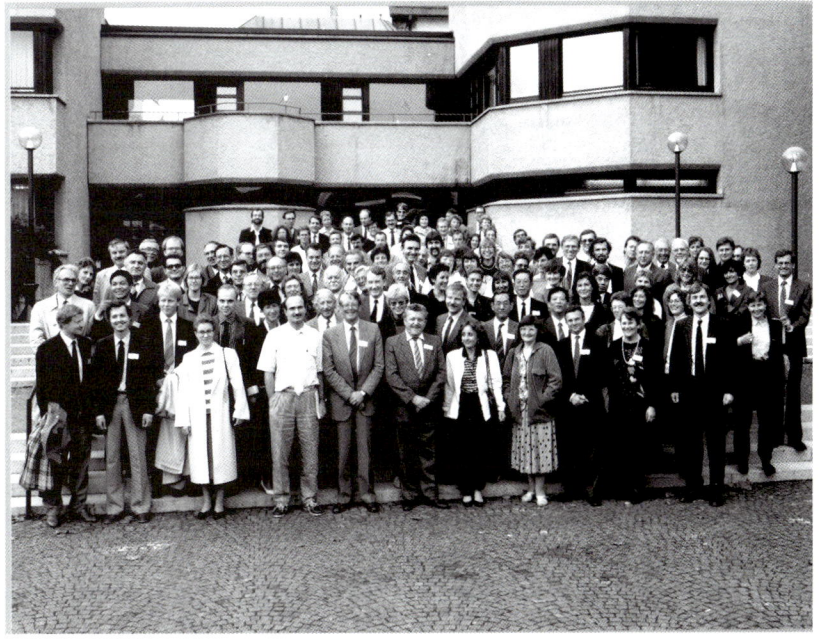

Later CPI Meetings

These were large and expensive meetings (see photograph). After the second meeting they moved away from Geneva and were hosted, organized and partially funded by individual MONICA Collaborating Centres (see list). Nine were held altogether. The Council had the key role to review, decide and plan the execution of the MONICA Project; to monitor and evaluate its

CPI-5, Augsburg 1988. Investigators were young and the world black and white

progress; to exchange experience and information among PIs and team members; to review and to change the recommendations made by the MSC; and to elect the new members of the MSC. The emphases changed over time. Early meetings were concerned with interpretation and changes to the Protocol and Manual, quality control issues, coding workshops, optional studies; later meetings were concerned with publications. The MONICA Data Centre staff and Steering Committee took the opportunity to meet with Principal Investigators who had questions or problems.

CPI-9

The final CPI was held in Milan in 1998. Its main objectives were to ensure MONICA's completion, decide future governance, revise publication rules, review progress with main hypotheses and decide on future MONICA collaborations. New publication rules, new authorship and citation rules were decided. These helped to speed up MONICA publication and to recognize contributions from authors. The composition of the MSC was also changed to include key advisers for finalizing the Project. The final structure of the MONICA Archive was revised and approved. The PIs also agreed upon the composition of the working groups appointed to prepare the final papers on the two main hypotheses of the Project. The CPI-9 also established the rules for voting and the quorum for changing the management and publication rules as well as the procedure for appointing future new members of the MSC by postal ballot. Last but not least, the CPI-9 approved the original outline of this MONICA Monograph and asked for it to be completed using the available funds.

MONICA Congresses and Symposia

The CPI meetings themselves were used as an opportunity to display posters from different centres. Three specific MONICA Congresses were also held, hosted by individual MONICA Collaborating Centres but numerous MONICA satellite meetings or sessions were also held within bigger international meetings in epidemiology, heart disease and stroke. The second and third MONICA Congresses were recorded in supplements to scientific journals (4, 5) and MONICA was responsible for, or a major contributor to, two other journal supplements (6, 7). The first was from a meeting organized by the National Institutes of Health in Washington. The most recent was from an International Epidemiological Association satellite meeting, at which major MONICA findings were presented (see table).

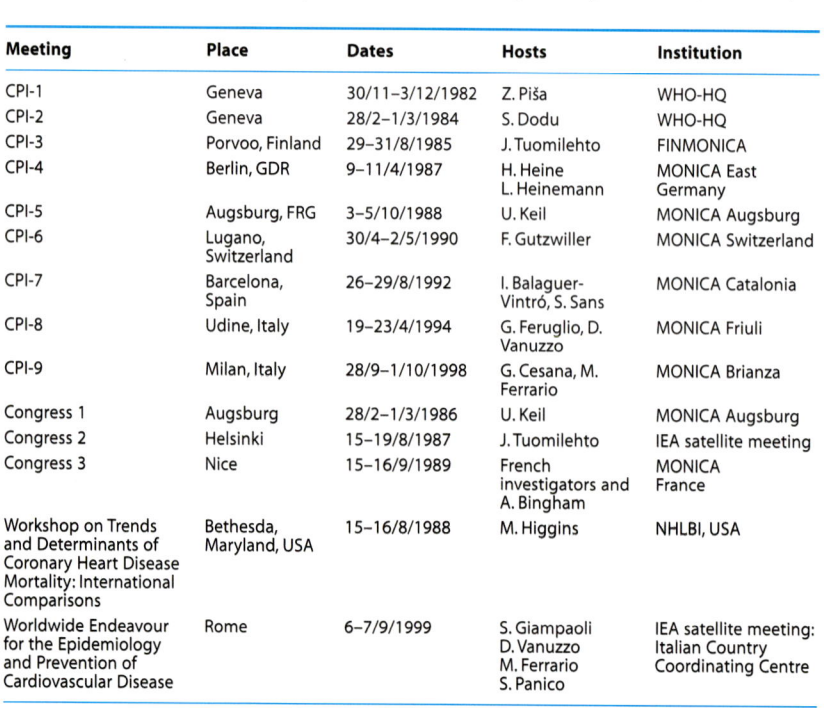

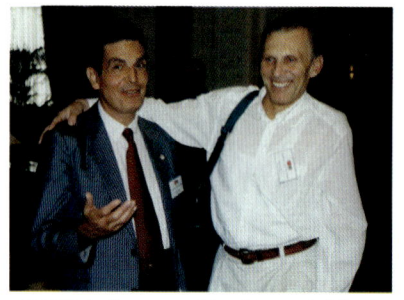

MONICA family meets—Diego Vanuzzo (Friuli) with Hermann Wolf (Halifax)

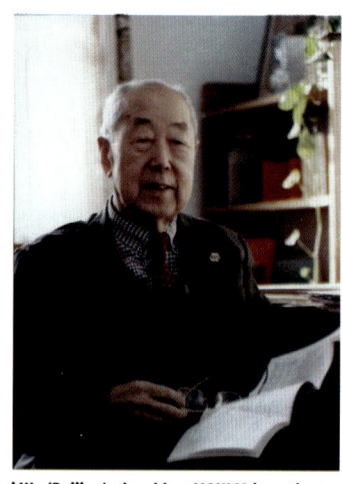

Yingkai Wu (Beijing), the oldest MONICA investigator

Meeting	Place	Dates	Hosts	Institution
CPI-1	Geneva	30/11–3/12/1982	Z. Piša	WHO-HQ
CPI-2	Geneva	28/2–1/3/1984	S. Dodu	WHO-HQ
CPI-3	Porvoo, Finland	29–31/8/1985	J. Tuomilehto	FINMONICA
CPI-4	Berlin, GDR	9–11/4/1987	H. Heine L. Heinemann	MONICA East Germany
CPI-5	Augsburg, FRG	3–5/10/1988	U. Keil	MONICA Augsburg
CPI-6	Lugano, Switzerland	30/4–2/5/1990	F. Gutzwiller	MONICA Switzerland
CPI-7	Barcelona, Spain	26–29/8/1992	I. Balaguer-Vintró, S. Sans	MONICA Catalonia
CPI-8	Udine, Italy	19–23/4/1994	G. Feruglio, D. Vanuzzo	MONICA Friuli
CPI-9	Milan, Italy	28/9–1/10/1998	G. Cesana, M. Ferrario	MONICA Brianza
Congress 1	Augsburg	28/2–1/3/1986	U. Keil	MONICA Augsburg
Congress 2	Helsinki	15–19/8/1987	J. Tuomilehto	IEA satellite meeting
Congress 3	Nice	15–16/9/1989	French investigators and A. Bingham	MONICA France
Workshop on Trends and Determinants of Coronary Heart Disease Mortality: International Comparisons	Bethesda, Maryland, USA	15–16/8/1988	M. Higgins	NHLBI, USA
Worldwide Endeavour for the Epidemiology and Prevention of Cardiovascular Disease	Rome	6–7/9/1999	S. Giampaoli D. Vanuzzo M. Ferrario S. Panico	IEA satellite meeting: Italian Country Coordinating Centre

References

1. *Proposal for the Multinational Monitoring of Trends and Determinants in Cardiovascular Disease and Protocol (MONICA PROJECT)*. WHO/MNC/82.1, 7 October 1982. CVD Unit, World Health Organization, Geneva. (See CD-ROM.)
2. *Multinational Monitoring of Trends and Determinants in Cardiovascular Diseases "MONICA PROJECT" Manual of Operations.* WHO/MNC/82.2 DRAFT MOO, November 1983. Cardiovascular Diseases Unit, World Health Organization, Geneva. (See CD-ROM.)
3. WHO MONICA Project. MONICA Manual. (1998–1999). Part I: Description and Organization of the WHO MONICA Project. Part 2: Organization and Management of the WHO MONICA Project. Available from URL: http://www.ktl.fi/publications/monica/manual/part1/i-2.htm, URN:*NBN:fi-fe19981148*. MONICA Web Publication 1.
4. *Acta Medica Scandinavica. Supplementum*, 1988, 728.
5. *Revue d'Epidémiologie et de Santé Publique*, 1990, 38(5–6): 389–550.
6. *International Journal of Epidemiology*, 1989, 18(Suppl 1):S1–S230.
7. *International Journal of Epidemiology*, 2001, 30(Suppl 1):S1–S72.

Marco Ferrario, Hugh Tunstall-Pedoe

#5 MONICA Steering Committee (MSC)

Early history (from SF)

As it was originally envisioned, what later became the MONICA Project was to include about a dozen centres. As the Project developed in the early 1980s, interest was widespread and included most of the countries in Europe (then still politically polarized into East and West) and many in Asia, the western Pacific, and the Americas. This demanded a larger administrative structure than had originally been foreseen.

The first meeting of what became the Council of Principal Investigators was held in Geneva from 30 November to 3 December 1982. One significant impediment to progress was the lack of a data analysis centre to coordinate such items as data format, transmission, quality control checks, and the like. The Principal Investigators decided to establish a 'steering committee' to form a 'ghost data centre' to work on these issues. The MONICA Steering Committee (MSC) was therefore created at the meeting; membership included representatives from WHO Headquarters (Zbyněk Píša, Martti Karvonen) and the WHO European Office, (Vadim Zaitsev); the Data Centre Chief (then vacant); Hugh Tunstall-Pedoe as Rapporteur; and three elected Principal Investigators (Pekka Puska, Stephen Fortmann and Alessandro Menotti).

The first meeting of the MSC was held two months later, from 9 to 10 February 1983, in Helsinki, Finland. Pekka Puska, from the host country, was elected Chair for this session. The meeting focused on quality control, completion of the protocol, and the structure of MONICA. By then negotiations between WHO and the Finnish government to establish the Data Centre (MDC) in Helsinki were at an advanced stage. It was anticipated that Jaakko Tuomilehto would become Chief of the MDC.

The second meeting of the MSC was held in Liège, Belgium from 8 to 9 September 1983, in conjunction with the Annual Meeting of the European Society of Cardiology. Since there was no local host, chairmanship of the MSC was rotated to another elected Principal Investigator, Stephen Fortmann. This meeting also focused on the urgent needs of settling the protocol and manual of operations, the criteria for centres to be admitted to the study, and the organization and governance of the study. The MDC had still not been formally established, because of financial issues, but Jaakko Tuomilehto attended as MDC Chief-designate.

The other main organizational challenge was the establishment of a coordinating centre. Several sites had been interested in serving this role, but WHO could not find the financial support. The Cardiovascular Diseases (CVD) Unit

- managed the Project between meetings of the Principal Investigators
- a mixture of elected, ex-officio and co-opted members
- 29 formal meetings over the years and over 100 telephone conferences
- 5-year commitment for elected members, the last 18 months as Chair

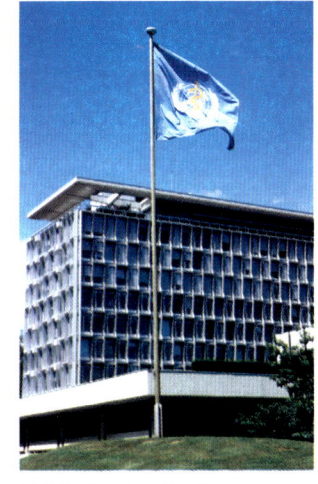

WHO Headquarters, Geneva

at WHO Headquarters in Geneva thus became the *de facto* coordinating centre, and remained so throughout the study.

The third MSC meeting in Geneva, 11–12 January 1984, was followed by the second meeting of the Principal Investigators, also in Geneva, 28 February–1 March 1984. Stephen Fortmann was asked to continue to chair the MSC to provide continuity during this challenging period when the Project was getting organized but funding was insufficient. At the PI meeting Pekka Puska asked to leave the MSC and Stefan Rywik was elected to replace him. (Alessandro Menotti also later resigned owing to pressure of other work.) This established the tradition, later codified, of electing one new member of the MSC (and also a reserve member) at each meeting of the PIs. Another change occurred at this time, with Zbyněk Píša retiring as Chief of the CVD Unit and being replaced by Silas Dodu.

Stephen Fortmann remained Chair of the MSC until the third PI Meeting in Porvoo, Finland, 29–31 August 1985. From then on, chairmanship of the MSC went by custom, but also by formal election within the MSC, to the most senior of the elected PIs and lasted until the next meeting of the PIs, when this person would leave the MSC and a replacement would be elected. Financial constraints continued to plague the study, so meetings of the PIs, which should have been held annually, took place at 18-month intervals. Service on the MSC therefore lasted four to five years and chairmanship about one and a half years.

Later history (from HTP)

The MONICA Steering Committee continued to meet in Geneva between meetings of Principal Investigators and also met immediately before, during and immediately after the PI meetings. It was an exhausting schedule for those involved. In 1987 MONICA adopted electronic mail. Electronic mail, along with FAX machines, telephone conferences, and the Internet later revolutionized the way in which MONICA and the MONICA Steering Committee conducted business (see #11 *Communications in MONICA*). By early 2002 the MONICA Steering Committee had met 29 times in formal sessions but had also conducted 102 telephone conferences.

The core MONICA personnel on the MONICA Steering Committee were strengthened by the appointment of consultants (see #6 *MONICA Management Centre (MMC)*) and, in Geneva, by staff members from the Cardiovascular Diseases Unit, who attended the meetings, as well as by staff from the MONICA Data Centre. Support for these meetings was provided by Mary-Jane Watson who provided valuable continuity and tireless devotion over two decades. Although it sometimes had a large number of members, the MONICA Steering Committee benefited from a useful mix of fixed and changing members.

Chairmanship of the MSC was a demanding commitment. While most Chairs were pleased to give it up after eighteen months or so, this nonetheless marked the end of their involvement with the MSC unless they were re-elected. Several of them remarked on how strange it felt, after five years of work, to be no longer involved in telephone conferences or deluged with MSC e-mail. The Editorial Advisory Group of this Monograph has been one way of re-involving ex-Chairs with the current MONICA Steering Committee.

In addition to dealing with internal MONICA business, the MSC also tried to use its visits to Geneva to impress on WHO officials the importance of continued funding for the project. Cardiovascular disease was erroneously considered by many in the 1980s and early 1990s to be a problem only of the developed world (see #14 *MONICA and the Prevention of Cardiovascular Disease*). This misguided notion was unfortunately reinforced by the lack of MONICA centres in the developing world (see #10 *Recruitment of Populations* for the explanation). WHO was itself in the throes of severe financial difficulties over the MONICA decade that spanned from the middle of the 1980s to the middle of the 1990s. Annual dues were missing from prominent defaulters, and there were wild fluctuations in the value of currencies. The MSC achieved less than it hoped in this respect. However, a fund was established in Geneva with donations from commercial sources which helped to support MONICA manuscript groups, data analyses and publications. What support there was from Geneva proved to be crucial in the longer-term.

Formal constitution and workings of the MONICA Steering Committee are described in the MONICA Manual (1).

Key personnel

Current (December 2002): Kjell Asplund (Chair), Philippe Amouyel (Publications Coordinator), Andrzej Pająk, Alun Evans, Hugh Tunstall-Pedoe (Rapporteur), Shanthi Mendis (MONICA Management Centre), Kari Kuulasmaa (MONICA Data Centre), Aushra Shatchkute (WHO, Copenhagen), Annette Dobson (statistical consultant).

Previous elected members: Robert Beaglehole, Marco Ferrario, Stephen Fortmann, Felix Gutzwiller, Michael Hobbs, Ulrich Keil, Alessandro Menotti, Pekka Puska, Stefan Rywik, Susana Sans.

Former Chiefs and Responsible Officers of CVD/HQ Geneva: Ingrid Martin, Ivan Gyarfas, Siegfried Böthig, Silas Dodu, Zbyněk Píša. *Former WHO, Copenhagen:* Vadim Zaitsev. *Former Data Centre:* Jaakko Tuomilehto.

Former consultants: Martti Karvonen, Ron Prineas, Manning Feinleib, Fred Epstein, Zbyněk Píša, Dale Williams.

In attendance: Mary-Jane Watson.

Reference

WHO MONICA Project. MONICA Manual. (1998–1999). Part I: Description and Organization of the WHO MONICA Project. Part 2: Organization and Management of the WHO MONICA Project. Available from URL: http://www.ktl.fi/publications/monica/manual/part1/i-2.htm, URN:*NBN:fi-fe19981148*. MONICA Web Publication 1.

Stephen Fortmann, Hugh Tunstall-Pedoe

#6 MONICA Management Centre (MMC)

Administrative centre

Cardiovascular Diseases, Management of Noncommunicable Diseases,
World Health Organization,
1211 Geneva 27, Switzerland
T +41 22 791 2733; F +41 22 791 4151

Description

The Cardiovascular Diseases Unit at the World Health Organization Headquarters in Geneva, under the leadership of its Chief, Dr Zbyněk Píša, had a crucial role in initiating what was to become the WHO MONICA Project in 1979. It was subsequently embarrassed by its success, as the number of centres nominated as candidates was several times greater than expected. Attempts were made to find funding for a coordinating centre in a number of potential countries. After these failed it was decided to set up a MONICA Data Centre, which was housed in Helsinki, but to retain the Management Centre in Geneva. This decision was welcomed by participants from many central and eastern European countries. In the 1980s Europe was ideologically divided and a western coordinating centre could have created problems for them. Not only was the World Health Organization neutral ground, but in addition, the Cardiovascular Diseases Unit and its parent Division of Noncommunicable

- initiated what became MONICA in 1979
- administrative centre for two decades despite reorganization and financial constraints
- neutral focus when the world was ideologically divided

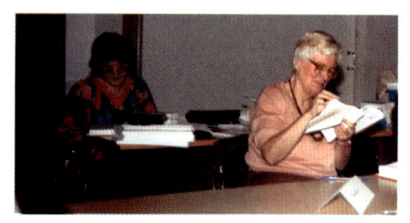

Diseases were staffed predominantly by medical officers from the socialist republics. Although medical officers changed over time, continuity was provided for almost the whole of the MONICA Project by the then Administrative Assistant, Mary-Jane Watson, a point of contact for very many MONICA investigators, although increasingly involved in other things later on. Secretarial continuity was provided by Margaret Hill.

Initially the Management Centre was responsible for almost everything, funding meetings of the Principal Investigators in Geneva, organizing MONICA Steering Committee meetings and partially funding the MONICA Data Centre. This latter role subsequently diminished as the Data Centre acquired its own funding. While MONICA had secretarial support in Geneva, it never had a full-time administrator or medical officer. Over the years, extraneous sources of funding financed the Data Centre and meetings of the Council of Principal Investigators, and data issues began to predominate. The role of the Management Centre, which was limited by its finances, centred on servicing the MONICA Steering Committee (which met increasingly infrequently), its regular telephone conferences, and in organizing the distribution of MONICA Memos (see #88 *MONICA Memos*).

The MONICA Management Centre initially had a stimulating role to play in the recruitment of candidate MONICA Collaborating Centres. Later it had the converse unenviable role of dealing with the fallout when some MCCs were failing. While some withdrew gracefully, others refused to walk off when shown the red card by the MONICA Steering Committee, and attempted to bring pressure through national representatives.

At its initiation the WHO MONICA Project was a joint project of the World Health Organization Headquarters in Geneva, and the European Regional Office in Copenhagen (EURO). Although this did not continue, the chronic diseases officer in EURO subsequently remained as a long-term member of the MONICA Steering Committee and coordinated an optional study (see #46 *MONICA Optional Psychosocial Substudy (MOPSY)*).

One of the key roles of the MONICA Management Centre was the recruitment and appointment of consultants to the project. These participated in the meetings of Principal Investigators, and later in the MONICA Steering Committee and worked on the project between these meetings.

Apart from future Principal Investigators, leading figures in the early days of the creation of MONICA, brought together by the Management Centre, were Zbyněk Píša (Czechoslovakia, now Czech Republic, Chief CVD Unit), his successor Silas Dodu (Ghana, Chief CVD Unit), George Lamm (Hungary, European Office), Tom Strasser (Yugoslavia, Medical Officer, CVD Unit), Martti Karvonen (Finland, consultant), Ron Prineas (USA, consultant), Manning Feinleib (USA, consultant), Fred Epstein (Switzerland, consultant), and later Dale Williams (USA, consultant). After MONICA was established, continuity in Geneva was maintained by Siegfried Böthig (GDR, now Germany, Chief CVD), Ivan Gyarfas (Hungary, Chief CVD) and Ingrid Martin (GDR, now Germany, Responsible Officer CVD). What was originally the Cardiovascular Diseases Unit in Geneva underwent reorganization and changes of building over the MONICA years. The present officer for Cardiovascular Diseases, in its reorganized structure, is Shanthi Mendis (Sri Lanka, Responsible Officer CVD).

The formal functions of the MONICA Management Centre are laid down in the MONICA Manual (*1*).

Key personnel

Responsible Officer: Shanthi Mendis (2000–). *Former Responsible Officers:* Zbyněk Píša (1979–1983), Silas Dodu (1983–1985), Siegfried Böthig (1985–1989), Ivan Gyarfas (1989–1996), Ingrid Martin (1996–2000). *Administrative Assistant:* Mary-Jane Watson. *Secretarial:* Margaret Hill.

Reference
WHO MONICA Project. MONICA Manual. (1998–1999). Part I: Description and Organization of the Project. Section 2: Organization and Management. Available from URL: http://www.ktl.fi/publications/monica/manual/part1/i-2.htm, *URN:NBN:fi-fe19981148*.
MONICA Web Publication 1.

Hugh Tunstall-Pedoe, Shanthi Mendis

#7 MONICA Data Centre (MDC)

Background and tasks
It was clear from the outset of the study, that each MONICA Collaborating Centre (MCC) would be responsible for the collection, management and analysis of its own data for local purposes. It was also accepted that a central facility would be needed to collect data from the MCCs to analyse them in testing the main hypotheses. The role of and requirements for such a facility, later known as the MONICA Data Centre (MDC), were defined in 1982 by a group of external consultants as the following:

- to function as the central repository and manager of core data received from the MCCs, (see #36 *Data Transfer, Checking and Management*) (*1*)
- to undertake quality control of data (*1, 2*)
- to undertake interim and final statistical analyses (*2, 3*)
- to provide data sets to investigators carrying out other studies approved by the Steering Committee
- to consult with MCCs on data collection, data management, data processing and statistical analysis.

In addition to these functions, the MDC was closely involved in:

- preparation of data collection methods and instruments (*1*)
- archiving of the Project's data (*4*)
- management of the Project in close collaboration with the Steering Committee and the Management Centre.

The MDC was not involved in management or analysis of data from the Optional Studies.

- emphasized quality assurance of data
- exploited advances in technology such as e-mail and the Internet
- published MONICA quality assessment and other reports on the Web
- provided a base for visiting workers and manuscript groups
- processed large volumes of data safely and accurately

Administrative centre
International CVD Epidemiology Unit,
Department of Epidemiology and Health Promotion,
National Public Health Institute (KTL),
Mannerheimintie 166,
00300 Helsinki, Finland
T +358 9 4744 8640; F +358 9 4744 8338

The MDC was established in 1984 in the Department of Epidemiology of the National Public Health Institute (KTL) in Helsinki, Finland. KTL had local and international experience in cardiovascular disease epidemiology, but had never been involved in the coordination of data from a multinational project. The initial skills required for its tasks were acquired quickly through visits to places that already had such experience. Visits by consultants to the MDC assisted with the further development of skills. Particularly helpful was the collaboration with Dale Williams and his co-workers then at the Collaborative Studies Coordinating Center at Chapel Hill, North Carolina.

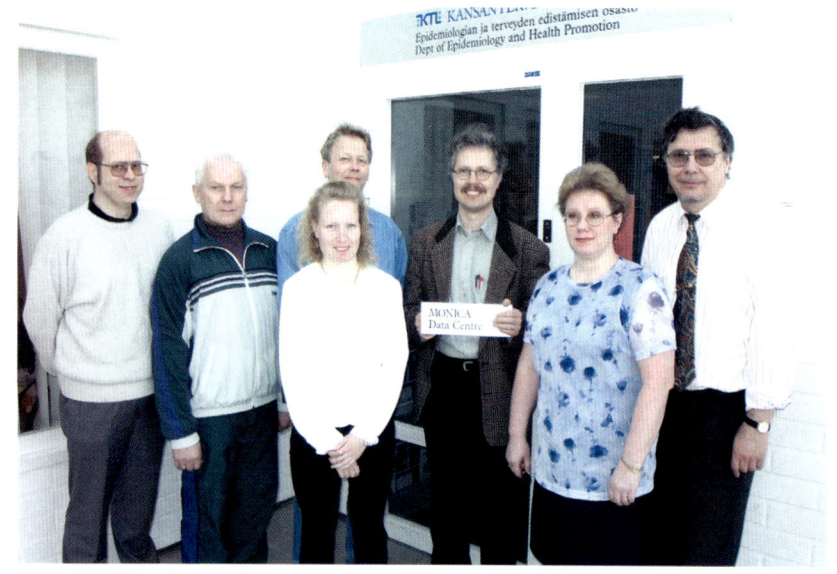

MONICA Data Centre staff 2001: Markku Mähönen, Zygimantas Cepaitis, Hanna Tolonen, Esa Ruokoski, Kari Kuulasmaa, Tuula Virmanen-Ojanen and Vladislav Moltchanov

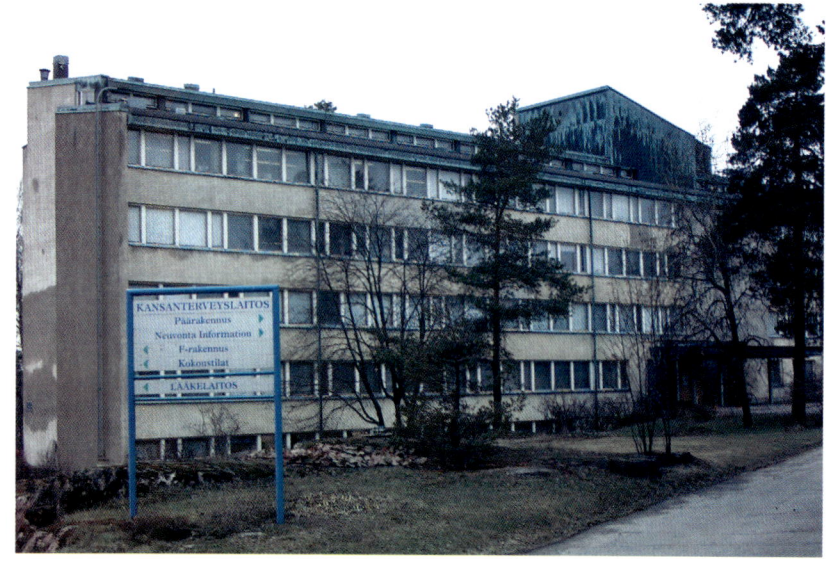

KTL—host organization of the MDC in Helsinki

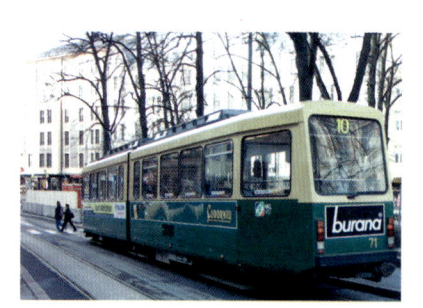

Tram 10 served the MDC from central Helsinki

Personnel

In the beginning, the MDC staff consisted of the Chief (epidemiologist), an epidemiologist, a statistician, a database administrator and a secretary. It soon became clear that while more resources were needed for data management and statistical computing, the need for medical and epidemiological expertise could be filled by experts from the Steering Committee and the MCCs. For the next fifteen years, the number of full-time staff at the MDC varied between four and seven persons. Crucial for the performance of the MDC was close collaboration with the MCCs, the Quality Control Centres, the Management Centre and the Steering Committee. Collaboration with the MCCs was not limited to the preparation and transfer of the study data. Numerous visits, lasting from a few days to several months, were made to the MDC by experts from the MCCs to work on statistical computing, planning and writing of the Project's reports and publications. Also important was the careful work of many MCCs in checking the MCC specific statistical computing which the MDC had undertaken for the collaborative reports and publications.

Funding

The MDC was established by a contract between WHO and KTL. Although it was projected that the MDC would be needed for 15 years, the contracts had to be renewed annually. The first contract stipulated that the costs would be divided roughly fifty-fifty between the two parties: KTL was to provide two persons, an office and computing facilities, while WHO provided a fixed amount of money. The WHO contribution remained at the same level throughout the 1980s. However, soon after the start, the effective contribution of WHO decreased by a third because of exchange rate fluctuations. KTL responded by providing an additional full-time person in 1988. In the early 1990s, the financial contribution from WHO gradually ceased, and for six years the main source of funding outside KTL was the National Heart Lung and Blood Institute in the USA. In 1996–99, the time of the last bits of data transfer, the final quality assessments and the preparation of the final results, the main funding outside KTL came from the European Union through its 4th framework research grant (BIOMED). See Acknowledgements.

Continuing activity

The unit of KTL established for the MDC is now called the International Cardiovascular Disease Epidemiology Unit. Its main activities include:

- further analysis of the MONICA data
- running the Data Centre for the EU-funded MORGAM study, in which cohorts examined by MONICA and some other risk-factor surveys are followed-up for cardiovascular diseases. A subcomponent of the study is a nested case-cohort study on genetic issues
- planning of coordinated population risk-factor surveys for European countries.

Key personnel

Kari Kuulasmaa (Chief, 1987–, ST, E) 1984–; Jaakko Tuomilehto (Former Chief, E) 1984–86; Matti Romo (E) 1984; Markku Mäkinen (SA, DBA) 1984–85; Liisa Palonen (S) 1984–88; Jorma Torppa (DBA, SC, SA) 1985–97; Eija Kalliala (SA) 1985–86; Esa Ruokokoski (SA, DBA, SC) 1986–98; Tuula Virman-Ojanen (S) 1987–; Juha Akkila (SC) 1988–89; Juha Pekkanen (E) 1988–89; Anna-Maija Rajakangas (SC, DBA) 1989–95; Anna-Maija Koivisto (SC) 1989–91; Vladislav Moltchanov (SC) 1991–98; Anu Molarius (SC, E) 1992–99; Markku Mähönen (E) 1993–; Zygimantas Cepaitis (DBA, SC, SA) 1994–; Hanna Tolonen (SC, E) 1996–. (ST = statistics, SA = systems analysis, DBA = data base administration, SC = statistics and statistical computing, E = epidemiology, SE = secretary.)

References
MONICA Web Publications are also accessible on the Monograph CD-ROM

1. WHO MONICA Project. MONICA Manual. (1998–1999) Part V: Data Transfer and Analysis. Section 1: Data Transfer to the MONICA Data Centre. Available from URL: http://www.ktl.fi/publications/monica/manual/part5/v-1.htm URN:*NBN:fi-fe19981160*. MONICA Web Publication 1.
2. MONICA Quality assessment reports and data books were published at http://www.ktl.fi/publications/monica/. MONICA Web Publications 2–18.
3. List of collaborative publications available at http://www.ktl.fi/monica/public/publications.htm and see #86 *Abstracts of MONICA Publications*.
4. At the time of publication of this Monograph, the full archived data are still confidential. Their use is subject to the MONICA publication rules, which are available in the MONICA Manual Part I: Description and Organization of the Project. Section 2: Organization and Management of the WHO MONICA Project. Available at http://www.ktl.fi/publications/monica/manual/part1/1-2.htm. URN:*NBN:fi-fe19981148*. A subset of MONICA data is available on the Monograph CD-ROM.

Kari Kuulasmaa

#8 MONICA Quality Control Centres (MQCs)

MONICA Quality Control Centres (MQCs), were the centres nominated by WHO in consultation with the MSC to provide expertise on specified areas of the core project. There were four Quality Control Centres with specific tasks. The Centre for Health Services was not established until near the end, while the other three were set-up at the inception of MONICA and had more in common. At first they were concerned with training, testing and external quality control—circulating test materials to centres to ascertain and monitor their performance. Later they were also concerned with the quality of collaborative data arriving in the MONICA Data Centre and with analysis and publication of the results. The latter tasks were also a concern for the groups that were established to look at the quality of data for other factors such as blood pressure, obesity and smoking. Because there was no external quality control of these items, they were not the concern of formal MQCs. Internal quality control was one of the responsibilities of the MCCs. See MONICA Quality assessment reports (*1*) which give an idea of the range of quality assurance issues that were addressed in MONICA. See also #12 *Quality Assurance*, sections on specific data items and #88 *MONICA Memos*, which show how many external quality control exercises

- training and testing were essential for successful monitoring of trends
- event registration, ECG coding, and lipid measurement were the initial concerns
- training and testing material (external quality control) were possible for these
- as data became available, quality assessment groups addressed other issues

took place, particularly in the early years of MONICA. Also see relevant parts of the MONICA Manual, such as Part IV, sections 3 and 4 (*2, 3*).

The terms of reference of the MQCs are listed together at the end of this section. Some centres had terms of reference that were specific to them. These are listed first. The aims and terms of reference are edited from MONICA Manual Part I, Section 2 (*4*).

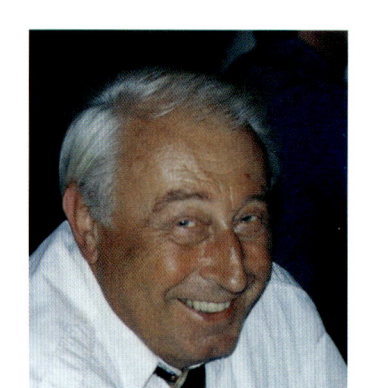

A. MONICA Quality Control Centre for Lipid Measurements

WHO Collaborating Centre for Blood Lipid Research in Atherosclerosis and Ischaemic Heart Disease (usually known as the WHO Lipid Reference Centre)
Laboratory for Atherosclerosis Research
Institute for Clinical and Experimental Medicine (IKEM)
Videnska 800, PO Box 10
14000 Prague 4, Czech Republic

Aim

To ensure comparability of data collection in the MONICA Project by testing the performance of centres in lipid measurements.

Specific terms of reference

In close cooperation with the MSC and MMC, the Prague Centre will provide the following services:

1. Procure quality control pools for lipid measurements at the MCCs.
2. Establish and execute a reference programme for testing the total cholesterol, HDL-cholesterol and thiocyanate methods.
3. Ensure comparability at regular intervals against the WHO Collaborating Centre for Blood Lipid Standardization at the Centers for Disease Control, Atlanta, Georgia, USA.

Key personnel

Responsible Officer: Rudolf Poledne. *Former Responsible Officer:* Dušan Grafnetter.

Dušan Grafnetter, former head of MQC for Lipids

B. Quality Control Centre for ECG Coding

National Institute of Cardiology
IX Haman Kato Ut 29
PO Box 88
1450 Budapest, Hungary

Aim

To standardize the interpretation of ECG according to Minnesota coding in order to improve diagnostic performance in assigning MONICA ECG categories.

Specific terms of reference

In close cooperation with the MSC, the MMC and the MQC for Event Registration, Dundee (Dundee Centre), the MONICA Quality Control Centre for ECG Coding, Budapest (Budapest Centre) will provide the following services:

1. Preparation of standard sets of ECG tracings for distribution to centres to assess differences in ECG coding. Official MONICA reference codes will be established in consultation with the Dundee Centre using the algorithm produced by the Dundee Centre.
2. Reports, including statistical analysis and commentary, will be prepared and circulated. The attention of each centre will be drawn to their weak points and suggestions for improved performance will be put forward.

3. The Budapest Centre will provide the official Minnesota reference codes for the ECG tracings included in the sets of specimen case histories elaborated by the Dundee Centre and will agree the official MONICA categories with Dundee.
4. The Budapest Centre will provide consultation services and organize training courses in ECG coding as needed and appropriate.
5. The Budapest Centre will maintain a programme of standardization for its own ECG coding activities with the Minnesota Coding Laboratory at the University of Minnesota, Minneapolis, whilst such a link remains in existence, but will also establish an external panel of expert coders, or task force, that will provide and code test material and standardize the Centre.

Key personnel
Responsible Officer: Peter Ofner. *Former Responsible Officer:* András Mádai.

C. Quality Control Centre for Event Registration
Cardiovascular Epidemiology Unit
Ninewells Hospital and Medical School
University of Dundee
Dundee DD1 9SY, Scotland

Aim
To standardize the coding and classification of coronary and stroke events according to the MONICA Protocol in order to improve comparability and stability within and between centres, thereby maximizing the chances of detecting true time trends in event rates and minimizing the likelihood of spurious trends.

Specific terms of reference
In close cooperation with the MSC, the MMC and the MQC Budapest, the Dundee Centre is responsible for the following areas:

1. Preparation and circulation of sample case histories and other material covering both coronary and stroke events, to be followed up with general commentaries and specific reports.
2. Developing an operational definition for coronary and stroke events leading to diagnostic algorithms and, where appropriate, computer programs based on these.

Key personnel
Responsible Officer: Hugh Tunstall-Pedoe. Kristin Barrett, Colin Brown.

D. Quality Control Centre for Health Services
Department of Public Health
University of Western Australia
Western Australia 6907, Australia

Aim
To develop methods for the collection and quality assessment of standardized data on the provision of health services and selected aspects of medical and surgical care for the management of cardiovascular disease in MONICA Collaborating Centres.

Specific terms of reference
In close cooperation with the MSC, MDC, MMC and MQC for Event Registration, the Perth Centre is responsible for the following areas:

1. Developing and testing, in consultation with the MONICA Data Centre and the Steering Committee, the data instruments to ensure collection of comparable data for health services assessment within the WHO MONICA Project.

Key personnel
Responsible Officer: Michael Hobbs. Konrad Jamrozik.

Common terms of reference, applying to more than one MONICA Quality Control Centre

1. Respond to queries on their area of expertise, provide consultation services and organize training courses and workshops where appropriate.
2. Provide periodic summary reports on the performance of the various centres drawing attention to their weak points and making suggestions for improvement.
3. Assist the MMC in taking appropriate action when the performance of an individual centre is unsatisfactory.
4. Present status and progress reports at regular intervals to the MSC.
5. Respect confidentiality of all data received from MCCs.
6. Communicate directly with individual MCCs on technical matters, or through the MONICA Memo system.
7. Collaborate with the MDC, MSC and MCCs in preparing reports on the quality of event data sent to the MDC and its interpretation.
8. Assisting in the revision of the appropriate section of the MONICA Manual and in the preparation of manuscripts.

References
MONICA Web Publications are also accessible on the Monograph CD-ROM

1. MONICA Quality assessment reports. MONICA Web Publications 2–18. Available from URL: http://www.ktl.fi/publications/monica/index.htm
2. WHO MONICA Project. MONICA Manual. (1998–1999). Part IV: Event Registration. Section 3: Event registration quality assurance methods. Available from URL: http://www.ktl.fi/publications/monica/manual/part4/iv-3.htm URN:*NBN:fi-fe19981158*. MONICA Web Publication 1.
3. WHO MONICA Project. MONICA Manual. (1998–1999). Part IV: Event Registration. Section 4: ECG coding quality assurance methods. Available from URL: http://www.ktl.fi/publications/monica/manual/part4/iv-4.htm URN:*NBN:fi-fe19981159*. MONICA Web Publication 1.
4. WHO MONICA Project. MONICA Manual. (1998–1999). Part I: Description and Organization of the Project. Section 2: Organization and Management. Available from URL: http://www.ktl.fi/publications/monica/manual/part1/i-2.htm URN:*NBN:fi-fe19981148*. MONICA Web Publication 1.

Hugh Tunstall-Pedoe

#9 MONICA Reference Centres (MRCs)

MONICA Reference Centres dealt with optional studies carried out within the framework of the WHO MONICA Project. See #43–#49. They coordinated and advised on their specific areas of expertise as follows:

- acted as resource centres in areas in which they had special expertise or interest
- helped to develop common protocols and provide a focus for the relevant optional studies
- coordinated any collaborative studies and planned any joint analyses
- advised their collaborators on any methodological or quality control problems whenever necessary
- organized data management for the respective optional study
- kept the MMC informed through six-monthly reports

- initiatives to collaborate on subjects and items beyond the MONICA core
- difficult or expensive to measure, or not cross-culturally standardized
- often inadequately resourced
- MONICA's Cinderella subjects, but some successes (see #43–#49)

- followed international developments in their respective fields, helped with necessary contacts with other related studies and advised centres on possible additional activities in the field in question.

This listing is taken from the latest MONICA Manual. Some of these reference centres are no longer operational, others are still working on data analyses and publications and some have changed their provenance. In the absence of central funding it is not surprising that they did not all succeed in fulfilling their terms of reference and some changed their sites and responsible officers over the years. See #43–#49.

MRC Nutrition (MRC-NUT) (See #44)

Department of Chronic Diseases and Environmental Epidemiology
National Institute of Public Health and the Environment
PO Box 1
NL-3720 BA Bilthoven, The Netherlands

Responsible Officer: Daan Kromhout. *Former Responsible Officer:* Guy De Backer (Ghent), Pirjo Pietinen (Helsinki).

MRC Vitamins and Polyunsaturated Fatty Acids (See #45)

Vitamin Unit
Institute for Biochemistry and Molecular Biology
University of Bern
Bühlstrasse 28
3000 Bern 9, Switzerland

Responsible Officer: Fred Gey. Now transferred to Alun Evans (Belfast).

MRC Physical Activity (MOSPA) (See #47)

Behavioral Epidemiology and Evaluation Branch
Division for Health Education
Centers for Disease Control
Atlanta, Georgia 30333, USA

Responsible Officer: Deborah Jones. *Former Responsible Officer:* Daniel Brunner (Tel Aviv), Kenneth Powell, Diane Jones (also CDC, Atlanta).

MRC Psychosocial Substudy (MOPSY) (See #46)

Office of Chronic Diseases, WHO Regional Office for Europe
8 Scherfigsweg
DK—2100 Copenhagen

Responsible Officer: Aushra Shatchkute. *Former Responsible Officer:* Vadim Zaitsev.
Data Centre: Ursula Härtel, GSF-MEDIS Institute, Neuherberg-Munich.

MRC Drugs (MRC-DRG) (See #48)

Bremer Institut für Präventionsforschung und Sozialmedizin (BIPS)
St Jürgen Str. 1
D—2800 Bremen 1

Responsible Officer: Eberhard Greiser. *Former Responsible Officer:* K Øydvin (Oslo).

MRC Haemostatic Factors and CHD (MRC-HFC) (See #49)

Division of Epidemiology
The Queen's University of Belfast
Mulhouse Building
Grosvenor Road
Belfast BT12 6BJ

Responsible Officer: John Yarnell. *Data Coordinator:* Evelyn McCrum (Belfast). *Laboratories:* Gordon Lowe, Ann Rumley (Dept of Medicine, Glasgow), Michael Brown (Dept Haematology, Frenchay Hospital, Bristol).

Coordinating Officer for Optional Studies: Siegfried Böthig (Zwickau, Germany).

Hugh Tunstall-Pedoe

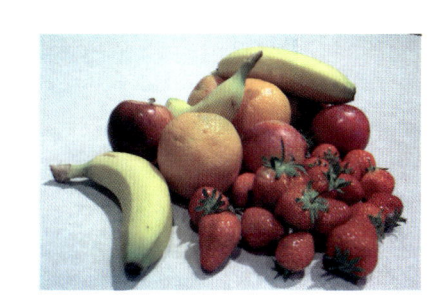

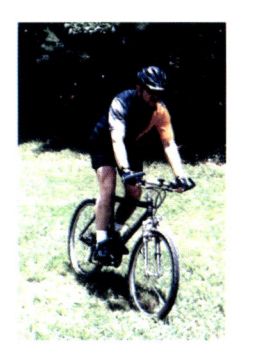

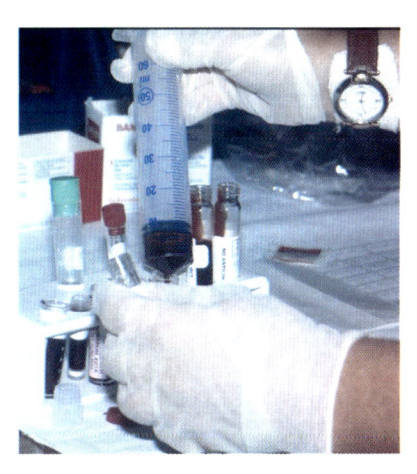

#10 Recruitment of Populations

- interest in MONICA, when announced, was much greater than expected
- entry criteria were demanding, but took time to apply
- medical, epidemiological, and funding requirements were substantial
- beyond the capacity of most developing countries
- paradoxically, that is where the cardiovascular disease explosion is now occurring (see #14)

Requirement for recruitment

Trends in morbidity, mortality and risk factors in one population cannot necessarily be extrapolated elsewhere. Following the American experience, the World Health Organization MONICA Project was set up to monitor what happened in many different populations in order to elucidate the underlying patterns. What had happened in the United States might be atypical. Realization of what was occurring there had come too late to make critical observations at the onset of the decline (1). MONICA needed data from different populations and countries at different stages of the rise and fall of cardiovascular disease, and particularly coronary heart disease, mortality. See #1 *Background to the WHO MONICA Project*. It was hoped to recruit populations with differing levels of coronary and stroke mortality, where predicted trends were increasing in some and decreasing in others. Therefore, geographic, cultural, social and material diversity of populations was to be welcomed.

Constraints on recruitment

To produce usable data however, there were constraints on which populations could be considered. The populations had to be relatively stable, living within well-defined geographic or administrative boundaries. Medical services for coronary heart disease and stroke had to be available within the area, and sufficiently advanced to provide proper diagnostic facilities to facilitate case-ascertainment of acute events. MONICA registers were to use existing diagnostic data on non-fatal events, and medico-legal data on fatal events. While cardiovascular clinical expertise was needed within the population, the MONICA Collaborating Centre (which could be based at some distance from it) also needed to have access to expertise in cardiovascular epidemiology in order to understand and conform to the common protocol, to be able to set up disease registers and to mount population surveys. Population demographic and routine mortality data for the population concerned had to be available.

Unfortunately these requirements, a consequence of the need to validate diagnoses and calculate event rates and trends, made recruitment of populations from developing countries problematic. In the early 1980s, most of the world's population was not living in countries that could provide death certificates or population denominator data needed for the calculation of mortality statistics (2). This, as well as the need for long-term commitment of resources, explains most of the geographical distribution of the eventual MONICA populations, see graphics G1 and G2. There were no populations from South America or Africa, and few populations from Asia. The lack of populations from North America had other explanations. Strongly involved in the early planning of MONICA, the National Heart, Lung and Blood Institute (NHLBI) ran an exploratory study, the Community Cardiovascular Surveillance Program (CCSP), in the USA and then continued with a parallel but different study to MONICA, the Atherosclerosis Risk in Communities, ARIC study (3).

Funding

The most fundamental requirement for recruitment (although never stated in the MONICA Protocol) was that the potential MONICA Collaborating Centres, which volunteered the populations that interested them, had to be self-funding. The World Health

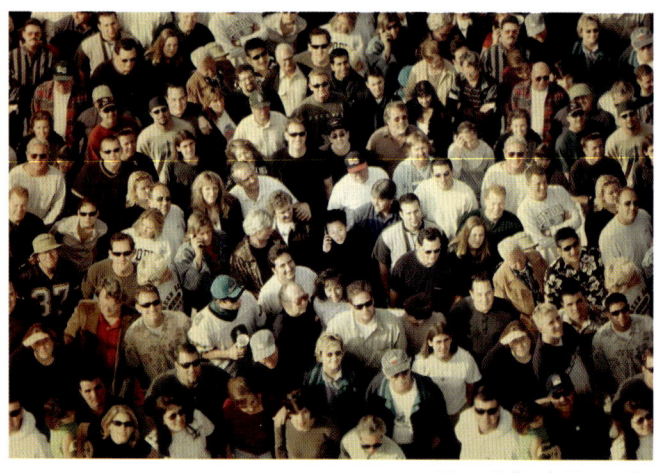

38 populations in 21 countries

Organization funded coordination, but not registration or population surveys within the populations concerned—see population pages #51–#83 where sources of funding are listed. Although 10-year funding was not necessarily always guaranteed at the start, recruitment was only feasible if that possibility had not been definitely excluded. Unlike a centrally funded drug trial therefore, where almost every detail can be rigidly enforced, MONICA was always an association of independently funded investigators who had agreed to work together. MONICA would not have been possible without the prior existence of many experienced groups around the world with an interest in the same problem, able to make the long-term commitment and to find local funds. Some recruits were relatively inexperienced but brought with them their enthusiasm to learn and participate as well as stable funding.

How big a population—Reporting Units and Reporting Unit Aggregates

Much time was spent in the early stages discussing population sizes. It was calculated that in order to establish trends with a satisfactory degree of precision over a 10-year period, a candidate population would need to be experiencing 300 coronary deaths a year in men in the target age-range of 25–64. This target was found to be a problem. It meant a large population even where disease rates were high, and an enormous one where they were low, and implied that trends in coronary disease in women and in stroke would not be measurable. On this basis, few populations would have qualified. However, if trends in rates were larger than expected, they would be detected with smaller numbers. The number was later changed to 200. The Data Book shows that although many MONICA populations were below even that target they still made a contribution (4).

Later a different statistical viewpoint prevailed. It was not necessary for trends within each population to be measured with great precision. For testing hypotheses across populations it was desirable to have many populations that were as heterogeneous as possible—differing from each other, but internally homogeneous. In order to produce large enough populations some MONICA Collaborating Centres had designated populations that were made up of different components. It was decided that each of these components should be identifiable as a Reporting Unit (RU), and coded thus on the relevant data records. A subsequent decision could be made as to how these were put together as Reporting Unit Aggregates (RUAs) (5). Precision of estimated trends within populations was therefore not the real issue for MONICA collaborative analyses. However, it could be for individual investigators in small centres who might spend ten years recording trends in event rates without ever knowing precisely which way they were going (see graphic G15 which shows estimated trends and 95% confidence intervals for coronary-event rates). This problem was particularly true for trends in coronary disease in women and for trends in stroke.

How many populations?

In the very early planning stages it was envisaged that MONICA would consist of perhaps 10–15 populations, however, it finished up with two to three times that number. Such a response was an embarrassing success for the World Health Organization as it made MONICA a more costly study than had been planned. Looking back, it is clear that 10–15 populations would have been a great improvement on the previous American experience, but with each population being one data point, the number of these points would have been less than ideal for the regression analyses that were eventually used, although number is not the only criterion. (Compare the hypothesis testing analyses in this Monograph for coronary events: 38 points and for stroke 15 points. See graphics G69–G77.)

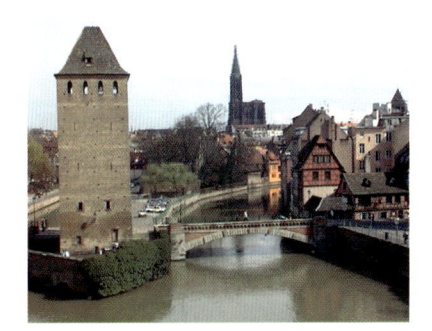

Strasbourg

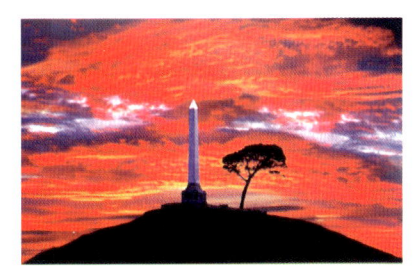

Auckland

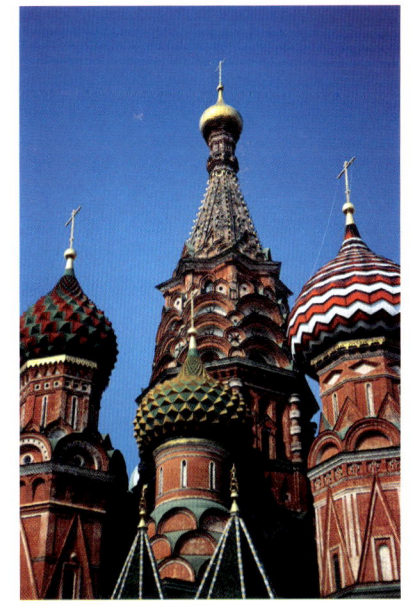

Moscow

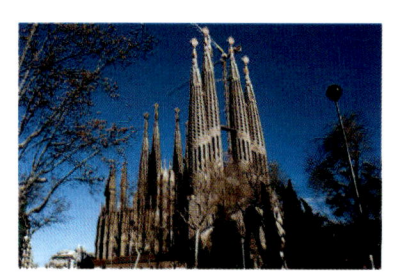

Barcelona

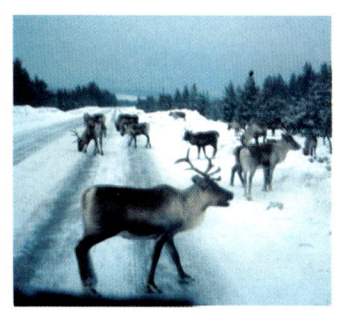

Northern Sweden

Recruits on probation: candidate MONICA Collaborating Centres

In the early days, suitable populations, with the promise of funding, were welcomed to MONICA through their Principal Investigators. However, they still had to qualify by providing results of pilot or feasibility studies and a local Manual of Operations translated into English (see #19 *Other Documents Used in MONICA*). After some centres had begun registration and others had yet to do so, the Council of Principal Investigators decided that to qualify, coronary-event registration had to be started by October 1984. This meant that the full calendar year with which the latest starters began their trend analyses for coronary events was 1985, see graphic G8. Full participants in MONICA who continued to fulfil the requirements for continuing participation were designated MONICA Collaborating Centres. Fellow travellers, who ran in parallel but did not qualify in time to be included in the Project, or lapsed from full participation, were designated Associate Collaborating Centres. These funded their own participation at Principal Investigator Meetings and their data were not centrally analysed. This Monograph is mainly concerned with those MONICA Collaborating Centres that provided sufficient data to help test the original MONICA hypotheses on trends.

References

1. Havlik RJ, Feinleib M, eds. *Proceedings of the Conference on the Decline in Coronary Heart Disease Mortality, October 24–25, 1978*. Washington, DC: National Heart, Lung and Blood Institute, 1979, NIH publication No.79–1610, DHES.
2. Uemura K, Píša Z. Recent trends in cardiovascular disease mortality in 27 industrialized countries. *World Health Statistics Quarterly*, 1985, 38:142–162. PMID: 4036160.
3. The ARIC Investigators. The Atherosclerosis Risk in Communities (ARIC) Study: design and objectives. *American Journal of Epidemiology*, 1989, 129:687–702. PMID:2646917.
4. Mähönen M, Tolonen H, Kuulasmaa K, for the WHO MONICA Project. MONICA coronary event registration data book 1980–1995. (October 2000). Available from URL: http://www.ktl.fi/publications/monica/coredb/coredb.htm, URN:NBN:fi-fe20001204. MONICA Web Publication 25.
5. WHO MONICA Project. MONICA Manual. (1998–1999). Part I: Description and Organization of the Project. Section 1: Objectives and Outline Protocol. Available from URL: http://www.ktl.fi/publications/monica/manual/part1/i-1.htm, URN:NBN:fi-fe19981147. MONICA Web Publication 1.

Jaakko Tuomilehto, Zbyněk Píša, Hugh Tunstall-Pedoe

#11 Communications in MONICA

Introduction

MONICA investigators had to communicate and transfer data and manuscripts across the world by various means. Looking back, it is difficult to imagine MONICA being successfully completed without the means of communication that developed as the project progressed.

Communication groups

Within MONICA there was a worldwide network of communications across the study structure, not all the elements of which are shown in the organization chart in #3. The different groups were:

- the Council of Principal Investigators (CPI)
- the MONICA Steering Committee (MSC)
- Manuscript Groups, and others.

MONICA Collaborating Centres (MCCs), the MONICA Management Centre (MMC), the MONICA Data Centre (MDC) and MONICA Quality Control Centres (MQCs) were in frequent, often daily communication with each other, back and forth.

- a research network which created an international 'MONICA family'
- over two decades experienced and exploited the communications revolution
- e-mail, FAX, and the Internet carried an otherwise under-resourced international project to completion
- MONICA Investigators pioneered the new technologies in their own institutions

Forms of communication

These ranged from formal meetings and working visits to telephone conferences and MONICA Memos (see below).

Early formal conferences of investigators

The WHO MONICA Project began with a series of meetings of would-be investigators, planned months beforehand, with written invitations, agendas, conference documents, minutes and conference reports. These could not take place more than once or twice a year. Planning communications came by normal surface mail and airmail. Large institutions had TELEX machines but these were rarely used. Telephone use was limited by its cost. Some people were happy to receive international calls but not to initiate them.

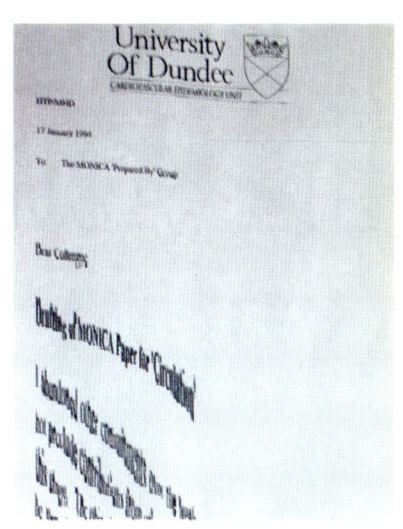

MONICA Steering Committee meetings

The meetings of Principal Investigators were large, very costly and infrequent. It was decided to set up a MONICA Steering Committee that would meet every few months. It had a designated membership of continuing and rotating members. It met frequently during the early stages of MONICA, and less frequently thereafter. Agendas, documents and minutes came by mail. Meetings were costly and difficult to arrange. The MONICA Steering Committee had had 29 formal face-to-face meetings by the end of 2001 but these had become increasingly infrequent, because of the expense and, conversely, because of the advent of cheaper methods of communication.

Faulty Fax from 1994 preserved on Kari Kuulasmaa's office wall

Telephone conferences

With reductions in the price of telephone calls the MONICA Steering Committee began to arrange monthly or two-monthly telephone conferences. The main difficulty was arranging times and dates when everyone could participate—the Committee covers many different time-zones. By the end of 2002 the MONICA Steering Committee had held 105 telephone conferences.

MONICA Memos

The MONICA Management Centre in Geneva introduced a system of MONICA Memos (MNM) to circulate and request information. The contents varied, but they always had a covering letter from the Chief of the CVD Unit and an opening statement as to what action was required, by what deadline, and where the response was to go. Planning and sending a MONICA Memo and getting a reply took several weeks at first. There were comments about delays at MONICA Meetings. Nonetheless, the MONICA Memo system was invaluable and over 400 were circulated between January 1983 and December 2002. A Memo could vary in length from one sheet of A4 paper to a large set of tables or a draft paper for approval. Reproduction and distribution of MONICA Memos was a major function of the Management Centre and could not have been assumed by anyone else. The covering letter from WHO gave them official status. They were not to be ignored. Some were distributed widely to a general mailing list while others contained unpublished data for Principal Investigators alone. (See #88 *MONICA Memos* and also the Monograph CD-ROM part 2.) There were eventually three varieties:

A—confidential, B—not confidential, and C—electronic (see below).

FAX

After the mid-1980s, MONICA entered the electronic age. "Do you have access to a FAX machine?" became a routine question. Initially this meant seeking help from another department, hundreds of metres away in the same institution, or through a post-office or shop. Output was often a slippery piece of paper, difficult to write on, darkening or fading when exposed to daylight, and documents could be unreadable even when newly received. Later every small department got its own machine.

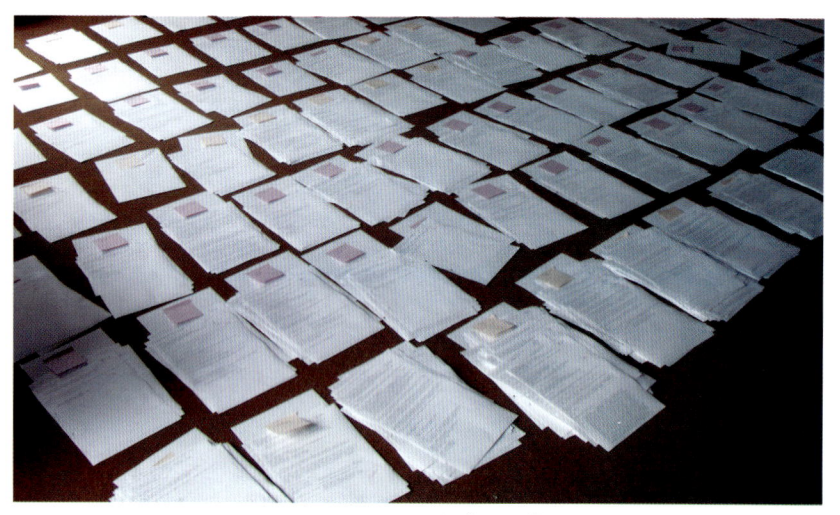

E-mail

The MONICA Steering Committee started using electronic mail in 1987 and has circulated thousands of messages since then. MONICA investigators were often way ahead of academic or medical colleagues in this respect. Difficulties with 'attachments' were initially very common and unfortunately still occur. For eastern European centres where ordinary mail could take weeks, this was a major advance, starting often through amateur networks.

Sorting E-mails on the Monograph, Dundee June 2001

The World Wide Web

The final step in rapid communication occurred when the MONICA Data Centre in Helsinki started a website for the WHO MONICA Project in 1996: http://www.ktl.fi/monica/. The public website describes and identifies the project, listing its sites and key personnel and MONICA publications. Linked to it however are password-protected pages which contain much of the ongoing business of MONICA. The MSC page contains minutes and agendas of telephone conferences and documents for discussion. MONICA manuscript groups had their own web pages for draft documents. Even the data analyses performed in the MONICA Data Centre were published on the manuscript groups' web pages. For example, the graphics in this Monograph were developed between Helsinki and Dundee. Updated versions were placed on an internal web page from Helsinki and an e-mail message sent to Dundee where they were downloaded and commented upon by e-mail. This could be done several times in one day. Differences in time-zone and working hours were often advantageous, with late-night comments from Dundee acted on in Helsinki while Dundee was at breakfast. The latest MONICA Memos have been distributed through the web.

MONICA collaborators, through the cross-fertilization of ideas, and demands of the project, have been ahead of their national colleagues in using new technology. However, the price paid for rapid communication of information is that there is too much of it from different sources, and documents can be overlooked. "I have not received it", is the face-saving plea of a busy colleague sent a FAX or e-mail, now buried. Recent communications however, show that some MONICA Collaborating Centres still have notepaper with their TELEX address proudly displayed!

Hugh Tunstall-Pedoe

#12 Quality Assurance

A major concern for any large-scale, long-term multi-centre collaborative study is to collect data of appropriate quality that is highly comparable across the many participating centres that are collecting the data and over the several years of the study's duration. This issue was especially important for the MONICA Project as it was being planned for 30–40 MONICA Collaborating Centres (MCCs) in 24 countries over four continents with even more numerous, often separated populations under study. It involved data collection activities from three separate screening activities over a 10-year period, plus those required for other important data components such as coronary and stroke-event registration, monitoring of coronary care, and collection of routine mortality and demographic information.

To address this fundamental issue, the MONICA Project created and operated a carefully constructed Quality Assurance programme. This programme was developed by the MONICA Steering Committee (MSC) and was implemented with considerable energy by the MONICA Management Centre (MMC), the MONICA Data Centre (MDC), the MONICA Quality Control Centres (MQC) and selected members of the MSC. Quality Assurance was based on:

- the use of standardized data collection methods and procedures
- training of the data collection and data processing personnel in the use of standardized methods
- quality control at various stages of data collection and processing, and at various levels of the Project
- retrospective assessment of the quality of the data that was eventually attained and the documentation of shortcomings and centre-specific features in the data.

The data collection standards as well as instructions for the training and internal quality control in the centres are described in the MONICA Manual (1) Three MONICA Quality Control Centres were created at the start. Each was responsible for training MCC data collection personnel and for assisting the MSC with monitoring the performance of the individual MCCs in the relevant areas. The three MQCs were:

- MONICA Quality Control Centre for Lipid Measurement, responsible for the quality of the total cholesterol, HDL-C and triglycerides measurements,
- MONICA Quality Control Centre for Event Registration, responsible for the quality of the registration and coding of coronary and stroke events, and
- MONICA Quality Control Centre for ECG Coding, responsible for the quality of the coding of electrocardiograms.

(See #8 *MONICA Quality Control Centres (MQCs)*.)

After the experience of the initial population surveys, two training seminars were organized for those in the centres responsible for the local training of survey teams. These were held in Helsinki in 1991 and in Gargnano, Italy, in 1993.

The MSC assessed the overall quality of the data collection process and the transmission of data to the MDC on a routine basis. These reviews covered a number of issues. Scores on individual items and overall scores were reviewed with the MQC leadership at MSC meetings.

- not additional, but fundamental to MONICA procedures
- built in to all stages of the monitoring process
- MONICA Quality assessment reports published on the Internet

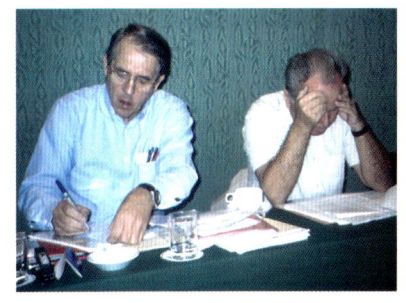

Dale Williams at a CPI Meeting (Zbyněk Píša on his left)

The quality of the data attained, together with a description of any shortcomings and centre-specific characteristics, were documented separately for each major data item in MONICA Quality assessment reports. These were produced periodically, and some of the problems identified could still be remedied. The final MONICA Quality assessment reports were published on the World Wide Web (2). They are an invaluable source of information for anyone analysing the MONICA data.

Perhaps most important was the fact that a carefully constructed and implemented Quality Assurance programme was used by the MONICA Project. This programme received constant ongoing attention from the MSC and all the central agencies and committees. Further, it was supported by the MCCs in their efforts to contribute high quality, useful data.

References
MONICA Web Publications are also accessible on the Monograph CD-ROM
Quality Assurance is so pervasive in MONICA that it is invidious to name specific documents. It is referred to in specific sections of this Monograph but see also:

1. WHO MONICA Project. MONICA Manual. (1998–1999). Available from URL: http://www.ktl.fi/publications/monica/manual/index.htm, URN:NBN:fi-fe19981146. MONICA Web Publication 1.
2. MONICA Quality assessment reports. MONICA Web Publications 2-18. Available from URL: http://www.ktl.fi/publications/monica/index.htm

Dale Williams, Kari Kuulasmaa

#13 Ethics and Confidentiality

Introduction

In the 1980s ethical issues were not of major concern to MONICA as it was following well-established procedures. Unlike recruitment for trials of powerful new drugs or procedures, the physical risk to people involved in MONICA's disease registration or population surveys was immeasurably small. Even so, there were ethical issues of consent and confidentiality. MONICA investigators had to satisfy local ethical requirements for research in each population in which they worked. These requirements were sometimes illogically inconsistent in different countries. Recent attempts at international standardization through measures such as the European Convention on Human Rights may be beneficial in the long-term but much will depend on how they are interpreted. Just now it would be difficult to initiate a new MONICA Project in many former participating countries because of doubts about what newly framed legislation on confidentiality, medical records, and civil rights actually means. The issues involved in population surveys and in coronary or stroke event registration will now be considered separately.

- MONICA did not use invasive, intrusive or hazardous procedures
- it did collect confidential personal medical information
- twenty years ago it was accepted as in the public interest
- MONICA followed ethical guidelines and was generally welcomed
- concern over civil rights is now making similar research more difficult to carry out

Disease registration

In order to calculate trends in event rates and survival, the investigator must be able to include information on all the possible events that come to the attention of the medical and medico-legal systems. This means obtaining access to case notes, pathology and biochemistry reports, both in hospitals and in the community. These need to be merged with information from death certificates and death records, eyewitness accounts of sudden deaths and post-mortem reports. In the case of 'hot pursuit' some information will be obtained directly from living patients, with permission given face to face. In the case of 'cold pursuit' and for fatal cases, this is not practical. (See #20 *Registration of Coronary Events, Hot and Cold Pursuit.*) Registration and the linking of records in MONICA were usually approved by privacy and ethical committees who were satisfied that the researchers were of good standing, would keep the information securely, and use it only for medical research. They could even make it a condition that no direct contact be made with living patients or relatives. Medical records belonged to the medical and medico-legal organizations concerned. Newer ideas implying that records belong to the patient and may not be used for any purpose without individual written permission threaten the completeness of disease registration. Patients refusing permission would be undermining the need for comprehensiveness. Results would be biased and incomplete. Refusal of some would tend to devalue the remaining contributions of the majority who did take part.

Population surveys

These cannot be done without the explicit cooperation of the participant. Ethical concerns involve the researchers' access to the sampling frame, and the way in which the original written invitation is phrased. Does it accurately state what is involved? Does it make unjustified promises of personal benefit to the participant? What follow-up recruitment methods are justified if there is no response? On arrival at the clinic the participant had to have a full explanation and give written consent to the survey procedures. This included venepuncture for blood specimens. Potential problems here were what to do if any of the individual findings was seriously abnormal and who, if anybody, should receive a report. Non-participation, or non-response is a well-recognized problem in such surveys. (See #29 *Recruitment and Response Rates.*)

Data management

Individual medical or risk-factor information is necessary for the event registration and population survey components of MONICA. Records of individuals are maintained, although the analyses are carried out on whole groups. It is essential to maintain the individuality and integrity of each record without compromising confidentiality. This is usually done by keeping the MONICA medical information entirely separate, but with a unique personal number, which can be cross-linked with a confidential file elsewhere containing identification information such as names and addresses. The latter is needed for several reasons. One is that the research is much more powerful and cost-effective if it involves 'following-up' participants for their future mortality and morbidity. The researcher then needs to be able to link MONICA records with subsequent hospital or death-certificate data. This cannot be done without personal identifiers. It is also important to be able to check whether records have been inadvertently duplicated. In addition, research participants have the right to know what information is held about them on computer.

MONICA, in distributing anonymous records through the MONICA Database for further analyses by collaborators, has taken care to remove potentially over-specific information. Actual birth-dates were removed from the records before they were distributed, although it seems inconceivable that anyone would seriously wish to identify individuals on that basis.

Many MONICA Investigators, with permission, took specimens of urine, blood and sometimes other tissues for immediate analysis, but then stored what was left for further analyses of possible new risk factors in the future. Some research ethics committees now want researchers to specify exactly what tests are to be done when a specimen is requested, which would limit such activity. A particular problem arises with specimens containing DNA, unique genetic material, a problem now facing many researchers and research committees. The DNA profile of an individual has implications for their blood-relatives as well

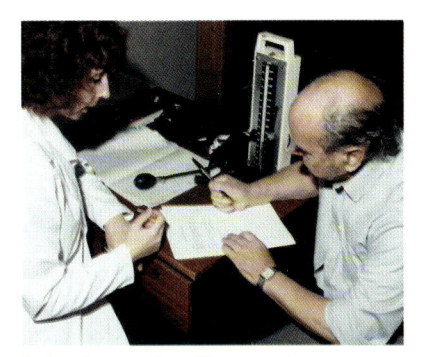

Explanation precedes written consent

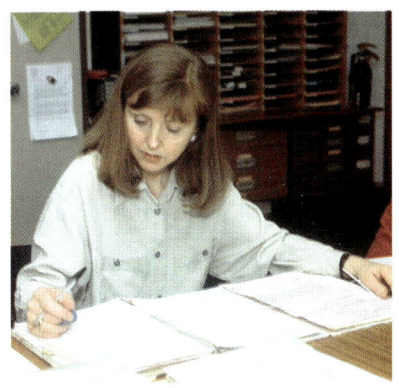

MONICA preserved confidentiality of medical records

as themselves. There are also potential problems of 'ownership' of biological material which might have commercial implications, such as patent rights.

Conclusion

MONICA investigators conformed to best practice in their own countries. In the two decades of the MONICA Project the MONICA Steering Committee and MONICA Data Centre have not been made aware of any breaches of confidentiality, or of ethical complaints arising from this huge study.

Increasing sophistication, both of medical research and of the general public have made issues of ethics and confidentiality increasingly prominent. It is important for the future that non-commercial research in public health for the public good such as MONICA is not prevented, or seriously frustrated, by over-zealous legislators, by over-promotion of individuals' rights without concern for their responsibilities, or by sensational publicity leading to a breakdown of public trust. Much will depend on the good sense of the public and on such research continuing to be seen as for the public good rather than private gain.

Alun Evans, Hugh Tunstall-Pedoe

#14 MONICA and the Prevention of Cardiovascular Disease

- by seeking to explain trends in CVD MONICA planned to control them
- MONICA trained professionals and sensitized others to the importance of CVD and cardiovascular risk factors, and their surveillance
- most CVD now occurs in the developing world where it is rapidly increasing
- MONICA has shown that the increase in the epidemic can be reversed

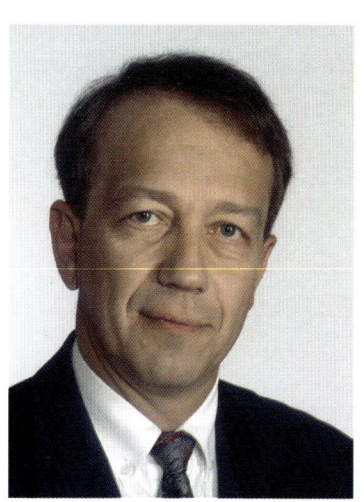

Pekka Puska

Questions for prevention

The ultimate aim of the MONICA Project was to serve prevention. It was designed to cast light on crucial questions from the 1980s whether trends in mortality are more influenced by primary prevention (attack rates) or by treatment (case fatality). Are trends in attack rates in the population driven by changes in risk factors—a key question in primary prevention?

Already during the design of the project a number of problems were encountered. These were related to our ability to measure changes both in risk factors and in disease rates. These questions concerned sample sizes, age groups and possible time-lags. Although these problems surfaced again in the analysis of the results, the MONICA Project has nevertheless provided significant answers to its original questions.

Answers and new questions

According to the results, both primary prevention and treatment influence mortality trends. The pattern varies in different populations. A high proportion of pre-hospital deaths puts great emphasis on primary prevention. Trends are influenced by risk factors—allowing for some time-lag. The degree to which risk-factor changes can explain trends remains, unfortunately, somewhat unclear. Like all research, MONICA provided answers, but raised many new questions. As a result, the project is likely to inspire further research into prevention.

Other benefits

The WHO MONICA Project has served global cardiovascular disease (CVD) prevention in other important ways, but indirectly. MONICA has been a model for how a huge multi-component, multinational project can be implemented and managed, how standardized data can be collected, data analysed, communication organized, and so on. Further, MONICA became, as one of its founders predicted, a gold standard 'model for good housekeeping' in monitoring trends in CVD rates and respective risk factors. Countries and programmes that had nothing to do with MONICA use and refer to 'MONICA methodology' in their work. MONICA has shown the way in CVD monitoring, a cornerstone for prevention.

Growing global burden of CVD

During the twenty years that MONICA was carried out, a significant change took place in the global burden of CVDs. When MONICA was started, CVDs were predominantly seen as the burden of industrialized countries. Indeed, most of the MONICA centres were in that part of the world. At the end of the MONICA period, estimates showed that CVDs had rapidly increased in the developing world, and that the epidemic continues to increase. Today the majority of the CVD deaths in the world are in developing countries. Every third death in the world is cardiovascular (1). Coronary heart disease is the number one killer in the world. CVDs are increasingly attacking economically disadvantaged countries and population groups, thus contributing to poverty and hindering economic development.

CVD prevention—key for global health

Thus, CVD prevention is a crucial issue of contemporary global public health. Fortunately, as MONICA results show, quite dramatic reductions in CVD attack rates are possible. The greatest reduction was by as much as 6.5% per year over a 10-year period in North Karelia, Finland. This is a province in which systematic long-term prevention has been implemented.

Our challenge is not merely to predict and to monitor the trends, but to influence them. Even modest changes in CVD trends can have a huge public health impact. And many MONICA centres show that quite substantial changes can take place in ten years—both up and down. These kinds of changes have nothing to do with genetics; they are the result of environmental changes, and especially of lifestyle changes. Prevention is possible and it pays off.

MONICA's place in the history of CVD prevention

The WHO MONICA project has without any doubt significantly contributed to global prevention efforts. This has occurred because of its scientific contributions, and through the provision of a good foundation for future monitoring and surveillance efforts. One challenge for prevention is to create meaningful, coordinated global efforts to reverse the unfavourable trends that we see in a large part of the world. The focus should be on broad instructions to reduce the numbers of people affected by the few well-proven risk factors that relate closely to certain lifestyles. This calls for global leadership by WHO, and strong collaboration between governments, public health experts, and other partners.

Reference

1. Murray CJ, Lopez AD. Mortality by cause for eight regions of the world: Global Burden of Disease Study. *Lancet*, 1997, 349:1269–1276. PMID 9142060.

Pekka Puska

Director, Noncommunicable Disease Prevention and Health Promotion, World Health Organization, Geneva. Previously Principal Investigator of FINMONICA 1982–87, first Chair of MONICA Steering Committee

#15 Reminiscences of MONICA's Rapporteur

- Multinational Monitoring of Trends and Determinants in Cardiovascular Disease
- "you will have to call it the MONICA Project!"
- "quality control, quality control, I have never heard of such a study for quality control!"
- "—did MONICA really say that?"

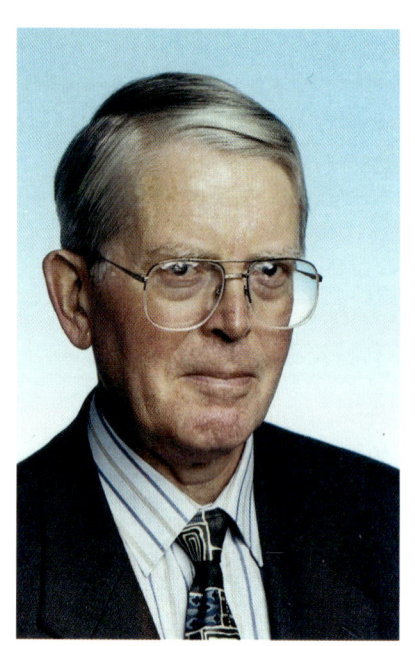

Hugh Tunstall-Pedoe was MONICA's Rapporteur from 1979

European Myocardial Infarction Community Registers

I first met Zbyněk Píša, MONICA's godfather, in 1969 in the office of Professor Jerry Morris at the London School of Hygiene and Tropical Medicine. Setting up a heart attack register was one of Jerry Morris's dreams, foreshadowed in his book on *Uses of Epidemiology* (1). It was finally happening thanks to the European Heart Attack Registers. These were being coordinated by Zbyněk Píša, the officer responsible for chronic diseases at the World Health Organization Regional Office in Copenhagen. I had been recruited, as a young trainee cardiologist, to set up a register in the London Borough (suburb) of Tower Hamlets. The dream was coming true. We needed a community perspective to explain why population mortality rates continued to rise when coronary care units (CCUs) were being championed as halving heart-attack mortality.

Months later I attended a World Health Organization Working Group Meeting in Copenhagen. Zbyněk Píša told me that, as the English-language participant, I was to write up the proceedings—in WHO terminology I was the Rapporteur. I had brought my family with me for a holiday. I never did so again. Diagnostic criteria for definite myocardial infarction were based on a WHO document of 1959 (2). This provided, with illustrations, two electrocardiographic criteria: development of new Q waves, and evolution and disappearance of an injury current in three stages. A footnote said that an injury current was not necessary if new Q waves were observed. I questioned whether evolution of an injury current was also sufficient—otherwise it was illogical and redundant. Nobody knew. I summoned up courage and inserted 'and/or' between the two criteria where they have remained ever since (3, 4). Diagnostic criteria are not just descriptions—they have to be watertight and to be able to classify potential cases consistently, something often forgotten even now (5).

Quality control

At the next meeting I suggested circulating test case-histories, to see whether coding was consistent. I was asked to do so. Results showed major disagreements on certain items, and failure by some participants to understand why these were included. One group claimed that all their coronary deaths occurred in hospital. It was a minority in the other centres. The explanation given by the group was that nobody was dead until a doctor said so: there were no doctors outside the hospital. Jerry Morris chaired this meeting. He insisted that we start again using only data collected after key items had been more specifically defined. However, earlier data re-emerged in the final publication. Looking back now it was rather primitive—bundles of incomplete record forms being sent to and fro across Europe. Although we had defined definite and possible myocardial infarction, the latter including some very borderline cases, results were pooled in the final analyses. Zbyněk Píša, by this time in Geneva, asked me to write a chapter on methods for a monograph on *Myocardial Infarction Community Registers* (3). I did so, stating what had worked, what had not, and identifying problems. The chapter was acknowledged, but the monograph appeared without it. I was told later that my chapter was "not quite what was wanted". By this time I was working on another WHO study with coronary end-points, the European factory study, with Professor Geoffrey Rose (6). I published my critique of heart attack registers in a cardiology journal, its title honouring Jerry Morris (7).

Preparations for MONICA

In 1979 Zbyněk Píša asked me to send him reprints of this critique to be used as a working document for a small meeting that followed the Bethesda *Conference on the Decline of Coronary Heart Disease Mortality* (8). The plan was to revive heart attack registration so as to study trends over time. That year I spent several weeks in Minneapolis at the then Laboratory of Physiological Hygiene, Stadium Gate 27, where the Minnesota Heart Survey was being launched to monitor trends in coronary disease and risk factors. This was the home of the *Seven Countries Study* (9), and of Minnesota coding of the electrocardiogram (10), as well as the joint parent of *Cardiovascular Survey Methods* (11). Immediately after Zbyněk Píša's small meeting in September 1979 he asked me to be Rapporteur at another meeting taking place two months later in Geneva, and to draft the outline of a protocol for a study of trends by listing the subject headings in preparation for this. So began my involvement with a series of meetings leading to MONICA. Ron Prineas from Minneapolis was a consultant at these early meetings. We used the European *Myocardial Infarction Community Registers* (3), the *Minnesota Field Survey Manual* (12) and *Cardiovascular Survey Methods* (11) to plan the study. In 1981 I moved to Scotland and helped to initiate Scottish MONICA, fortunately for me, as England did not participate.

Development of the protocol and the name

Attendance at early meetings changed but the Chair, Fred Epstein, and the Rapporteur, I myself, did not change. There was creative tension between his ambitious wish to relate trends in cardiovascular disease to 'changes in known risk factors, daily living habits, health care and major socioeconomic features measured at the same time in defined communities . . .' (13) and my wish to define what was feasible and measurable. The group discussed the title of the project. I suggested 'determinants' for risk factors and argued for 'multinational' rather than 'international'. Zbyněk Píša had doubts about 'multinational' but the long title was being spelled out as *Multinational Monitoring of Trends and Determinants in Cardiovascular Disease*, when Tom Strasser, a Medical Officer in the CVD Unit (subsequently with the World Hypertension League in Geneva) cried, "In that case you will have to call it the MONICA Project!" The short name and the long name remained.

'MONICA' was a marvellous name. It was one of the first studies to be given an acronym. Others copied it. Many knew about MONICA years before we produced any results, because the name intrigued them. In 1998 during the summer 'silly season' when there was little news, press reports of the initial results of MONICA that we had presented at the European Congress of Cardiology in Vienna, mischievously suggested that there was no connection at all between coronary risk factors and coronary risk. The name MONICA was so topical for other reasons to do with the American presidency that I was able to use it to obtain very rapid publication of an article refuting the media misrepresentation (14).

Fred Epstein was a charming and accomplished Chairman. He knew that meetings could not draft documents. When we reached a controversial subject, and four different speakers had produced five opinions on what we should do, he would say "Thank you everybody. We will now move on to the next topic. We can safely leave what you have said with our excellent Rapporteur". I would then struggle to produce a proposal that was sensible and feasible. By the next meeting former protagonists had forgotten their previous positions, and would suggest minor changes in wording. It took months of work, with visits to Geneva between meetings. I was once there to consult on psychosocial studies and measuring medical care. The WHO expert on the latter told me that we could not record quality of coronary care, because medical intervention in chronic disease generally made outcomes worse—an orthodox view around 1980, just as the extraordinary coronary care and secondary prevention revolutions were beginning. Luckily, we ignored his advice.

Ten years had made a big difference to the science of such studies. Monitoring of trends meant trying to detect small changes. Quality control was

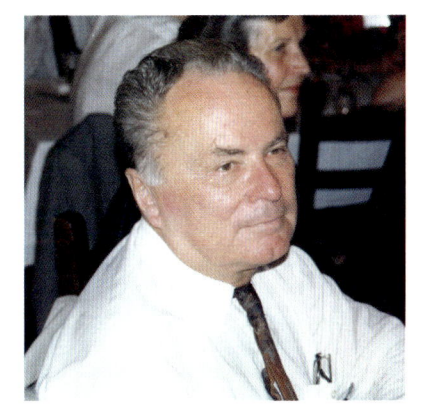

Zbyněk Píša initiated what became MONICA

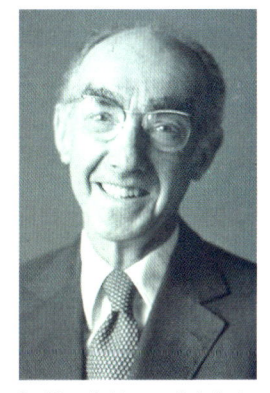

Fred Epstein (deceased) chaired early MONICA meetings

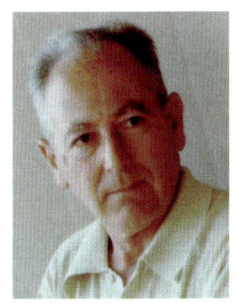

Tom Strasser (deceased) gave MONICA its name

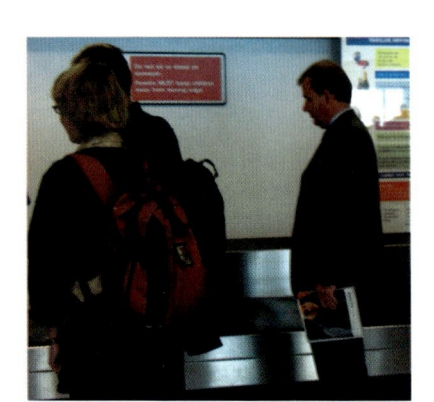

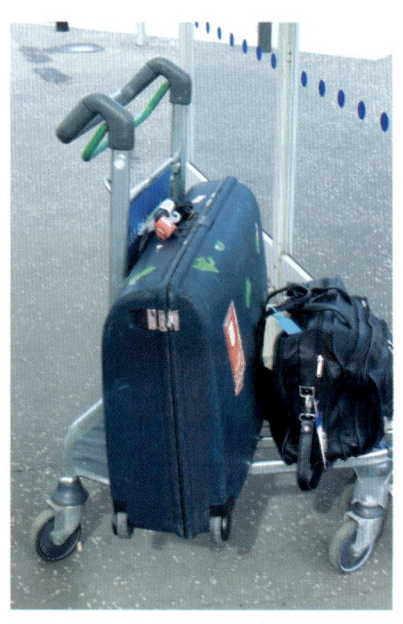

essential. Training and testing were fundamental. I was again struggling with diagnostic criteria which, this time, were more quantitative (*4*), and with preparing and marking endless series of test case-histories, see #88 *MONICA Memos*. Early meetings of Principal Investigators were preoccupied with quality assurance, with announcing results of quality control exercises, and with coding workshops. I remember a cry from the floor once, "Quality control, quality control, I have never heard of such a study for quality control!" It was not mutiny as the centre concerned followed decisions carefully, once they were made.

Early years

We spent a long time waiting for results to accrue in the Data Centre in Helsinki and to pass our numerous checks. The first collaborative population survey results on risk factors were published in 1988 and 1989 (*15, 16*). Although there was concern about aspects of quality control and response rates, population surveys were a well-established epidemiological routine. Results from coronary-event registration, however, took considerably longer. In 1990, as head of the Quality Control Centre for Event Registration I reviewed data then available in the MONICA Data Centre in Helsinki, and reported back to MONICA Collaborating Centres in a MONICA Memorandum (*17*). It was 'crunch time' for MONICA. Data from only a handful of MONICA centres were publishable, the majority having overlooked an important protocol requirement. They had submitted only cases satisfying MONICA diagnostic criteria, not those clinically diagnosed as myocardial infarction or coronary deaths that failed the criteria. (A similar problem existed with stroke.) This meant that numbers of MONICA coronary events, if fatal, were smaller than numbers of coronary deaths in local statistics. A similar situation applied to non-fatal myocardial infarction. We needed fully coded details of all false-positives to be made available, to prove that reported cases were not being overlooked (*13, 18*). Round the world, MONICA Investigators had to go back several years and send in record forms for the missing false-positive cases. Everybody did so with good grace. The first cross-sectional paper on coronary events was published in *Circulation* in 1994. It was a paper with a worldwide impact and has been cited since more than 500 times (*4*).

Maturity

Following the publication of cross-sectional results came years of data accumulation, discussion of data quality, and of centres failing to meet deadlines for essential data. Some discussions were interminable and slow to resolve. After one MONICA Steering Committee meeting I suggested to the then Chair that I re-circulate the minutes from the previous year to see if anyone noticed the difference. He was not amused. Eventually we parted company or lost contact with failing centres. We were then able to concentrate on the long-term data we had, and how it should be analysed.

Finding that the *Lancet* was interested in publishing our 10-year results by fast-tracking made an enormous difference. Some MONICA papers had spent months or years with particular journals, or had received referees' comments that disheartened the original authors, who moved on to other things. Knowing that editors were interested and waiting was a great stimulus, although the papers concerned still needed an enormous effort both in submission and in dealing rapidly with referees' comments (*19–21*). Although the main results papers of MONICA were well received, a problem has always been that tables with 30 rows or more for different populations, and numerous columns, are difficult to read. Editors prefer tables to figures. Figures usually appear in black and white, too small for individual results to be read with ease. Most readers of the papers would not study the tables carefully and this would be true even of many statisticians and epidemiologists. While preparing the main results papers for MONICA, however, we showed superb colour slides at scientific meetings. But these were too transient for the audience to identify specific populations, and were not published.

This Monograph provides the opportunity to celebrate the MONICA Project at 23 years, to make our results and data available in one place to scientists, students and teachers, and to publish our coloured graphics for general study. Publication marks the end of a classic era. MONICA was launched when individuals and funding bodies were sympathetic to a ten-year commitment to answer a major problem. We are now in an era of rapid results, 'more bangs to the buck', and multiple career moves. MONICA finally took over twenty years, a third of my life and proportionately more of the lives of those who are younger. MONICA investigators refer to the MONICA family with the men questioning whether MONICA was a wife or a mistress. Either way it is improbable that we will see her again—despite many of us suspecting that twenty years of data on trends would have helped to answer many of the questions that were left unresolved by ten.

References
MONICA Web Publications are also accessible on the Monograph CD-ROM

1. Morris JN. *Uses of Epidemiology*, London, Livingstone, 1957.
2. *Hypertension and coronary heart disease: classification and criteria for epidemiological studies.* Geneva, World Health Organization, 1959 (WHO Technical Report Series, No. 168).
3. World Health Organization Regional Office for Europe. *Myocardial infarction community registers*, Copenhagen, 1976 (Public Health in Europe 5).
4. Tunstall-Pedoe H, Kuulasmaa K, Amouyel P, Arveiler D, Rajakangas AM, Pajak A, for the WHO MONICA Project. Myocardial infarction and coronary deaths in the World Health Organization MONICA Project. Registration procedures, event rates, and case-fatality rates in 38 populations from 21 countries in four continents. *Circulation*, 1994, 90:583–612. PMID: 8026046. MONICA Publication 16.
5. The Joint European Society of Cardiology/American College of Cardiology Committee. Myocardial infarction redefined—a consensus document of the Joint European Society of Cardiology/American College of Cardiology Committee for the Redefinition of Myocardial Infarction. *European Heart Journal*, 2000:1502–1513.
6. World Health Organization European Collaborative Group. Multifactorial trial in the prevention of coronary heart disease. 1. Recruitment and initial findings. *European Heart Journal*, 1980, 1:73–80. PMID: 7026247.
7. Tunstall-Pedoe H. Uses of coronary heart attack registers. *British Heart Journal*, 1978, 40:510–515. PMID: 656216.
8. Havlik RJ, Feinleib M, eds. *Proceedings of the Conference on the Decline in Coronary Heart Disease Mortality, October 24–25, 1978*. Washington, DC: National Heart, Lung and Blood Institute, 1979, NIH publication No.79-1610, DHES.
9. Keys A. *Seven Countries: A Multivariate Analysis of Death and Coronary Heart Disease*, Cambridge, Mass. and London, England, Harvard University Press, 1980.
10. Prineas RJ, Crow RS, Blackburn H. *The Minnesota Code Manual of Electrocardiographic Findings: Standards and Procedures for Measurement and Classification*, Littleton, Mass. and Bristol, England, John Wright, 1982, ISBN 0-7236-7053-6.
11. Rose GA, Blackburn H, Gillum RF, Prineas RJ. *Cardiovascular Survey Methods.* 2nd ed. Geneva, World Health Organization, 1982 (Monograph series No. 56).
12. Laboratory of Physiological Hygiene. *Survey Manual of Operations 1981–82*, Minneapolis, Minn., University of Minnesota, 1981.
13. WHO MONICA Project. MONICA Manual. (1998–1999). Available from URL: http://www.ktl.fi/publications/monica/manual/index.htm, URN:*NBN:fi-fe19981146*. MONICA Web Publication 1.
14. Tunstall-Pedoe H. Did MONICA really say that? *British Medical Journal*, 1998, 317:1023–1023. PMID: 9765191.
15. Pajak A, Kuulasmaa K, Tuomilehto J, Ruokokoski E, for the WHO MONICA Project. Geographical variation in the major risk factors of coronary heart disease in men and women aged 35–64 years. *World Health Statistics Quarterly*, 1988, 41:115–140. PMID: 3232405. MONICA Publication 3.
16. The WHO MONICA Project. A worldwide monitoring system for cardiovascular diseases: Cardiovascular mortality and risk factors in selected communities. *World Health Statistics Annual*, 1989, 27–149. ISBN 92 4 067890 5. ISSN 0250–3794. MONICA Publication 11.
17. MONICA MEMO 177 of 15.02.90. Eligibility of MCCs for publication of Coronary Event Data. Internal MONICA Document distributed to all Principal Investigators. (See CD-ROM.)

18. Mähönen M, Tolonen H, Kuulasmaa K, Tunstall-Pedoe H, Amouyel P, for the WHO MONICA Project. Quality assessment of coronary event registration data in the WHO MONICA Project. (January 1999). Available from URL: http://www.ktl.fi/publications/monica/coreqa/coreqa.htm, URN:*NBN:fi-fe19991072*. MONICA Web Publication 2.
19. Tunstall-Pedoe H, Kuulasmaa K, Mähönen M, Tolonen H, Ruokokoski E, Amouyel P, for the WHO MONICA Project. Contribution of trends in survival and coronary-event rates to changes in coronary heart disease mortality: 10-year results from 37 WHO MONICA Project populations. *Lancet*, 1999, 353:1547–1557. PMID: 10334252. MONICA Publication 36.
20. Kuulasmaa K, Tunstall-Pedoe H, Dobson A, Fortmann S, Sans S, Tolonen H, Evans A, Ferrario M, Tuomilehto J, for the WHO MONICA Project. Estimation of contribution of changes in classic risk factors to trends in coronary-event rates across the WHO MONICA Project populations. *Lancet*, 2000, 355:675–687. PMID: 10703799. MONICA Publication 38.
21. Tunstall-Pedoe H, Vanuzzo D, Hobbs M, Mähönen M, Cepaitis Z, Kuulasmaa K, Keil U, for the WHO MONICA Project. Estimation of contribution of changes in coronary care to improving survival, event rates, and coronary heart disease mortality across the WHO MONICA Project populations. *Lancet*, 2000, 355:688–700. PMID: 10703800. MONICA Publication 39.

Hugh Tunstall-Pedoe

Administrative Data

#16 Routine Mortality Data

One of the primary purposes of MONICA was to assess the validity of routine mortality data from death certificates. This is because there were concerns that trends in death rates from coronary heart disease and stroke were artificially affected by changes in reporting and coding practices, changes in the International Classification of Diseases (ICD) (see *Glossary*), and changes in diagnostic accuracy (*1*, *2*). In addition, death certificate coding may vary between countries leading to artificial differences in death rates, one explanation for the so-called 'French paradox'.

Therefore MONICA collected annual numbers of deaths, for selected causes of death by age and sex, in the study populations. The causes of death included the main groups of cardiovascular deaths, related categories to which coronary or stroke deaths might be attributed (e.g. hypertensive disease or diabetes mellitus), other major causes of mortality (e.g. cancers and respiratory diseases), causes with shared aetiology (e.g. lung cancer as a marker of smoking-related disease), and poorly specified causes such as 'Signs, Symptoms and Ill-defined Conditions' and 'Sudden death, cause unknown'.

Comparison of routine mortality data and deaths classified according to the MONICA criteria are reported for coronary events by Tunstall-Pedoe et al. (*3*), and for stroke by Asplund et al. (*4*) on methods, and Thorvaldsen et al. (*5*) on results. Overall the results confirm the validity of the routine data for broad categories of deaths from stroke (ICD-9:430–438) (*5*). For coronary heart disease, deaths coded to ICD-8 or -9: 410–414 generally meet the MONICA criteria but mortality rates calculated from all deaths that meet the MONICA criteria were somewhat higher than rates based on the official statistics, with considerable variations between populations (*3*, *6*). See also graphics G19 and G20.

Routine mortality data were used in testing the observed MONICA mortality and coronary-event rates, but are given special attention in this Monograph in Graphics G3–G6 and also in three MONICA Publications (*7–9*).

- the alleged declines in coronary deaths sparked off the MONICA Project
- routine mortality statistics were subjected to case-by-case scrutiny
- stroke deaths were usually validated by such scrutiny
- trends in coronary deaths were usually confirmed
- some low coronary-death rates were revised upwards by MONICA investigators

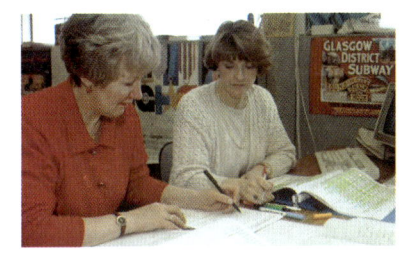

Extracting death certificate data from printout (Glasgow)

References

1. Havlik RJ, Feinleib M, eds. *Proceedings of the Conference on the Decline in Coronary Heart Disease Mortality, October 24–25, 1978*, Washington, DC: National Heart, Lung and Blood Institute, 1979, NIH publication No. 79-1610, DHES.
2. Malmgren R, Warlow C, Bamford J, Sandercock P. Geographical and secular trends in stroke incidence. *Lancet*, 1987, 1:1196–1200. PMID: 2890819.
3. Tunstall-Pedoe H, Kuulasmaa K, Amouyel P, Arveiler D, Rajakangas AM, Pajak A, for the WHO MONICA Project. Myocardial infarction and coronary deaths in the World Health Organization MONICA Project. Registration procedures, event rates, and case-fatality rates in 38 populations from 21 countries in four continents. *Circulation*, 1994, 90:583–612. PMID: 8026046. MONICA Publication 16.
4. Asplund K, Tuomilehto J, Stegmayr B, Wester PO, Tunstall-Pedoe H. Diagnostic criteria and quality control of the registration of stroke events in the WHO MONICA project. *Acta Medica Scandinavica. Supplementum*, 1988, 728:26–39. PMID: 3202029. MONICA Publication 5.
5. Thorvaldsen P, Asplund K, Kuulasmaa K, Rajakangas AM, Schroll M, for the WHO MONICA Project. Stroke incidence, case fatality, and mortality in the WHO MONICA Project. *Stroke*, 1995, 26:361–367. PMID: 7886707. MONICA Publication 19.
6. Tunstall-Pedoe H, Kuulasmaa K, Mähönen M, Tolonen H, Ruokokoski E, Amouyel P, for the WHO MONICA Project. Contribution of trends in survival and coronary-event rates to changes in coronary heart disease mortality: 10-year results from 37 WHO MONICA Project populations. *Lancet*, 1999, 353:1547–1557. PMID: 10334252. MONICA Publication 36.

7. Tuomilehto J, Kuulasmaa K, Torppa J, for the WHO MONICA Project. WHO MONICA Project: geographic variation in mortality from cardiovascular diseases. Baseline data on selected populations, characteristics and cardiovascular mortality. *World Health Statistics Quarterly*, 1987, 40:171–184. PMID: 3617777. MONICA Publication 1.

8. The WHO MONICA Project. A worldwide monitoring system for cardiovascular diseases: Cardiovascular mortality and risk factors in selected communities. *World Health Statistics Annual*, 1989, 27–149. ISBN 92 4 067890 5. ISSN 0250-3794. MONICA Publication 11.

9. Stewart AW, Kuulasmaa K, Beaglehole R, for the WHO MONICA Project. Ecological analysis of the association between mortality and major risk factors of cardiovascular disease. *International Journal of Epidemiology*, 1994, 23:505–516. PMID: 7960374. MONICA Publication 17.

Annette Dobson

#17 Demographic Data

Use of population demographic data in MONICA

Data on the size of the study populations were one of the core data components of the WHO MONICA Project. They were used as the denominators for the calculation of coronary and stroke-event rates.

Requirements for the data

Demographic data had to be available for the same populations, defined by residence in the chosen administrative/geographic areas, in which the coronary and stroke registration, and the population surveys were carried out. The best routinely available mid-year estimates of the population were to be sent annually by the MONICA Collaborating Centres (MCCs) to the MONICA Data Centre (MDC). These were to be broken down by sex and 5-year age group for the 25–64 years age range, and optionally for the 65–74 age group (*1*).

Altogether, data were collected for 79 population units during 1980–1997. The period for different populations ranged from 7 to 16 years.

Sources of the data

The two main sources of the data were:

- computerized population registers, which usually provided reliable and accurate population figures, and
- systems based on decennial or other censuses with annual intercensal estimates, the quality of which depended on many factors.

The intercensal estimates were often provided by the national or regional authorities. In some cases, the population figures were available for census years only, and the intercensal estimates were produced by local agencies, the MCC or the MDC.

Quality of the data

Although bias (errors) in estimating populations sizes result in proportionately the same bias in calculating event rates, the quality of demographic data is seldom questioned in epidemiological studies. MONICA, however, applied strict quality control to the data:

- the data, which were received in the MDC on paper forms, were keyed. Checking for data-entry errors was done by scanning sums of rows and columns of the forms
- description of the details of local sources of data and the procedures used to process the data were obtained in collaboration with the MCCs

- population numbers are essential data for calculating disease rates
- emphasis is usually placed on counting the disease numerator
- errors in the denominator matter just as much
- the MDC tested the credibility of demographic data and challenged it

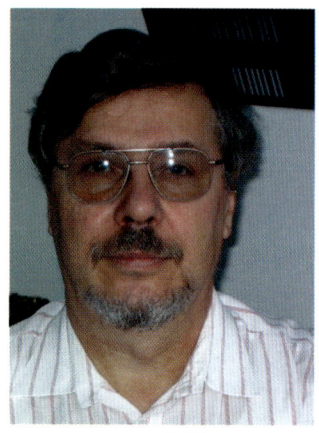

Vladislav Moltchanov

- a special method was developed to check the internal consistency of the data for all reported years for each population.

These quality control procedures revealed major problems in the data for some populations. Some of the problems were due to inadequate intercensal estimation, and many of the problems could be remedied. Where intercensal estimation was based on census data only, the estimates were often accurate only for 2–3 years after the last census year. In two countries the official statistics were corrected after feed-back from the MONICA Project. More details about the demographic data and their quality control can be found in the MONICA Quality assessment report (*2*).

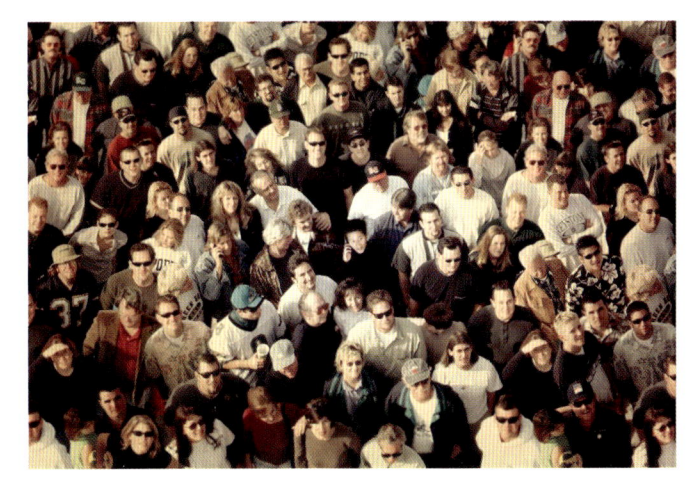

Population composition varies by time and place

References
MONICA Web Publications are also accessible on the Monograph CD-ROM

1. WHO MONICA Project. MONICA Manual. (1998–1999). Part II: Annual Statistics. Section 1: Population Demographics and Mortality Data Component. (December 1998). Available from URL: http://www.ktl.fi/publications/monica/manual/part2/ii-htm, URN:*NBN:fi-fe19981149*. MONICA Web Publication 1.
2. Moltchanov V, Kuulasmaa K, Torppa J, for the WHO MONICA Project. Quality assessment of demographic data in the WHO MONICA Project. (April 1999). Available from URL: http://www.ktl.fi/publications/monica/demoqa/demoqa.htm, URN:*NBN:fi-fe19991073*. MONICA Web Publication 3.

Vladislav Moltchanov

#18 Health Services

With the realization that rapidly changing management of acute and sub-acute coronary heart disease could affect both the short and longer-term outcome of coronary events and possibly their frequency, MONICA Principal Investigators resolved in 1988 to collect additional data about the health services available for coronary heart disease in addition to the coronary care recorded in specific events, see #24 *Acute Coronary Care*.

Qualitative information relating to access to a range of services, diagnostic procedures and treatments was collected for the period 1980–92 from virtually all Reporting Units. The data collected included information on access to the following (see MONICA Manual Form UA (*1*)):

- emergency departments, ambulance services, cardiac surgery, cardiology
- echocardiography, coronary angiography, radionuclide imaging
- coronary artery bypass grafts (CABG), percutaneous transluminal coronary angioplasty (PTCA), thrombolytic drugs.

Evidence of the progressive improvement in the coverage of MONICA populations by ambulances with cardiac defibrillators and staff trained in their use, is one example of the findings to emerge from these data.

Further information on hospital utilization for coronary heart disease, and for coronary artery revascularization procedures (CARPs, that is coronary artery bypass grafts—CABG, and percutaneous transluminal coronary angioplasty—PTCA) was collected from MCCs with access to appropriate administrative statistical systems or procedure registers. Fifteen centres provided usable data but with varying periods of coverage. The data demonstrated large differences between populations in the rate of previous and new CARPs, not

- MONICA studied acute manifestations of coronary disease and stroke
- coronary care when recorded was linked to the coronary-event registration
- the health services study recorded relevant administrative data

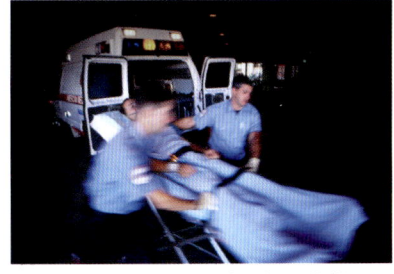

More ambulancemen/paramedics with defibrillators during MONICA

explained by variations in coronary-event rates, and more likely to reflect availability of resources available in different healthcare systems. See MONICA Manual Forms UB (Hospital Separations), UC (Hospital Aggregate Bed Days), UD (Procedure Reporting Form) (1).

The Health Services component of MONICA was designated a core item and therefore the subject of the fourth MONICA Quality Control Centre, see #8 *MONICA Quality Control Centres (MQCs)*. This occurred late on in MONICA. Some MCCs were unable to comply. In addition, the population denominators for these administrative data were often different from those that the MCCs used as Reporting Units or Reporting Unit Aggregates (RUAs) for their other analyses. The data were not used in testing either of the main hypotheses. Results have figured in MONICA internal presentations and in conference abstracts but there are, as yet, neither Data Books nor formal publications.

Reference
MONICA Web Publications are also available on the Monograph CD-ROM
1. WHO MONICA Project. MONICA Manual. (1998–1999). Part II: Annual Statistics. Section 2: Health services data component. Available from URL: http://www.ktl.fi/publications/monica/manual/part2/ii-1.htm URN:*NBN:fi-fe19981150*. MONICA Web Publication 1.

Michael Hobbs

#19 Other Documents Used in MONICA

Introduction

- MONICA Collaborating Centres (MCCs) were assessed by external quality control
- next their core data were analysed in the MONICA Data Centre (MDC)
- the MDC and MONICA Steering Committee (MSC) needed further information for detailed quality assessment
- this was provided by additional questionnaires

Preceding sections described paper records, containing statistical data for their populations, sent in by MONICA Collaborating Centres (MCCs) for each calendar year. The exchange of paper and electronic records on MONICA data between the MONICA Data Centre and the MCCs is described in #36 *Data Transfer, Checking and Management* and in detail in the MONICA Manual (1), including the inventories and communication logs designed to prevent errors. The purpose of this section is to describe documents not featuring in the MONICA Manual. MONICA Memos are described in #11 *Communications in MONICA*, listed in #88 *MONICA Memos*., and are reproduced in the second CD-ROM They make a chronological list of MONICA's preoccupations as it developed, including most of the documents described below. In each case the first relevant Memo is listed, not the later ones.

Annual Progress Reports
(MONICA Memo 12, 6 June 1983)

MCCs were required to send annual progress reports to the MONICA Management Centre (MMC). Other MONICA centres, MQCs and MDC were required to provide six-monthly reports. These were a source of information about what was, and was not happening in different centres, and of any problems the Principal Investigator wished to report. Early sets of progress reports were circulated as MONICA Memos. Later MONICA concentrated on the timely delivery, quality and completeness of data reaching the MONICA Data Centre, a more fundamental indicator of what was happening. So progress reports figured less prominently.

MONICA Local Manuals
(MONICA Memo 15, 12 August 1983)

At the start, candidate MCCs were required to provide their locally written Manual of Operations and Record Forms, translated into English where necessary, showing that they had conducted pilot studies, particularly on coronary-event registration, and would conform with the MONICA Protocol. These were to be approved by two members of the MONICA Steering Committee, see #10 *Recruitment of Populations*. This exercise had its limitations. Manuals were heavy documents, difficult to move round the world, and tedious to review. Investigators could readily duplicate parts of the existing MONICA protocol and manual of operations. Reviewers found it easier to detect definite errors than omissions in the text. Descriptions of pilot studies were sometimes cursory. Later, when some MCCs were failing, the question arose as to whether this exercise could have been done better. The task of reviewing 30 or more manuals had been formidable.

Local record form formats and questionnaires continued to be collected for the Data Centre as these were revised.

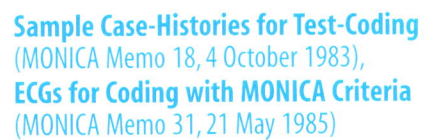

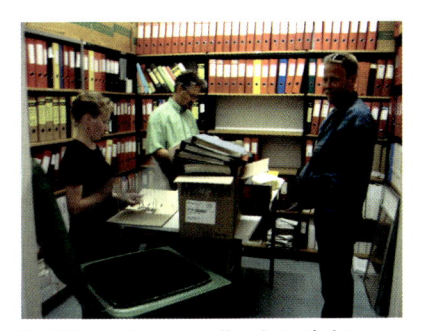

The MDC stored paper as well as electronic data

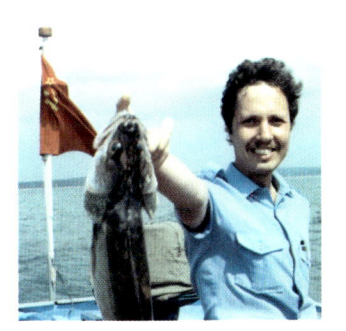

Sample Case-Histories for Test-Coding
(MONICA Memo 18, 4 October 1983),
ECGs for Coding with MONICA Criteria
(MONICA Memo 31, 21 May 1985)

Testing and training material from two of the MQCs could be sent on paper as MONICA Memos to the MCCs who sent their codings back to the MQC. The MQCs returned to them their individual scores and remarks and an overall assessment and commentary would appear later in a further MONICA Memo. This was an iterative process that created further training and testing material with standard answers, and accounted for many of the early MONICA Memos. In a similar manner, quality control specimens were distributed to participating laboratories for lipid (and early-on for thiocyanate) analysis.

Kari Kuulasmaa site-visiting Novosibirsk, River Ob 1987

Sample Selection Description
(MONICA Memo 50, 6 July 1985)

Although many MCCs used simple random sampling for their population surveys, this was not true of all of them. Information in the MONICA Data Centre on what sampling procedures and what sampling frames were being used was inadequate. This and Memo 68 addressed these issues, see #28 *Sampling*.

Annual Hospital Enzyme Use Reporting Form
(MONICA Memo 56, 16 August 1985)

MONICA devoted considerable effort to the standardization of the coding of electrocardiograms, see #22 *Minnesota Coding of the Electrocardiogram*, but cardiac enzyme results were potentially more important in the diagnosis of definite myocardial infarction, see #23 *Diagnosing Myocardial Infarction and Coronary Death*. MONICA investigators had no control over which enzyme tests were done in their local hospitals, in their standardization, or in changes of these over time—a possible source of both between-population bias, and of spurious trends over time within populations. This Memo and form were an attempt to record what was happening in each local hospital, in terms of which tests were used and their designated normal values. It addressed an important issue but was abandoned except as a local option. The information was potentially valuable within each MCC, but not helpful to the MONICA Data Centre, as the central pooling record for coronary events did not record which hospital, enzymes or isoenzymes were involved in a particular case.

Site Visit Procedures
(MONICA Memo 68, 20 March 1986)

Originally, review of Manuals was to be supplemented by site visits. These were costly in time and other resources, so original plans to visit every centre proved impracticable. Many of the site visits that did take place were precipitated by serious problems or were opportunistic with the visitor calling in at the local MONICA centre when travelling nearby for another reason. There was a difficult balance between critically reviewing the procedures of a multifaceted study on site, encouraging the local team, and meeting civic dignitaries and leading medical people to reinforce the team and its need for support and resources. Event registration was continuous, but population surveys were intermittent, so what could be reviewed varied according to timing. Finally, site visitors needed to be fully briefed beforehand. After initial experiences it was decided to design a detailed questionnaire for MCCs which covered all the questions that should figure in a site visit. Results of this proved invaluable. While designed as a preliminary for site visits, it indicated whether or not they might be necessary.

Coronary and Stroke Event Registration Procedures
(MONICA Memo 117, 17 December 1987)
and Population Survey Procedures 1991 and 1995

After the MDC had started collecting data, it became apparent that information on the local manuals and site visit forms was still insufficient to enable proper assessment of the quality of the data coming from different MCCs. Detailed questionnaires on coronary and stroke event registration procedures (sent as a Memo) as well as on population survey procedures (sent directly to MCCs by the MDC) were prepared centrally and then completed by each MCC. The first survey procedure questionnaire in 1991 was used to document procedures in the completed initial and middle surveys, and what was planned for remaining surveys. In the second round in 1995, information on the now completed middle and final surveys was corrected or confirmed.

Together with the site visit forms, the procedure questionnaires provided information that was unavailable elsewhere and was used by different Quality Assessment groups (2).

References
MONICA Web Publications are also available on the Monograph CD-ROM

1. WHO MONICA Project. MONICA Manual. (1998–1999). Part V: Data Transfer and Analysis. Section 1: Data Transfer to the MONICA Data Centre. Available from URL: http://www.ktl.fi/publications/monica/manual/partv/v-1.htm URN:*NBN:fi-fe19981160*. MONICA Web Publication 1.

2. MONICA Quality assessment reports. Available from URL: http://www.ktl.fi/publications/monica/ URN:*NBN:fi-fe19991072*. MONICA Web Publications 2–18.

Hugh Tunstall-Pedoe

Coronary-Event Registration and Coronary Care

#20 Registration of Coronary Events, Hot and Cold Pursuit

The ideal
Registration of disease is simple if:

- all sufferers from the condition seek medical help
- the medical services always anticipate the diagnosis
- there is a universally accepted set of diagnostic criteria
- full diagnostic tests are done on every case and results are unequivocal
- all cases are processed by one central medical organization in each population
- information is kept in a form that can be readily transcribed, copied or downloaded
- there are no legal or ethical constraints on such a transfer for medical research.

The reality
In reality there are problems in coronary-event registration

- coronary events can be fatal or non-fatal, each involving different medical services
- most deaths occur suddenly outside hospital
- medico-legal procedures and investigation of sudden deaths vary between populations
- a proportion of victims of non-fatal myocardial infarction do not seek medical help
- a proportion of those seeking help are misdiagnosed and/or inadequately investigated
- clinicians do not follow a standardized set of diagnostic criteria
- information may be needed from several different sources
- medical records may be disorganized and fragmentary
- access may be limited for reasons of confidentiality or by organizational constraints.

Registration
Each centre was responsible for carrying out pilot studies to ascertain the best methods for identifying cases in their chosen population. Following notification or discovery of a case (see Hot and Cold pursuit below), the medical and/or medico-legal records were obtained. The final common path for all the MONICA registers was to extract and transcribe a small number of important data items from these onto a coding record form. The contents of this could be analysed locally and forwarded to the MONICA Data Centre along with an inventory. Every coronary event was allocated a unique local reference number along with the date of registration and the MONICA Collaborating Centre code. Coronary events can be recurrent. Each event was defined as lasting for 28 days from the onset. After this time any new event led to a new record, so the register was of coronary events, rather than of people (1, 2).

- coronary-event registers record how many events occur
- this implies a comprehensive record of events managed in hospitals
- —but also of deaths (and possibly other events) occurring outside

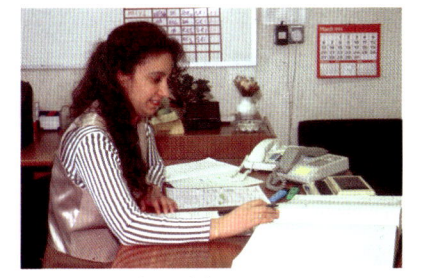

Disease registration—listing the cases

Registration methods

Notification and investigation of fatal cases usually involved access to the local medico-legal authority and to death certificates. Because coronary deaths are usually sudden, occurring outside hospital, notification usually occurred when the victim was already dead. Details were collected after a variable delay. Discovery of non-fatal cases could use either of two methods, or a combination of them, which we have labelled 'hot' and 'cold pursuit'.

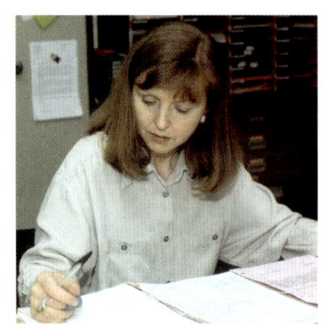

Hot pursuit

In its pure form, hot pursuit involves discovering cases through the emergency and admission medical services, and obtaining information by direct interview or by extracting case notes while the patient is still in care. Apart from the ambulance and general practitioner services, the emergency rooms, admitting wards, coronary-care units, biochemical and electrocardiographic services can all be used to identify cases. Hot pursuit is useful for obtaining information, for example on timing, which may not be routinely recorded in the notes. Informed consent can be obtained from patients under care. It is costly in time and human resources however, because many alleged coronary cases turn out to be false-positives, and full diagnostic and 28-day survival data are not available just after admission. Patients and their medical records may be moved around and out of the hospital, being chased by the registration team in 'hot pursuit'.

Extracting information using cold pursuit

Cold pursuit

Cold pursuit is the antithesis of hot pursuit. There is no involvement with acute medical services. Instead potential cases are identified through the diagnoses on listings of hospital discharge records. These lists are used to identify cases for registration whose records are then obtained from the hospital records department. Because hospital diagnoses of myocardial infarction often disagreed with the MONICA criteria for definite myocardial infarction, an excess of coronary cases was screened. In some populations case note review was extended to other diagnoses such as unstable angina, or all emergency admissions with coronary heart disease. Cold pursuit generally involved fewer cases being reviewed and less work than did hot pursuit (3–5). On the other hand it is difficult to combine it with obtaining consent from the patients. See #13 *Ethics and Confidentiality*.

References
MONICA Web Publications are also accessible on the Monograph CD-ROM

1. WHO MONICA Project. MONICA Manual. (1998–1999). Part IV: Event Registration. Section 1: Coronary Event Registration Data Component. Available from URL: http://www.ktl.fi/publications/monica/manual/part4/iv-1.htm URN:*NBN:fi-fe19981154*. MONICA Web Publication 1.
2. Mähönen M, Tolonen H, Kuulasmaa K, Tunstall-Pedoe H, Amouyel P, for the WHO MONICA Project. Quality assessment of coronary event registration data in the WHO MONICA Project. (January 1999). Available from URL: http://www.ktl.fi/publications/monica/coreqa/coreqa.htm, URN:*NBN:fi-fe19991072*. MONICA Web Publication 2.
3. Tunstall-Pedoe H. Problems with criteria and quality control in the registration of coronary events in the MONICA study. *Acta Medica Scandinavica. Supplementum*, 1988, 728:17–25. PMID: 3202028. MONICA Publication 4.
4. Tunstall-Pedoe H. Diagnosis, measurement and surveillance of coronary events. *International Journal of Epidemiology*, 1989, 18(3 suppl 1):S169–173. PMID: 2807699. MONICA Publication 10.
5. Tunstall-Pedoe H, Kuulasmaa K, Amouyel P, Arveiler D, Rajakangas AM, Pająk A, for the WHO MONICA Project. Myocardial infarction and coronary deaths in the World Health Organization MONICA Project. Registration procedures, event rates, and case-fatality rates in 38 populations from 21 countries in four continents. *Circulation*, 1994, 90:583–612. PMID: 8026046. MONICA Publication 16.

Hugh Tunstall-Pedoe

#21 Coronary-Event Registration Record Form

Registration record form

Initially it was decided to keep the coronary-event record form as simple as possible, omitting a number of data items that had been used previously in the European Myocardial Infarction Registers (1). Many of these were later reincorporated into the Acute Coronary Care record form although this was not used continuously (see #24 *Acute Coronary Care*). Items recorded as 'core' in this and other MONICA records were fundamental to the study, but additional material could be added for local or MONICA optional studies (see #43 *Optional Studies—Beyond the Core*). All central 'core' items had a standard format and set of definitions for cross-cultural validity.

- age and sex of the victim
- date and place of the event
- hospital case or sudden death
- evidence to reach a diagnostic category
- survival to four weeks

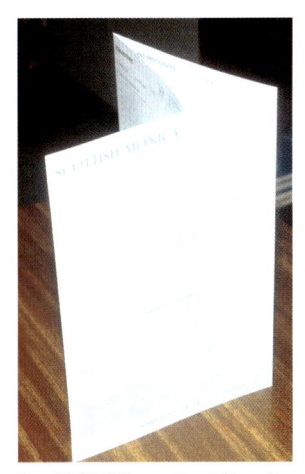

Identifying the record

As in all the record forms, the core data items first identified which form was being used and then the MONICA Collaborating Centre, the Reporting Unit, and the Serial Number (2). The serial number incorporated a check digit which enabled algorithms to be run to detect errors in data entry—entering the serial number wrongly was an error to be avoided.

Characterization of the person

The victim was characterized by date of registration, sex, date of birth and date of onset of the acute attack that was being registered. Other identification was withheld. Because even this information might conceivably identify unique individuals, and therefore breach confidentiality, date of birth is modified when making MONICA data available through the MONICA sample database. (See #13 *Ethics and Confidentiality*.)

Scottish MONICA record—6 sides of A4

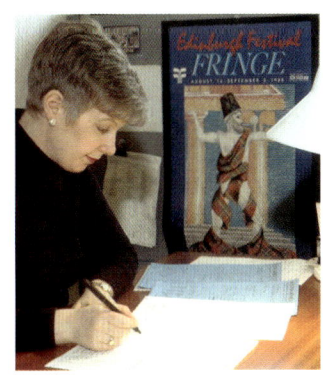

Medical and diagnostic data

Further items that were coded included whether this was a hospital case, medically unattended, or managed elsewhere and whether the victim survived for 28 days or not so that the event could be classified as a non-fatal or fatal case. Key items were recorded next that determined the diagnostic category, from symptoms, electrocardiographic findings, serum enzymes and necropsy findings (see #23 *Diagnosing Myocardial Infarction and Coronary Death*). These four items were the subject of a diagnostic algorithm described in the MONICA Manual (2).

The diagnoses on the discharge record or the death certificate were important for comparing MONICA diagnoses with local diagnoses. Previous myocardial infarction determined whether this was a first or recurrent event, while a history of chronic ischaemic heart disease, recorded later in the form was helpful in allocating a 'possible' category to deaths (2, 3).

A number of codes were reserved for fatal cases: date of death, survival time, and necropsy details. The same record was used for extracting hospital records of myocardial infarction and for deaths occurring outside hospital; in the latter situation several items might be coded as not relevant or not known.

Coding coronary records

Treatment by thrombolysis

Treatment was coded in the acute coronary care record which was used intermittently, and linked to the coronary-event record (see Graphic G11 and #24 *Acute Coronary Care*). However, thrombolytic therapy was added to the coronary-event record during the study when it was becoming common, largely because there was concern at that time that really rapid and effective thrombolysis might downgrade definite myocardial infarction to possible by reducing the amount of heart muscle destroyed or infarct size, and thereby interfere with the diagnostic criteria for definite infarction.

Quality control

Coding of all the items was checked by external quality control using test case-histories, and by internal quality control, using duplicate coding. Some of the code items were very straightforward, whereas others were the subject of considerable discussion and needed a full description of all the options (2, 4, 5).

References
MONICA Web Publications are also accessible on the Monograph CD-ROM

1. World Health Organization Regional Office for Europe. *Myocardial infarction community registers*, Copenhagen, 1976 (Public Health in Europe 5).
2. WHO MONICA Project. MONICA Manual. (1998–1999). Part IV: Event Registration. Section 1: Coronary Event Registration Data Component. Available from URL: http://www.ktl.fi/publications/monica/manual/part4/iv-1.htm URN:*NBN:fi-fe19981154*. MONICA Web Publication 1.
3. Tunstall-Pedoe H, Kuulasmaa K, Amouyel P, Arveiler D, Rajakangas AM, Pająk A, for the WHO MONICA Project. Myocardial infarction and coronary deaths in the World Health Organization MONICA Project. Registration procedures, event rates, and case-fatality rates in 38 populations from 21 countries in four continents. *Circulation*, 1994, 90:583–612. PMID: 8026046. MONICA Publication 16.
4. WHO MONICA Project. MONICA Manual. (1998–1999). Part IV: Event Registration. Section 3: Event registration quality assurance methods. Available from URL: http://www.ktl.fi/publications/monica/manual/part4/iv-3.htm URN:*NBN:fi-fe19981158*. MONICA Web Publication 1.
5. Mähönen M, Tolonen H, Kuulasmaa K, Tunstall-Pedoe H, Amouyel P, for the WHO MONICA Project. Quality assessment of coronary event registration data in the WHO MONICA Project. (January 1999). Available from URL: http://www.ktl.fi/publications/monica/coreqa/coreqa.htm URN:*NBN:fi-fe19991072*. MONICA Web Publication 2.

Hugh Tunstall-Pedoe

#22 Minnesota Coding of the Electrocardiogram (ECG)

The problem

The electrocardiogram is used by clinicians in the diagnosis of acute myocardial infarction. The pattern on the graph registered by each normal or sinus beat does not change appreciably in a healthy person. During acute myocardial infarction, however, specific changes occur in the parts of the electrocardiogram that reflect the electrical depolarization and repolarization of the main heart muscle mass. These are called the QRS complex and the T wave. An 'injury current' appears between them in the ST segment. The QRS complex changes with the development of 'pathological' Q waves. The T wave can change from positive to negative. The sequence of changes is characteristic in a classical case and can be observed from the onset of the event until a few days later.

The classical ECG progression may not be observed. The first graph in the event may show 'changes' which could be new or old. Delays may censor out the early progression while later progression may be lost through failure to record further graphs, or death. The infarction may not show up because it is not big enough, affects a part of the heart that is poorly represented in the standard recordings, or because previous damage conceals the effect. Technical problems include: muscle tremor, poor electrical contact, badly placed electrodes creating spurious change in consecutive graphs, interference and artefacts on the graph, differences in response of ECG machines, and poor standardization.

- Minnesota coding of the ECG standardizes a clinical diagnostic procedure
- ECG reading is subject to considerable observer variation
- Minnesota coding reduces, but cannot abolish, this variability
- coding was the subject of training and of external quality control procedures

Clinical reading of the electrocardiogram

The human brain recognizes patterns. Clinicians 'eyeball' a sequence of electrocardiograms without artificial aid, although sequential ECGs can be analysed by computer if recorded on the same or compatible machines. Eyeballing was used for the European Heart Attack Registers. The protocol contained a simple diagram of the classical ECG changes in infarction (*1, 2*). 'Eyeballing' is a qualitative judgement, subject to variation and therefore to cross-sectional and longitudinal biases.

The Minnesota code

This code is a standardized quantitative method of analysing individual electrocardiograms developed at the then School of Physiological Hygiene, Stadium Gate 27 in Minneapolis (*3, 4*). It was originally developed for cross-sectional population surveys and then used in follow-up studies to confirm infarction when a normal baseline electrocardiogram was followed by an abnormal one. These coding rules were extended to coronary-event registration. The technique is quantitative but poses problems for the epidemiologist similar to those experienced by the clinician in the availability and technical quality of recordings and the frequent absence of an early baseline graph in the sequence. This differs from the situation in field surveys where the timing and nature of any electrocardiogram is pre-determined by the investigator.

Minnesota coding involves use of a magnifying lens or loupe with a graticule for accurate measurement, plus a transparent plastic ruler. Coding is normally carried out by two 'blinded' observers independently, with a third arbitrating when the codes disagree (*3*).

Minnesota coding in MONICA

In MONICA, considerable resources were devoted to making ECG coding quantitative through the use of the Minnesota code, a major departure from earlier European coronary registers (*1*). Register staff photocopied any available graph recorded shortly before the onset of myocardial infarction; the first one recorded in the event; a late pre-discharge record; and others on consecutive days following hospital admission. This made a total of four. Minnesota coding for MONICA involved Q and QS codes (code 1), ST depression (code 4), T wave inversion and flattening (code 5), ST elevation (code 9-2) and suppression codes (various). A coding record format was prepared in Dundee along with a computer algorithm for deriving MONICA ECG categories. Principal Investigators decided not to incorporate Minnesota codes themselves into the core coronary-event record sent to the MONICA Data Centre, but to retain such codes locally. The four ECGs in each event were coded separately although special rules were being developed in the 1980s to assess significant serial change (*3*).

Quality Assurance

A MONICA Quality Control Centre for ECG coding was established in Budapest, Hungary. Training and testing material were circulated and training exercises were held. Results of formal exercises were used to 'score' MONICA Collaborating Centres. These exercises identified potential problems, although a good performance on test material did not guarantee similar performance in local cases. Observer variation could be random or systematic. Some random variation is inevitable. Systematic variation results in biased over or under-diagnosis of infarction. Retaining photocopies of ECGs enabled MONICA Collaborating Centres to carry out routine duplicate coding under good working conditions, and to go back and look for a drift in coding frequencies over time, see #08 *MONICA Quality Control Centres (MQCs)*, and #88 *MONICA Memos*.

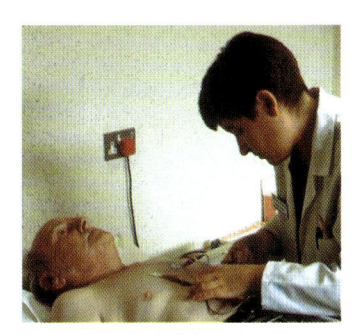

Accurate placement of electrodes

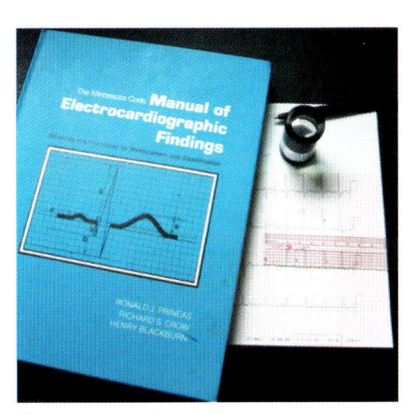

Minnesota coding tools

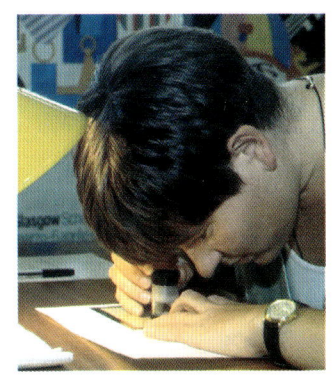

Minnesota coding

References
MONICA Web Publications are also accessible on the Monograph CD-ROM

1. World Health Organization Regional Office for Europe. *Myocardial infarction community registers*, Copenhagen, 1976 (Public Health in Europe 5).
2. *Hypertension and coronary heart disease: classification and criteria for epidemiological studies.* Geneva, World Health Organization, 1959 (WHO Technical Report Series, No. 168).
3. Prineas RJ, Crow RS, Blackburn H. *The Minnesota Code Manual of Electrocardiographic Findings: Standards and Procedures for Measurement and Classification*, Littleton, Mass. and Bristol, England, John Wright, 1982, ISBN 0-7236-7053-6.
4. Blackburn H. *If it isn't fun*, Minneapolis, 2001, ISBN 1-887268-03-0.
5. WHO MONICA Project. MONICA Manual. (1998–1999). Part IV: Event Registration. Section 4: ECG coding quality assurance methods. Available from URL: http://www.ktl.fi/publications/monica/manual/part4/iv-4.htm URN:*NBN:fi-fe19981159*. MONICA Web Publication 1.

Hugh Tunstall-Pedoe

#23 Diagnosing Myocardial Infarction and Coronary Death

Problem

Textbooks describe typical cases of a disease. To record the frequency of a disease it is necessary to define it to include less typical or borderline cases. Only in rare genetic diseases is it possible to separate cases from non-cases with absolute assurance. Diagnosis may be in doubt because the evidence is available but inconclusive, or because evidence is incomplete. Case definition implies a diagnostic classification. MONICA had to lay down definitions and diagnostic classifications that could be standardized in populations with different social and medical-care systems and that would reliably reflect trends over time.

- MONICA standardized existing clinical criteria
- symptoms, ECG findings and blood tests all contributed in life
- previous history and post-mortem findings were added in fatal cases
- different criteria produce different event rates and case fatality from the same data

European Myocardial Infarction Registers

This previous WHO study had formulated a diagnostic classification for definite and possible acute myocardial infarction, and for definite, possible and 'insufficient data' coronary deaths. Despite the attempt to define 'definite myocardial infarction', the eventual results were published combining it with 'possible myocardial infarction'. The latter, however, ranged from cases that almost satisfied criteria for definite, to episodes of prolonged chest pain with equivocal and even negative electrocardiographic and cardiac enzyme results, which did not have an obvious non-coronary explanation (*1*). Myocardial infarction was classified on the basis of the symptoms, the electrocardiogram and the cardiac enzyme results during the episode. Fatal coronary events were classified on the basis of any of these findings in life, any previous history of coronary disease, and findings at post-mortem examination.

The MONICA definition and classification
Living cases

MONICA took over the previous WHO definition and classification from the European Registers. However, it made them more objective by adopting some rules taken from large field trials carried out in the United States. MONICA defined a group of cases labelled 'ischaemic cardiac arrest' but these were too infrequent to be significant. The definition of chest pain was slightly modified. The electrocardiogram was made quantitative by the adoption of strict Minnesota coding

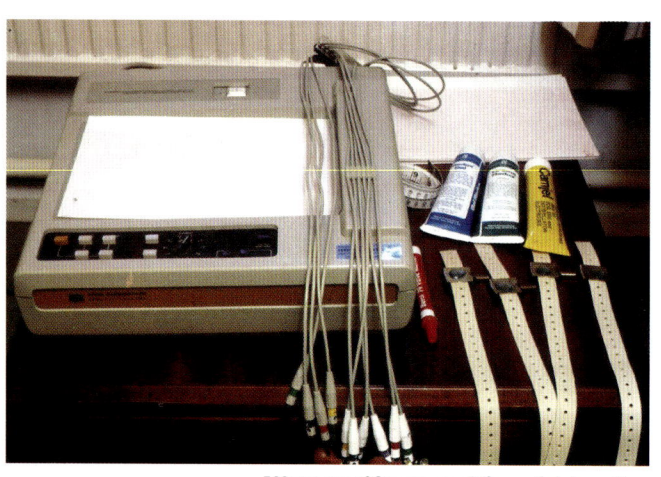

ECG was one of five sources of diagnostic information

rules. (See #22 *Minnesota Coding of the Electrocardiogram.*) (*2*) Attempts were made to standardize classification of cardiac enzyme results. Although 'abnormal' was defined as 'twice the upper limit of normal', MONICA had no control over how normal levels were defined locally, nor which enzymatic tests were employed, introduced or discontinued during the study. Assays were not internationally standardized at that time or since. Because the performance of ECG machines is internationally standardized, as is the Minnesota code, the ECG was the most objective criterion for identifying definite infarction. However, only a minority of definite infarcts had the full unequivocal electrocardiographic progression allowing classification on ECG alone—most become definite because of the accompanying rise in (unstandardized) cardiac enzymes. See discussion in #19 *Other Documents Used in MONICA.*

To monitor the frequency of non-fatal myocardial infarction MONICA investigators decided to use the 'definite' category. Some MONICA Collaborating Centres incorporated some of the 'possible' sub-groups into their local analyses (*3*). This increased the numbers, and the attack rates for non-fatal events, thereby also reducing the 28-day case fatality. The effects are similar to those brought about by the recent redefinition of myocardial infarction, which is based overwhelmingly on assay of cardiac troponins (*4*).

Fatal cases

Diagnostic rules and classification were unchanged from the European registers. Apart from delayed deaths from myocardial infarction, coronary deaths were usually sudden but this was not a diagnostic criterion. A definite case was where myocardial infarction or coronary thrombosis was found at postmortem, while possible cases showed evidence of coronary heart disease at postmortem or in the clinical history without an alternative explanation for the death. The 'insufficient data' group, subsequently renamed 'unclassifiable' included deaths in which there was no evidence of another cause of death, but no good evidence of coronary heart disease either. The frequency with which this classification had to be used is a comment on the standard of death certification in different countries, as it was used in 22% of coronary deaths overall in MONICA and in over 40% in some populations (*5*).

Quality control

The MONICA Quality Control Centre in Dundee circulated test case-histories for coding to MONICA Collaborating Centres. This was done frequently at the start of MONICA, less often thereafter. MCCs were encouraged to translate test case histories, to keep a bank of training and testing materials, and to code and classify a proportion of their local coronary-event records in duplicate to understand observer bias and variation (*6*). The diagnostic classification for each case was allocated locally before the transfer of data to the MONICA Data Centre. A computer algorithm was developed in Dundee and used to check such coding on the materials received in Helsinki.

References
MONICA Web Publications are also accessible on the Monograph CD-ROM
1. World Health Organization Regional Office for Europe. *Myocardial infarction community registers*, Copenhagen, 1976 (Public Health in Europe 5).
2. Prineas RJ, Crow RS, Blackburn H. *The Minnesota Code Manual of Electrocardiographic Findings: Standards and Procedures for Measurement and Classification*, Littleton, Mass. and Bristol, England, John Wright, 1982, ISBN 0-7236-7053-6.
3. Salomaa V, Dobson A, Miettinen H, Rajakangas AM, Kuulasmaa K, for the WHO MONICA Project. Mild myocardial infarction—a classification problem in epidemiologic studies. WHO MONICA Project. *Journal of Clinical Epidemiology*, 1997, 50:3–13. PMID: 9048685. MONICA Publication 24.

4. The Joint European Society of Cardiology/American College of Cardiology Committee. Myocardial infarction redefined—a consensus document of the Joint European Society of Cardiology/American College of Cardiology Committee for the Redefinition of Myocardial Infarction. *European Heart Journal*, 2000:1502–1513.

5. Tunstall-Pedoe H, Kuulasmaa K, Amouyel P, Arveiler D, Rajakangas AM, Pająk A, for the WHO MONICA Project. Myocardial infarction and coronary deaths in the World Health Organization MONICA Project. Registration procedures, event rates, and case-fatality rates in 38 populations from 21 countries in four continents. *Circulation*, 1994, 90:583–612. PMID: 8026046. MONICA Publication 16.

6. WHO MONICA Project. MONICA Manual. (1998–1999). Part IV: Event Registration. Section 3: Event registration quality assurance methods. Available from URL: http://www.ktl.fi/publications/monica/manual/part4/iv-3.htm URN:*NBN:fi-fe19981158*. MONICA Web Publication 1.

Hugh Tunstall-Pedoe

#24 Acute Coronary Care

Introduction

The WHO MONICA Second Hypothesis tested the association, across the participating populations, between 10-year trends in case fatality (percentage of attacks that were fatal within 28 days) and 10-year trends in acute coronary care in the attack. (See #2 *MONICA Hypotheses and Study Design*.) The problem posed for the MONICA investigators was to derive a satisfactory indicator of acute coronary care that could be used in exploring this second hypothesis. It was hoped to include indicators of the severity of the attack in individual cases, in case these changed over time. Unlike trials of drugs where individuals are randomly allocated to treatments, the associations implied by the above hypothesis were to be tested at a population level, performing what is technically described as an ecological analysis (*1*).

- acute coronary care was emphasized when MONICA began
- long-term treatment is now thought to be as important

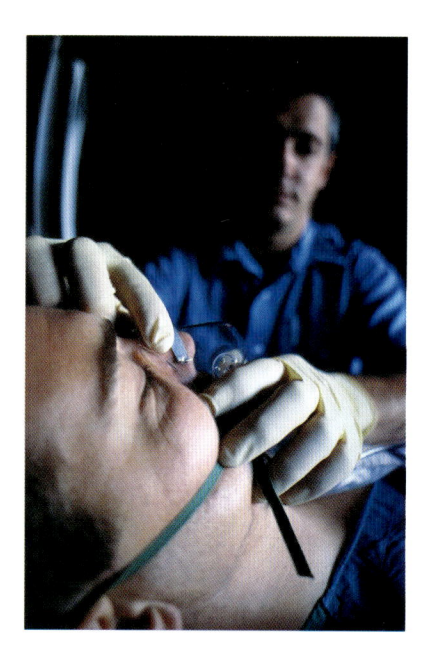

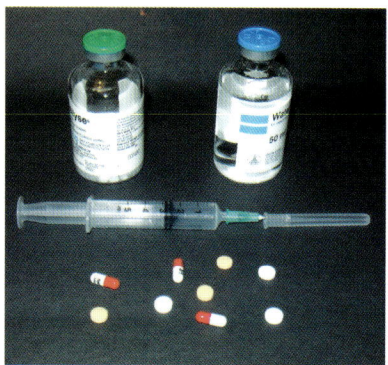

Methods

During the planning stage, in the early 1980s when many clinical trials of treatments had been small-scale and the results contradictory, there was considerable discussion as to what constituted good acute coronary care. Eventually a detailed event-based document was used which was linked to the associated individual coronary-event record (*2*). It recorded medication and cardiovascular interventions for three different time periods in relation to the onset of the index attack: before the onset, from the onset to discharge or death (if within 28 days), and at discharge in survivors.

During the period of MONICA, from the mid-1980s to the mid-1990s, a revolution occurred in acute coronary care, as well as in the management of subacute CHD and in the secondary prevention of CHD, as the results of large randomized controlled trials were reported which changed the behaviour of physicians both in their acute treatment of myocardial infarction and in use of long-term medication afterwards and in angina pectoris. MONICA was designed too early to fully take account of this phenomenon, or it might have included a study of the use of medication more than 28 days after myocardial infarction. With up to 50% of cases of myocardial infarction occurring in patients with a history of coronary heart disease already diagnosed, the medications prescribed before the onset, and at discharge were indirect indicators of levels of secondary prevention in the population.

The study required that the Acute Coronary Care record be added to routine registration towards the beginning and also towards the end of event-registration. Some centres used the record continuously, others did so only from the late 1980s when the MONICA Principal Investigators recommended continuous recording. Recording of coronary care was therefore most comprehensive at the end of the MONICA period. Because of the debate about what should be done, there were variable delays among the MONICA centres in the times at which they started to record coronary care, with different centres beginning to record details of coronary care at different times. Graphic G11 shows the first period of coronary care recording (3). Coronary care was to be recorded in 500 consecutive cases in each centre, but many of these were fatal cases or cases classified as possible non-fatal myocardial infarction, a category not included in the hypothesis-testing analyses.

Results

Most MONICA Collaborating Centres were able to obtain good data on medication between the onset of the event and discharge from hospital in non-fatal definite acute myocardial infarction, and also at discharge from hospital. These cases were also those in which medication before the onset of the attack was most likely to be recorded in hospital case-notes. In fatal cases and in possible myocardial infarction, when patients were not admitted to hospital at all, or more briefly than in definite cases, information was less reliable. Indeed, in many populations information on cases of sudden death outside hospitals was often unobtainable (3).

The MONICA Second Hypothesis was therefore tested using information on the treatment of definite non-fatal myocardial infarction. Results of comparisons of treatment in two different time periods are shown in graphics G57–G68. Despite the small numbers (by MONICA standards) of coronary care records in some centres in the first period, when drug usage was low, increases were so dramatic that this mattered less than it might have done. Inadequacies of the data (3) were taken into account in defining a quality control score (4).

Results of the testing of the Second Hypothesis are published (5). Results are shown in graphic G77. The analyses covered only eight of the drugs and procedures involved in the acute coronary care record, incorporated into a treatment score. See #25 *Treatment Scores*. Details of other MONICA diagnostic categories, other drugs and procedures, and of other periods not covered by the hypothesis testing are available from the Data Book (6) and in manuscripts awaiting publication.

References
MONICA Web Publications are also accessible on the Monograph CD-ROM

1. WHO MONICA Project. MONICA Manual. (1998–1999). Part I: Description and Organization of the Project. Section 1: Objectives and outline protocol. Available from URL: http://www.ktl.fi/publications/monica/manual/part1/i-1.htm, URN:*NBN:fi-fe19981146*. MONICA Web Publication 1.

2. WHO MONICA Project. MONICA Manual. (1998–1999). Part IV. Event Registration. Section 1: Coronary event data registration component. Available from URL: http://www.ktl.fi/publications/monica/manual/part4/iv-1.htm, URN:*NBN:fi-fe19981154*. MONICA Web Publication 1.

3. Mähönen M, Cepaitis Z, Kuulasmaa K, for the WHO MONICA Project. Quality assessment of acute coronary care data in the WHO MONICA Project. (February 1999). Available from URL: http://www.ktl.fi/publications/monica/accqa/accqa.htm, URN:*NBN:fi-fe19991081*. MONICA Web Publication 4.

4. Tunstall-Pedoe H, Mähönen M, Cepaitis Z, Kuulasmaa K, Vanuzzo D, Hobbs M, Keil U, for the WHO MONICA Project. Derivation of an acute coronary care quality score for the WHO MONICA Project. (February 2000). Available from URL: http://www.ktl.fi/publications/monica/carpfish/appendc/accqscore.htm, URN:*NBN:fi-fe976569*. MONICA Web Publication 23.

5. Tunstall-Pedoe H, Vanuzzo D, Hobbs M, Mähönen M, Cepaitis Z, Kuulasmaa K, Keil U, for the WHO MONICA Project. Estimation of contribution of changes in coronary care to improving survival, event rates, and coronary heart disease mortality across the WHO MONICA Project populations. *Lancet*, 2000, 355:688–700. PMID: 10703800. MONICA Publication 39.

6. Mähönen M, Cepaitis Z, Kuulasmaa K, for the WHO MONICA Project. MONICA acute coronary care data book 1981–1995. (December 2001). Available from URL: http://www.ktl.fi/publications/monica/accdb/accdb.htm, URN:*NBN:fi-fe20011304*. MONICA Web Publication 29.

Diego Vanuzzo

#25 Treatment Scores

Introduction

In order to test the WHO MONICA Project Second Hypothesis (see #2 *MONICA Hypotheses and Study Design*) an index was needed of effective coronary care to be used analogously to the risk-factor score in the First Hypothesis (see #35 *Risk-Factor Scores*). Such scores were not available. MONICA had to develop its own. Early attempts within our data to develop indicators of severity by finding which coronary-care record items went with a good or bad outcome were frustrating. MONICA was population-based. Most coronary deaths occur suddenly outside hospital or soon after arrival, often before observation of clinical status or effective treatments—victims received no or little treatment in the attack. Information on those or previous treatments was often missing through inaccessibility or non-existence of records. The best retrospective indicator of bad outcome was no treatment, or missing information. In hospital, the longer a severe case survived, the more medication and different drugs were administered. Death went both with no medication and a lot of medication, and death itself censored the information available for a severity score. Restriction to delayed deaths would exclude the majority of deaths.

- MONICA developed a simple indicator or score for population coronary care
- it reflected what went on in acute events before and after arrival in hospital
- it focused on a small number of evidence-based treatments

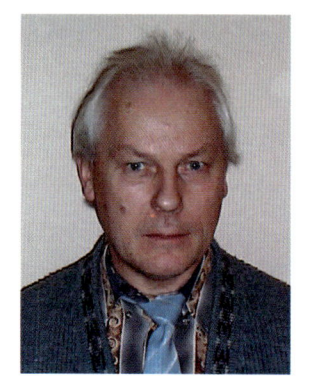

Zygimantas Cepaitis—coronary care analyses in the MDC

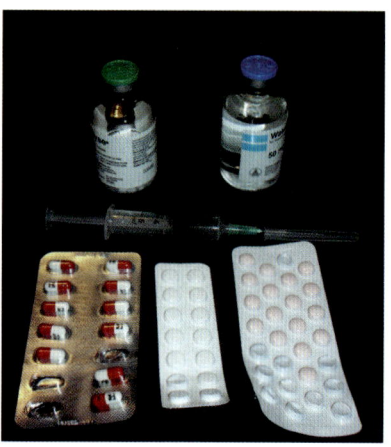

Treatment scores incorporated 8 treatments, 7 of them drugs

Methods

What was eventually agreed was a score based on indicators of the adoption, within the population, of evidence-based coronary care. In order to avoid loss of information this was based on cases of definite non-fatal myocardial infarction. These would have a full period of hospitalization recorded, and had a high degree of cross-population comparability. In addition to drugs and procedures administered during 'acute coronary care', it was also decided to add medication and procedures preceding the attack. This gave a crude indication of the level of secondary prevention in the community in those cases with a history of coronary heart disease (almost 50% in some populations). The indicator was crude because of the potential selection bias of having a recurrent event but it was better than no indicator at all and the same for all centres.

Results

The score was restricted to a small number of drugs and procedures already shown to be unequivocally effective through large randomized controlled trials. These were beta blockers, antiplatelet drugs (aspirin) and angiotensin converting enzyme (ACE) inhibitors used immediately before the onset, and also (scored separately) within the attack, plus two more—previous coronary artery reperfusion procedures (coronary artery bypass grafting-CABG and/or percutaneous transluminal angioplasty-PTCA) and use of thrombolytic drugs in the attack, making eight in all. Timing of the start of care was a data item in the coronary care record, but quality was variable. It was often not known. Therefore delay from onset to administration of thrombolytic therapy was not a score component, although thrombolytic therapy was. During the MONICA period these eight seemed to be the key treatments whose adoption indicated good coronary care, although others have emerged since.

Debate took place within the group working on the Second Hypothesis as to whether to have a simple score by adding up the treatments, or to make it more sophisticated by weighting each drug or procedure by its presumed impact. Both were done, but on examining the results it was found that the very simple 'equivalent treatment' and the more complex 'weighted treatment' scores were very highly correlated, as were almost all of the treatments. Both predicted population outcomes for case fatality, but also, we found, for trends in event rates and coronary deaths. Results of the simple Equivalent Treatment Score for two different time periods are shown in graphics G65–G68 and the components from which it is derived in the preceding graphics G57–G64. Its use in the Second Hypothesis is illustrated in G77a–G77c. Further information is available from the acute coronary care record (*1*), the MONICA Quality assessment report (*2*), the Data Book (*3*), the definitive publication in *Lancet* (*4*) and two appendices to this paper published on the MONICA Website (*5, 6*).

References
Monica Web Publications are also available on the Monograph CD-ROM

1. WHO MONICA Project. MONICA Manual. (1998–1999). Part IV. Event Registration. Section 1: Coronary event data registration component. Available from URL: http://www.ktl.fi/publications/monica/manual/part4/iv-1.htm, URN:*NBN:fi-fe19981154*. MONICA Web Publication 1.

2. Mähönen M, Cepaitis Z, Kuulasmaa K, for the WHO MONICA Project. Quality assessment of acute coronary care data in the WHO MONICA Project. (February 1999). Available from URL: http://www.ktl.fi/publications/monica/accqa/accqa.htm, URN:*NBN:fi-fe19991081*. MONICA Web Publication 4.

3. Mähönen M, Cepaitis Z, Kuulasmaa K, for the WHO MONICA Project. MONICA acute coronary care data book 1981–1995. (December 2001). Available from URL: http://www.ktl.fi/publications/monica/accdb/accdb.htm, URN:*NBN:fi-fe20011304*. MONICA Web Publication 29.

4. Tunstall-Pedoe H, Vanuzzo D, Hobbs M, Mähönen M, Cepaitis Z, Kuulasmaa K, Keil U, for the WHO MONICA Project. Estimation of contribution of changes in coronary care to improving survival, event rates, and coronary heart disease mortality across the WHO MONICA Project populations. *Lancet*, 2000, 355:688–700. PMID: 10703800. MONICA Publication 39.

5. Hobbs M, Mähönen M, Jamrozik K, for the WHO MONICA Project. Constructing an evidence-based treatment score for relating changes in treatment to changes in mortality, coronary events and case fatality in the WHO MONICA Project. (February 2000). Available from URL: http://www.ktl.fi/publications/monica/carpfish/appendb/wts.htm, URN:*NBN:fi-fe976568*. MONICA Web Publication 22.

6. Vanuzzo D, Pilotto L, Pilotto L, Mähönen M, Hobbs M, for the WHO MONICA Project. Pharmacological treatment during AMI and in secondary prevention: the scientific evidence. (February 2000). Available from URL: http://www.ktl.fi/publications/monica/carpfish/appenda/evidence.htm, URN:*NBN:fi-fe976567*. MONICA Web Publication 21.

Hugh Tunstall-Pedoe

Stroke Registration

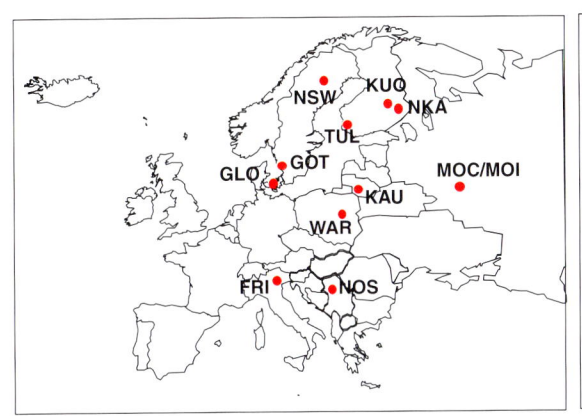

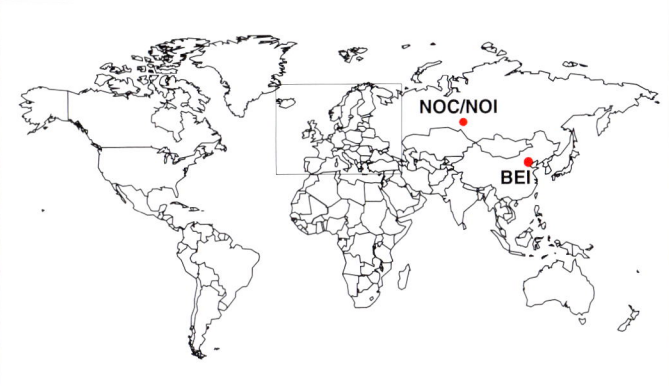

#26 Registration of Stroke Events

Populations

Long-term trends of stroke occurrence were recorded in 15 of the MONICA populations. Although fewer than half of the MONICA centres participated in the stroke component, this has been, by far, the largest epidemiological study of stroke based on individual data ever performed.

All 15 populations recorded strokes in the 35–64 year age range. Eight also included 65–74 year-old stroke victims. The MONICA stroke study is community-based, so all events were registered irrespective of whether the patients were admitted to hospital or not.

Registrations

Strokes were recorded in a uniform manner in the MONICA populations. Data gathered included information on previous strokes, where the patient was treated, what diagnostic procedures were performed, concomitant cardiac events, survival and cause of death. The stroke was recorded as fatal if the patient died within 28 days. If there were repeated strokes occurring within 28 days of the first one they were counted as a single event (1).

Data quality

To ensure good quality of the stroke data:

- the centres were compared on how they coded series of test cases
- five key indicators of the quality of the stroke registers were developed and applied to the data provided by the MONICA centres
- data submitted to the MONICA Data Centre in Helsinki were checked for completeness, logical consistency and possible duplicate registrations of the same event before they were entered into the stroke database (2–6).

- less than half of MONICA populations registered stroke
- but it was still the largest stroke study ever undertaken
- half the centres included the 65–74 age group
- strokes were registered regardless of admission to hospital

References
MONICA Web Publications are also accessible on the Monograph CD-ROM
1. WHO MONICA Project. MONICA Manual. (1998–1999). Part IV: Event Registration. Section 2: Stroke event registration data component. Available from URL: http://www.ktl.fi/publications/monica/manual/part4/iv-2.htm URN:*NBN:fi-fe19981155*. MONICA Web Publication 1.

2. Asplund K, Tuomilehto J, Stegmayr B, Wester PO, Tunstall-Pedoe H. Diagnostic criteria and quality control of the registration of stroke events in the WHO MONICA project. *Acta Medica Scandinavica. Supplementum*, 1988, 728:26–39. PMID: 3202029. MONICA Publication 5.

3. Asplund K, Bonita R, Kuulasmaa K, Rajakangas AM, Feigin V, Schädlich H, Suzuki K, Thorvaldsen P, Tuomilehto J, for the WHO MONICA Project. Multinational comparisons of stroke epidemiology. Evaluation of case ascertainment in the WHO MONICA Stroke Study. World Health Organization Monitoring Trends and Determinants in Cardiovascular Disease. *Stroke*, 1995, 26:355–360. PMID: 7886706. MONICA Publication 18.

4. Thorvaldsen P, Asplund K, Kuulasmaa K, Rajakangas AM, Schroll M, for the WHO MONICA Project. Stroke incidence, case fatality, and mortality in the WHO MONICA project. *Stroke*, 1995, 26:361–367. PMID: 7886707. MONICA Publication 19.

5. WHO MONICA Project. MONICA Manual. (1998–1999). Part IV: Event Registration. Section 3: Event registration quality assurance methods. Available from URL: http://www.ktl.fi/publications/monica/manual/part4/iv-3.htm URN:*NBN:fi-fe19981158*. MONICA Web Publication 1.

6. Mähönen M, Tolonen H, Kuulasmaa K, for the WHO MONICA Project. Quality assessment of stroke event registration data in the WHO MONICA Project. (November 1998). Available from URL: http://www.ktl.fi/publications/monica/strokeqa/strokeqa.htm URN:*NBN:fi-fe19991080*. MONICA Web Publication 5.

Kjell Asplund

#27 Diagnosis of Stroke

Is it a stroke or not?

In MONICA, the diagnosis of stroke was based entirely on clinical symptoms and signs, using the WHO definition (see box).

- stroke itself is a clinical diagnosis based on symptoms and signs
- modern imaging techniques help decide what sort of stroke has occurred

WHO definition of stroke (*1*)
Rapidly developing clinical signs of focal (or global) disturbance of cerebral function lasting more than 24 hours (unless interrupted by surgery or death) with no apparent cause other than a vascular origin.

The clinical presentation of stroke is highly variable, so it was necessary to define a number of symptoms and signs that are accepted as being typical for a stroke (such as sudden onset of weakness of limbs, difficulties with speech and certain visual disturbances). Symptoms that were not specific enough to be used as diagnostic for the MONICA Project were also listed (for instance, sudden onset of dizziness or confusion) (*1, 2*).

The reliance on clinical symptoms and signs alone has made the long-term monitoring of stroke in the MONICA populations independent of the rapid technical development in stroke diagnosis that has occurred since the first MONICA registrations were done in 1982 (introduction of computerized tomography (CT) scanners and magnetic resonance cameras). Patients with transient brain (ischaemic) attacks (TIAs) or bleeding inside the head caused by trauma or tumours have not been included.

What subtype of stroke?

Stroke is a heterogeneous group of cerebrovascular disorders. Without the new imaging technologies, it is not possible to distinguish with certainty a brain infarct from an intracerebral haemorrhage. In many MONICA centres, particularly in east Europe, access to CT scanning for stroke patients has been very limited. As a result, it has not been possible to undertake a study of stroke subtypes as part of the MONICA study (*2, 3*). An exception is subarachnoid haemorrhage, a sudden bleeding between the meninges on the surface of the brain, which can be diagnosed by a spinal tap (lumbar puncture). As a result, one of the MONICA stroke reports was devoted to subarachnoid haemorrhage (*4*).

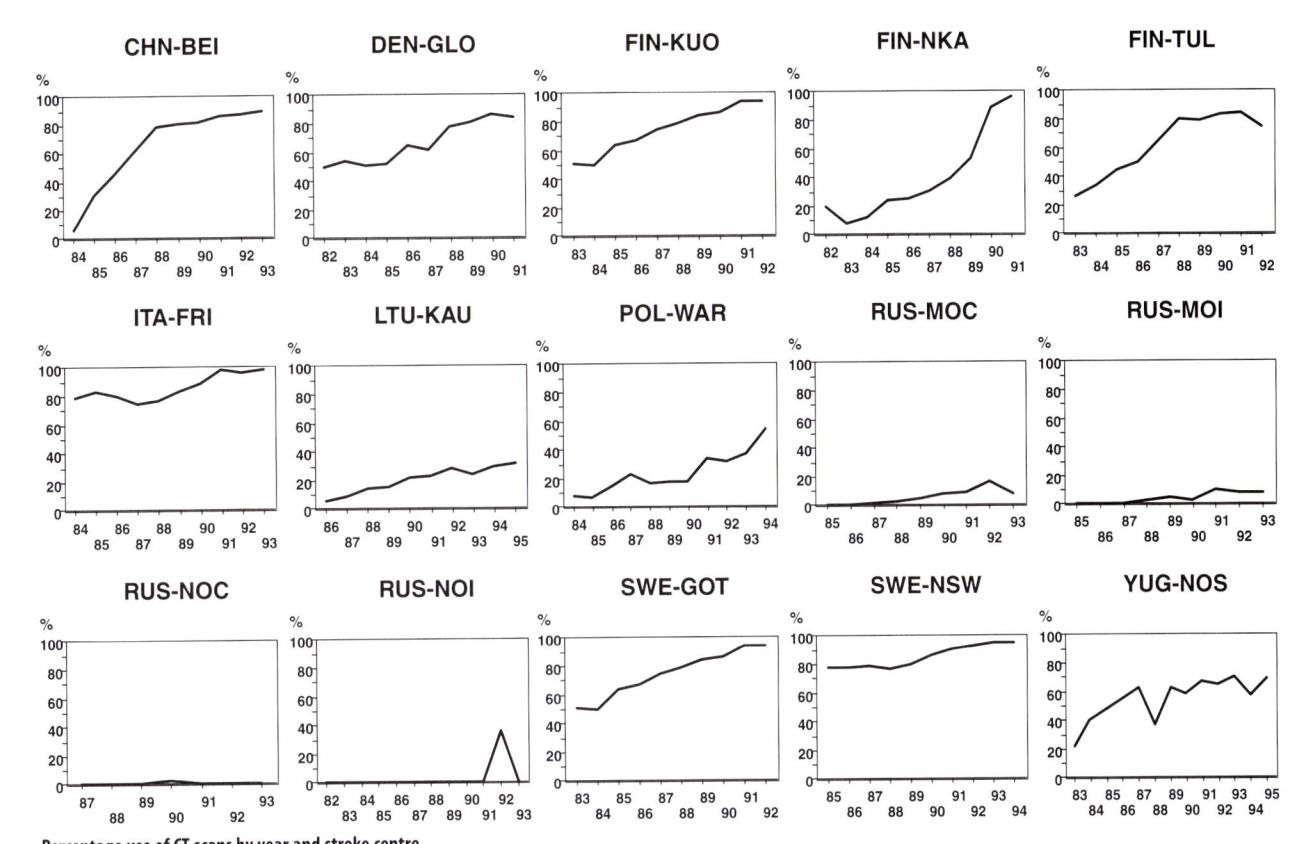

Percentage use of CT scans by year and stroke centre

References
MONICA Web Publications are also accessible on the Monograph CD-ROM

1. WHO MONICA Project. MONICA Manual. (1998–1999). Part IV: Event Registration. Section 2: Stroke event registration data component. Available from URL: http://www.ktl.fi/publications/monica/manual/part4/iv-2.htm, URN:*NBN:fi-fe19981155*. MONICA Web Publication 1.

2. Asplund K, Rajakangas AM, Kuulasmaa K, Thorvaldsen P, Bonita R, Stegmayr B, Suzuki K, Eisenblätter D, for the WHO MONICA Project. Multinational comparison of diagnostic procedures and management of acute stroke—the WHO MONICA Study. *Cerebrovascular Diseases*, 1996, 6:66–74. PMID: nil. MONICA Publication 21.

3. Mähönen M, Tolonen H, Kuulasmaa K, for the WHO MONICA Project. Quality assessment of stroke event registration data in the WHO MONICA Project. (November 1998). Available from URL: http://www.ktl.fi/publications/monica/strokeqa/strokeqa/htm, URN:*NBN:fi-fe19991080*. MONICA Web Publication 5.

4. Ingall T, Asplund K, Mähönen M, Bonita R, for the WHO MONICA Project. A multinational comparison of subarachnoid hemorrhage epidemiology in the WHO MONICA stroke study. *Stroke*, 2000, 31:1054–1061. PMID: 10797165. MONICA Publication 40.

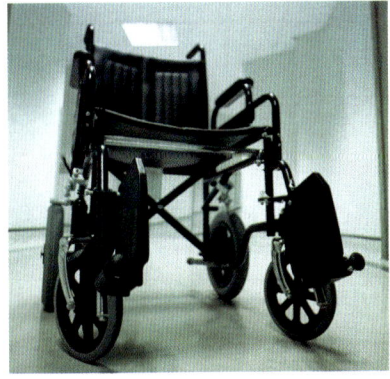

One third of stroke victims remain disabled

Kjell Asplund

Population Surveys

#28 Sampling

Why sampling?
The study populations used in the MONICA Project ranged in size from less than 100 000 to almost 1 million. Together they amounted to more than 10 million persons aged 25–64. For obvious reasons, the risk factors could not be measured in all of these individuals. Instead random samples were investigated.

Sample size
The size of the consecutive independent population samples required for the study were calculated on the basis that changes from 60% to 40% in smoking prevalence, 3 mmHg in diastolic blood pressure and 0.3 mmol/l in total cholesterol should be detectable at a significance level of 5%. For blood pressure and cholesterol, this required samples of 200 persons. For smoking, only 100 people were required. Therefore, the minimum sample size was set at 200 persons in each 10-year age/sex group. The total sample size in each population survey would therefore be 1200 or 1600, depending on whether or not the optional 25–34 year age group was included. Actual sample sizes were most commonly between one and two thousand, but as large as 3000 in some populations. Larger sample sizes made possible local comparisons between subgroups of the population, such as geographic sub-regions or socioeconomic classes.

It became apparent during the project that the precision of the risk-factor estimates depends not only on sample size but also on the quality of the data. As the sample size is increased, the sampling error diminishes and measurement bias, which does not depend on the sample size, becomes relatively more important (see Figure). With good quality assurance the measurement bias can be kept small but it cannot be avoided completely. Its actual magnitude and direction are usually unknown. The MONICA Quality assessments of blood pressure and cholesterol measurements (1, 2) suggest that a sample size of 200–300 for any subgroup of interest may be optimal for population estimates. This agrees well with the sample size required by the MONICA study as a whole, where 10-year age/sex groups were defined as the subgroups of interest.

Sampling frames
The sampling frame is the list from which the sample is drawn. The sampling frames used in MONICA are discussed elsewhere. See #29 *Recruitment and Response Rates* (3).

Sample selection
To ensure that the surveys were representative of the geographically defined target populations throughout the 10-year period, the samples for the different surveys were independent. This meant that the samples for the second or the third survey were selected irrespective of whether or not individuals were included

- men and women were chosen at random from population lists
- —then recruited, with consent, into the population surveys
- there was a need to balance numbers of subjects against careful measurement in each one

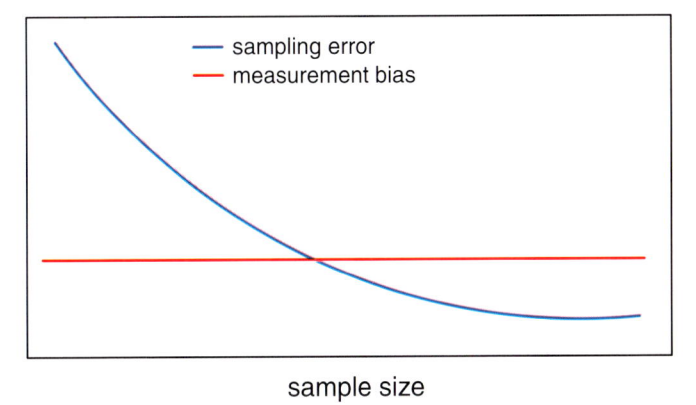

Numbers improve precision—not bias

in previous surveys. In most populations the samples were stratified by sex and 10-year age group (4). Within each stratum, single-stage sampling was recommended and was used in about two-thirds of the populations (3). For the others, multistage sampling was used because it was more practical for logistical or other reasons related to the feasibility of conducting the survey. Sometimes multistage sampling was used because it was not feasible to create a sampling frame of individuals drawn from the entire population.

References
MONICA Web Publications are also accessible on the Monograph CD-ROM

1. Kuulasmaa K, Hense HW, Tolonen H, for the WHO MONICA Project. Quality assessment of data on blood pressure in the WHO MONICA Project. (May 1998). Available from URL: http://www.ktl.fi/publications/monica/bp/bpqa.htm, URN:*NBN:fi-fe19991082*. MONICA Web Publication 9.
2. Ferrario M, Kuulasmaa K, Grafnetter D, Moltchanov V, for the WHO MONICA Project. Quality assessment of total cholesterol measurements in the WHO MONICA Project. (April 1999). Available from URL: http://www.ktl.fi/publications/monica/tchol/tcholqa.htm, URN:*NBN:fi-fe19991083*. MONICA Web Publication 10.
3. Wolf HK, Kuulasmaa K, Tolonen H, Ruokokoski E, for the WHO MONICA Project. Participation rates, quality of sampling frames and sampling fractions in the MONICA Surveys. (September 1998). Available from URL: http://www.ktl.fi/publications/monica/nonres/nonres.htm, URN:*NBN:fi-fe19991076*. MONICA Web Publication 7.
4. Kuulasmaa K, Tolonen H, Ferrario M, Ruokokoski E, for the WHO MONICA Project. Age, date of examination and survey periods in the MONICA surveys. (May 1998). Available from URL: http://www.ktl.fi/publications/monica/age/ageqa.htm, URN:*NBN:fi-fe19991075*. MONICA Web Publication 6.

Kari Kuulasmaa

#29 Recruitment and Response Rates

Introduction

Since the risk-factor profile of the MONICA target populations was estimated by sample surveys, the question that needed to be addressed was how representative were the random samples of the respective target populations? The major factors determining representativeness are:

- *Quality of the sampling frame.* The list from which the sample is to be drawn should contain all the members of the target population and nobody else.
- *Response rate.* All individuals who are randomly selected should provide data for the study, i.e. the ideal response rate would be 100%.

- anyone invited to participate in a survey is entitled to refuse
- low participation increases the potential for biased survey results
- comparing responders with non-respondents proved difficult
- so actual biases could not be estimated

Sampling frames

One way of assessing the quality of the sampling frame lies in the percentage of selected persons that could be located, i.e. that had not moved away or died before an attempt was made to contact them. Typical sampling frames used by the MONICA Collaborating Centres (MCCs) were population registers, electoral lists, and lists of public health insurance plans. A few sampling frames were known to have quality problems (up to 30% of the sample was not contacted despite repeated attempts by mail, telephone, or home visits) but they were the best available choice for the respective MCC.

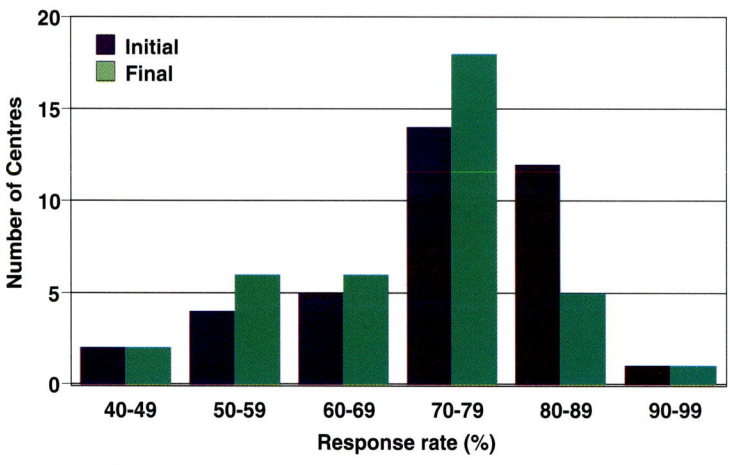

Response rates in initial and final surveys

Response rates

The measure that is most important for assessing the extent to which a sample is representative is the percentage of randomly selected persons that provided data for the study (response rate). Response rates can be defined in more than one way. Two parallel definitions were used in MONICA (*1*). Figure 1 shows the distribution of response rates for all collaborating centres during the initial and final survey using one of these definitions. In the final survey more MCCs had lower response rates.

Card confirming survey appointment

Non-response bias

If non-response were a random phenomenon, responders would still be representative. Non-response creates bias where responders and non-respondents (non-responders) are systematically different for the factors being studied. Theoretically, it is possible to assess the potential for bias of the risk-factor estimates by collecting relevant information from non-respondents. Simple information like age and sex may be available from the sampling frame, and, by simple, even telephone questionnaire, smoking status, but data dependent on full participation such as blood pressure and blood cholesterol are not available. MONICA designed a 'non-respondent' record to be completed for such persons. However it was not successful (*2*). It could not be used on people that could not be located. But even people who were located usually refused to provide information, confirming that they meant "no", when they refused to participate in the first place.

References
MONICA Web Publications are also accessible on the Monograph CD-ROM

1. Wolf HK, Kuulasmaa K, Tolonen H, Ruokokoski E, for the WHO MONICA Project. Participation rates, quality of sampling frames and sampling fractions in the MONICA Surveys. (September 1998). Available from URL: http://www.ktl.fi/publications/monica/nonres/nonres.htm, URN:*NBN:fi-fe19991076*. MONICA Web Publication 7.
2. WHO MONICA Project. MONICA Manual. (1998–1999). Part III: Population Survey. Section 1: Population Survey Data Component. Available from URL: http://www.ktl.fi/publications/monica/manual/part3/iii-1.htm URN:*NBN:fi-fe19981151*. MONICA Web Publication 1.

Andrzej Pająk, Hermann Wolf

#30 Questionnaire Design and Contents

Questionnaire items

The MONICA population survey data consist of both physical measurements made during clinical examinations, and data gathered through questionnaires. The detailed specifications of the data that were to be gathered by the MONICA Collaborating Centres (MCCs) and submitted to the MONICA Data Centre (MDC) were defined in the data transfer formats in the MONICA Manual (*1*). In the beginning, the questionnaire items covered

- marital status
- education
- smoking
- awareness and treatment of hypertension.

- MONICA used standardized questionnaires
- they were translated into local languages
- some centres used self-administered questionnaires and some used interviewers
- later MONICA surveys involved supplementary and added items

In 1989, before the MCCs submitted their middle survey data to the MDC, some items were added, including:

- exposure to other people's tobacco smoke (passive smoking)
- awareness and treatment of high cholesterol
- measurement of blood pressure and cholesterol in the past year
- use of aspirin to prevent or treat heart disease
- menopausal status and use of estrogens for menopausal symptoms
- use of contraceptive pills.

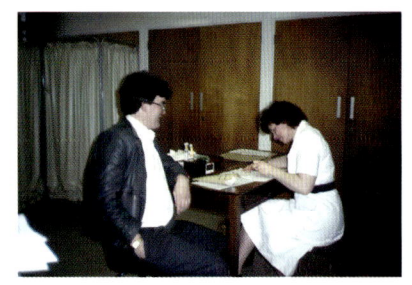

Questionnaires could be self-completed or by interview

MCCs that had already included such questions were now able to submit the results to the MDC. Other MCCs could include these items in their final surveys. Availability of data about these items from the different MCCs is documented in the relevant MONICA Quality assessment reports (*2*).

Smoking questionnaire

For data about smoking, MONICA used many items from the questionnaire contained in *Cardiovascular Survey Methods* (*3*), although some additional items were not added to the questionnaire until 1989. Drawing on experience gained from using questionnaires during test exercises conducted during MONICA training seminars, some of the questions were further refined during the MONICA Project. The final MONICA questionnaire on smoking is contained in the Manual (*1*).

Questionnaires used by the MCCs

Each MCC had to prepare its questionnaires in its own local language or languages. The design varied according to whether the questionnaire was self-administered or interviewer-administered—for example it could be posted to the participant in advance with an appointment to bring it completed for checking at a subsequent survey clinic. Some MCCs used a simple questionnaire, which included only the 'core' items required for the MONICA data, whereas others used many more questions for local purposes or for the MONICA optional studies, see #43–#49 *Optional Studies*.

Questionnaire items were specified in the data transfer formats in the form of interview questions and answers so that it was quite easy to prepare a survey questionnaire that corresponded to the requirements of these formats. Sometimes local questions differed from MONICA questions. This could be because the MCCs wanted to maintain continuity with earlier or parallel surveys, or similarly because their initial MONICA survey contained local questions about a certain issue before MONICA had adopted it as a core item and specified the data transfer formats. Compatibility of the local questionnaire items to the MONICA standard was routinely assessed in the relevant MONICA Quality assessment reports (*2*).

References
MONICA Web Publications are also accessible on the Monograph CD-ROM

1. WHO MONICA Project. MONICA Manual. (1998–1999). Part III: Population Survey. Section 1: Population survey data component. (December 1997) Available from URL: http://www.ktl.fi/publications/monica/manual/part3/iii-1.htm, URN:*NBN:fi-fe19981151*. MONICA Web Publication 1.
2. MONICA Quality assessment reports. Available from: http://www.ktl.fi/publications/monica/index.html. MONICA Web Publications 2–18.
3. Rose GA, Blackburn H, Gillum RF, Prineas RJ. *Cardiovascular Survey Methods*, 2nd *ed*. Geneva, World Health Organization, 1982 (Monograph series No. 56).

Hanna Tolonen, Kari Kuulasmaa

#31 Smoking

Introduction

Cigarette smoking is one of the three classic risk factors identified in Framingham and other cohort studies. Unlike blood pressure, blood cholesterol, height and weight, which are continuously distributed quantitative variables, smoking is a categorical variable—either you smoke or you do not. To establish population trends in smoking prevalence large numbers of subjects need to be studied. Among the many components of cigarette smoke, it is not known exactly which accelerate the development of coronary disease. Therefore it is difficult to know what to measure. Cigarettes differ in their composition in different countries and at different times, as do the way in which they are smoked. Using the prevalence of daily cigarette smoking is therefore a crude method of measuring changes in the exposure of the population to the products of burning tobacco. Historical studies suggested that *ab-initio* unmixed pipe or cigar smoking might be less hazardous than cigarette smoking. However, this may not be the case for those who changed to these from cigarettes and who still inhale. It is therefore arguable whether to define an ex-smoker as someone who has stopped smoking completely or who has stopped smoking cigarettes.

When MONICA was launched there was concern that smoking was becoming socially unacceptable. Smokers might increasingly be shamed into concealing what they were doing. Answering questionnaires falsely could create a bias in the result that could increase with progressive under-reporting over time.

Methods

A standardized questionnaire was adopted from *Cardiovascular Survey Methods* (*1, 2*). Participating centres had to translate it into their local languages so that it could either be completed by an interviewer, or filled in by participants in the survey themselves, with the results being subsequently checked at a clinic. See #30 *Questionnaire Design and Contents*. A standard assay for serum or plasma thiocyanate was organized for general use on the blood samples taken to measure blood cholesterol (*3*). Centres were also encouraged to use expired-air carbon monoxide and serum cotinine as additional biochemical tests of smoke exposure.

Quality assessment issues

Some centres continued to use local smoking questionnaires for reasons of continuity (*4*). The initial standard questionnaire was found to be inadequate when it came to compiling information about smokers who smoked only on some days of the week. Additional questions were added after the first survey (*2*). Serum thiocyanate, an assay that is easy to standardize, produced bizarre results when compared across populations. It had poor specificity and sensitivity for cigarette smokers. It also showed strange between-population differences for levels in non-smokers and these levels were inconsistent over time. It was therefore abandoned as a core data item. MONICA Collaborating Centres were encouraged to use expired-air carbon monoxide and serum cotinine for validation. However, few of them used these methods on the majority of their subjects. Since MONICA was initiated there has been increasing interest in passive smoking. While it is difficult to study, it was nonetheless studied as a local option by many MCCs, who used questionnaires and the same biochemical methods. Standard questions on passive smoking were added to the core study in 1989, see #30 *Questionnaire Design and Contents*.

- cigarette smoking is a classic coronary risk factor
- unlike blood pressure and cholesterol it is assessed by questionnaire
- irregular smokers cause problems for coding
- problems with biochemical validation
- widespread interest in passive smoking

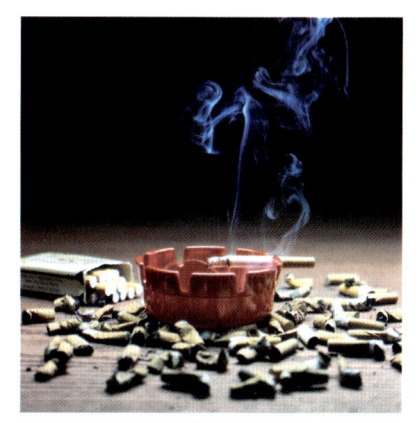

What happened to smoking rates in MONICA populations?

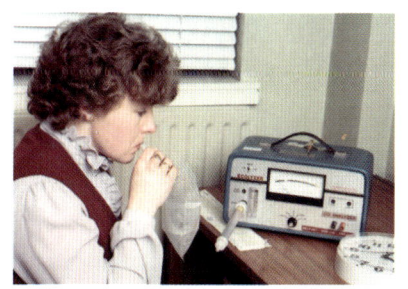

Exhaled carbon monoxide reflects recent active smoking

Results

MONICA final analyses have concentrated on the prevalence of cigarette smoking, where a smoker is defined as one who smokes daily. It is probable that the need for biochemical validation was overestimated at the beginning. Population surveys are relatively non-threatening to the participants compared with face-to-face discussions with their doctors about smoking, where they may be tempted to deceive. Where biochemical validation was analysed in the surveys it suggested that there were relatively few people who were deceitful about their smoking habits. It was unlikely that the prevalence of smoking deception changed appreciably between the three surveys. The results of smoking prevalence and trends in smoking habits are shown in graphics G36–G39 and have been published (5). Other results are in the Data Book (6).

References
MONICA Web Publications are also accessible on the Monograph CD-ROM

1. Rose GA, Blackburn H, Gillum RF, Prineas RJ. *Cardiovascular Survey Methods.* 2nd ed. Geneva, World Health Organization, 1982 (Monograph series No. 56).
2. WHO MONICA Project. MONICA Manual. (1998–1999). Part III: Population Survey. Section 1: Population Survey Data Component. Available from URL: http://www.ktl.fi/publications/monica/manual/part3/iii-1.htm, URN:*NBN:fi-fe19981151*. MONICA Web Publication 1.
3. WHO MONICA Project. MONICA Manual. (1998–1999). Part III: Population Survey. Section 3: Standardization of thiocyanate measurements. Available from URL: http://www.ktl.fi/publications/monica/manual/part3/iii-3.htm, URN:*NBN:fi-fe19981153*. MONICA Web Publication 1.
4. Molarius A, Kuulasmaa K, Evans A, McCrum E, Tolonen H, for the WHO MONICA Project. Quality assessment of data on smoking behaviour in the WHO MONICA Project. (February 1999). Available from URL: http://www.ktl.fi/publications/monica/qa30.htm, URN:*NBN:fi-fe19991077*. MONICA Web Publication 8.
5. Molarius A, Parsons RW, Dobson AJ, Evans A, Fortmann SP, Jamrozik K, Kuulasmaa K, Moltchanov V, Sans S, Tuomilehto J, Puska P, for the WHO MONICA Project. Trends in cigarette smoking in 36 populations from the early 1980s to the mid 1990s: findings from the WHO MONICA Project. *American Journal of Public Health*, 2001, 91:206–212. PMID: 11211628. MONICA Publication 42.
6. Tolonen H, Kuulasmaa K, Ruokokoski E, for the WHO MONICA Project. MONICA population survey data book. (October 2000). Available from URL: http://www.ktl.fi/publications/monica/surveydb/title.htm, URN:*NBN:fi-fe20001206*. MONICA Web Publication 27.

Alun Evans, Hugh Tunstall-Pedoe

#32 Blood Pressure

Introduction

- blood pressure is a major coronary and cerebrovascular risk factor
- standardized measurement is essential in population studies
- quality assessment scores of BP measurements were used in collaborative analyses
- high validity of BP data for cross-sectional and longitudinal analyses

Blood pressure (BP) is known to fluctuate in individuals from moment to moment reflecting physiological responses to internal and external stimuli. Nevertheless, distributions of BP values in whole populations can be validly characterized by measurements taken on a single occasion in a representative sample of individuals (1). Single-occasion BP measurements in individuals have been shown to be strong indicators of coronary and cerebrovascular risk (2). Furthermore, small changes in the average BP values of a population—usually considered irrelevant in a clinical setting—may be of considerable importance to public health (3). MONICA required an exceptionally high level of standardization for the measurement of BP (4). This was necessary to ensure between-population, or cross-sectional, comparability of BP levels. More important, for testing MONICA hypotheses, it was required for a valid longitudinal assessment of the (probably) small BP changes occurring within each population over the 10-year study period.

Quality assurance

The assessment of the quality of BP measurements is particularly challenging as there is no 'gold-standard' reference to which individual measurements can be related (and they cannot be stored for re-examination like blood specimens or electrocardiograms). A standardized quality assurance protocol for blood pressure measurement was devised for MONICA (5). It addressed the following issues:

- quality assurance before surveys (e.g. measurement devices used, training and certification of nurses or technicians, etc.)
- quality control during surveys (e.g. cuff sizes, time of day, room temperature, etc.)
- quality indicators based on recorded BP values (e.g. missing measurements, last digit preference (6), time trends etc.)
- change in any of the above over time, that is, from one survey to another.

Detailed MONICA Quality assessment reports on BP measurements are available for the baseline survey (5) and for the entire project (7).

Summary scores of the quality of BP measurements were generated for each centre. Scores that indicated a poor quality of measurement resulted in the subsequent exclusion of the respective centre from some collaborative analyses (8). Quality indicators were also used in sensitivity analyses to assess the potential impact that a poor quality of measurement would have on the results of the study (9).

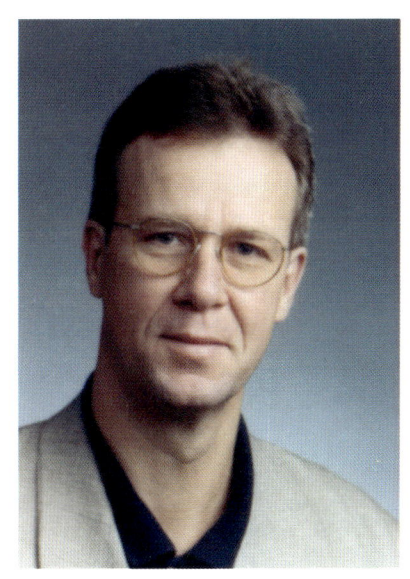

Hans-Werner Hense

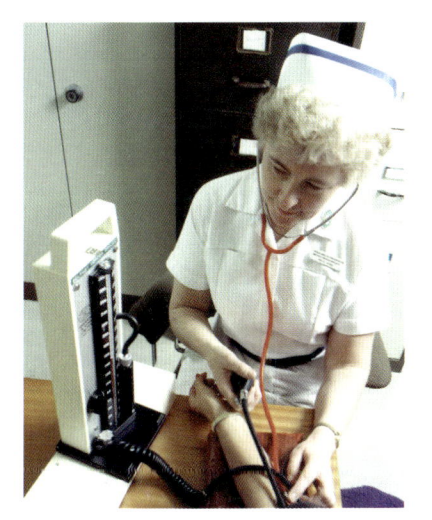

Methods

In the population surveys two blood pressure measurements were made under carefully specified conditions before venepuncture (4). The mean of the two readings was used to characterize the individual concerned. The MONICA protocol preceded the widespread use of automatic blood-pressure recording devices, which have not been validated for long-term epidemiological surveys. MCCs were divided between those using the standard mercury sphygmomanometer and those using the random-zero mercury sphygmomanometer.

Random-Zero sphygmomanometer (Belfast)

Results

Systolic blood pressure was used for testing the risk-factor or First MONICA Hypothesis (9) as well as for graphics G40–G43, although diastolic blood pressure analyses appear in the survey Data Book (10). Graphics G40–G43 show very considerable variations in blood pressure levels between different populations—they were shown to be particularly high in Finnish populations. Blood pressure levels appear to be falling in considerably more populations than those in which it is rising.

References
MONICA Web Publications are also accessible on the Monograph CD-ROM

1. Kannel W. Clinical misconceptions dispelled by epidemiological research. *Circulation*, 1995, 92:3350–3360. PMID: 7586324.
2. MacMahon S, Peto R, Cutler J, Collins R, Sorlie P, Neaton J, Abbott R, Godwin J, Dyer A, Stamler J. Blood pressure, stroke, and coronary heart disease. Part 1: Prolonged differences in blood pressure: prospective observational studies corrected for regression dilution bias. *Lancet*, 1990, 335:764–774. PMID: 1969518.
3. Rose G. Sick individuals and sick populations. *International Journal of Epidemiology*, 1985, 14:32–38. PMID: 3872850.
4. WHO MONICA Project. MONICA Manual. (1998–1999). Part III: Population Survey. Section 1: Population Survey Data Component. Available from URL: http://www.ktl.fi/publications/monica/manual/part3/iii-1.htm, URN:*NBN:fi-fe19981151*. MONICA Web Publication 1.
5. Hense HW, Koivisto AM, Kuulasmaa K, Zaborskis A, Kupsc W, Tuomilehto J, for the WHO MONICA Project. Assessment of blood pressure measurement quality in the baseline surveys of the WHO MONICA project. *Journal of Human Hypertension*, 1995, 9:935–946. PMID: 8746637. MONICA Publication 20.

6. Hense HW, Kuulasmaa K, Zaborskis A, Kupsc W, Tuomilehto J, for the WHO MONICA Project. Quality assessment of blood pressure measurements in epidemiological surveys. The impact of last digit preference and the proportions of identical duplicate measurements. WHO Monica Project. *Revue d'Epidémiologie et de Santé Publique*, 1990, 38:463–468. PMID: 2082452. MONICA Publication 14.

7. Kuulasmaa K, Hense HW, Tolonen H, for the WHO MONICA Project. Quality assessment of data on blood pressure in the WHO MONICA Project. (May 1998). Available from URL: http://www.ktl.fi/publications/monica/bp/bpqa.htm, URN:*NBN:fi-fe19991082*. MONICA Web Publication 9.

8. Wolf HK, Tuomilehto J, Kuulasmaa K, Domarkiene S, Cepaitis Z, Molarius A, Sans S, Dobson A, Keil U, Rywik S, for the WHO MONICA Project. Blood pressure levels in the 41 populations of the WHO MONICA Project. *Journal of Human Hypertension*, 1997, 11:733–742. PMID: 9416984. MONICA Publication 31.

9. Kuulasmaa K, Tunstall-Pedoe H, Dobson A, Fortmann S, Sans S, Tolonen H, Evans A, Ferrario M, Tuomilehto J, for the WHO MONICA Project. Estimation of contribution of changes in classic risk factors to trends in coronary-event rates across the WHO MONICA Project populations. *Lancet*, 2000, 355:675–687. PMID: 10703799. MONICA Publication 38.

10. Tolonen H, Kuulasmaa K, Ruokokoski E, for the WHO MONICA Project. MONICA population survey data book. (October 2000). Available from URL: http://www.ktl.fi/publications/monica/surveydb/title.htm, URN:*NBN:fi-fe20001206*. MONICA Web Publication 27.

Hans-Werner Hense

#33 Cholesterol

Introduction

Cholesterol, otherwise known as total cholesterol (TC), blood, serum or plasma cholesterol is one of the core classic risk factors in MONICA, and the only one measured in the laboratory. Levels of change in average or mean cholesterol values in the population that are of importance to the epidemiologist are of the same magnitude as those that may occur as the result of laboratory drift (inconsistency in a laboratory's standardization) over the same time. They may even be smaller than those occurring through random variation between one reading and the next in the same individual. Measurement of genuine, as against spurious, trends in total cholesterol in populations over time was therefore a severe challenge for MONICA, as total cholesterol was measured locally rather than in one central collective laboratory. Total cholesterol, which does show seasonal variation (higher in winter in many populations), does not vary appreciably with time of day or fasting/non-fasting status, nor does HDL-cholesterol (see *Glossary, Abbreviations and Nicknames*). Other lipid measurements and fractions do vary and are assayed by lipid clinics after a prolonged fast, a procedure that is not generally practical for epidemiological field surveys.

- quality of total cholesterol determinations is a key issue in detecting time trends in risk factors
- in most MONICA populations mean levels are decreasing, with some relevant exceptions

Methods

Comparability of cholesterol measurements is influenced by the conditions operating over several steps of the measurement procedure, which can be divided into two stages: the pre-analytic stage (conditions under which blood is drawn, specimen handling and storage before analysis) and the analytic stage (methods used for determination, reagents, analysers, etc). Potential hazards were well known at the start of MONICA through previous extensive research, particularly that carried out in the Lipid Research Clinics in the USA (*1*). A section of the MONICA Manual was devoted to potential problems and to standardization of procedures (*2*). Earlier versions of this were influenced by lipid laboratories working with lipid clinics rather than on population surveys. This was later amended.

Quality assurance

Potential sources of between-population pre-analytical variability or bias in MONICA were the use or non-use of a tourniquet, the posture of the subjects during venepuncture, the comparability of seasonal periods when the surveys were carried out, the duration, temperature and other conditions of storage of samples at different stages of the measurement process, and the material (plasma or serum) used for lipid determinations (3, 4). Some centres took specimens from participants who were fasting but most used non-fasting subjects. Blood was taken during routine survey visits throughout the day, scheduled, in accordance with the Manual, to follow rather than precede blood-pressure measurement, in case the use of a needle caused anxiety and influenced blood pressure.

Enzymatic methods were recommended and were generally adopted by most laboratories, using the same brand of reagents (2). However, different methods and procedures for total-cholesterol determinations were permitted in MONICA, to allow for laboratories that wished to be consistent with previous or ongoing studies. Collaborating laboratories were required to standardize their measurement methods and to participate in a blind external quality control system, run by the World Health Organization Regional Lipid Reference Centre in Prague, Czech Republic, which was designated as the MONICA Quality Control Centre for Lipid Measurements (see #8 *MONICA Quality Control Centres (MQCs)*). However, using the same logic, they were permitted to continue with standardization on the Centers for Disease Control (CDC) laboratory in Atlanta, Georgia, USA, if they had already done so. Laboratories were expected to begin processing the external quality control material for a three-month run-in period before, and then throughout each population survey, as well as using a rigid system of internal quality control (2).

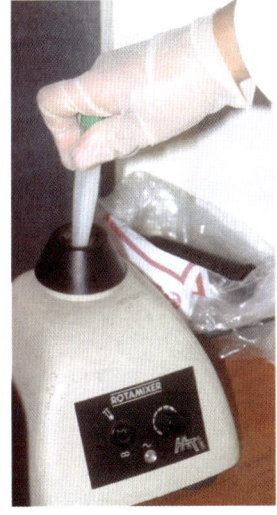

Mixing blood

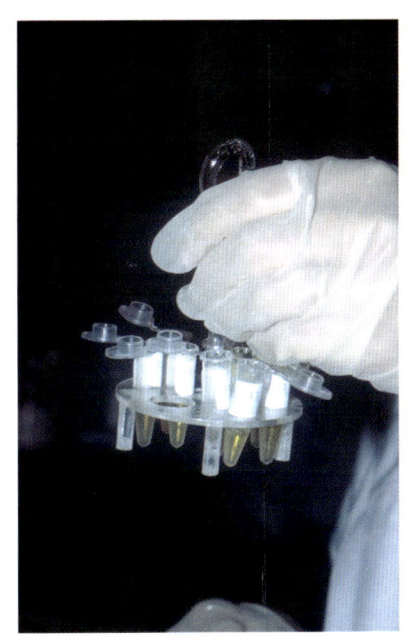

Results

Cholesterol was of prime concern for MONICA in view of its role in the *Framingham* and *Seven Countries Study*. The latter suggested that it was the key determinant of international differences in coronary heart disease rates, and therefore possibly of trends (5, 6). Data on total cholesterol gathered from the initial population surveys were of unacceptable quality in a small number of centres. However, many centres failed the external quality control tests for HDL-cholesterol (4, 7). The latter was an optional item, not featuring in the MONICA hypotheses, and was not used in collaborative analyses when these measurements were found to be inadequately standardized.

MONICA was concerned with longitudinal results within populations, rather than with cross-sectional results between populations, although the MONICA study did create a unique opportunity for the latter. Centres were urged to be consistent in their pre-analytical procedures in order to prevent bias between surveys, but at the same time to improve the accuracy and precision of their laboratory performance. Correction of bias detected through the external quality control was permitted only if very specific criteria were met (4), but the results of external quality control contributed in the final analysis to the weighting of the quality score (8–10). See #40 *Statistical Analysis*.

Separating serum—is the label correct?

Results of the initial survey featured in *World Health Statistics Annual 1989* (11). Mean total cholesterol levels in the MONICA populations in the initial and final surveys are shown in graphics G44 and G45; trends in total cholesterol and

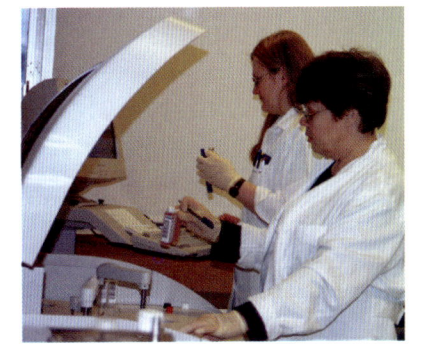

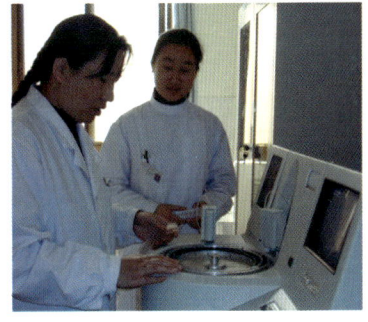

Techniques were standardized from Reykyavik . . . across to Beijing

POPULATION SURVEYS

their geographical distribution are shown in graphics G46 and G47. Changes in total cholesterol were usually downwards, were small, but often statistically significant, and made a considerable contribution to the improvement in risk-factor scores observed in many populations (8–10). Trends in men and women were generally comparable. Those populations which showed an increase in total cholesterol included some whose quality scores made their results questionable, see graphic G56.

References
MONICA Web Publications are also available on the Monograph CD-ROM

1. Lipid Research Clinics Program. *Manual of Laboratory Operations: Lipid and lipoprotein analysis*, Bethesda, Md: National Institutes of Health, 1974,1. Revised 1982. DHEW Publication NIH 75-628.
2. WHO MONICA Project. MONICA Manual. (1998–1999). Part III: Population Survey. Section 2: Standardization of Lipid Measurements. Available from URL: http://www.ktl.fi/publications/monica/manual/part3/iii-2.htm. URN:*NBN:fi-fe19981146*. MONICA Web Publication 1.
3. Döring A, Pająk A, Ferrario M, Grafnetter D, Kuulasmaa K, for the WHO MONICA Project. Methods of total cholesterol measurement in the baseline survey of the WHO MONICA Project. *Revue d'Epidémiologie et de Santé Publique*, 1990, 38:455–461. PMID: 2082451. MONICA Publication 13.
4. Ferrario M, Kuulasmaa K, Grafnetter D, Moltchanov V, for the WHO MONICA Project. Quality assessment of total cholesterol measurements in the WHO MONICA Project. (April 1999). Available from URL: http://www.ktl.fi/publications/monica/tchol/tcholqa.htm, URN:*NBN:fi-fe19991083*. MONICA Web Publication 10.
5. Dawber TR. *The Framingham Study. The Epidemiology of Atherosclerotic Disease*, Cambridge, Mass., Harvard University Press, 1980.
6. Keys A. *Seven Countries: A Multivariate Analysis of Death and Coronary Heart Disease*, Cambridge, Mass. and London, England, Harvard University Press, 1980.
7. Marques-Vidal P, Ferrario M, Kuulasmaa K, Grafnetter D, Moltchanov V, for the WHO MONICA Project. Quality assessment of data on HDL-cholesterol in the WHO MONICA Project. (June 1999). Available from URL: http://www.ktl.fi/publications/monica/hdl/hdlqa.htm, URN:*NBN:fi-fe19991137*. MONICA Web Publication 11.
8. Dobson A, Evans A, Ferrario M, Kuulasmaa KA, Moltchanov VA, Sans S, Tunstall-Pedoe H, Tuomilehto JO, Wedel H, Yarnell J, for the WHO MONICA Project. Changes in estimated coronary risk in the 1980s: data from 38 populations in the WHO MONICA Project. World Health Organization. *Annals of Medicine*, 1998, 30:199–205. PMID: 9667799. MONICA Publication 32.
9. Evans A, Tolonen H, Hense HW, Ferrario M, Sans S, Kuulasmaa K, for the WHO MONICA Project. Trends in coronary risk factors in the WHO MONICA Project. *International Journal of Epidemiology*, 2001, 30(Suppl 1):S35–S40. PMID: 11211628. MONICA Publication 43.
10. Kuulasmaa K, Tunstall-Pedoe H, Dobson A, Fortmann S, Sans S, Tolonen H, Evans A, Ferrario M, Tuomilehto J, for the WHO MONICA Project. Estimation of contribution of changes in classic risk factors to trends in coronary-event rates across the WHO MONICA Project populations. *Lancet*, 2000, 355:675–687. PMID: 10703799. MONICA Publication 38.
11. The WHO MONICA Project. A worldwide monitoring system for cardiovascular diseases: Cardiovascular mortality and risk factors in selected communities. *World Health Statistics Annual*, 1989, 27–149. ISBN 92 4 067890 5. ISSN 0250-3794. MONICA Publication 11.

Marco Ferrario

#34 Height, Weight and Waist Circumference

Introduction

Nobody foresaw during the planning stages of the MONICA Project that obesity would become a worldwide health problem in the 21st century (1).

Methods

Yet provisions were made in the MONICA Manual (2) to measure height and weight in an accurate way, using beam-balance scales and height rules (also known as stadiometers). Shoes had to be removed, as well as outer garments and all the small objects that people carry in their pockets, so as to avoid exaggerated heights and weights. Self-reported height and weight were not acceptable.

- obesity is a risk factor that can be measured in several different ways
- in many populations obesity was increasing as other risk factors and CHD declined
- abdominal obesity was monitored, but not from the start of MONICA

Abdominal obesity

Mid-way through the Project, growing scientific evidence was pointing to abdominal obesity as an independent risk factor for coronary heart disease (3). Consequently, measurements of waist and hip circumference were added to the middle and final population surveys (2).

Indicators

Body mass index (BMI) or Quetelet index (weight in kilograms divided by the square of the height in metres), was used to express relative weight.

Overweight was defined as BMI ≥25 kg/m^2; obesity as BMI ≥30 kg/m^2.

Waist circumference and the ratio of waist to hip circumference were used to indicate abdominal obesity.

Measuring height

Quality assurance

It was recommended that weight measurements should be rounded to the nearest 200 grams. Height, waist and hip measurements were rounded to the nearest centimetre. The majority of centres complied with the protocol. Deviations from the protocol and problems encountered are listed in the MONICA Quality assessment reports (4, 5). Beam-balance scales were not always practical for survey teams moving from place to place. Equipment used for measuring height could also vary in sophistication.

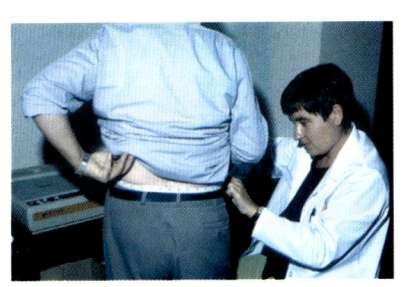

Measuring waist circumference

Findings

Obesity results from an imbalance between energy intake and expenditure although the factors involved can be complex (6, 7). In MONICA, while there was no clear geographical pattern for men, there was a clearer one for women (see graphics G48–G51). BMI was rising in most male populations in MONICA and in women the tendency was also towards an increase. This trend was unique to this risk factor. The data shown in the graphics are published. Social gradients appear to be widening (8–10).

Abdominal obesity is not featured in the graphics, but it increased with age, especially in women, but with geographical variations. While abdominal obesity is more common than a high BMI, they do not always go together (11–13).

The increase in obesity was paradoxical for MONICA (8):

- rising BMI often went with a decline in the mean blood pressure and blood cholesterol in the population
- rising BMI was associated with falling coronary-event rates across populations.

Implications for the future

It is unclear whether and when the epidemic in obesity will impact on cardiovascular disease—it has serious implications especially for the incidence of diabetes mellitus (8). The 'weightings' for BMI in our risk-factor score were small. Perhaps waist circumference would have been more powerful (See #35 *Risk-Factor Scores*). A surveillance programme is needed. These issues are setting the agenda for research in epidemiology and public health in the new century.

References
MONICA Web Publications are also accessible on the Monograph CD-ROM

1. International Obesity Task Force. Website available at: URL: http://www.iotf.org
2. WHO MONICA Project. MONICA Manual. (1998–1999). Part III: Population Survey. Section 1: Population Survey Data Component. Available from URL: http://www.ktl.fi/publications/monica/manual/part3/iii-1, URN:*NBN:fi-fe19981151*. MONICA Web Publication 1.
3. Björntorp P. The associations between obesity, adipose tissue distribution and disease. *Acta Medica Scandinavica. Supplementum*, 1988, 723:121–134. PMID: 3293356.

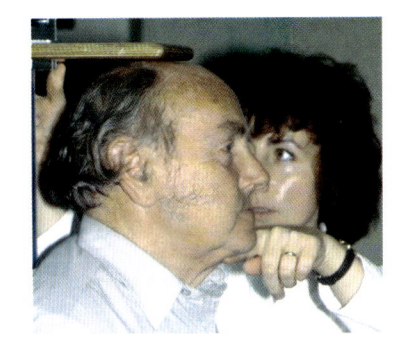

4. Molarius A, Kuulasmaa K, Sans S, for the WHO MONICA Project. Quality assessment of weight and height measurements in the WHO MONICA Project. (May 1998). Available from URL: http://www.ktl.fi/publications/monica/bmi/bmiqa20.htm, URN:*NBN:fi-fe19991079*. MONICA Web Publication 12.

5. Molarius A, Sans S, Kuulasmaa K, for the WHO MONICA Project. Quality assessment of data on waist and hip circumferences in the WHO MONICA Project. (October 1998). Available from URL: http://www.ktl.fi/publications/monica/waisthip/waisthipqa.htm, URN:*NBN:fi-fe19991091*. MONICA Web Publication 13.

6. Molarius A, Seidell JC, Kuulasmaa K, Dobson AJ, Sans S, for the WHO MONICA Project. Smoking and relative body weight: an international perspective from the WHO MONICA Project. *Journal of Epidemiology and Community Health*, 1997, 51:252–260. PMID: 9229053. MONICA Publication 27.

7. Sans S and Evans A. Are cardiovascular disease trends driven by gadflies? (letter) *International Journal of Epidemiology*, 2001, 30:624–625. PMID:11416095.

8. Kuulasmaa K, Tunstall-Pedoe H, Dobson A, Fortmann S, Sans S, Tolonen H, Evans A, Ferrario M, Tuomilehto J, for the WHO MONICA Project. Estimation of contribution of changes in classic risk factors to trends in coronary-event rates across the WHO MONICA Project populations. *Lancet*, 2000, 355:675–687. PMID: 10703799. MONICA Publication 38.

9. Tolonen H, Kuulasmaa K, Ruokokoski E, for the WHO MONICA Project. MONICA population survey data book. (October 2000). Available from URL: http://www.ktl.fi/publications/monica/surveydb/bmi/table634_summary.htm, URN:*NBN:fi-fe20001206*. MONICA Web Publication 27.

10. Molarius A, Seidell JC, Sans S, Tuomilehto J, Kuulasmaa K, for the WHO MONICA Project. Educational level, relative body weight, and changes in their association over 10 years: an international perspective from the WHO MONICA Project. *American Journal of Public Health*, 2000, 90:1260–1268. PMID: 10937007. MONICA Publication 41.

11. Molarius A, Seidell JC, Sans S, Tuomilehto J, Kuulasmaa K, for the WHO MONICA Project. Waist and hip circumferences, and waist-hip ratio in 19 populations of the WHO MONICA Project. *International Journal of Obesity and Related Metabolic Disorders*, 1999, 23:116–125. PMID: 10078844. MONICA Publication 35.

12. Molarius A, Seidell JC, Sans S, Tuomilehto J, Kuulasmaa K, for the WHO MONICA Project. Varying sensitivity of waist action levels to identify subjects with overweight or obesity in 19 populations of the WHO MONICA Project. *Journal of Clinical Epidemiology*, 1999, 52: 1213–1224. PMID: 10580785. MONICA Publication 37.

13. Molarius A, Seidell JC, Sans S, Tuomilehto J, Kuulasmaa K, for the WHO MONICA Project. Varying sensitivity of waist action levels to identify subjects with overweight or obesity in 19 populations of the WHO MONICA Project—tables and figures for waist action level 1. (December 1999). Available from URL: http://www.ktl.fi/publications/monica/waction/waction.htm, URN:*NBN:fi-fe19991138*. MONICA Web Publication 19.

Susana Sans

#35 Risk-Factor Scores

What is a risk-factor score?

MONICA used risk-factor scores (also called risk scores) to summarize the combined effect in individual survey participants of their:

- summarizes the combined effect of the classic risk factors
- facilitates the testing of the First MONICA (risk-factor) Hypothesis
- different scores for the two sexes, for coronary disease and for stroke

- daily cigarette-smoking status,
- systolic blood pressure,
- total cholesterol, and
- body mass index (BMI)

in determining their estimated risk of contracting coronary heart disease or suffering a stroke. The risk score was derived from a linear combination of the risk factors.

Risk score for coronary events

For coronary events the risk score was derived from the Nordic Risk Assessment Study which had the following features (*1, 2*):

- baseline risk-factor levels and follow-up data from different Nordic studies
- 110 751 (62 150 men, 48 601 women) at baseline
- 1650 (1422 men and 228 women) died from coronary heart disease during follow-up.

Coefficients for the coronary-event risk score are given in Table 1.

Risk score for stroke events

The risk score for stroke events was derived from Finnish follow-up data (3):

- baseline risk-factor levels from Finnish risk-factor surveys conducted in 1982 and 1987
- 14 902 (7195 men and 7705 women) at the baseline
- 553 (299 men and 234 women) fatal and non-fatal stroke events during follow-up.

The coefficients for the stroke risk score are given in Table 2 (3).

Regression dilution

For risk factors, which have large within-person variation compared with the between-person variation, the regression coefficients underestimate their true effect (4). To compensate for this regression dilution, the risk-score coefficients for systolic blood pressure and total cholesterol can be multiplied by 1.5 (4–6).

Interpretation of the risk scores

The differing mean risk scores for different populations reflect estimated relative event rates on a logarithmic scale. The difference in scores between two populations is an estimate of the ratio of their projected event rates. The trends in risk score estimate the relative changes in event rates.

Results

Population levels and trends in the coronary risk-factor scores are shown in graphics G52–G55 and contribute to graphics G69–G70. The stroke risk-factor scores contribute to graphics G73–G74. The scoring is different for men and women. Tables 1 and 2 show that in seven out of eight comparisons risk-factor coefficients are higher for men. These are the only graphics in MONICA in which comparison of the sexes is misleading. They are not being measured to the same standard—the mathematical model in each sex is different.

Table 1. Coefficients for the coronary-event risk score

Risk factor	Men	Women
Daily smoking (0/1)	0.807	0.851
Systolic blood pressure (mmHg)	0.014	0.020
Total cholesterol (mmol/l)	0.290	0.250
BMI (kg/m^2)	0.049	0.007

Table 2. Coefficients for the stroke risk score

Risk factor	Men	Women
Daily smoking (0/1)	0.607	0.409
Systolic blood pressure (mmHg)	0.011	0.010
Total cholesterol (mmol/l)	0.055	–0.004
BMI (kg/m^2)	0.054	0.043

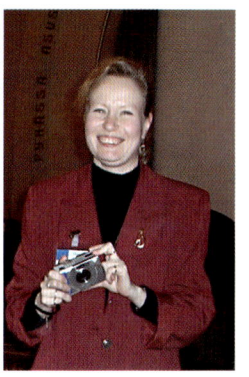

Hanna Tolonen has a break from this Monograph

References

MONICA Web Publications are also accessible on the Monograph CD-ROM

1. Dobson A, Evans A, Ferrario M, Kuulasmaa KA, Moltchanov VA, Sans S, Tunstall-Pedoe H, Tuomilehto JO, Wedel H, Yarnell J, for the WHO MONICA Project. Changes in estimated coronary risk in the 1980s: data from 38 populations in the WHO MONICA Project. World Health Organization. *Annals of Medicine*, 1998, 30:199–205. PMID: 9667799. MONICA Publication 32.
2. Kuulasmaa K, Tunstall-Pedoe H, Dobson A, Fortmann S, Sans S, Tolonen H, Evans A, Ferrario M, Tuomilehto J, for the WHO MONICA Project. Estimation of contribution of changes in classic risk factors to trends in coronary-event rates across the WHO MONICA Project populations. *Lancet*, 2000, 355:675–687. PMID: 10703799. MONICA Publication 38.
3. Tolonen H, Kuulasmaa K, Asplund K, Mähönen M, for the WHO MONICA Project. Do trends in population levels of blood pressure and other cardiovascular risk factors explain trends in stroke event rates?—methodological appendix. (May 2002). Available from URL: http://www.ktl.fi/publications/monica/stroke_h1/appendix.htm, URN:NBN:fi-fe20021258. MONICA Web Publication 30.
4. Clarke R, Shipley M, Lewington S, Youngman L, Collins R, Marmot M, Peto R. Underestimation of risk associations due to regression dilution in long-term follow-up of prospective studies. *American Journal of Epidemiology*, 1999, 150:341–353. PMID:10453810.
5. MacMahon S, Peto R, Cutler J, Collins R, Sorlie P, Neaton J, Abbott R, Godwin J, Dyer A, Stamler J. Blood pressure, stroke, and coronary heart disease. Part 1: Prolonged differences in blood pressure: prospective observational studies corrected for regression dilution bias. *Lancet*, 1990, 335:764–774. PMID: 1969518.
6. Law MR, Wald NJ, Wu T, Hackshaw A, Bailey A. Systematic underestimation of association between serum cholesterol concentration and ischaemic heart disease in observational studies: data from the BUPA study. *British Medical Journal*, 1994, 308: 363–366. PMID: 8124143.

Hanna Tolonen

Data Handling, Quality Assessment and Publication

#36 Data Transfer, Checking and Management

From magnetic tapes to Internet

When the MONICA Project was started, computing and data transfer facilities were quite different from what they are today. In most MONICA Collaborating Centres (MCCs), computing and data management were done with big mainframe computers each occupying a whole room. The capacity of these computers was negligible in comparison with any modern portable PC. The computing facilities also varied a lot between the MCCs. In some centres, programs were still entered into the computer using punched paper tapes, while some already had visual terminals or PCs. When the MONICA Data Centre (MDC) was established in 1984, the National Public Health Institute (KTL), where it was located, had a brand new VAX computer with 2MB of central memory. The development of computing facilities at the MDC has fortunately been considerably faster than the accumulation of MONICA data.

At the start of the Project, the most feasible media for transferring data from the MCCs to the MONICA Data Centre were paper forms or magnetic tapes. For data on individual coronary or stroke events as well as survey data, MONICA chose magnetic tape which had well-defined storage standards. After a few years, when floppy disks were capable of storing sufficient quantities of data, MONICA began to use them. In recent years most of the data have been transferred over the Internet by e-mail. Throughout the study, aggregated yearly population and mortality data were submitted to the MDC on paper forms. The details of the data transfer procedures are described in Part V of the MONICA Manual *(1)*, while the fixed formats for data records are described in the parts of the Manual dealing with the different data components. Over the years, the MONICA Data Centre received almost one thousand data shipments containing almost 5000 separate files with over 3.2 million data records.

Data checking

A basic feature of the transfer process from the MCCs was that it included not only individual patient records but also inventories showing what was included, and what was not included, and the reasons for non-inclusion *(1)*. Every data file received by the MDC was routinely checked for correctness and consistency. The specifications used for checking can be found in the MONICA Quality assessment reports *(2)*. The so-called Computer Generated Error Correction Form *(1)* was printed and sent back to the MCC for correction or elucidation. The MCCs retained control over their data and therefore the MDC was allowed to make corrections only when specifically empowered to do so by the MCC. This procedure limited the risk of disagreement between the data sets held

- data were strictly managed to minimize potential for error
- MCCs needed to retain control of their data
- MCCs and MDC had to ensure that their databases did not diverge through action in one place and not the other

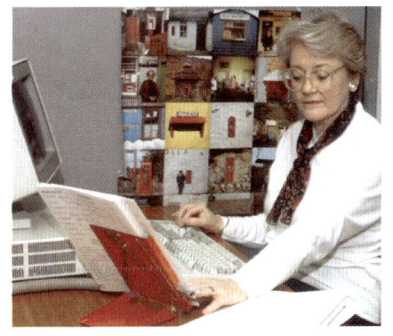

MONICA data were keyed into a microcomputer twice

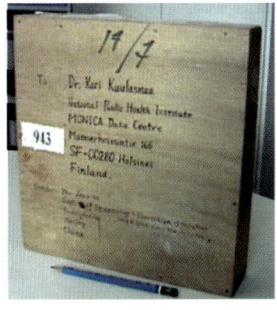

First computer tape from Beijing

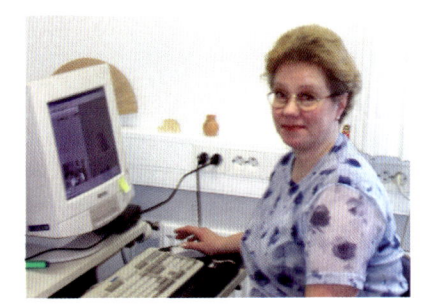

Tuula Virmanen-Ojanen logged data transfers to and from the MDC

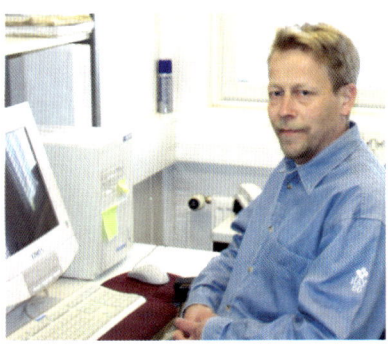

Esa Ruokokoski wrote the data processing software

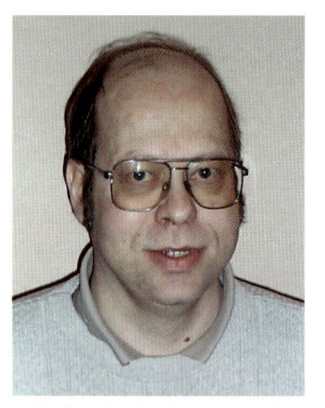

Physician Markku Mähönen examined coronary and stroke data

by the MDC and the MCCs. About 3000 error correction forms were circulated this way.

Data management

The first plan for data management in the MDC was based on the use of SAS (a statistical data analysis package). It soon became obvious that given the amount of data expected and the need for fast access to individual records, more powerful tools were needed. We therefore adopted a relational database engine, the RDB/VMS, which had been used successfully in another project in KTL. It was a good choice: during the next 15 years we faced very few problems with the database system.

References
MONICA Web Publications are also accessible on the Monograph CD-ROM
1. WHO MONICA Project. MONICA Manual. (1998–1999). Part V: Data Transfer and Analysis. Section 1: Data Transfer to the MONICA Data Centre. Available from URL: http://www.ktl.fi/publications/monica/manual/part5/v-1.htm, URN:*NBN:fi-fe19981160*. MONICA Web Publication 1.
2. The MONICA Quality assessment reports are available at http://www.ktl.fi/publications/monica/index.htm. MONICA Web Publications 2–18.

Esa Ruokokoski, Markku Mähönen

#37 Event Rates, Case Fatality and Trends

Event rates

- rates involve a numerator, a denominator, and a time period
- denominator for event or mortality rates is the general population
- denominator for case fatality is cases of disease (here coronary or stroke events)
- comparison of groups with different age composition is aided by age standardization

Several different event rates were used in MONICA. Before describing them it is necessary to explain briefly, for the uninitiated, what is meant by an 'event rate' in general. More events are likely to happen in a big population over a long time interval than in a small one over a short period. In order to compare two populations and discount these differences, we standardize the time interval, most frequently to one year, and compensate for differences in size by expressing the rate against a common convenient number, such as rate per 100 000. Many registration staff in MONICA spent their time registering coronary and stroke events as accurately as they could (*1, 2*). These were the numerators for event rates. They might not have realized that accurate denominators, population numbers, are essential for the accurate calculation of event rates (*3*). This is why the annual demographic data were so important, as changes in numbers of events year by year could result from real changes in disease rates, or simply from changes in population size (See #17 *Demographic data*). Disease rates are very strongly related to age. Standardization of disease rates to rate per 100 000 per year does not overcome the problem of differing age structures in different populations. This is overcome by age standardization (See #39 *Age Standardization*).

Event rates used in MONICA were:

- attack rates based on all defined events both fatal and non-fatal
- non-fatal event rates
- MONICA fatal event rates (also known as MONICA CHD or stroke mortality rates)
- official mortality rates based on routine death certification
- first event rates for coronary or stroke events in subjects without a previous event.

All these event rates used the same population denominators. In the case of first event rates this is arguable because the true denominator, those without a previous history, was not known. This quibble would not have made a big difference to the result.

Case fatality

For both coronary and stroke events, survival status was determined at 28 days from the onset of the event:

If (Date of death)-(Date of onset) < 28 the event was fatal, if 28 or more non-fatal

Case fatality, unless otherwise qualified, was defined at 28 days and reported as the percentage of events that were fatal within this period. Case fatality varies with age and therefore with the age composition of the groups being considered. To standardize for age when analysing case fatality we used our own weightings, see #39 *Age Standardization*. Case fatality was split up into different components in particular MONICA publications, such as pre-hospital, hospital-related, 24-h and post 24-h (*4–6*).

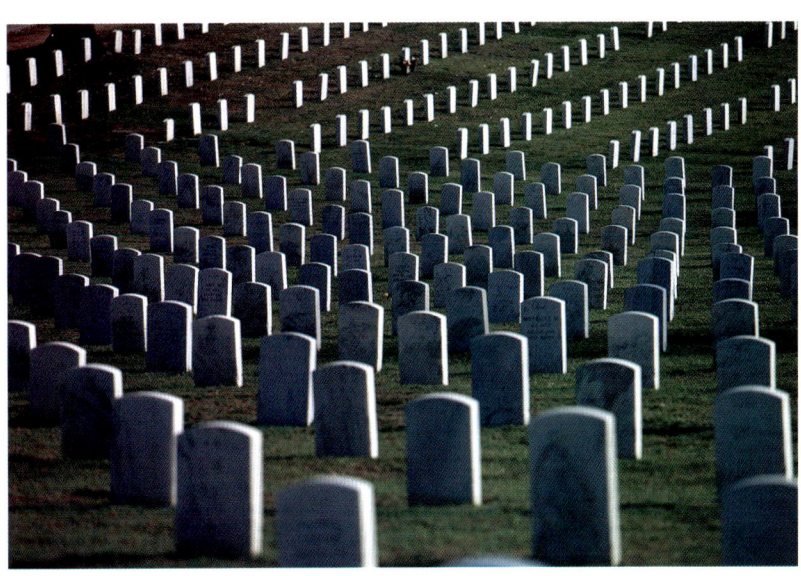

Coronaries and strokes can be 40% of all deaths

Trends in event rates and case fatality

Graphics G14 and G27 show that event rates did not usually change in a uniform manner for any population over the years, but trends had to be summarized somehow. The mathematical assumption for rates was that they changed by a constant proportion over time, rather than a constant amount, so the model is log-linear rather than linear (that is like compound interest). For the purpose of summarizing case fatality, it was also assumed that any change was log-linear over time. Case fatality did not vary very greatly between populations whereas event rates varied five-fold. It should be recognized that our mathematical summary model would place two populations side by side in the rankings if their event rates both fell by forty percent, even if the starting rates were very different (*7*).

References
MONICA Web Publications are also accessible on the Monograph CD-ROM

1. Mähönen M, Tolonen H, Kuulasmaa K, Tunstall-Pedoe H, Amouyel P, for the WHO MONICA Project. Quality assessment of coronary event registration data in the WHO MONICA Project. (January 1999). Available from URL: http://www.ktl.fi/publications/monica/coreqa/coreqa.htm, URN:*NBN:fi-fe19991072*. MONICA Web Publication 2.

2. Mähönen M, Tolonen H, Kuulasmaa K, for the WHO MONICA Project. Quality assessment of stroke event registration data in the WHO MONICA Project. (November 1998). Available from URL: http://www.ktl.fi/publications/monica/strokeqa/strokeqa.htm, URN:*NBN:fi-fe19991080*. MONICA Web Publication 5.

3. Moltchanov V, Kuulasmaa K, Torppa J, for the WHO MONICA Project. Quality assessment of demographic data in the WHO MONICA Project. (April 1999). Available from URL: http://www.ktl.fi/publications/monica/demoqa/demoqa.htm, URN:*NBN:fi-fe19991073*. MONICA Web Publication 3.

4. Mähönen M, Tunstall-Pedoe H, Rajakangas AM, Cepaitis Z, Kuulasmaa K, Dobson A, Keil U, for the WHO MONICA Project. Definitions of case fatality for coronary events in the WHO MONICA Project. (February 2000). Available from URL: http://www.ktl.fi/publications/monica/carpfish/appendd/cfdef.htm, URN:*NBN:fi-fe976570*. MONICA Web Publication 24.

5. Chambless L, Keil U, Dobson A, Mähönen M, Kuulasmaa K, Rajakangas AM, Lowel H, Tunstall-Pedoe H, for the WHO MONICA Project. Population versus clinical view of case fatality from acute coronary heart disease: results from the WHO MONICA Project 1985–1990. *Circulation*, 1997, 96:3849–3859. PMID: 9403607. MONICA Publication 29.

6. Tunstall-Pedoe H, Vanuzzo D, Hobbs M, Mähönen M, Cepaitis Z, Kuulasmaa K, Keil U, for the WHO MONICA Project. Estimation of contribution of changes in coronary care to improving survival, event rates, and coronary heart disease mortality across the WHO MONICA Project populations. *Lancet*, 2000, 355:688–700. PMID: 10703800. MONICA Publication 39.

7. Tunstall-Pedoe H, Kuulasmaa K, Mähönen M, Tolonen H, Ruokokoski E, Amouyel P, for the WHO MONICA Project. Contribution of trends in survival and coronary-event rates to changes in coronary heart disease mortality: 10-year results from 37 WHO MONICA project populations. *Lancet*, 1999, 353:1547–1557. PMID: 10334252. MONICA Publication 36.

Hugh Tunstall-Pedoe

#38 Population Prevalence and Trends

Survey data

Risk-factor surveys produce data on continuous variables like blood pressure and weight, and categorical variables like smoking status. We can also categorize continuous variables using cut-off points. When reporting survey results, different types of variables require different presentations.

- mean levels of systolic blood pressure, total cholesterol and BMI in the population
- proportions of daily smokers in the populations
- changes in risk-factor levels over time

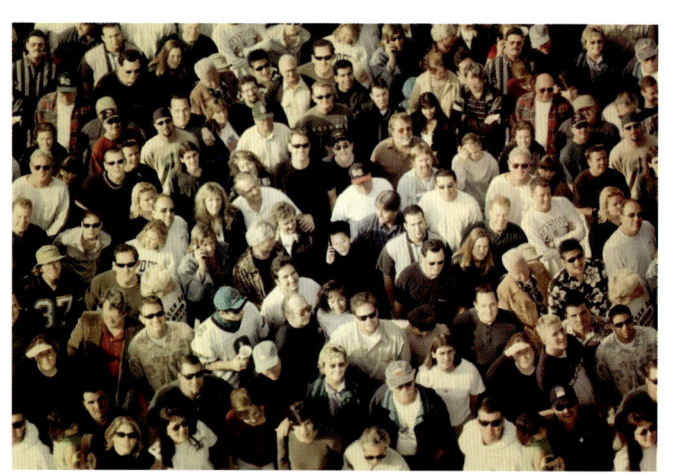

Prevalence

The prevalence of a risk factor—the proportion of survey respondents having a defined condition—such as hypertension, is used to present results for categorized variables. See for example graphics G36 and G37 for the prevalence of daily cigarette smoking. The formula for calculating age-standardized prevalence rates is given in the MONICA Population Survey Data Book (*1*).

Population mean

The mean is used to describe the level of a continuous variable, such as systolic blood pressure, in the population. See for example graphics G40 and G41 for the mean systolic blood pressure. The formula for calculating the age-standardized population mean is also given in the MONICA Population Survey Data Book (*1*).

What proportion smoke—what is the average blood pressure?

Trends

The prevalences and means are used to describe cross-sectional results. When we have several surveys in the same population, separated in time, we can see the changes in the prevalences and mean values over time. See for example graphic G46 for the 10-year trend in total cholesterol. The trends were calculated from the pooled data from two or three surveys using linear regression analysis, with the persons' dates of examination as the explanatory variable (*2*).

References
MONICA Web Publications are also accessible on the Monograph CD-ROM

1. Tolonen H, Kuulasmaa K, Ruokokoski E, for the WHO MONICA Project. MONICA population survey data book. (October 2000). Available from URL: http://www.ktl.fi/publications/monica/surveydb/title.htm, URN:*NBN:fi-fe20001206*. MONICA Web Publication 27.
2. Kuulasmaa K, Dobson A, for the WHO MONICA Project. Statistical issues related to following populations rather than individuals over time. *Bulletin of the International Statistical Institute*: *Proceedings of the 51st Session*, *1997 Aug 18–26, Istanbul, Turkey*, Voorburg: International Statistical Institute, 1997, Book 1:295–298. Also available from URL: http://www.ktl.fi/publications/monica/isi97/isi97.htm. PMID: nil. MONICA Publication 28.

Hanna Tolonen

#39 Age Standardization

Why do we need to standardize for age?

Young people have much lower cardiovascular disease (CVD) event rates than older people. Therefore, crude event rates calculated simply from numbers of events and the size of the population depend strongly on the proportions of people of different ages in the population. If age-specific event rates are the same in two populations, but their age composition differs, then crude event rates will also be different—misleading if the true explanation is overlooked. A similar problem arises when using crude event rates to follow a population over time—change may reflect that in age-composition of the population rather than change in rates within specific age groups.

Therefore age standardization is used to enable comparisons of event rates to be made between different populations, or the same population over time, by removing the confounding effect of differences or changes in the age distribution.

The risk factors measured in MONICA: blood pressure, total cholesterol, smoking and BMI also vary between age groups. Therefore, age standardization is also used to adjust the prevalences and mean values of the risk factors, when wide age ranges are used for comparison between populations, or for following trends.

Age standardization is important when summary results are shown for wide age groups. However, because age standardization produces a summary value that conceals the effect of age, it may also conceal important differences with age within and between groups. Age-specific results still need to be examined. For the main MONICA publications results have usually been standardized for the 35–64 age group, but in some data books results are also given by 10-year age groups.

- age standardization facilitates comparison of groups of differing age composition
- a world standard population was used in MONICA for event rates and risk-factor prevalence, but a different standard for case fatality

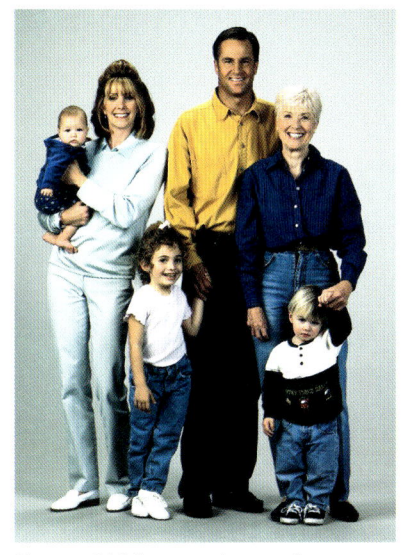

Disease and risk factors vary by age and sex

How to standardize for age

Simple (direct) age standardization is done by:

- first   partition the population into narrow age groups
- next   calculate the event rates, prevalences or mean values within each of them
- finally   take a weighted mean of these values using a 'standard' weighting (*1*).

The result is that rates are re-calculated as if they had arisen from populations with the same 'standard' age-composition.

It is important for the comparability of the results that the same weights are used for all populations throughout the study. The weights are often chosen in such a way that they reflect the age distribution of the average or total study population.

Weights for event rates, population prevalences and mean values

The natural choices for the age standardization weights for the MONICA Project were the nominal (and now historical) 'World population' or the 'European population', two standard or reference populations defined previously and used in cancer epidemiology and by WHO in the *World Health Statistics Annual (2)*. These standard populations were compared with the composition of MONICA populations in the early 1980s. In the 25–64 year age group, the age distribution of the pooled MONICA population was reasonably close to that of both standard populations, although this was not true for all MONICA populations in some of whom the influence of the Second World War was still visible. Many European populations were closer to the World than to the European population, and because MONICA was global, the 'World population' was adopted as the standard or reference population for MONICA. Its weights in the 35–64 age group were:

Age group	35–39	40–44	45–49	50–54	55–59	60–64
Weight	6	6	6	5	4	4

(which means results for each age group are multiplied by the stated factor, results are added together and then divided by 31).

For risk factors, where the variation with age was smaller than in event rates, 10-year age groups were used for age standardization. More details of age standardization of event rates, prevalences and mean values in MONICA can be found in the Data Books (3, 4). Trends in event rates were calculated from age-standardized annual rates. Trends in risk factors were calculated separately for each 10-year age group, and then age-standardized by taking a weighted mean of the trends in the 10-year age groups.

Weights for case fatality

Case fatality in MONICA is the 28-day (or other short-term) death rate percent in those who have had a coronary or stroke event, rather than in the general population. Inevitably older age groups predominate. In order to reflect this the weights for age-standardizing case fatality were taken from the age distribution of coronary and stroke events in pooled MONICA data (5):

Age group	35–44	45–54	55–64
Weight	1	3	7

(which means results for each age group are multiplied by the stated factor, results are added together, and then divided by 11).

References
MONICA Web Publications are also accessible on the Monograph CD ROM

1. Armitage P, Berry G. *Statistical methods in Medical Research*, 2nd ed. Oxford, Blackwell Scientific Publications, 1987.
2. Waterhouse J, Muir CS, Correa P, Powell J, eds. *Cancer incidence in five continents*, Lyon, IARC, 1976 (Vol. 3, pl 456).
3. Mähönen M, Tolonen H, Kuulasmaa K, for the WHO MONICA Project. MONICA Coronary event registration data book 1980–1995. (October 2000). Available from URL: http://www.ktl.fi/publications/monica/coredb/coredb.htm, URN:*NBN:fi-fe20001204*. MONICA Web Publication 25.
4. Tolonen H, Kuulasmaa K, Ruokokoski E, for the WHO MONICA Project. MONICA population survey data book. (October 2000). Available from URL: http://www.ktl.fi/publications/monica/surveydb/title.htm, URN:*NBN:fi-fe20001206*. MONICA Web Publication 27.
5. Tunstall-Pedoe H, Kuulasmaa K, Amouyel P, Arveiler D, Rajakangas AM, Pajak A, for the WHO MONICA Project Myocardial infarction and coronary deaths in the World Health Organization MONICA Project. Registration procedures, event rates, and case-fatality rates in 38 populations from 21 countries in four continents. *Circulation*, 1994, 90:583–612. PMID: 8026046. MONICA Publication 16.

Hanna Tolonen

#40 Statistical Analysis
—relating changes in risk factors and treatment to changes in event rates

Populations versus individuals

MONICA was designed to answer questions for populations rather than individuals, see #2 *MONICA Hypotheses and Study Design* (*1*). This means that the number used for statistical analysis consisted of fewer than 40 populations rather than the many millions of people within those populations. With such a 'small' study it is difficult to obtain unequivocal answers. Furthermore, the large amount of variation between people within each population means that trends in populations cannot be estimated very reliably.

Statistical variation

The challenge for MONICA was to reduce variability as much as possible and then to estimate both within-population and between-population variability carefully. Rigorous training of research staff in standard measurement techniques and an obsessive level of quality assessment were used to reduce both systematic and random variations in data about individual people within populations. Standardized methodology set out in the MONICA Manual (*1*) was used to minimize differences in measurements between study populations.

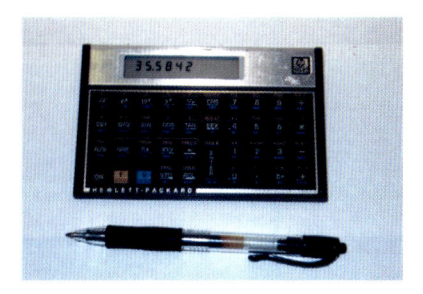

Estimating changes in populations

Linear regression was used to estimate the average annual (or average 10-year) change in each risk factor or risk score in a population, see #38 *Population Prevalence and Trends*. Variations from year to year over the 10 years of the study meant that it would not have been possible to estimate reliably any non-linear effects. Changes in event rates, case fatality and types of treatment in each population over 10 years were similarly calculated (in the former cases using a log-linear model, see #37 *Event Rates, Case Fatality and Trends*). Age standardization was used to take account of differences in age structure between populations, see #39 *Age Standardization*. For each estimate of change in the population we also calculated a standard error that reflected the precision of the estimate.

Relating changes in populations

To calculate the magnitude of the effects of population changes in risk-factor levels and treatment on population changes in event rates, we used linear regression and correlation, taking into account the variability in all the estimates. As standard statistical theory does not apply to this situation, we had to develop new methods (*2–4*). In the main analyses we also weighted the data according to quality scores for each variable and considered the time lag between changes in risk factors and outcomes (*5–8*).

What is now known from MONICA?

Predictably from a study with so few 'subjects' (i.e. populations) the final results had wide confidence intervals. Also the proportion of the variation in population changes in event rates 'explained' by population changes in risk factor and treatment levels varied. Nevertheless the MONICA findings for populations are consistent with results for individuals and they support population-level approaches to the control of cardiovascular disease.

- MONICA used standard statistical procedures for many analyses
- in hypothesis testing it developed techniques which allowed for precision and quality scores of data items

Hypothesis testing was beyond basic calculator statistics

References
MONICA Web Publications are also accessible on the Monograph CD-ROM

1. WHO MONICA Project. MONICA Manual. (1998–1999). Available from URL: http://www.ktl.fi/publications/monica/manual/index.htm, URN:*NBN:fi-fe19981146*. MONICA Web Publication 1.

2. Kuulasmaa K, Dobson A, for the WHO MONICA Project. Statistical issues related to following populations rather than individuals over time. *Bulletin of the International Statistical Institute: Proceedings of the 51st Session, 1997 Aug 18–26, Istanbul, Turkey*, Voorburg: International Statistical Institute, 1997, Book 1; 295–298. Also available from URL: http://www.ktl.fi/publications/monica/isi97/isi97.htm. PMID: nil. MONICA Publication 28.

3. Dobson A, Filipiak B, Kuulasmaa K, Beaglehole R, Stewart A, Hobbs M, Parsons R, Keil U, Greiser E, Korhonen H, Tuomilehto J. Relations of changes in coronary disease rates and changes in risk factor levels: methodological issues and a practical example. *American Journal of Epidemiology*, 1996, 143:1025–1034. PMID: 8629609. MONICA Publication 22.

4. Dear KBG, Puterman ML, Dobson AJ. Estimating correlations from epidemiological data in the presence of measurement error. *Statistics in Medicine*, 1997, 16:2177–2189. PMID: 9330427

5. Kuulasmaa K, Tunstall-Pedoe H, Dobson A, Fortmann S, Sans S, Tolonen H, Evans A, Ferrario M, Tuomilehto J, for the WHO MONICA Project. Estimation of contribution of changes in classic risk factors to trends in coronary-event rates across the WHO MONICA Project populations. *Lancet*, 2000, 355:675–687. PMID: 10703799. MONICA Publication 38.

6. Tunstall-Pedoe H, Vanuzzo D, Hobbs M, Mähänen M, Cepaitis Z, Kuulasmaa K, Keil U, for the WHO MONICA Project. Estimation of contribution of changes in coronary care to improving survival, event rates, and coronary heart disease mortality across the WHO MONICA Project populations. *Lancet*, 2000, 355:688–700. PMID: 10703800. MONICA Publication 39.

7. Kuulasmaa K, Dobson A, Tunstall-Pedoe H, Fortmann S, Sans S, Tolonen H, Evans A, Ferrario M, Tuomilehto J, for the WHO MONICA Project. Estimation of contribution of changes in classical risk factors to trends in coronary-event rates across the WHO MONICA Project populations: methodological appendix to a paper published in the *Lancet*. (February 2000). Available from URL: http://www.ktl.fi/publications/monica/earwig/appendix.htm, URN:*NBN:fi-fe19991356*. MONICA Web Publication 20.

8. Tunstall-Pedoe H, Mähänen M, Cepaitis Z, Kuulasmaa K, Vanuzzo D, Hobbs M, Keil U, for the WHO MONICA Project. Derivation of an acute coronary care quality score for the WHO MONICA Project. (February 2000). Available from URL: http://www.ktl.fi/publications/monica/carpfish/appendc/accqscore.htm, URN:*NBN:fi-fe976569*. MONICA Web Publication 23.

Annette Dobson

#41 Preparation of Manuscripts and Presentations

- a protracted process to produce a quality product

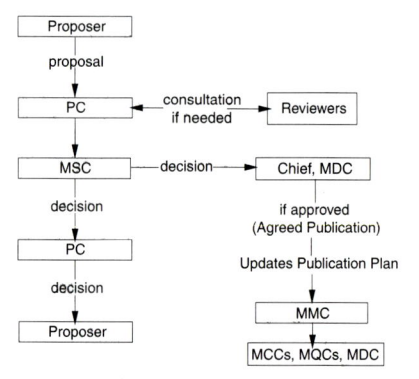

From manuscript proposal to approval

The MONICA Project has published 45 collaborative papers in scientific journals (December 2002) and several others are in preparation. An additional 30 publications, many reporting and commenting on the quality of MONICA data, others methodological, are published on the MONICA Website. The number of articles published by individual MONICA centres (or from collaborations between small numbers of centres) is not easy to estimate but runs into many hundreds if not a thousand or more.

To write an article on data from a multinational study like MONICA is a major undertaking. Different scientific cultures and personalities come together to produce a common product. All participating centres must accept that their data have been used and interpreted correctly and must give their approval.

In the past this has required a firm structure for producing MONICA publications. A set of publication rules was established (*1*). One of the members of the MONICA Steering Committee has served as Publications Coordinator, encouraging authors and ensuring that they adhere to the publication rules that the MONICA collaborators have adopted. The figures illustrate (in an abbreviated form) the long route from the original idea for writing an article to the final submission to a scientific journal.

The preparation and approval of an oral presentation of MONICA data at a scientific meeting has followed a similar, although simplified, procedure.

The strict MONICA publication rules have sometimes been cumbersome. There can be considerable delays at various stages leading up to the final manuscript. Nevertheless, the MONICA publication structure has had several strengths:

- only important scientific questions are dealt with
- articles are written by leading experts in cardiovascular epidemiology
- articles are written in an exciting multinational atmosphere
- very thorough quality checks are made of the data
- the tight review process ensures high quality of the final product.

To keep track of all articles that have been proposed and to monitor their progress, the MONICA Data Centre in Helsinki has maintained a database of all proposed articles, their manuscript groups and their status from Step1 (approved but not yet started) to Step 7 (published).

MONICA Publication rules have undergone some changes over the years. Initially authorship of papers was attributed to 'WHO MONICA Project' with the group that prepared it appearing as a footnote on the title page. Next, the group responsible for preparing the publication appeared after the Project name on the authorship line—although those citing the papers tended to leave the names off. More recently, in recognition of the considerable effort required by authors to work on collaborative papers, and in response to journal editors who increasingly want named people to be answerable for papers, even those from large studies, the authors have been named first 'x, y, z, for the WHO MONICA Project' and that is how the MONICA family now wants its papers to be cited. MONICA's authorship rules have not always been followed by journals—some have had to publish corrections to their own ill-advised corrections. (See #85 and #86 *MONICA Publication List/Abstracts of Publications*.) Publication rules are likely to be modified further in the future as access to the MONICA database is progressively relaxed and outsiders are encouraged to participate.

From manuscript to publication

The MONICA Steering Committee and MONICA Data Centre have always been on the lookout for those ready to work on MONICA collaborative papers, hoping that the MONICA Collaborating Centres contained would-be authors who were underoccupied. Experience has shown however that the best identifier of a potential MONICA author is somebody who is already writing papers locally for major international journals. Considerable knowledge of the Project and persistence is needed to lead a major paper. These are seldom completed in one short-term burst of enthusiasm. Despite that, authorship of MONICA collaborative articles is widespread. There are approximately 70 authors from 16 or more countries, thereby participating in MONICA's objective of 'multinational monitoring' (2).

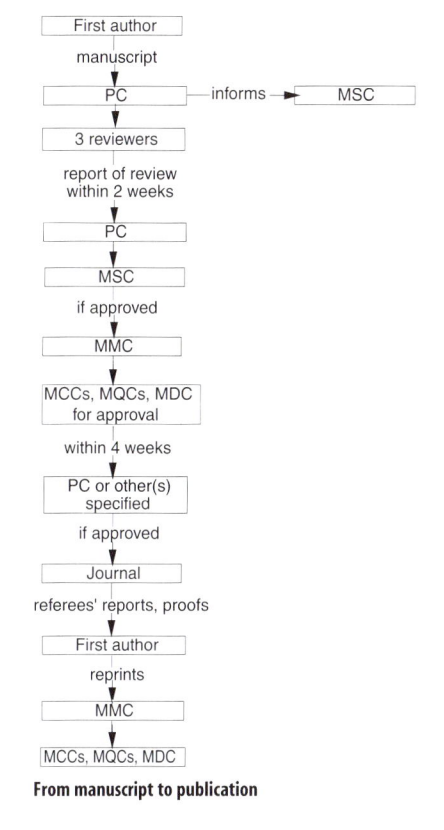

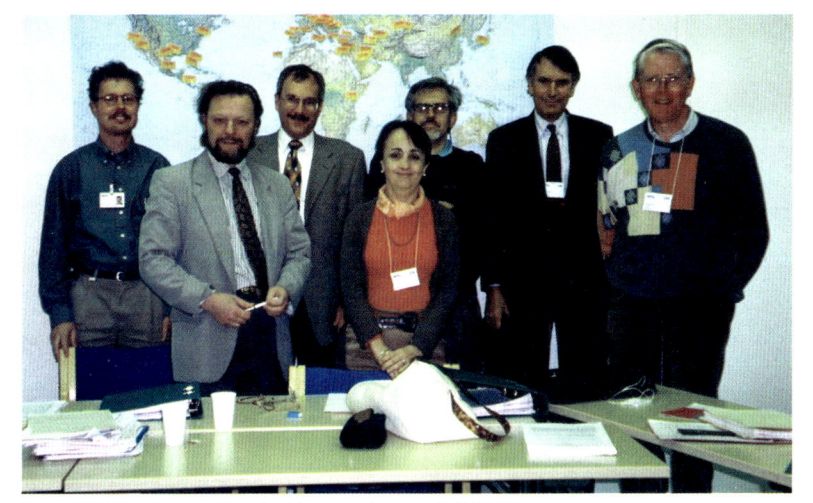

The EARWIG (First Coronary Hypothesis) manuscript group in Helsinki

References
MONICA Web Publications are also accessible on the Monograph CD-ROM

1. WHO MONICA Project. MONICA Manual. (1998–1999). Part I: Description and Organization of the Project. Section 2: Organization and Management of the WHO MONICA Project. Available from URL: http://www.ktl.fi/publications/monica/manual/part1/ i-2.htm#s7, URN:NBN:fi-fe19981148. MONICA Web Publication 1. See Paragraph 7: Publication rules.
2. MONICA Collaborative Publications, available on the Website: http://www.ktl.fi/monica/public/publications.htm, also on Monograph CD-ROM and See #85 and #86.

Kjell Asplund

#42 Making Graphics for MONICA

- MONICA developed its own house-styles for displaying multi-centre results
- these are demonstrated in the graphics pages of this Monograph

Presenting results from a multi-centre study

In MONICA, each Reporting Unit Aggregate (RUA) is considered as one independent population. When preparing a presentation or publication from collaborative MONICA data there can be over 30 RUAs in one presentation or publication. Presenting results from these populations in an easily readable and understandable format is not easy. It is difficult enough to present results for a single population independently—much more difficult to show comparisons and relations between 30 or more different ones.

One figure tells more than 1000 words

Multi-centre results can always be put into a table, listing populations and their results. When the number of populations increases, the size of the table also increases. Big tables like this require a huge effort from the reader. It is not easy to make out the difference between populations and their results from a table in small print with many different rows and columns and hundreds of cells.

Figures are a good way to present results of any study. From a figure, the general pattern is seen and comparisons between groups or populations are much easier to understand than from tables. But figures too can be confusing if they are not well prepared and too many different things are included.

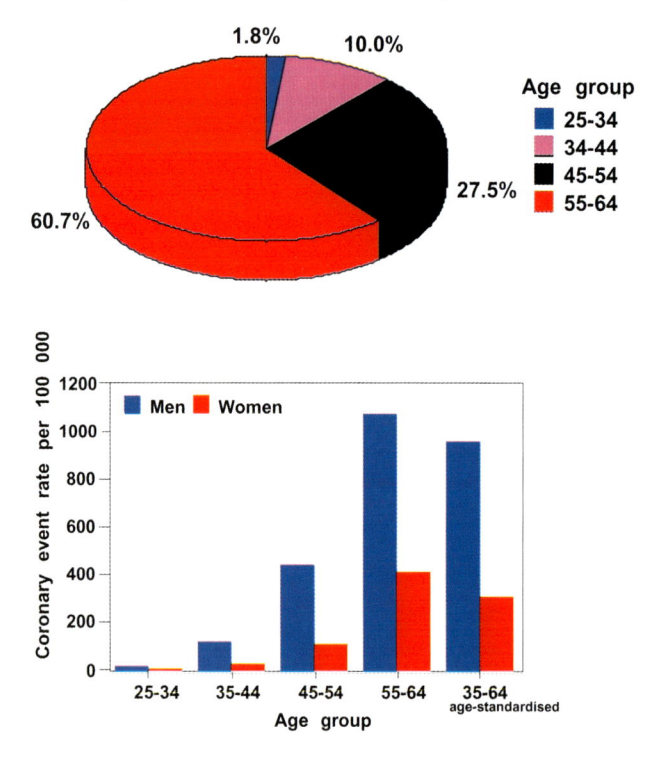

Figure 1. Results from one population

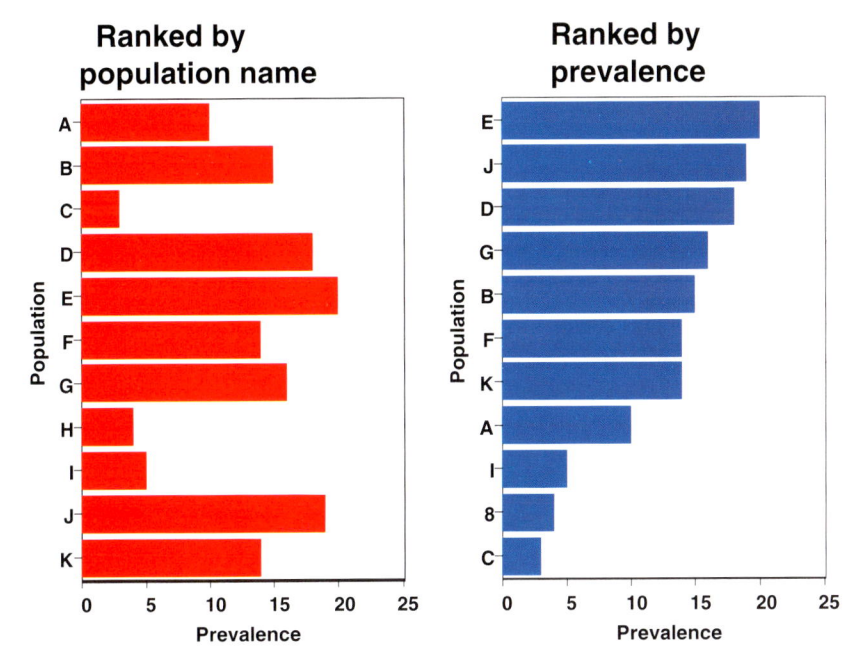

Figure 2. Results from several populations in two formats

Limitations of graphics from a multi-centre study

When presenting results from one population, the sexes and/or age groups can easily be compared using only one figure (Figure 1). Putting 30 populations in one figure won't allow the comparison of age groups or sexes in the same figure.

Formats for graphical presentations in MONICA

Comparing graphically, for example, the event rates, smoking prevalence, average systolic blood pressure, trends in obesity, or any other results from the 30+ MONICA populations we always followed the same general rules:

- results are for the 35–64 year age group
- age-standardized
- men and women presented separately in their own figures
- but often results by sex are placed side by side, or vertically on the same page to allow comparison.

To allow the reader to assess the difference between prevalences and changes in populations, the populations are usually ranked according to the prevalence or the change. Listing by population name makes it easier to identify specific populations but the difference between populations and how they compare is less clear. See Figure 2. Also compare the risk-factor graphics G36–G56 with those for coronary care, G57–G67.

Hanna Tolonen

MONICA Optional Studies

#43 Optional Studies—Beyond the Core

See #9 *MONICA Reference Centres (MRCs)* for further information

Core versus optional

When MONICA was launched it had the ambitious objective 'to assess the extent to which trends in cardiovascular disease . . . are related to changes in known risk factors, daily living habits, health care, or major socioeconomic features . . .'. It then qualified this with 'Collaborating centres will wish to cover all these areas, but the basic protocol covers key items only, leaving the rest as local options'. This ambitious manifesto, tempered by alarm as to what it might involve, and rapid compromise, demonstrates the dilemma posed by MONICA. Key items, subsequently labelled core items, were fundamental to the MONICA hypotheses. For these, there were standard protocols and methods of measurement that were usable by all participating centres. There were other factors for which standard, cross-cultural protocols and procedures were not available, or would be too expensive for general use. Collecting core data items for ten years or so was a formidable challenge, even without adding others. However, if we stopped at core items, there was a risk that the study would be criticized for being traditional and boring. It would lack spice and excitement if others were not added. Yet adding in costly, unproven and non-standardized factors would detract from the core, perhaps even affecting its quality, and would inhibit widespread participation. (*1*)

- interchange between core and optional items
- interchange between local options and collaborative options
- MONICA 'add-on' studies have done much good work

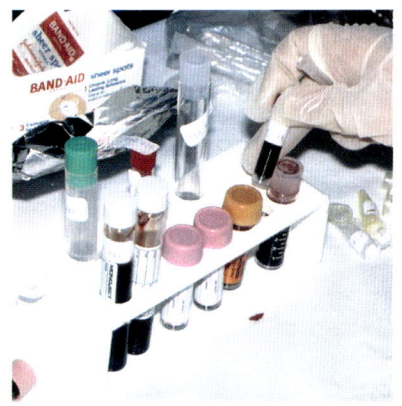

Blood contains more than cholesterol

Interchange between core and optional

Local investigators were free to add additional questions or data items to their registration or population survey records. 'Local options' were of no concern to the MONICA Project as such, so that it was core items alone that were forwarded to the Data Centre in Helsinki. However, some items considered 'optional' at the start were subsequently added late as 'core items' to the registration and survey record forms, in particular questions relating to new coronary care drugs, additional questions on smoking and passive smoking, but also waist and hip circumference. There was also a tendency to go the other way if there were problems. This was true of serum thiocyanate and HDL-cholesterol, neither of which was fundamental to the MONICA hypotheses, nor actually core items, but for which protocols, procedures and data formats were specified at the start. Subsequent analysis of the data (thiocyanate), and quality control performance (HDL-cholesterol) showed that results should not be used for cross-sectional and longitudinal trends within MONICA centres as a whole, although they were potentially usable locally (*2–4*). Although psychosocial studies were generally considered optional, data items on marital and educational status were 'core', and analysed as such in a MONICA Quality assessment report (*5*).

Problems of collaboration in optional studies

Where there was sufficient interest in a particular option, MONICA investigators were encouraged to develop common methods and data sets for voluntary collaboration within MONICA. This applied particularly to some areas considered fundamental to coronary disease—diet, exercise and psychosocial factors. Launched later than the core study, and usually unable therefore to generate anything more than cross-sectional data, the MONICA optional studies were not given the attention or resources of core items, unless external funding was found. It needed an enthusiastic well-resourced coordinator to make an optional study succeed. Coordinators of topics such as drugs, diet, and physical activity changed at least once during MONICA, whereas psychosocial studies were subdivided.

Publication lists from individual populations record the variety of local options that were added by individual investigators, as will a bibliographic search of the literature for the newer risk factors. Some investigators published independent studies of risk factors (for example diet, vitamins) that colleagues elsewhere pursued in MONICA collaborative optional studies. Some centres concentrated on the core protocol. Some gave this less attention than other items that could be added in, particularly to population surveys. Many optional studies involved interdisciplinary and interdepartmental collaborations. The number of publications arising from multi-centre collaboration in optional studies is small compared with the number of single centre publications in the same areas. Heavy commitment of time, resources and funding to the core study, lack of involvement of the MONICA Data Centre, lack of time at Principal Investigators Meetings, all made the MONICA collaborative optional studies the Cinderella of MONICA. Yet paradoxically, MONICA investigators, usually using the MONICA framework, are major contributors to the literature on newer non-classic risk factors.

The following sections, #44–#49, are devoted to brief accounts of some of the MONICA optional studies. Individual investigators describe their local options in their own population pages and among their publications, or on their websites. See #51–#83.

References
MONICA Web Publications are also accessible on the Monograph CD-ROM

1. WHO MONICA Project. MONICA Manual. (1998–1999). Part I: Description and Organization of the Project. Section 1: Objectives and Outline Protocol. Available from URL: http://www.ktl.fi/publications/monica/manual/part1/I-1.htm, URN:*NBN:fi-fe19981147*. MONICA Web Publication 1.

2. WHO MONICA Project. MONICA Manual. (1998–1999). Part III: Population Survey. Section 2: Standardization of lipid measurements. Available from URL: http://www.ktl.fi/publications/monica/manual/part3/iii-2.htm, URN:*NBN:fi-fe19981152*. MONICA Web Publication 1.

3. WHO MONICA Project. MONICA Manual. (1998–1999). Part III: Population Survey. Section 3: Standardization of thiocyanate measurements. Available from URL: http://www.ktl.fi/publications/monica/manual/part3/iii-3.htm, URN:*NBN:fi-fe19981153*. MONICA Web Publication 1.

4. Marques-Vidal P, Ferrario M, Kuulasmaa K, Grafnetter D, Moltchanov V, for the WHO MONICA Project. Quality assessment of data on HDL cholesterol in the WHO MONICA Project. (June 1999). Available from URL: http://www.ktl.fi/publications/monica/hdl/hdlqa.htm, URN:*NBN:fi-fe19991137*. MONICA Web Publication 11.

5. Molarius A, Kuulasmaa K, Moltchanov V, Ferrario M, for the WHO MONICA Project. Quality assessment of data on marital status and educational achievement in the WHO MONICA Project. (December 1998). Available from URL: http://www.ktl.fi/publications/monica/educ/educqa.htm, URN:*NBN:fi-fe19991078*. MONICA Web Publication 14.

Hugh Tunstall-Pedoe

#44 MONICA Optional Study on Nutrition

See #9 *MONICA Reference Centres (MRCs)* for further information

The collection of dietary data was optional in the MONICA project. Between 1982 and 1985 several meetings were held to discuss what dietary survey method should be used (*1*). The three-day record was selected as the preferred method. Between 1982 and 1989 dietary survey data were collected using either three or seven-day records in nine European MONICA centres. This survey was later carried out between 1994 and 1996 by seven centres. In total about 7000 men aged 45–64 participated in the different surveys. Guy de Backer, University of Ghent, Belgium coordinated the optional study on nutrition until 1994. In 1995 that responsibility was transferred to Daan Kromhout, RIVM, Bilthoven, The Netherlands.

The aim of the dietary surveys was to study trends in diet in relation to trends in cardiovascular (CVD) morbidity and mortality. Complete data are available from only six centres. It is therefore not possible to study associations between trends in diet and trends in CVD morbidity and mortality at the population level. The available data will be used to describe changes in dietary pattern during a 10-year period and to study prospectively diet-CVD relationships in about 5000 men aged 45–64 at baseline and followed up for CVD morbidity and mortality since 1982–1989. The dietary record data collected in the Caerphilly Study in the period 1979–1983 were added to the data collected by the nine MONICA centres surveyed in that period. The emphasis in data analysis will be on fish and plant foods and on fatty acids and antioxidants in relation to CVD occurrence.

In the period 1995–1999 an inventory was made about the way dietary data were collected, coded and transformed from foods to nutrients in the different MONICA centres. A database was prepared that presented dietary data in a standardized way. In addition, two grant proposals were prepared for the European Union, one in the context of the FAIR Programme and another one for the 5th Framework Programme. Neither proposal was funded. Two nutritional epidemiologists worked on the database in the period 1995–1999. A post-doctoral researcher worked on preparation of the database during 2002. Thereafter data analysis can start.

- nutritional intake is difficult and expensive to measure
- national and cultural differences make standardized measurements difficult to achieve

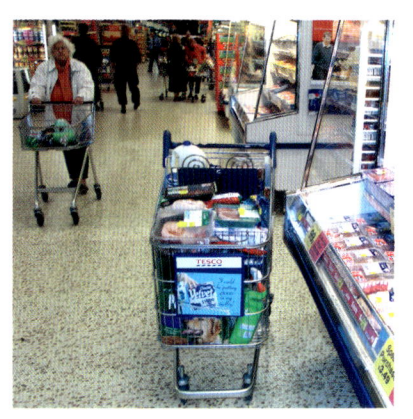

People change what they eat

Reference
Haveman-Nies A, Bokje E,Ocké M, Kromhout D. MONICA Optional Study on Nutrition: the dietary assessment methodology. RIVM report 261753001/2002. Available from URL: http://www.rivm.nl//bibliotheek/rapporten/261753001.pdf.

Daan Kromhout

#45 MONICA Optional Study on Antioxidant Vitamins and Polyunsaturated Fatty Acids (PUFA)

See #9 *MONICA Reference Centres (MRCs)* for further information

The vitamin-antioxidant hypothesis became the subject of intense interest shortly after MONICA was launched. One of the champions of this hypothesis was Fred Gey who lobbied for MONICA participation in a study organized from his base in the laboratory of a Swiss drug company (Hoffmann-La Roche). This company provided funding for recruitment of subjects, specimen collection, storage and transfer of specimens, laboratory assay and data analysis. This

- the vitamin-antioxidant hypothesis became prominent during MONICA
- centrally funded, this study produced results and publications

substudy produced results and publications (*1, 2*). Coordination of vitamin studies was transferred to the University of Bern when Fred Gey moved there. On his retirement from there it was transferred to the Belfast Centre for work on other analytes from the original specimens.

References
1. Gey KF, Stahelin HB, Puska P, Evans AE. Relationship of plasma level of vitamin C to mortality from ischemic heart disease. *Annals of the New York Academy of Sciences*, 1987, 498:110–123. PMID: 3497600.
2. Gey KF, Puska P. Plasma vitamins E and A inversely correlated to mortality from ischaemic heart disease in cross-cultural epidemiology. *Annals of the New York Academy of Sciences*, 1989, 570:268–282. PMID: 2629597.

Hugh Tunstall-Pedoe

#46 MONICA Optional Psychosocial Substudy (MOPSY)

See #9 *MONICA Reference Centres (MRCs)* for further information

Aims
The aims of the MONICA Psychosocial study were:

- to clarify the relationship between 10-year trends in certain psychosocial factors and corresponding trends in the incidence of cardiovascular disease, in order to provide estimates of the relative importance of psychosocial risk factors and standard risk factors in predicting and controlling cardiovascular disease in populations
- to foster cooperation for the development of a battery of standardized, internationally comparable methods for the assessment of psychosocial factors related to health.

Psychosocial variables under study
In addition to the core MONICA data, the centres participating in the MONICA Psychosocial Study were also obtaining information for the defined populations under study on the following psychosocial variables:

- type A coronary-prone behaviour pattern
- health knowledge and attitudes
- work characteristics
- life stress (life events)
- vital exhaustion and sleep disturbances
- other psychological variables
- social support
- socioeconomic characteristics on an aggregated level
- social and geographical mobility.

Hypotheses to be tested
The central null hypotheses to be tested were parallel to those of the core MONICA project:

1. For the participating centres there is no relationship between changes in psychosocial risk factors and changes in the incidence of coronary heart disease (CHD) (fatal plus non-fatal cases) over a 10-year period.

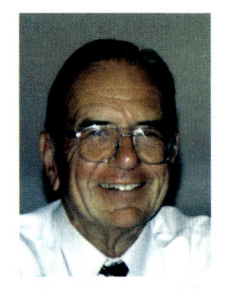

Fred Gey promoted the vitamin-antioxidant hypothesis

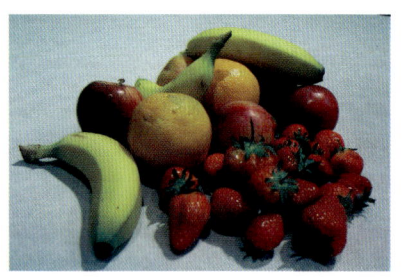

How do fruit and vegetables help the heart?

- coordinated from the European Office of WHO
- produced hypotheses, protocols and local publications
- problems of standardization of questionnaires

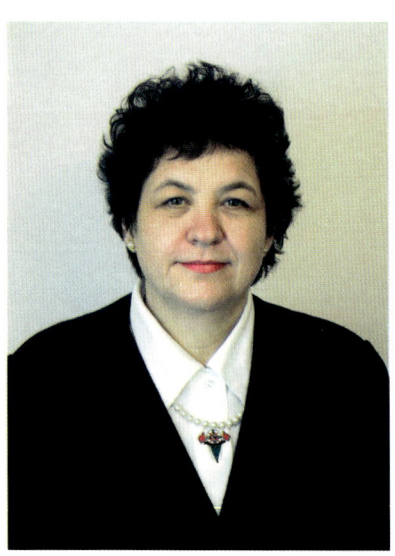

Aushra Shatchkute

2. For the participating centres there is no relationship between changes in psychosocial risk factors and changes in the incidence of classical coronary risk factors.

Within the MONICA centres the following general hypotheses were proposed for testing:

1. Different levels of psychosocial risk factors in individuals are not related to differences in the prevalence of CHD morbidity (for example measured by ECG, angina pectoris questionnaire). To be tested in the cross-sectional studies.
2. Different levels of psychosocial risk factors in individuals are not related to different risks of CHD mortality and morbidity. To be tested in cross-sectional and cohort studies.
3. Different levels of psychosocial risk factors are not related to prevalence and incidence of the classical coronary risk factors. To be tested in cross-sectional and cohort studies.

A Data Management Centre was established at the MEDIS Institute in Munich, Germany (Institut für Medizinische Informatik und Systemforschung). Nineteen centres sent data for central processing at the Centre.

However, international comparability has been limited through the lack of standardized questionnaires. Therefore, for the second and third surveys, a manual of operations with recommendations for standardized measurements was introduced.

The main achievements of the MONICA Psychosocial Substudy were the establishment of an international network to study CVD psychosocial risk factors, and the elaboration of standardized questionnaires to assess these factors. This group of studies produced considerable discussion, and some common questionnaires, but most activity in this area seems to have been at a local rather than at a multi-centre collaborative level. Many MCCs have published data on social deprivation and its relation to risk factors and cardiovascular disease.

Aushra Shatchkute

#47 MONICA Optional Study of Physical Activity (MOSPA)

See #9 *MONICA Reference Centres (MRCs)* for further information

The reference centre for physical activity was initially in Tel Aviv, but this group encountered problems with implementing the core protocol. The enthusiasm of the CDC Atlanta group for their developing questionnaire, and offer of free data analyses, at the Council of Principal Investigators Meeting in Lugano in 1990, led many MCCs to incorporate it as an 'add-on' to their middle and/or final MONICA population surveys.

The WHO MONICA Optional Study of Physical Activity (MOSPA) questionnaire was developed by the Centers for Disease Control and Prevention (CDC) with the assistance of several experts and individuals involved with the WHO MONICA Project. The instrument was put into its final form on 4 December 1987 and distributed in MONICA MEMO 115 (see #88 *MONICA Memos* and the MONICA CD-ROM). The MOSPA questionnaire is divided up into four activity categories or domains. Physical activity questions cover occupational, travel to work, household, and leisure-time physical activity.

- physical activity is easy to recognise but not so easy to measure
- a standard questionnaire was eventually used by several MONICA centres
- introduced too late for the study of 10-year trends

Cycling—USA

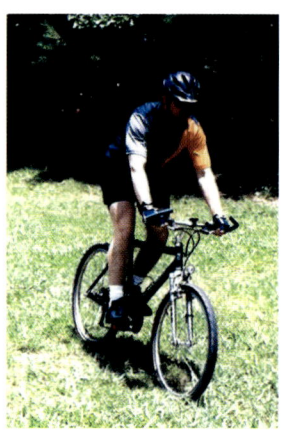

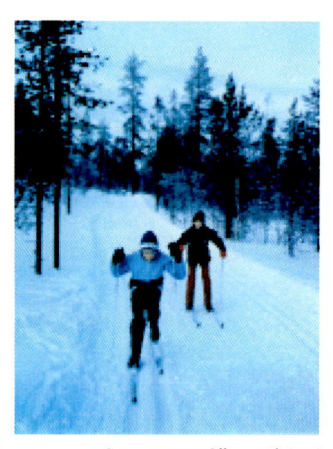

Cross-country skiing—Finland

Since it was included among the Collection of Physical Activity Questionnaires for Health-Related Research (1) we continue to receive requests for the questionnaire and supporting documentation.

As the MOSPA Data Management Centre, the CDC (Atlanta, USA) developed the MOSPA algorithm, edited and analysed data sets from MOSPA participating sites, and submitted a comprehensive physical activity report to each MOSPA site. In 1997, the following MOSPA sites received analyses of minutes/week and MET (metabolic equivalent task) minutes/week for light, moderate, vigorous and overall intensity levels for each physical activity domain: MOSPA-Augsburg, MOSPA-Catalonia, MOSPA-East Germany, MOSPA-Friuli, Pol-MOSPA-Krakow, Pol-MOSPA-Warsaw, Scottish MOSPA, Sino-MOSPA Beijing, and Siberian MOSPA.

Reference

1. Pereira MA, FitzerGerald SJ, Gregg EW, Joswiak ML, Ryan WJ, Suminski RR, Utter AC, Zmuda JM. A collection of Physical Activity Questionnaires for health-related research. *Medicine and Science in Sports and Exercise*, 1997, 29(6Suppl):S1–S205. PMID 9243481. (the CDC questionnaire is on pages S162–S169).

Deborah Jones

#48 MONICA Optional Study on Drugs

See #9 *MONICA Reference Centres (MRCs)* for further information
Earlier activity in this area was carried out in Oslo

- MONICA concluded at its end that drug usage influences cardiovascular disease
- yet it failed to plan measurements of drug use in the population as a core item
- hence the MONICA Optional Study on Drugs

Although drugs are of major medical, social and economic importance in the context of cardiovascular disease, the MONICA core study included only minimum information about drug utilization. Several PIs, however, considered this topic important enough to acquire more detailed information beyond the core during the MONICA population surveys, using their own methods, but within the framework of the MONICA Optional Study on Drugs. The Bremen Institute for Prevention Research and Social Medicine (BIPS) was appointed the Reference Centre for Drug Epidemiology (MRC-Drugs) for this optional study because of its previous activities and experience in this field. The MRC-Drugs asked each MCC about drug data acquisition and availability for the joint analysis, which started in 1997 and was based on survey data from 26 regional surveys from 12 MCCs in seven countries. This made a total of 39 260 survey participants, aged 35–64 years. The first results of investigations into antihypertensive drug treatment and its relation to hypertension control and myocardial infarction have recently been published (1). Further analyses are planned. Among others, these analyses will focus on specific antihypertensive drug groups and on serum lipid-reducing drug treatment.

Reference

Janhsen K. *Joint Analysis of the MONICA Optional Study on Drugs: Antihypertensive Drug Treatment in an International Comparison and its Relations to Hypertension Control and Myocardial Infarction.* [Doctoral dissertation]. Bremen, University of Bremen, 2001.

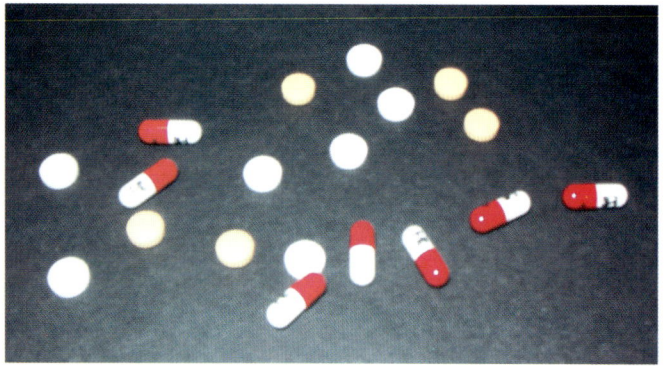

Eberhard Greiser, Katrin Janhsen

#49 MONICA Optional Study on Haemostatic Risk Factors

See #9 *MONICA Reference Centres (MRCs)* for further information

This study was funded by the British Heart Foundation. During the final MONICA population survey (1991–1997), samples were collected, using a standardized protocol, from men and women aged 45–64 years in 12 populations, eleven of them European. Laboratory analyses took place in Bristol and in Glasgow. Results were available for 3250 subjects (Bristol samples) and 2372 subjects (Glasgow samples). Mean population levels of haemostatic risk factors were adjusted for age, smoking habit and body mass index. In general, populations with a high incidence of CHD had higher levels of haemostatic risk factors. Correlations between coronary-event rates current at the time of the surveys and population levels of haemostatic factors were significant in the case of the vWf antigen for men and women ($r = 0.69$ and 0.88) and for nephelometric fibrinogen ($r = 0.78$) for men and D-dimer ($r = 0.84$) for women.

C reactive protein is being measured in the populations; DNA has been collected and may be used to genotype risk factors of interest. Results are being prepared for formal publication.

- association between population levels of CHD and von Willebrand's factor

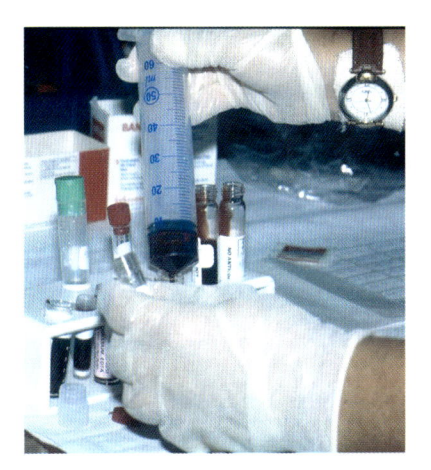

References
1. Yarnell J, McCrum E, Evans A, Rumley A, Lowe G. Haemostatic cardiovascular risk factors in the WHO MONICA Project: an international comparison. *Blood Coagulation and Fibrinolysis*, 1999, 10:No.8, 015(Abs). (PMID: nil).
2. Yarnell JWG, Sweetnam PM, Rumley A, Lowe GDO. Lifestyle and hemostatic risk factors for ischemic heart disease. The Caerphilly Study. *Arteriosclerosis Thrombosis and Vascular Biology*, 2000, 20:271–279. PMID: 10634829.

John Yarnell, Evelyn McCrum, Alun Evans

MONICA Populations

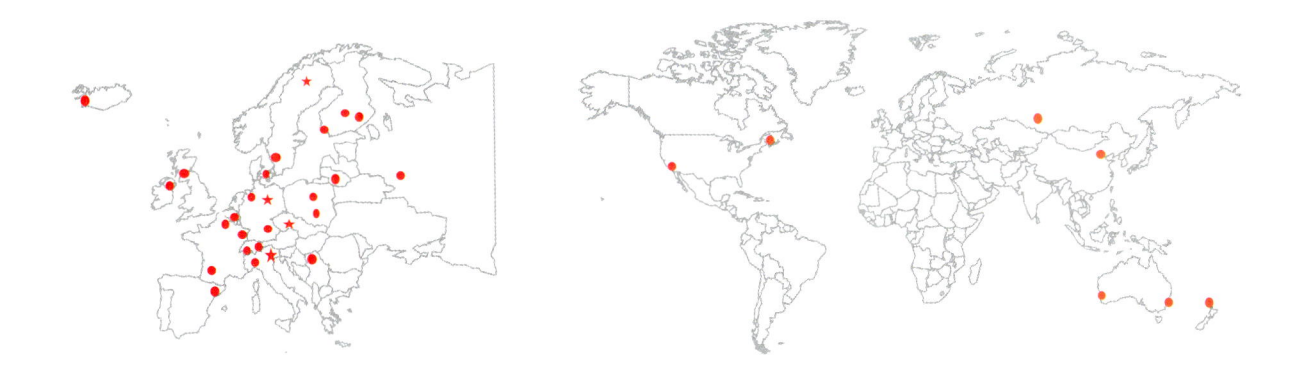

#50 Introduction to Population Pages

Population name (7 character population name, 2 digit population name)
MCC Number: MCC Name
Number of Reporting Units

Population names are those previously agreed. See *Appendix*, MONICA Manual (*1*).

> In their own words:
> - who they are
> - what they are
> - what they contributed
> - what made them special

Map
The maps locate the MONICA populations for an international readership (but see the disclaimer on page ii). A red spot denotes a single location. A red star indicates scattered populations or a large territory in one RUA.

Administrative Centre
This is the institution of the MCC and the Principal Investigator. It may be situated at a distance from the population being studied. Institution names, telephone, FAX and e-mail addresses are all subject to change and are updated, when notified, on the MONICA public Website (*2*).

Population
Description of the target population for registration and population surveys. Population size is from the MONICA demographic assessment (*3*).

Funding
Local sources of funding. Activity within the MCCs was not funded by WHO which funded coordination work only.

Dates
Registration activity and surveys did not always correspond with data that were used in the collaborative analyses. The latter timings are shown in the introductory graphics pages of this Monograph and are also available from MONICA Quality assessment reports on the different activities such as coronary-event registration, coronary care, stroke-event registration and population surveys (*4–7*).

Additional description
Other activities linked to MONICA.

Local research interests and continuing activity
Self-explanatory.

Key personnel
As identified by the Principal Investigator.

Selected publications
Chosen locally, but verified on PUBMED wherever possible. Does not include MONICA collaborative publications, see #85 and #86 *MONICA Publication List and Abstracts*.

References
MONICA Web Publications are also accessible on the Monograph CD-ROM

1. WHO MONICA Project. MONICA Manual. (1998–1999). Available from URL: http://www.ktl.fi/publications/monica/manual/index.htm, URN:*NBN:fi-fe19981146*. MONICA Web Publication 1. Part I. Appendix 2.

2. http://www.ktl.fi/monica/public/address.htm

3. Moltchanov V, Kuulasmaa K, Torppa J, for the WHO MONICA Project. Quality assessment of demographic data in the WHO MONICA Project. (April 1999). Available from URL: http://www.ktl.fi/publications/monica/demoqa/demoqa.htm, URN:*NBN:fi-fe19991073*. MONICA Web Publication 3.

4. Mähönen M, Tolonen H, Kuulasmaa K, Tunstall-Pedoe H, Amouyel P, for the WHO MONICA Project. Quality assessment of coronary event registration data in the WHO MONICA Project. (January 1999). Available from URL: http://www.ktl.fi/publications/monica/coreqa/coreqa.htm, URN:*NBN:fi-fe19991072*. MONICA Web Publication 2.

5. Mähönen M, Cepaitis Z, Kuulasmaa K, for the WHO MONICA Project. Quality assessment of acute coronary care data in the WHO MONICA Project. (February 1999). Available from URL: http://www.ktl.fi/publications/monica/accqa/accqa.htm, URN:*NBN:fi-fe19991081*. MONICA Web Publication 4.

6. Mähönen M, Tolonen H, Kuulasmaa K, for the WHO MONICA Project. Quality assessment of stroke event registration data in the WHO MONICA Project. (November 1998). Available from URL: http://www.ktl.fi/publications/monica/strokeqa/strokeqa.htm, URN:*NBN:fi-fe19991080*. MONICA Web Publication 5.

7. Kuulasmaa K, Tolonen H, Ferrario M, Ruokokoski E, for the WHO MONICA Project. Age, date of examination and survey periods in the MONICA surveys. (May 1998). Available from URL: http://www.ktl.fi/publications/monica/age/ageqa.htm, URN:*NBN:fi-fe19991075*. MONICA Web Publication 6.

Hugh Tunstall-Pedoe

#51 Australia-Newcastle (AUS-NEW, AN)

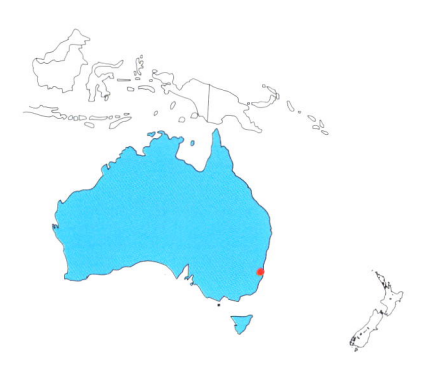

- high coronary-event rates, especially in women
- declining risk-factor levels
- declining coronary deaths, definite myocardial infarction and case fatality
- less severe events are increasing

MCC 11: Newcastle
Five Reporting Units merged into one Reporting Unit Aggregate (RUA).

Administrative centre
Centre for Clinical Epidemiology and Biostatistics, University of Newcastle,
New South Wales 2308, Australia
Current contact: Professor Annette Dobson,
School of Population Health,
University of Queensland, Herston, Brisbane Q 4006, Australia
T +61 7 3365 5346; F +61 7 3365 5442
E-mail: a.dobson@sph.uq.edu.au.

Population
Residents aged 25–69 of the Hunter Region of New South Wales, 120 km north of Sydney on Australia's east coast; total population of 445 000 in 1991, many descended from British industrial immigrants. Closure of shipyards and steelworks in the last two decades caused economic depression. Coalmining, farming and viniculture occur inland. Health services improved with a new hospital, and specialist services, including cardiac surgery. Health services and the education sector are major employers in Newcastle.

Funding
Jointly with Perth: 1. National Heart Foundation of Australia. 2. National Health and Medical Research Council. 3. Commonwealth Department of Health. *Local:* 4. BHP Company and Hunter Area Health Service.

Dates
Coronary-event registration: 1985–1993. Coronary care: 1985, 1988–93. Risk-factor surveys: 1983, 1988/89, 1994. No stroke registration.

Additional description
The three Australasian MONICA Centres collaborated. Nested case-control studies were conducted on active and passive smoking, alcohol consumption and diabetes. John Malcolm (PhD), Scott Kinlay (PhD), Anne Russell (M.Med Stat), Khaldoon Al Roomi (PhD), Kate (Boyle) D'Este (PhD) and Patrick McElduff (PhD) researched MONICA-related projects.

Continuing activity
Elements of MONICA continue in the hospital-based Hunter Heart and Stroke Register and the programme of the new National Cardiovascular Monitoring Unit of the Australian Institute of Health and Welfare. This encompasses risk factors, acute events and treatment, using data from national health surveys, hospitals and death certificates, and use of pharmaceuticals.

Key personnel
Former PI: Stephen Leeder. PI: Annette Dobson. Associate PIs: Richard Heller, Robert Gibberd. Project Manager: Hilary Alexander. Data Managers/Statisticians: Paula (Steele) Colley, Janet Fisher, Patrick McElduff. Secretaries/ECG Coders: Sue Luxon, Colleen Griffith. Research Nurses: Julie Hanson, Denise Mowbray, Denise Marks, Robyn Gannon.

Selected publications
1. Heller RF, Dobson AJ, Alexander HM, Steele PL, Malcolm JA. Changes in drug treatment and case-fatality of patients with acute myocardial infarction. Observations from the Newcastle MONICA Project, 1984/5 to 1988/90. *The Medical Journal of Australia*, 1992, 157:83–86. PMID:1630395.
2. Dobson AJ, Jamrozik KD, Hobbs M, Heller RF, Steele PL, Parsons RW, Thompson P. Medical care and case fatality from myocardial infarction and coronary death in Newcastle and Perth. *Australian and New Zealand Journal of Medicine*, 1993, 23:12–18. PMID:8460967.
3. Heller RF, Steele PL, Fisher JD, Alexander HM, Dobson AJ. Success of cardiopulmonary resuscitation after heart attack in hospital and outside hospital. *British Medical Journal*, 1995, 311:1332–1336. PMID:7496282.
4. Boyle CA, Dobson AJ. The accuracy of hospital records and death certificates for acute myocardial infarction. *Australian and New Zealand Journal of Medicine*, 1995, 25: 316–323. PMID:8540872.

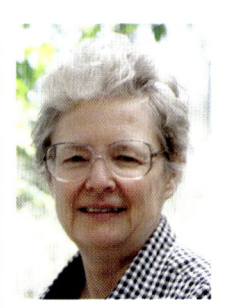

Annette Dobson

5. Chun BY, Dobson AJ, Heller RF. The impact of diabetes on survival among patients with first myocardial infarction. *Diabetes Care*, 1997, 20:704–708. PMID:9135930.
6. McElduff P, Dobson AJ. How much alcohol and how often? Population based case-control study of alcohol consumption and risk of a major coronary event. *British Medical Journal*, 1997, 314:1159–1164. PMID: 9146388.
7. McElduff P, Dobson AJ, Jackson R, Beaglehole R, Heller RF, Lay-Yee R. Coronary events and exposure to environmental tobacco smoke: a case-control study from Australia and New Zealand. *Tobacco Control*, 1998, 7:41–46. PMID:9706753.
8. McElduff P, Dobson A, Beaglehole R, Jackson R. Rapid reduction in coronary risk for those who quit cigarette smoking. *Australian and New Zealand Journal of Public Health*, 1998, 22:787–791. PMID:9889444.
9. Dobson AJ, McElduff P, Heller R, Alexander H, Colley P, D'Este K. Changing patterns of coronary disease in the Hunter Region of New South Wales, Australia. *Journal of Clinical Epidemiology*, 1999, 52:761–771. PMID: 10465321.
10. McElduff P, Dobson AJ. Trends in coronary heart disease—has the socio-economic differential changed? *Australian and New Zealand Journal of Public Health*, 2000, 24:465–473. PMID:11109682.

Annette Dobson

#52 Australia-Perth (AUS-PER, AP)

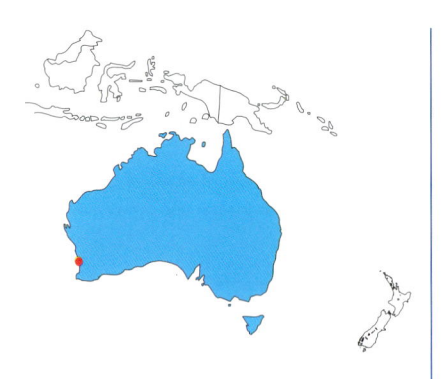

- lowest coronary mortality of all Australian big cities
- major decline in coronary deaths since 1967
- populations initially different for monitoring coronary event and risk-factor trends
- collaborative studies with Newcastle and Auckland
- studies of medical care with clinicians

MCC 10: Perth
Two Reporting Units, inner and outer Perth. Main results and Monograph graphics use risk-factor data from the inner city only (PERa) but coronary-event and coronary care data from both areas (PERb), as the outer city was not included in the first population survey.

Administrative centre
Department of Public Health, University of Western Australia,
Western Australia 6907, Australia
T +61 8 93801258; F +61 8 93801188
Website: http://www.publichealth.uwa.edu.au/research/
Site of MONICA Quality Control Centre for Health Services information.

Population
Perth is the capital of Western Australia with a population in 1991 of 1 189 000.

Funding
1. National Health & Medical Research Council.
2. National Heart Foundation of Australia.
3. Commonwealth Department of Health.
4. Health Department of Western Australia.

Dates
Coronary-event registration and coronary care together: 1984–93. Population surveys: 1980,* 1983, 1989, 1994. No MONICA stroke registration. * = not in MONICA database.

Additional description
Perth and Newcastle, two Australian MCCs, have respectively the lowest and highest coronary heart disease mortality of major Australian cities. Perth is an administrative and service centre with little heavy industry. The only city in Western Australia with a population over 25 000, it is more than 2000 km from major specialist medical services elsewhere. Its population is growing rapidly from substantial inward, and little outward, migration. Highly centralized medical services with sophisticated statistical systems, including record linkage, make it ideal for epidemiology and health services research.

Local research interests
Epidemiology and care of cardiovascular disease, including coronary heart disease. Abdominal aortic aneurysm. Peripheral vascular disease. Use of record linkage.

Continuing activity
Continuing cyclical registration of acute coronary events and stroke, and risk-factor surveys. Cohort studies of registered cases and survey participants. Application of record linkage to monitoring incidence, survival and treatment of selected cardiovascular conditions, particularly coronary artery revascularization.

Key personnel
Co–PIs: Michael Hobbs, Konrad Jamrozik. Others: Peter Thompson, Bruce Armstrong (until 1988).

Selected publications
Comprehensive list available on Vascular Epidemiology group page at: http://www.publichealth.uwa.edu.au/research/
1. Dobson AJ, Alexander HM, Leeder SR, Beaglehole R, Jackson RT, Stewart AW, Jamrozik KD, Martin CA, Hobbs MST. Risk factor levels and mortality of ischaemic heart disease in three Australasian centres. Auckland, Newcastle and Perth MONICA centres. *The Medical Journal of Australia*, 1988, 148:61–65. PMID:3257289.
2. Martin CA, Hobbs MS, Armstrong BK, de Klerk NH. Trends in the incidence of myocardial infarction in Western Australia between 1971 and 1982. *American Journal of Epidemiology*, 1989, 129:655–668. PMID:2923116.
3. Nidorf SM, Parsons RW, Thompson PL, Jamrozik K, Hobbs MS. Reduced risk of death at 28 days in patients taking a beta-blocker before admission to hospital with myocardial infarction. *British Medical Journal*, 1990, 300:71–74. PMID:1967956.
4. Hobbs MST, Jamrozik KD, Hockey RL, Alexander HM, Beaglehole R, Dobson AJ, Heller RF, Jackson R, Stewart AW. Mortality from coronary heart disease and incidence of acute myocardial infarction in Auckland, Newcastle and Perth. *The Medical Journal of Australia*, 1991, 155:436–442. PMID:1921812.
5. Thompson PL, Parsons RW, Jamrozik K, Hockey RL, Hobbs MS, Broadhurst R. Changing patterns of medical treatment in acute myocardial infarction. Observations from the Perth MONICA Project 1984–90. *The Medical Journal of Australia*, 1992, 157:87–92. PMID:1359390.
6. Dobson AJ, Jamrozik KD, Hobbs MS, Heller RF, Steele PL, Parsons RW, Thompson PL. Medical care and case fatality from myocardial infarction and coronary death in Newcastle and Perth. *Australian and New Zealand Journal of Medicine*, 1993, 23:12–18. PMID:8460967.
7. Parsons RW, Jamrozik KD, Hobbs MS, Thompson PL. Early identification of patients at low risk of death after myocardial infarction and potentially suitable for early hospital discharge. *British Medical Journal*, 1994, 308:1006–1010. PMID:8167512.
8. Beaglehole R, Stewart AW, Jackson R, Dobson AJ, McElduff P, D'Este K, Heller RF, Jamrozik KD, Hobbs MS, Parsons R, Broadhurst R. Declining rates of coronary heart disease in New Zealand and Australia, 1983–1993. *American Journal of Epidemiology*, 1997, 145:707–713. PMID:91259917.
9. McElduff P, Dobson AJ, Jamrozik K, Hobbs MS. Opportunities for control of coronary heart disease in Australia. *Australian and New Zealand Journal of Public Health*, 2001, 25:24–30. PMID:11297296.

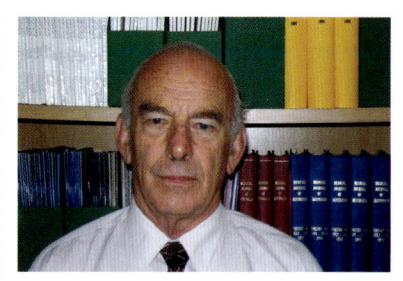

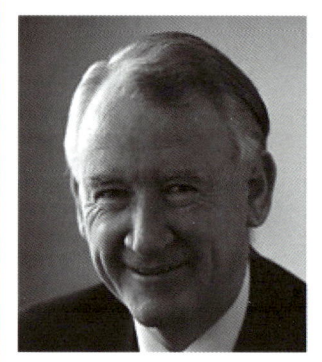

Michael Hobbs

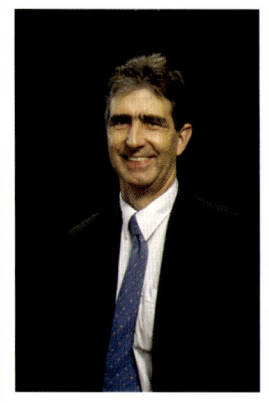

Konrad Jamrozik

Peter Thompson

Michael Hobbs, Konrad Jamrozik

#53 Belgium-Ghent/Charleroi (BEL-GCH, BE)

Belgium-Charleroi (BEL-CHA, BC)
Belgium-Ghent (BEL-GHE, BG)

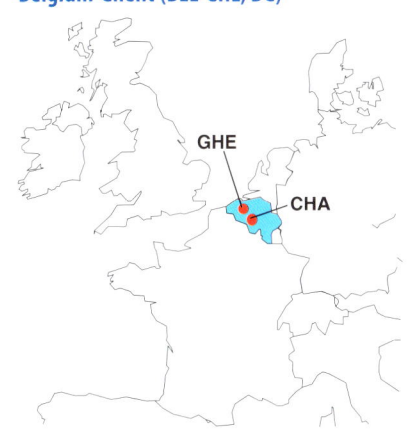

- contrasting Belgian populations only 100 km apart
- coronary-event rates 50% higher in Charleroi
- different risk-factor levels
- event rates falling in Ghent, rising in Charleroi

MCC 12: Ghent/Charleroi
Two geographically separate Reporting Units, Ghent and Charleroi; used separately for many analyses, amalgamated into one Reporting Unit Aggregate (RUA) for coronary care.

Description
The MONICA Project recruited two Belgian populations that were geographically close but with different economies, cultural traditions and languages. Event rates and trends over time were different. There was close collaboration between the two Principal Investigators and they were considered as one MONICA Collaborating Centre (MCC). The two Reporting Units are described separately. A third distinct Belgian population, Luxembourg, was entered initially as a separate MCC but did not produce data over a sufficient number of years for an analysis of trends. (See #84.)

Belgium-Charleroi (BEL-CHA, BC)

Administrative centre
Unité cardiovasculaire, École de Santé Publique CP 597, Université Libre de Bruxelles,
Route de Lennik, 808, B-1070 Bruxelles, Belgium
T +32 2 555 4087; F +32 2 555 4049

Population
Residents aged 25–69 of 15 municipalities, centred on the city of Charleroi. Charleroi was a major industrial centre in the nineteenth century. Its main industries were coal mining, iron and steel, and glass production. It became economically depressed in the 1930s, and remains so today, with many health problems and high unemployment, although it is slowly recovering. Since World War II, a significant Italian community has grown up. A cardiovascular prevention programme was launched in 1994. The total population in 1991 was 206 000.

Funding
1. 1983–1992: Fonds de la Recherche Scientifique Medicale (FRSM). 2. 1993–: Ministère de la Santé de la Communauté francaise de Belgique.

Dates
Coronary-event registration: 1983–92 (for MONICA database)*. Coronary care: 1986–1987, 1991–1992. Population surveys: 1985–1987, 1987–1990, 1990–1993. No stroke registration.

Continuing activity
*Coronary-event registration is continuing. A fourth population survey is being planned.

Key personnel
PI: Marcel Kornitzer. Others: L Berghmans, R Desqueuve, M Lannoy, MP Vanderelst, P Legrand, M Candeur, P de Smet.

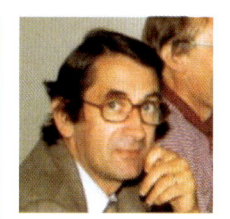

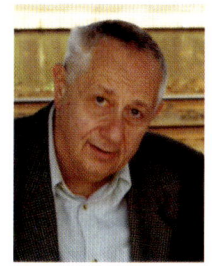

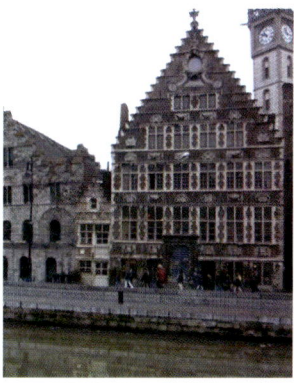

Belgium-Ghent (BEL-GHE, BG)

Administrative centre
Dept of Public Health, Ghent University, Ghent University Hospital,
2 Block A, De Pintelaan 185, B-9000 Gent, Belgium
T +32 92 403 627; F +32 92 404 994

Population
Once a major trading centre, in the 13th century Ghent was equal to Paris and larger than London. Its tradition of spinning and weaving reached a climax in the 19th century. It is now a relatively prosperous small city, with a total population in 1991 of 230 000. It is the capital of Eastern Flanders and is known for its financial services, iron and steel, and vehicle manufacture.

Funding
Belgian National Fund for Scientific Research.

Dates
Coronary-event registration: 1983–92. Coronary care: 1986–87, 1991–92. Population surveys: 1985–87, 1988–90, 1990–92. No stroke registration.

Continuing activity
Coronary-event registration continues. It has been extended to cover the 25–74 year age group, and to the region of Bruges. Further risk-factor surveys are planned.

Key personnel
PI: Guy De Backer. Others: S De Henauw, D De Bacquer, P Vannoote, N Popelier, F Van Onsem.

Selected publications
1. Berghmans L, Heyerick P, De Backer G, Kornitzer M, Fux M. Pilot project for registering myocardial infarctions in Belgium. *Acta Cardiologica*, 1985, 40:365–374. PMID:3876670.
2. Berghmans L, De Backer G, Kornitzer M, Dramaix M, Lagasse R, Payen R, Kittel F, Van Der Stichelen C, Derese A, Heyerick P. Comparison of the attack rates of acute myocardial infarction in two Belgian towns. *Acta Medica Scandinavica Supplementum*, 1988, 728:90–94. PMID:3202037.
3. De Craene I, De Backer G, Kornitzer M, De Henauw S, Bara L, Rosseneu M, Vercaemst R. Determinants of fat consumption in a general population. *Revue d'Epidémiologie et de Santé Publique*, 1990, 38:539–543. PMID:2082463.
4. De Henauw S, De Backer G. Preliminary results from the MONICA Ghent-Charleroi study. *Archives of Public Health*, 1991, 49:225–239. PMID:na.
5. De Henauw S, de Smet P, Aelvoet W, Kornitzer M, De Backer G. Misclassification of coronary heart disease in mortality statistics. Evidence from the WHO MONICA Ghent-Charleroi study in Belgium. *Journal of Epidemiology and Community Health*, 1998, 52:513–519. PMID:9876363.
6. De Henauw S, De Bacquer D, de Smet P, Kornitzer M, De Backer G. Trends in coronary heart disease in two Belgian areas: results from the MONICA Ghent-Charleroi study. *Journal of Epidemiology and Community Health*, 1999, 53:89–98. PMID:10396469.
7. De Henauw S, De Bacquer D, de Smet P, Kornitzer M, De Backer G. Trends and regional differences in coronary risk factors in two areas in Belgium: final results from the MONICA Ghent-Charleroi Study. *Journal of Cardiovascular Risk*, 2000, 7:347–357. PMID:11143765.

Guy De Backer, Stefaan De Henauw, Marcel Kornitzer

#54 Canada-Halifax County (CAN-HAL, CA)

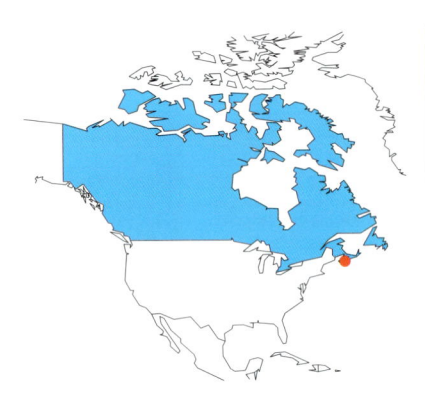

- the only Canadian population in MONICA
- coronary mortality close to Canadian average
- unusual increase in systolic blood pressure—but from a low level

MCC 15: Halifax
Single Reporting Unit.

Administrative centre
MONICA Research, QEII Centre for Clinical Research,
5790 University Ave, Halifax NS, B3H 1V7, Canada
T +1 902 473 4340; F +1 902 473 4497

Population
Residents aged 25–74 of the census division of Halifax County in Nova Scotia, Canada, incorporating the cities of Halifax, Dartmouth, Bedford, and the surrounding rural district. During the study period the population of Halifax County, which was 338 000 in 1991, was served by one tertiary care centre with cardiac intervention capabilities and three major hospitals, all within the core study area. In addition, there were three small acute hospitals in the rural area.

Funding
1. Heart and Stroke Foundation of Nova Scotia. 2. Health and Welfare Canada (NHRDP 6603). 3. Dalhousie University Internal Medicine Research Foundation. 4. Sun Life of Canada.

Dates
Coronary-event registration and coronary care: 1984–93. Population surveys: 1985–88, 1995. No stroke registration.

Additional description
Halifax County hosts five universities and colleges, and the provincial government. There are several federally funded research facilities there. The average educational level of the study population was high, with few manual labourers, and coronary disease rates were average for Canada, although they were much higher elsewhere in Nova Scotia.

Local research interests
Hypertension treatment in the community. Investigation and treatment of acute coronary syndromes. Long-term mortality of hospital survivors of myocardial infarction. Use of administrative databases for monitoring disease trends.

Continuing activity
Event registration and population surveys have ceased. A cohort follow–up study (over a 5-year period) of hospital survivors of myocardial infarction.

Key personnel
PI: Hermann Wolf. Co–PI: Ronald Gregor. Co–PI: Iqbal Bata. Former Co–PI: Ross MacKenzie. Health Record Technician: Brenda Brownell. Research Assistant: Kathy Webber. Data Manager: Petra Rykers.

Selected publications
1. Hoyt BK, Wolf HK. An electronic instrument for indirect blood pressure measurement. *Lancet*, 1984, 2:552–553. PMID:6147606.
2. Wolf HK, Rautaharju PM, Manton KG, Stallard E. Importance of electrocardiography for coronary risk factor surveys. (Letter to the Editor). *Lancet*, 1988, 2:633–634. PMID:2901014.
3. Gregor RD, Bata IR, Eastwood BJ, Garner JB, Guernsey JR, MacKenzie BR, Rautaharju PM, Wolf HK. Gender differences in the presentation, treatment and short-term mortality of acute chest pain. *Clinical and Investigative Medicine*, 1994, 17:551–562. PMID:7895419.
4. Eastwood BJ, Gregor RD, MacLean D, Wolf HK. Effects of recruitment strategy on response rates and risk factor profile in two cardiovascular surveys. *International Journal of Epidemiology*, 1996, 25:763–769. PMID:8921454.
5. Wolf HK, Hoyt B, Warren J. Is there an observer bias with random-zero blood pressure machines? *Blood Pressure Monitoring*, 1996, 1:439–442. PMID:10226272.
6. Bata IR, Eastwood BJ, Gregor RD, Guernsey JR, Klassen GA, MacKenzie BR, Wolf HK. Decreasing mortality from acute myocardial infarction: effects of attack rates and case severity. *Journal of Clinical Epidemiology*, 1997, 50:787–791. PMID:9253389.
7. Gregor RD, Bata IR, Eastwood BJ, Wolf HK. Ten-year trends of heart disease risk factors in the Halifax County MONICA Population. *Canadian Journal of Cardiology*, 1998, 14: 1017–1024. PMID:9738161.
8. Wolf HK, Andreou P, Bata IR, Comeau DG, Gregor RD, Kephart G, MacLean DR, Sketris I. Trends in the prevalence and treatment of hypertension in Halifax County from 1985 to 1995. *Canadian Medical Association Journal*, 1999, 161:699–704. PMID:10513276.
9. Bata IR, Gregor RD, Eastwood BJ, Wolf HK. Trends in the incidence of acute myocardial infarction between 1984 and 1993—The Halifax County MONICA Project. *Canadian Journal of Cardiology*, 2000, 16:589–595. PMID:10833538.
10. Gregor RD, Bata IR, Brownell B, Wolf HK. Trends in the in-hospital treatment of acute myocardial infarction between 1984 and 1993—The Halifax County MONICA Project. *Canadian Journal of Cardiology*, 2000, 16:596–603. PMID:10833539.

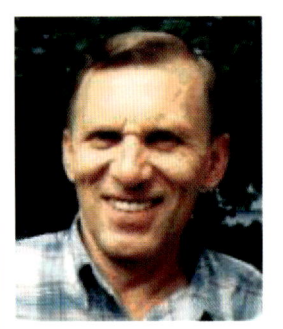

Hermann Wolf

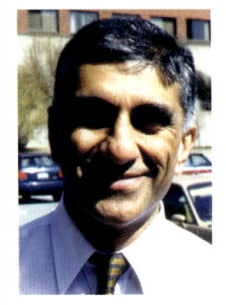

Iqbal Bata

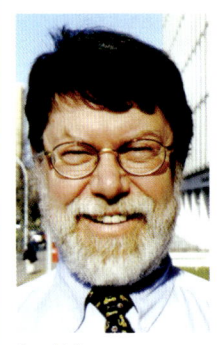

Ronald Gregor

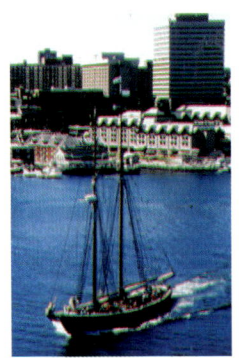

Halifax waterfront

Hermann Wolf, Ronald Gregor, Iqbal Bata

#55 China-Beijing (CHN-BEI, CN)

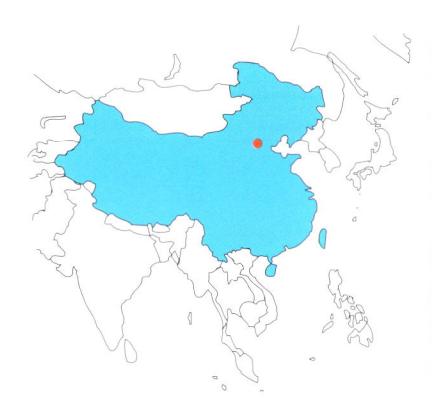

- with Novosibirsk, the only Asian populations in MONICA
- but MONICA was replicated across China
- low all-cause mortality, coronary-event rates and risk-factor scores
- highest male smoking rates, lowest cholesterol, and BMI of any population
- coronary-event rates increasing

MCC 17: Sino-MONICA-Beijing
Single Reporting Unit.

Administrative centre
Department of Epidemiology,
Beijing Institute of Heart, Lung & Blood Vessel Disease,
Andingmenwai, Beijing 100029, People's Republic of China
T +86 10 644 19738; F +86 10 644 19738

Population
Residents aged 25–74, of six separate urban and suburban districts and one rural county in the Beijing area, with a total population in 1991 of 686 000. Two-thirds of the population monitored between 1984 and 1993 were urban and one-third rural. Beijing, the capital of China, is a city with more than a thousand years of history. It has a population of 11 million. The lifestyle of the Beijing population has changed in the last 20 years, with dramatic economic developments. These have been accompanied by changes in cardiovascular risk factors and disease.

Funding
1. Ministry of Public Health of China. 2. World Health Organization.

Dates
Coronary-event registration and coronary care together: 1984–1993. Stroke registration: 1984–1993. (Collaborative trend estimates: 1987–1993.) Population surveys: 1984–1985, 1988–1989, 1993.

Additional description
While Beijing was the only Chinese population participating in the WHO MONICA project, a national collaboration (named Sino-MONICA) was organized and conducted from 1985 to 1993. It covered 16 Chinese provinces and used the same criteria and methods. This collaboration has provided valuable data for estimating the magnitude and trend of cardiovascular disease and risk factors in the different Chinese populations.

Local research interests
Stroke and risk factors. The discrepancy between the pathological studies of atherosclerosis in coronary arteries and the incidence rate of coronary events in China. The interaction between environmental risk factors and genetic characteristics for cardiovascular disease.

Continuing activity
Registration of coronary and stroke events in part of the Sino-MONICA populations. Cohort studies in those who participated in the risk-factor surveys.

Key personnel
PI: Zhaosu Wu. Former PI: Yingkai Wu. Co-PIs: Chonghua Yao, Dong Zhao.

Selected publications
1. Wu ZS, Hong ZG, Yao CH, Chen DY, Li N, Zhang M, Wu YY, Wu YK. Sino-MONICA-Beijing study: report of the results between 1983–1985. *Chinese Medical Journal* (English), 1987, 100:611–620. PMID:3129242.
2. Wu ZS, Yao CH, Chen DY, Li N, Shang M, Wu YY, Yao D, Wu GX, Wu YK. The Sino-MONICA-Beijing study: report on results between 1984 and 1986. *Acta Medica Scandinavica Supplementum*, 1988, 728:60–66. PMID: 3202033.
3. Yao CH, Wu ZS, Hong ZG, Xu XM, Zhang M, Wu YY, Yu SE, Wu YK. Risk factors of cardiovascular diseases in Beijing. *Chinese Medical Journal* (English), 1988, 101:901–905. PMID: 3150738.
4. Chen D, Roman GC, Wu GX, Wu ZS, Yao CH, Zhang M, Hirsch RP. Stroke in China (Sino-MONICA-Beijing study) 1984–1986. *Neuroepidemiology*, 1992, 11:15–23. PMID: 1608490.
5. Wu Y, Yao C, Wu Z, Zhang R, Zhang M, Wu G, Zhao D, Hong Z. Interim report of Sino-MONICA-Beijing for the years 1985–1989. *Chinese Medical Science Journal*, 1992, 7:125–129. PMID:1286179.
6. Yao C. [Sino-MONICA project: comparison of risk factors of cardiovascular diseases in 13 provinces or cities and the trend of their changes.] *Zhonghua Liu Xing Bing Xue Za Zhi*, 1993, 14:19–22. (Chinese). PMID:8504448.
7. Yao C, Wu Z, Wu Y. The changing pattern of cardiovascular diseases in China. *World Health Statistics Quarterly*, 1993, 46:113–118. PMID:8303905.
8. Zhao D, Wu ZS, Wang W, et al. [The epidemiological characteristics of acute coronary events in sixteen provinces of China]. *Chinese Journal of Epidemiology*, 1993, 14:10–12. (Chinese). PMID:8504446.
9. Wu GX, Wu ZS, He BL. [The epidemiological characteristics of stroke in sixteen provinces of China.] *Zhonghua Yi Xue Za Zhi*, 1994, 74:281–283, 325. (Chinese). PMID: 7953917.
10. Wu ZS, Yao CH, Zhao D, Wu G, Wang W. Study on trends and determinants in cardiovascular disease in China. Part I: morbidity and mortality monitoring. *Circulation*, 2001, 103:462–468. PMID:11157701.

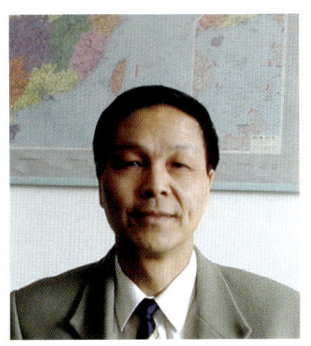

Zhaosu Wu

Zhaosu Wu

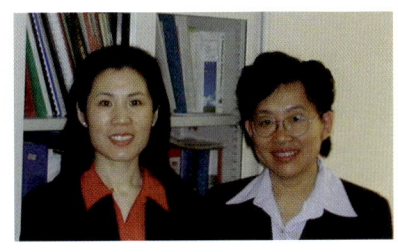

Dong Zhao and Chonghua Yao

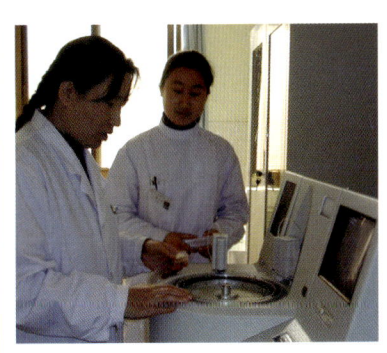

Cholesterol laboratory

#56 Czech Republic (CZE-CZE, CZ)

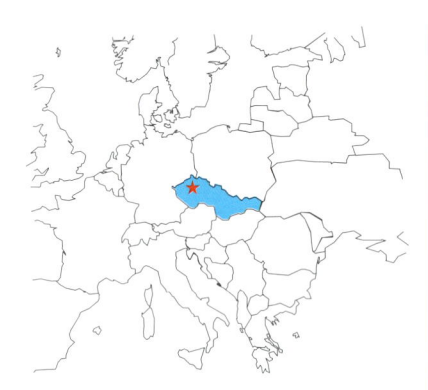

- a composite MONICA population from the Czech Republic
- coronary mortality rose and then fell in the MONICA decade
- home of one of MONICA's godfathers, Zbynek Píša

MCC 18: Czech-MONICA
Six geographically separate Reporting Units merged into one Reporting Unit Aggregate (RUA).

Administrative centre
Department of Preventive Cardiology, Institute for Clinical and Experimental Medicine, Vídenská 1958/9, 140 21 Prague 4, Czech Republic
T +420 2 4172 1574; F +420 2 4172 1574
Site of MONICA Quality Control Centre for Lipid Measurements.

Populations
Residents aged 25–64 of the six districts (Benešov, Cheb, Chrudim, Jindrichuv Hradec, Pardubice, Praha východ) representing the middle, south, east and west of Bohemia. Mixed rural and urban populations. High coronary mortality. Presented as one population. Total population in 1991 was 631 000.

Funding
1. Institute budget to1989. 2. Czech Ministry of Health Internal Grant Agency 1990–.

Dates
Coronary-event registration: 1984–1993. Coronary care: 1986–1987, 1991. Population surveys: 1985, 1988, 1992. No stroke registration.

Additional description
The MONICA core study, and studies linked with Czech MONICA (nutrition, psychosocial factors, trace elements genetics) were used for monitoring, investigation and interpretation of the changes in total and cardiovascular mortality, which occurred after the revolution in 1989. The MONICA and MONICA-linked Projects are the only source of data on the prevalence of different cardiovascular risk factors in the population of this country.

Local research interests
Longitudinal monitoring of the cardiovascular risk of the population over the period of increase and decline in total and cardiovascular mortality (classic and newer risk factors). Investigation of the health consequences of the economic and social transition in the country after 1989. Genetic studies, nutrition, psychosocial factors.

Continuing activity
Registration of coronary events has ceased. Population surveys continue (1997, 2000) as a new research project.

Key personnel
PI: Zdenka Škodová. Others: Zbyněk Píša, Rudolf Poledne, Zdenek Hejl, Petr Vojtíšek, Ružena Emrová, Zbynek Cícha, Lubomír Berka, Miloslav Hoke, Jaromíra Pikhartová, Kveta Hrdlicková, Eduard Wiesner, Dušan Grafnetter.

Selected publications
1. Škodová Z, Píša Z, Berka L, Cícha Z, Cerovská J, Emrová R, Hejl Z, Hrdlickova K, Hoke M, Pirkhartova J, et al. Myocardial Infarction Register in MONICA-Czechoslovakia Centre. *Acta Medica Scandinavica. Supplementum*, 1988, 728:79–83. PMID:3202035.
2. Škodová Z, Píša Z, Cerovská J, Grafnetter D, Wiesner E, Cícha Z, Pikhartova J, Berka L, Vorlicek J, Emrova R, et al. The effect of body fat distribution on cardiovascular risk factors in the population of the Czech Republic. *Cor et Vasa*, 1992, 34:189–198. PMID:1306415.
3. Škodová Z, Píša Z, Pikhartová J, Cícha Z, Vojtíšek P, Emrová R. Development of cardiovascular risk in the population of the Czech Republic. *Cor et Vasa*, 1993, 35:178–182. PMID:na.
4. Korunová V, Škodová Z, Dedina J, Valenta Z, Parízek J, Píša Z, Styblo M. Serum selenium in adult Czechoslovak (Central Bohemia) population. *Biological Trace Element Research*, 1993, 37:91–99. PMID:7688542.
5. Škodová Z, Píša Z, Valenta Z, Berka L, Hoke M, Cícha Z, Pikhartová J. Changes in cigarette smoking in the adult population of six districts of the Czech republic over the 1985–1992 period. *Cor et Vasa*, 1996, 38:11–17. PMID:na.
6. Bobák M, Škodová Z, Píša Z, Poledne R, Marmot M. Political changes and trends in cardiovascular risk factors in the Czech Republic 1985–1992. *Journal of Epidemiology and Community Health*, 1997, 51:272–277. PMID:9229056.
7. Bobák M, Hertzman C, Škodová Z, Marmot M. Socioeconomic status and cardiovascular risk factors in the Czech Republic. *International Journal of Epidemiology*, 1999, 28:46–52. PMID:10195663.
8. Hubácek JA, Rothe G, Pitha J, Škodová Z, Stanek V, Poledne R. Schmitz G. C (-260) → T polymorphism in the promoter of the CD14 monocyte receptor gene as a risk factor for myocardial infarction. *Circulation*, 1999, 99:3218–3220. PMID:10385492.
9. Poledne R, Škodová Z. Changes in nutrition, cholesterol concentration and cardiovascular disease mortality in the Czech population in the past decade. *Nutrition*, 2000, 16:785–786. PMID:10978865.
10. Bobák M, Škodová Z, Marmot M. Effect of beer drinking on risk of myocardial infarction: population based case-control study. *British Medical Journal*, 2000, 320:1378–1379. PMID:10818027.

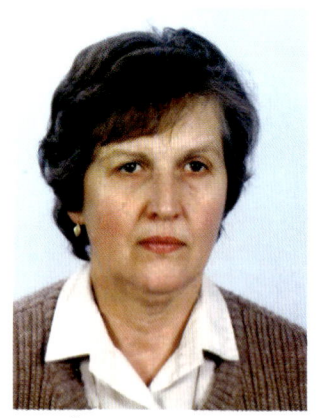

Zdenka Škodová

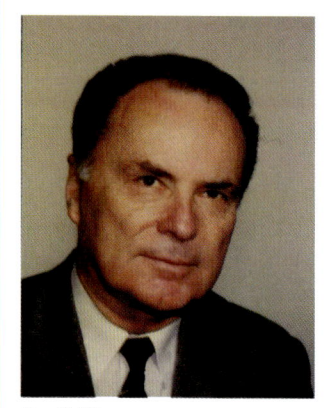

Zbyněk Píša

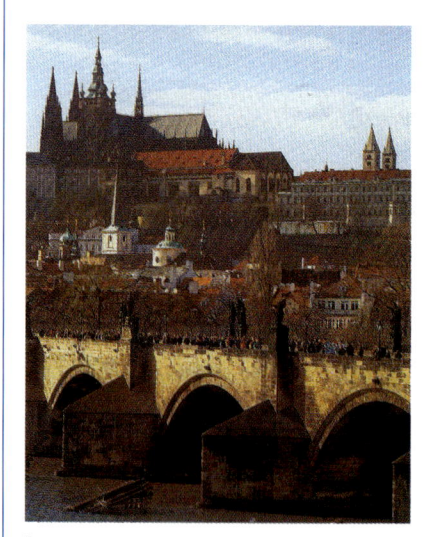

Prague

Zdenka Škodová, Zbyněk Píša

#57 Denmark-Glostrup (DEN-GLO, DN)

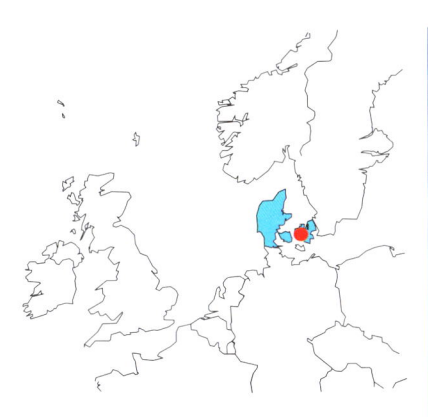

- Denmark's only MONICA population
- earlier risk-factor surveys go back to 1964
- Danish women have very high all-cause mortality

MCC 19: DAN-MONICA
Single Reporting Unit.

Administrative centre
Copenhagen County Centre for Preventive Medicine, Glostrup Hospital, University of Copenhagen, DK2600 Denmark
T +45 4323 3254; F +45 4323 3977
Coronary Heart Disease and Stroke Registers: Danish Institute of Public Health.

Population
Residents aged 25–74 of 11 municipalities in the urban county (Glostrup) of Copenhagen city. This county has hosted population studies continuously since 1964 from an epidemiological unit situated in a clinical environment. Over 30 000 men and women, one in ten of the total 1991 population of 326 000, have participated up to seven times in surveys based on random sampling and their date of birth.

Funding
1. Danish Heart Foundation. 2. Danish Medical Research Council.

Dates
Coronary and stroke-event registration: 1982–1991. Coronary care: 1987–1991. Population surveys: 1982–84, 1986/87, 1991/92.

Additional description
The Dan-MONICA population surveys used previous Glostrup Population Studies survey methods, employing Danish population registers to sample one year of birth for each 10–year age group. Participants have been re-surveyed after five and 10 years using the MONICA protocol plus additional items.

Local research interests
Stroke, dietary intake, physical activity, social status, gallstones.

Continuing activity
The Copenhagen county Centre for Preventive Medicine uses MONICA results in local clinical trials on risk-factor intervention in the community and in hospital settings. The Nationwide Danish Hospitalisation Register uses MONICA criteria for its validation of myocardial infarction. Register results show that high Danish mortality rates are not primarily from coronary disease or stroke.

Key personnel
PI* 1982–2000: Marianne Schroll. Coronary-event registration: Marianne Kirchhoff. Stroke-event registration: Per Thorvaldsen. Initial survey: Marianne Kirchhoff. Middle survey: Annette Sjøl. Final survey: Kristian Korsgaard Thomsen. Event database: Mette Madsen, Henrik Broennum–Hansen, Michael Davidsen. Risk-factor database: Svend Larsen. *Torben Joergensen now manages MONICA-related activities and data.

Selected publications
1. Thomsen KK, Larsen S, Schroll M. Cardiovascular risk factors and age: a cross-sectional survey of Danish men and women from the Glostrup Population Studies, 1991. *American Journal of Geriatric Cardiology*, 1995, 1:31–41. PMID:11416327.
2. Osler M, Kirchhoff M. Smoking knowledge and behaviour in Danish adults from 1982 to 1992. *Public Health*, 1995, 109:245–250. PMID:7667488
3. Kirchhoff M, Davidsen M, Broennum-Hansen H, Hansen B, Schnack H, Eriksen LS, Madsen M, Schroll M. Incidence of myocardial infarction in the Danish MONICA Population 1982–1991. *International Journal of Epidemiology*, 1999, 28:211–218. PMID:10342681.
4. Thorvaldsen P, Davidsen M, Broennum-Hansen H, Schroll M. Stable stroke occurrence despite incidence reduction in an aging population. Stroke trends in the Danish monitoring trends and determinants in cardiovascular disease (MONICA) Population. *Stroke*, 1999, 30:2529–2534. PMID:10582973.
5. Osler M, Gerdes LU, Davidsen M, Broennum-Hansen H, Madsen M, Joergensen T, Schroll M. Socioeconomic status and trends in risk factors for cardiovascular diseases in the Danish MONICA population, 1982–1992. *Journal of Epidemiology and Community Health*, 2000, 54:108–113. PMID:10715743.
6. Gerdes LU, Broennum-Hansen H, Madsen M, Borch-Johnsen K, Joergensen T, Sjoel A, Schroll M. Trends in selected biological risk factors for cardiovascular diseases in the Danish MONICA population 1982–1992. *Journal of Clinical Epidemiology*, 2000, 53:427–434. PMID:10785574.
7. Osler M, Jorgensen T, Davidsen M, Grønbæk M, Broennum-Hansen H, Madsen M, Gerdes LU, Schroll M. Socioeconomic status and trends in alcohol drinking in the Danish MONICA population, 1982–1992. *Scandinavian Journal of Public Health*, 2001, 29:40–43. PMID:11355715.
8. Broennum-Hansen H, Joergensen T, Davidsen M, Madsen M, Osler M, Gerdes LU, Schroll M. Survival and cause of death after myocardial infarction. The Danish MONICA study. *Journal of Clinical Epidemiology*, 2001, 54:1244–1250. PMID:11750193.
9. Broennum-Hansen H, Davidsen M, Thorvaldsen P. Long-term survival and causes of death after stroke. *Stroke*, 2001, 32:2131–2136. PMID:11546907.

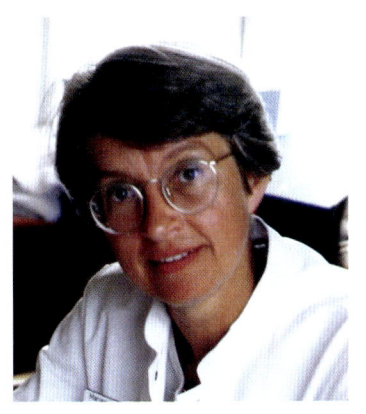

Marianne Schroll

Marianne Schroll

#58 Finland (FIN-FIN, FI)

Finland-Kuopio Province (FIN-KUO, FK)
Finland-North Karelia (FIN-NKA, FN)
Finland-Turku/Loimaa area (FIN-TUL, FU)

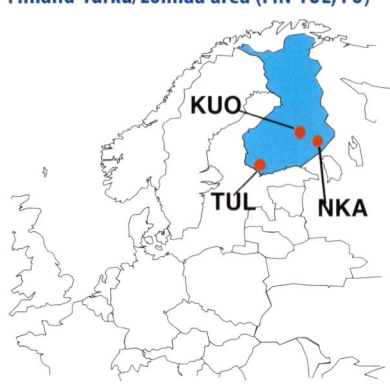

- very high coronary-event rates in men but major downward trends
- FINMONICA incorporated into national prevention strategy and ongoing population surveys
- base in National Public Health Institute (KTL) enabled observation to be combined with action
- administrative centre adjoined the MONICA Data Centre in Helsinki
- hosted 3rd Council of Principal Investigators in Porvoo, Finland, August 1985
- hosted 2nd MONICA Congress in Helsinki, Finland, August 1987, (*Acta Medica Scandinavica Supplementum*, 1988, 728)

MCC 20: FINMONICA
Three Reporting Units, separate for most analyses, merged for coronary care.

Administrative centre
Department of Epidemiology and Health Promotion, National Public Health Institute (KTL),
Mannerheimintie 166, 00300 Helsinki, Finland
T +358 9 47441; F +358 9 4744 8338

Finland-North Karelia (FIN-NKA, FN)
Residents of the rural province of North Karelia in eastern Finland, bordering Russia. North Karelia has high rates of unemployment and emigration. Its economy is based on forestry, farming, timber, paper and steel industries. Known for its exceptionally high rates of cardiovascular diseases since the Seven Countries Study in the 1950s, North Karelia has been the site of a community-based prevention programme, the North Karelia Project, since the early 1970s. Community registers for coronary and stroke events were set up, based in the main hospital at Joensuu, and risk-factor surveys were carried out. This experience was the background to the FINMONICA study, which therefore included North Karelia. The total population in 1991 was 174 000.

Finland-Kuopio Province (FIN-KUO, FK)
Residents of the rural province of Kuopio adjoining North Karelia to the west, in eastern Finland. Kuopio has the same economic base but with, in addition, a university and medical school established in Kuopio town in 1972. Kuopio province has similar disease problems and was the reference (control) community for the North Karelia Project in the 1970s, sharing the risk-factor surveys; but coronary and stroke registration were only set up with the FINMONICA study. The total population in 1991 was 257 000.

Finland-Turku/Loimaa area (FIN-TUL, FU)
Residents of Turku city and Loimaa town with neighbouring rural communities in southwestern Finland. Known to have the lowest cardiovascular mortality in Finland. Epidemiological studies of this area date back to the Seven Countries Study. A coronary-event register was set up in Turku in 1972. The area was included in FINMONICA to provide a contrast with the east. The local economy is relatively strong. The total population in 1991 was 200 000.

Funding
1. National Public Health Institute. 2. North Karelia Central Hospital, Kuopio University Hospital, City of Turku, Loimaa District Hospital. 3. Academy of Finland, Foundation for Cardiovascular Research.

Dates
Coronary-event registration: 1983–1992. Stroke-event registration, North Karelia: 1982–1991; Kuopio: 1983–1992; Turku: 1983–1992. Coronary care: September to December 1986, 1989 and 1992. Population surveys: 1982, 1987 and 1992.

Additional description
FINMONICA monitored the national action to reduce high rates of coronary heart disease and stroke in Finland. Five-yearly risk-factor surveys had previously been conducted in North Karelia and Kuopio in 1972 and 1977, and they are being continued, making the long-term analysis of risk-factor trends possible. The national personal identification number and computerized databases helped to ensure full coverage of event registration. Record linkage is used in prospective follow-up. Turku registered stroke at all ages, others registered stroke up to age 74.

Local research interests
FINMONICA included additional risk factors and cardiovascular and non-cardiovascular outcomes. Special interests have been smoking, diet, vitamins, electrolytes, socioeconomic factors, diabetes and other metabolic disorders, haemostatic factors.

Continuing activity
Coronary and stroke-event registration continued until 1998 in some but not all of the FINMONICA communities. Since then, coronary-event registration has continued in some but not all of the FINMONICA communities. Another risk-factor survey was carried out in all FINMONICA areas in 1997. The next one was completed in 2002. The risk-factor surveys have also been extended to cover several other geographic areas of Finland.

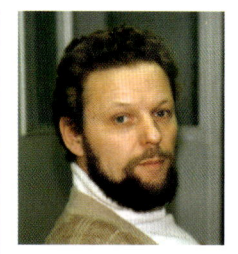

Key personnel
PI 1987–: Jaakko Tuomilehto. Former PI 1982–87: Pekka Puska. Both coronary and stroke-event registration: Pirjo Immonen-Räihä, Esko Kaarsalo, Markku Mähönen, Veikko Salomaa. Coronary-event registration: Antti Arstila, Matti Ketonen, Seppo Lehto, Heikki Miettinen, Harri Mustaniemi, Matti Niemelä, Pertti Palomäki, Kalevi Pyörälä, Tapio Vuorenmaa. Stroke-event registration: Erkki V. Narva, Kalervo Salmi, Cinzia Sarti, Juhani Sivenius. Population surveys: Erkki Vartiainen, Aulikki Nissinen, Pirjo Pietinen, Pekka Jousilahti. Data management, event-registration: Jorma Torppa.

Selected publications
A comprehensive list of all publications is available at: http://www.ktl.fi/eteo/publications
1. Pietinen P, Uusitalo U, Vartiainen E, Tuomilehto J. Dietary survey of the FINMONICA project in 1982. *Acta Medica Scandinavica Supplementum*, 1988, 728:167–177. PMID:3202027.
2. Marti B, Tuomilehto J, Korhonen HJ, Kartovaara L, Vartiainen E, Pietinen P, Puska P. Smoking and leanness: evidence for change in Finland. *British Medical Journal*, 1989, 298:1287–1290. PMID:2500198.

Jaakko Tuomilehto

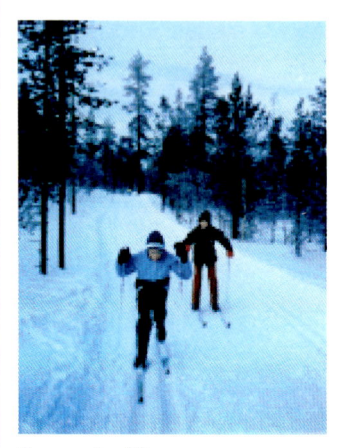

Cross-country skiing

3. Salomaa V, Korhonen HJ, Tuomilehto J, Vartiainen E, Pietinen P, Kartovaara L, Gref CG, Nissinen A, Puska P. Serum cholesterol distribution, measurement frequency and cholesterol awareness in three geographical areas of Finland. *European Heart Journal*, 1990, 11:294–301. PMID:2331997.
4. Marti B, Tuomilehto J, Salomaa V, Kartovaara L, Korhonen HJ, Pietinen P. Body fat distribution in the Finnish population: environmental determinants and predictive power for cardiovascular risk factor levels. *Journal of Epidemiology and Community Health*, 1991, 45:131–137. PMID:2072072.
5. Salomaa V, Jauhiainen M, Pietinen P, Korhonen HJ, Kartovaara L, Vartiainen E, Tuomilehto J. Five-year trend in serum HDL-lipoprotein cholesterol in the Finnish population aged 25–64 years. A suggestion of an increase. *Atherosclerosis*, 1991, 86:39–48. PMID:2064634.
6. Tuomilehto J, Korhonen HJ, Kartovaara L, Salomaa V, Stengård JH, Pitkänen M, Aro A, Javela K, Uusitupa M, Pitkäniemi J. Prevalence of diabetes mellitus and impaired glucose tolerance in the middle-aged population of three areas in Finland. *International Journal of Epidemiology*, 1991, 20:1010–1017. PMID:1800397.
7. Salomaa V, Arstila M, Kaarsalo E, Ketonen M, Kuulasmaa K, Lehto S, Miettinen H, Mustaniemi H, Niemelä M, Palomäki P, Pyörälä K, Torppa J, Tuomilehto J, Vuorenmaa T. Trends in the incidence of and mortality from coronary heart disease in Finland, 1983–1988. *American Journal of Epidemiology*, 1992, 136:1303–1315. PMID:1488958.
8. Tuomilehto J, Arstila M, Kaarsalo E, Kankaanpää J, Ketonen M, Kuulasmaa K, Lehto S, Miettinen H, Mustaniemi H, Palomäki P, Puska P, Pyörälä K, Salomaa V, Torppa J, Vuorenmaa T. Acute myocardial infarction (AMI) in Finland—baseline data from the FINMONICA AMI register in 1983–1985. *European Heart Journal*, 1992, 13:577–587. PMID:1618197.
9. Tuomilehto J, Sarti S, Narva EV, Salmi K, Sivenius J, Kaarsalo E, Salomaa V, Torppa J. The FINMONICA Stroke Register: Community-based stroke registration and analysis of stroke incidence in Finland, 1983–1985. *American Journal of Epidemiology*, 1992, 135:1259–1270. PMID:1626542.
10. Sarti C, Tuomilehto J, Sivenius J, Kaarsalo E, Narva EV, Salmi K, Salomaa V, Torppa J. Stroke mortality and case-fatality rates in three geographic areas of Finland from 1983 to 1986. *Stroke*, 1993, 24:1140–1147. PMID:8342187.
11. Palomäki P, Miettinen H, Mustaniemi H, Lehto S, Pyörälä K, Mähönen M, Tuomilehto J. Diagnosis of acute myocardial infarction by MONICA and FINMONICA diagnostic criteria in comparison with hospital discharge diagnosis. *Journal of Clinical Epidemiology*, 1994, 47:659–666. PMID:7722578.
12. Vartiainen E, Puska P, Jousilahti P, Korhonen HJ, Tuomilehto J, Nissinen A. Twenty-year trends in coronary risk factors in North Karelia and in other areas of Finland. *International Journal of Epidemiology*, 1994, 23:495–504. PMID:7960373.
13. Vartiainen E, Puska P, Pekkanen J, Tuomilehto J, Jousilahti P. Changes in risk factors explain changes in mortality from ischaemic heart disease in Finland. *British Medical Journal*, 1994, 309:23–27. PMID:8044063.
14. Mähönen M, Miettinen H, Pyörälä K, Molarius A, Salomaa V, Kuulasmaa K, for the FINMONICA AMI Register Study Team. Hospital discharge register data in the assessment of trends in acute myocardial infarction. *Annals of Medicine*, 1995, 27:547–554. PMID:8541030.
15. Salomaa V, Miettinen H, Palomäki P, Arstila M, Mustaniemi H, Kuulasmaa K, Tuomilehto J, for the FINMONICA AMI Register Study Group. Diagnostic features of acute myocardial infarction—changes over time from 1983 to 1990: results from the FINMONICA AMI register study. *Journal of Internal Medicine*, 1995, 237:151–159. PMID:7852917.
16. Vartiainen E, Sarti C, Tuomilehto J, Kuulasmaa K. Do changes in cardiovascular risk factors explain changes in mortality from stroke in Finland? *British Medical Journal*, 1995, 310:901–904. PMID:7719179.
17. Immonen-Räihä P, Arstila M, Tuomilehto J, Haikio M, Mononen A, Vuorenmaa T, Torppa J, Parvinen I. 21-year trends in incidence of myocardial infarction and mortality from coronary disease in middle-age. *European Heart Journal*, 1996, 17:1495–1502. PMID:8909905.
18. Jakovljevic D, Salomaa V, Sivenius J, Tamminen M, Sarti C, Salmi K, Kaarsalo E, Narva EV, Immonen-Räihä P, Torppa J, Tuomilehto J. Seasonal variation in the occurrence of stroke in a Finnish adult population. The FINMONICA Stroke Register. *Stroke*, 1996, 27:1774–1779. PMID:8841328.
19. Jousilahti P, Vartiainen E, Tuomilehto J, Puska P. Twenty-year dynamics of serum cholesterol levels in the middle-aged population of eastern Finland. *Annals of Internal Medicine*, 1996, 125:713–722. PMID:8929004.
20. Salomaa V, Miettinen H, Kuulasmaa K, Niemelä M, Ketonen M, Vuorenmaa T, Lehto S, Palomäki P, Mähönen M, Immonen-Räihä P, Arstila M, Kaarsalo E, Mustaniemi H, Torppa J, Tuomilehto J, Puska P, Pyörälä K. Decline of coronary heart disease mortality in Finland during 1983 to 1992: roles of incidence, recurrence and case-fatality. The FINMONICA MI Register Study. *Circulation*, 1996, 94:3130–3137. PMID:8989120.
21. Tuomilehto J, Rastenyte D, Sivenius J, Sarti C, Immonen-Räihä P, Kaarsalo E, Kuulasmaa K, Narva EV, Salomaa V, Salmi K, Torppa J, Tuomilehto J. Ten-year trends in stroke incidence and mortality in the FINMONICA Stroke Study. *Stroke*, 1996, 27:825–832. PMID:8623100.
22. Immonen-Räihä P, Mähönen M, Tuomilehto J, Salomaa V, Kaarsalo E, Narva EV, Salmi K, Sarti C, Sivenius J, Alhainen K, Torppa J. Trends in case-fatality of stroke in Finland during 1983 to 1992. *Stroke*, 1997, 28:2493–2499. PMID:9412639.
23. Jousilahti P, Vartiainen E, Tuomilehto J, Pekkanen J, Puska P. Role of known risk factors in explaining the difference in the risk of coronary heart disease between eastern and south-western Finland. *Annals of Medicine*, 1998, 30:481–487. PMID:9814835.
24. Kaarisalo MM, Immonen-Räihä P, Marttila RJ, Salomaa V, Torppa J, Tuomilehto J, for the FINMONICA MI and Stroke Register Teams. Stroke after Myocardial Infarction. *Cardiovascular Disease Prevention*, 1998, 1:200–206. PMID:na.
25. Kastarinen MJ, Salomaa VV, Vartiainen EA, Jousilahti PJ, Tuomilehto JO, Puska PM, Nissinen AM. Trends in blood pressure levels and control of hypertension in Finland from 1982 to 1997. *Journal of Hypertension*, 1998, 16:1379–1387. PMID:9746125.

Jaakko Tuomilehto

#59 France-Country Coordinating Centre

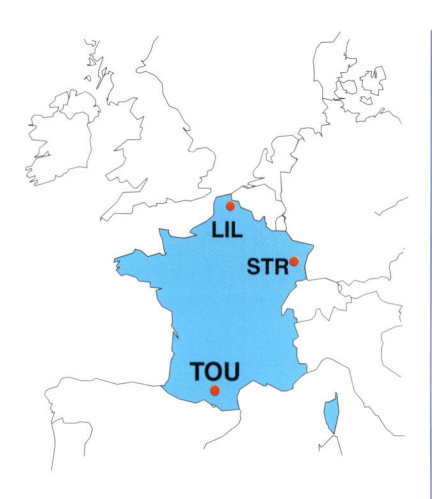

Administrative centre
Unité 258-INSERM, Hopital Paul Brousse, 16 av Paul Vaillant-Couturier, 94807 Villejuif Cedex, France
T +33 2 4559 5109; F +33 1 4726 9454

Description
The French Coordinating Centre, located in Unit 258 in Paris, initiated the national studies. It managed the French database and organized test case and ECG coding seminars. It also organized the 3rd International MONICA Congress in Nice (15–16 September 1989) and the publication of its proceedings in the Revue d'Epidémiologie et de Santé Publique. It initiated the ECTIM (case-control) Study and the PRIME (cohort) Study in cooperation with the three French Centres and the Belfast Centre. It currently coordinates the French simplified coronary heart disease registers.

Key personnel
PI: Pierre Ducimetière. Former PI: JL Richard. Others: A. Bingham. Formerly: T. Lang.

Selected publications (and see French MCCs)
1. Les Registres Français Des Cardiopathies Ischémiques. *L'infarctus du myocarde en France: données des trois registres des cardiopathies ischémiques de Lille, Strasbourg et Toulouse. Période 1985–1992*. Edité par la Fédération Française de Cardiologie, Oct. 1996. (French). PMID:na.
2. Les Registres Français Des Cardiopathies Ischémiques. *Facteurs de risque et comportements de prévention dans la population des trois registres MONICA–France. Enquête de population 1994–1997*. Edité par la Fédération Française de Cardiologie, Sept. 1998. (French). PMID:na
3. Lang T, Ducimetière P, Arveiler D, Amouyel P, Ferrières J, Ruidavets JB, Montaye M, Haas B, Bingham A. Is hospital care involved in inequalities in coronary heart disease morbidity and mortality in France? Results from the French WHO-MONICA Project in men aged 30–64. *Journal of Epidemiology and Community Health*, 1998, 52:665–671. PMID:10023467.

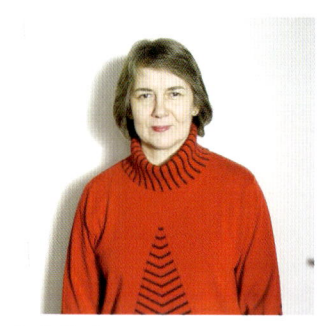

Pierre Ducimetière, Annie Bingham

- organized 3rd MONICA Congress in Nice
- publication in *Revue d'Epidémiologie et de Santé Publique*, 1990, 38.

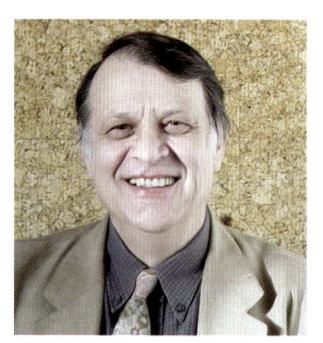

Pierre Ducimetière

Annie Bingham

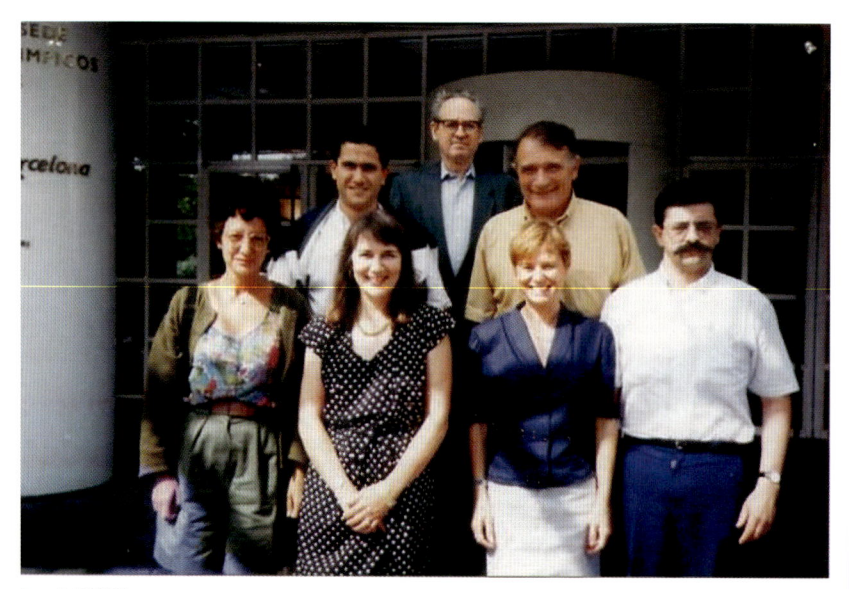

French MONICA group

#60 France-Lille (FRA-LIL, FL)

- the northernmost of the three French centres
- highest mortality rates in France
- north-south gradient challenges the so-called French Paradox

MCC 59: MONICA Lille
Single Reporting Unit.

Administrative centre
Department of Epidemiology and Public Health, INSERM U508,
Institut Pasteur de Lille, 1 rue Albert Calmette, B.P. 245, 59019 Lille Cedex, France
T +33 3 2087 7710; F +33 3 2087 7894
E-mail: philippe.amouyel@pasteur-lille.fr

Population
Residents aged 25–64 of the urban community of Lille in the Département du Nord, containing 86 administrative areas. The population is predominantly urban and the socioeconomic level is rather low. Mortality rates are high for all causes of death, and the highest for coronary heart disease in France. There is a university cardiology hospital located in Lille and 11 acute hospitals in the area, half of which are privately funded. The total population in 1991 was 1 068 000.

Funding
1. Comité National des Registres, Ministry of health. 2. INSERM (Institut National de la Santé et de la Recherche Médicale) 3. InVS (Institut de Veille Sanitaire). 4. University of Lille II. 5. Conseil Régional Nord-Pas-de-Calais. 6. Institut Pasteur de Lille.

Dates
Coronary-event registration: 1985–1994. Coronary care: 1986–1987, 1989, 1990–1994. Population surveys: 1986–1989, 1995/1996 (no middle survey). No stroke registration.

Additional description
All data are standardized across the three French centres with quality control procedures organized by the French coordinating centre. This fostered specific French studies and facilitated the estimation of trends in French coronary heart disease. The Lille Centre participated in the EUROASPIRE I and II Study (European Society of Cardiology), in a case-control study (ECTIM); and an on-going prospective study (PRIME) together with the two other French centres, and the UK-Belfast Centre.

Local research interests
Meteorology and air pollution; environmental risk factors. Genetics of coronary heart disease. Obesity, lipids and diabetes. Nutrition surveys.

Continuing activity
Registration continues with an extended age range of 35–75, as with the two other French centres. Cohort study (PRIME) continues.

Key personnel
PI: Philippe Amouyel. Co-PI: Michèle Montaye. Former Co-PIs: JL Salomez (1985–1989). MC Nuttens (1985–1989). G. Luc (1990) Population survey: D. Cottel.

Selected publications
1. Amouyel P, Arveiler D, Cambou JP, Montaye M, Ruidavets JB, Bingham A, Schaffer P, Richard JL. Myocardial infarction case-fatality gradient in three French regions: influence of acute coronary care. *International Journal of Epidemiology*, 1994, 23:700–709. PMID:8002182.
2. Dallongeville J, Marécaux N, Ducimetière P, Ferrières J, Arveiler D, Bingham A, Ruidavets JB, Simon C, Amouyel P. Influence of alcohol consumption and various beverages on waist girth and waist-to-hip ratio in a sample of French men and women. *International Journal of Obesity and Related Metabolic Disorders*, 1998, 22:1178–1183. PMID:9877253.
3. Meirhaeghe A, Helbecque N, Cottel D, Amouyel P. Beta2–adrenoceptor gene polymorphisms, body weight and physical activity. *Lancet*, 1999, 353:896–896. PMID:10093985.
4. Danet S, Richard F, Montaye M, Beauchant S, Lemaire B, Graux C, Cottel D, Marécaux N, Amouyel P. Unhealthy effects of atmospheric temperature and pressure on the occurrence of myocardial infarction and coronary deaths—a 10-year survey: the Lille WHO-MONICA project. *Circulation*, 1999, 100: E1–E7. PMID:10393689.
5. Montaye M, De Backer D, DeBacker G, Amouyel P. The EUROASPIRE Study Group Overweight and Obesity: A major challenge for coronary heart disease secondary prevention in clinical practice in Europe. *European Heart Journal*, 2000, 21:808–813. PMID:10781352.
6. Meirhaeghe A, Martin G, Nemoto M, Deeb S, Cottel D, Auwerx J, Amouyel P, Helbecque N. Intronic polymorphism in the fatty acid transport protein 1 gene is associated with increased plasma triglyceride levels in a French population. *Arteriosclerosis, Thrombosis, and Vascular Biology*, 2000, 20:1330–1334. PMID:10807750.
7. Cottel D, Dallongeville J, Wagner A, Ruidavets JB, Arveiler D, Ferrières J, Bingham A, Marécaux N, Amouyel P. The north-east-south gradient of coronary heart disease mortality and case-fatality rates in France are consistent with a similar gradient in risk factor clusters. *European Journal of Epidemiology*, 2000, 16:317–322. PMID:10959938.
8. Dallongeville J, Marecaux N, Cottel D, Bingham A, Amouyel P. Association between nutrition knowledge and nutritional intake in middle-aged men from Northern France. *Public Health and Nutrition*, 2001, 4:27–33. PMID:11255493.
9. Mediene-Benchekor S, Brousseau T, Richard F, Benhamamouch S, Amouyel P and the ECTIM study Group. Blood lipid concentrations and risk of myocardial infarction. *Lancet*, 2001, 358:1064–1065. PMID: 11589940.

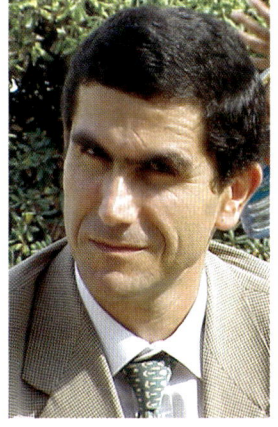

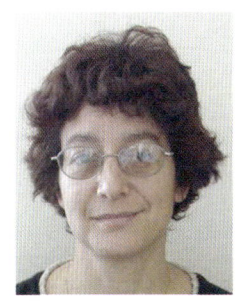

Philippe Amouyel

Philippe Amouyel

Michèle Montaye

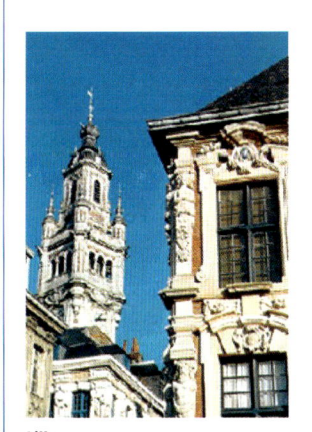

Lille

#61 France-Strasbourg (FRA-STR, FS)

- one of the three French MONICA centres, located in the north-east of the country
- high coronary-event and mortality rates for France
- studies of delays in hospitalization for patients suffering from an acute MI

MCC 54: MONICA Strasbourg
Single Reporting Unit (Bas-Rhin).

Administrative centre
Department of Epidemiology and Public Health, Faculty of Medicine
11, rue Humann, 67085 Strasbourg Cedex, France
T +33 3 9024 3195; F +33 3 9024 3189
E-mail: monica@medecine.u–strasbg.fr

Population
Residents aged 25–64 of the Bas-Rhin district of north-eastern France, across the Rhine from Germany. While the west of the district is rural with agriculture and viniculture, 42% of the population live in Strasbourg, a university city with high technology industry, a young expanding population, and low unemployment rates. However, compared with the French average, there is excess mortality from all causes, and from coronary heart disease. The total population in 1991 was 960 000.

Funding
1. INSERM (Institut National de la Santé et de la Recherche Médicale). 2. InVS (Institut National de Veille Sanitaire).

Dates
Coronary-event registration: 198(4*)5–1993. Coronary care: 1985, 1989–93. Population surveys: 1985–1987, 1995–1997. No middle survey. No stroke registration. (*Not in collaborative analyses.)

Additional description
The France-Strasbourg Centre is one of three French MONICA centres, actively collaborating with the support of the Coordinating Centre in Paris. The Strasbourg Centre has coronary-event rates similar to those observed in neighbouring MONICA centres such as France-Lille, Belgium, Germany and Switzerland. In the Bas-Rhin area, health insurance authorities have decided to promote a five-year preventive programme for cardiovascular disease that started in 2001.

Local research interests
Delivery of care, delays in hospitalization (pre-hospital phase). Physical activity, obesity; diet. Management of risk factors.

Continuing activity
Registration of coronary events continues. Cohort study (PRIME) continues.

Key personnel
PI: Dominique Arveiler. Co-PI: Paul Schaffer. Researchers: Bernadette Haas, Aline Wagner.

Selected publications
1. Simon C, Nuttens MC, Ruidavets JB, Bingham A, Schlienger JL, Saini J, Cambou JP, Richard JL, Romon M, Hedelin G. Blood pressure and dietary intake in a French population sample from three regions. *Revue d'Epidémiologie et de Santé Publique*, 1990, 38:531–538. PMID:2082462.
2. Schlienger JL, Simon C, Aby MA, Arveiler D, Schaffer P. [Lipid profile in adult population representative of a French district (Bas-Rhin)]. *Pathologie–Biologie* (Paris), 1991, 39:195–199. (French). PMID:2052423.
3. Fender M, Arveiler D, Facello A, Marine-Barjoan E, Uettwiller E, Jacques D, Veron C, Meyer V, Haas B, Hédelin G, Bingham A, Richard JL, Schaffer P. [Towards a decrease of myocardial infarction in the Bas-Rhin region? Results of the first six years of the MONICA Strasbourg register]. *Annales de Cardiologie et d'Angéiologie*, 1994, 43:373–379. (French). PMID:7993030.
4. Haas B, Arveiler D, Cambou JP, Amouyel P, Bingham A, Richard JL, Schaffer P. Therapeutic management of myocardial infarction: trends observed in the French MONICA Project between 1985 and 1991. *Revue d'Epidémiologie et de Santé Publique*, 1996, 44 Suppl.1:S53–S61. PMID:8935865.
5. Arveiler D. Epidemiology of coronary heart disease in women. *Archives des Maladies du Coeur et des Vaisseaux*, 1996, 89:25–31. PMID:na.
6. Hurlimann C, Arveiler D, Romier-Borgnat S, Montalvo O, Schaffer P. [Evaluation of delays before treatment of acute myocardial infarction: results of a survey conducted in Alsace]. *Archives des Maladies du Coeur et des Vaisseaux*, 1998, 91: 873–878. (French). PMID:9749179.
7. Lang T, Ducimetière P, Arveiler D, Amouyel P, Ferrières J, Ruidavets JB, Montaye M, Haas B, Bingham A. Trends and geographical disparities in coronary heart disease in France: are results concordant when different definitions of events are used? *International Journal of Epidemiology*, 1999, 28:1050–1058. PMID:10661647.
8. Eilstein D, Quénel P, Hédelin G, Kleinpeter J, Arveiler D, Schaffer P. [Air pollution and myocardial infarction. Strasbourg, France, 1984–89]. *Revue d'Epidémiologie et de Santé Publique*, 2001, 49:13–25. PMID:11226915.
9. Wagner A, Simon C, Ducimetière P, Montaye M, Bongard V, Yarnell J, Bingham A, Hédelin G, Amouyel P, Ferrières J, Evans A, Arveiler D. Leisure-time physical activity and regular walking or cycling to work are associated with adiposity and 5-year weight gain in middle-aged men: the PRIME Study. Interna-tional *Journal of Obesity and Related Metabolic Disorders*, 2001, 25:940–948. PMID:11443490.

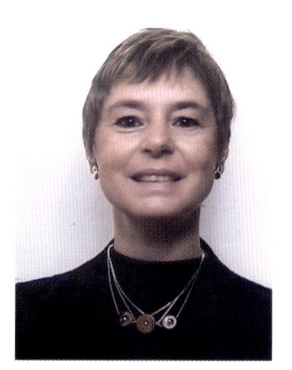

Dominique Arveiler

Paul Schaffer

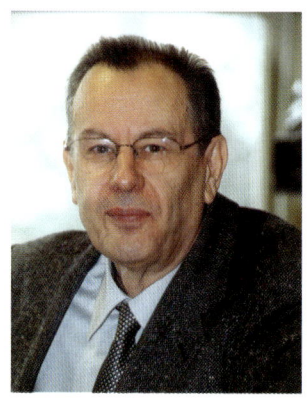

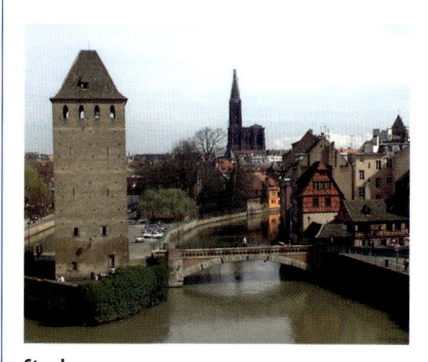

Strasbourg

Dominique Arveiler

#62 France-Toulouse (FRA-TOU, FT)

- lowest proportion of deaths from cardiovascular disease in MONICA
- low all-cause mortality
- average smoking and cholesterol levels, low blood pressure

MCC 55: MONICA Toulouse
Single Reporting Unit (Haute Garonne).

Administrative centre
Cardiovascular Epidemiology Unit, INSERM 558, Department of Epidemiology,
37 Allées Jules Guesde, 31073 Toulouse Cedex, France
T +33 5 6152 1870; F +33 5 6226 4240
E-mail: ferriere@cict.fr

Population
Residents aged 25–64 of the Haute-Garonne department, north of the Pyrénées, southwestern France. Haute-Garonne is a rural department with a total population in 1991 of 939 000, 71% of whom live in the city of Toulouse. Toulouse is known for aeronautical, aerospace and other high technology industries. It is located in a sunny, hot, rural area. The region has low all-cause mortality rates.

Funding
1. InVS (Institut de Veille Sanitaire). 2. INSERM (Institut National de la Santé et de la Recherche Médicale).

Dates
Coronary-event registration: 1985–1993. Coronary care: 1986 and 1989–1993. Population surveys: 1985–87, 1988–91, 1994–96. No stroke registration.

Additional description
The three French centres carried out the only cardiovascular epidemiological studies in France and facilitated the detailed analysis of the reported low mortality from coronary heart disease in France, called the French Paradox. (See French collaborative and WHO MONICA Project publications). Several hypotheses, genetic and/or environmental, have been put forward to explain low CHD rates in southern Europe. Research teams have been created exploiting advances in molecular biology, and improved standardization in the recording of environmental factors, such as nutrition and physical activity.

Local research interests
Public health: comprehension, application and dissemination of guidelines for cardiovascular disease-prevention in the population. Underlying causes of low coronary disease rates in the region. Studies of management of myocardial infarction management, specifically the role of invasive cardiology.

Continuing activity
Registration continues.

Key personnel
PI: Jean Ferrières. Co-PI: Jean-Bernard Ruidavets. Former PI: Jean-Pierre Cambou. Researchers: Pedro Marques-Vidal, Thierry Lang.

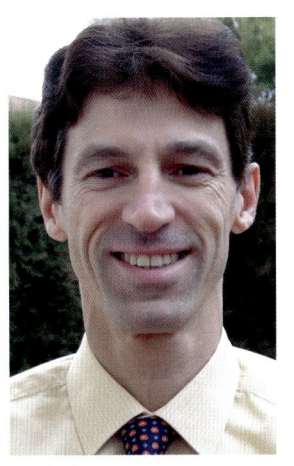

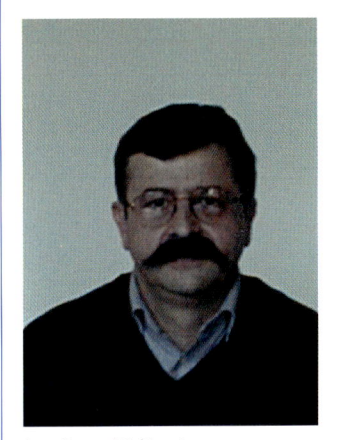

Selected publications
1. Ferrières J, Cambou JP, Ruidavets JB, Pous J. Trends in acute myocardial infarction prognosis and treatment in southwestern France between 1985 and 1990 (The MONICA Project-Toulouse). *American Journal of Cardiology*, 1995, 75:1202–1205. PMID:7778539.
2. Marques-Vidal P, Ducimetière P, Evans A, Cambou JP, Arveiler D. Alcohol consumption and myocardial infarction: a case-control study in France and Northern Ireland. *American Journal of Epidemiology*, 1996, 143:1089–1093. PMID:8633596.
3. Ferrières J, Ruidavets JB. Association between resting heart rate and hypertension treatment in a general population. *American Journal of Hypertension*, 1999, 12:628–31. PMID:10371373.
4. Ferrières J, Ruidavets JB, Fauvel J, Perret B, Taraszkiewicz D, Fourcade J, Niéto M, Chap H, Puel J. Angiotensin I-converting enzyme gene polymorphism in a low-risk European population for coronary artery disease. *Atherosclerosis*, 1999, 142:211–216. PMID: 9920524.
5. Ferrières J, Elias A, Ruidavets JB, Cantet C, Bongard V, Fauvel J, Boccalon H. Carotid intima-media thickness and coronary heart disease risk factors in a low-risk population. *Journal of Hypertension*, 1999, 17:743–748. PMID:10459870.
6. Danchin N, Vaur L, Genès N, Etienne S, Angioï M, Ferrières J, Cambou JP. Treatment of acute myocardial infarction by primary coronary angioplasty or intravenous thrombolysis in the "real world": one-year results from a nationwide French survey. *Circulation*, 1999, 99:2639–2644. PMID:10338456.
7. Marques-Vidal P, Ruidavets JB, Cambou JP, Ferrières J. Incidence, recurrence and case-fatality rates for myocardial infarction in coronary heart disease mortality in south-western France, 1985–1993. *Heart*, 2000, 84:171–175. PMID:10908254.
8. Ruidavets JB, Teissedre PL, Ferrières J, Carando S, Bougard G, Cabanis JC. Catechin in the Mediterranean diet: vegetable, fruit or wine? *Atherosclerosis*, 2000, 153:107–117. PMID:11058705.
9. Marques-Vidal P, Ruidavets JB, Cambou JP, Ferrières J. Trends in hypertension prevalence and management in south-western France, 1985–1996. *Journal of Clinical Epidemiology*, 2000, 53:1230–1235. PMID: 11146269.

Jean Ferrières

Jean Ferrières

Jean Bernard Ruidavets

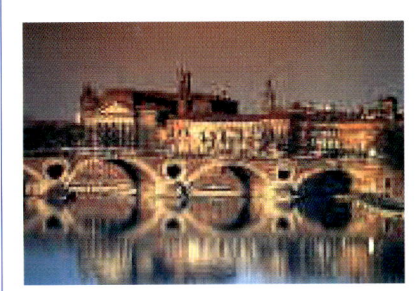

Toulouse

#63 Germany-Augsburg (GER-AUG, GA)

Germany-Augsburg Rural (GER-AUR, GR)
Germany-Augsburg Urban (GER-AUU, GU)

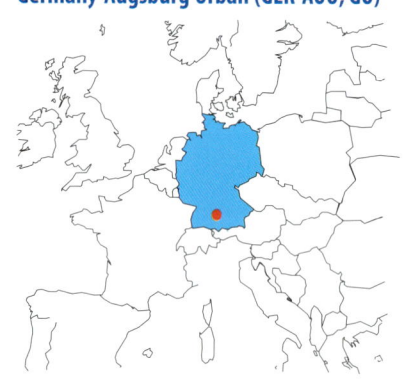

- the MONICA population in Bavaria
- relatively low coronary-event rates
- case fatality above average and failed to fall
- hosted First MONICA Congress in March 1986
- hosted Fifth Council of Principal Investigators in October 1988

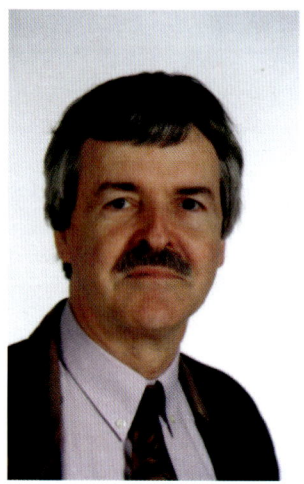

Ulrich Keil

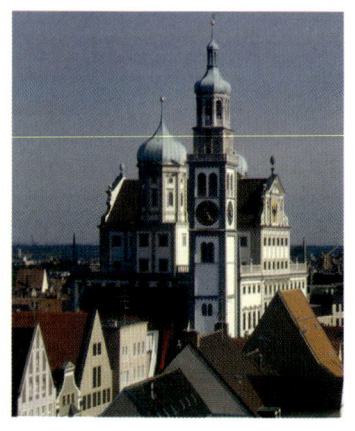

Augsburg

MCC 26: Augsburg
Two Reporting Units, separate for most analyses, merged for coronary care.

Administrative centres
Institute of Epidemiology and Social Medicine, University of Münster,
Domagkstrasse 3, D-48129 Münster, Germany
T +49 251 83 55396; F +49 251 83 55300.
E-mail: keilu@uni-muenster.de
and
Institute of Epidemiology, GSF-Research Centre for Environment and Health,
D-85758 Neuherberg, Germany

Population
Augsburg MONICA, Bavaria, south Germany, with a total population in 1991 of 575 000, is in almost equal halves: city of Augsburg (Reporting Unit 1) and the less urban Landkreis Augsburg and Landkreis Aichach-Friedberg (Reporting Unit 2). Manufacturing and services support the economy. Coronary-event registration of residents aged 25–74, used hot pursuit in 26 hospitals in and around the study area; but 70% of admissions were to Augsburg's central hospital. Each population survey recruited 5000 participants by random cluster-sampling; initial survey age 25–64, middle and final surveys, 25–74. Response rates were 75–80%.

Funding
1. GSF Forschungszentrum für Umwelt und Gesundheit, München. 2. Bundesministerium für Bildung und Wissenschaft, Bonn. 3. Pharmazeutische Industrie. 4. Stifterverband für die Deutsche Wissenschaft, Essen.

Dates
Coronary-event registration and coronary care: 1985–1995. Population surveys: 1984/85, 1989/90, 1994/95. No stroke registration.

Additional description
Founded by the Romans, Augsburg has been prominent in Germany since medieval times. It is the third largest city in Bavaria. The MONICA-Augsburg Project stimulated awareness of cardiovascular disease, and additional health research in the area. The local medical community were supportive of MONICA, but were worried initially by the high community case-fatality from myocardial infarction (found in all populations) and subsequently by the failure of hospital case-fatality to decline.

Local research interests
Population versus clinical view of case fatality. Left ventricular hypertrophy. Nutrition, alcohol, fibrinogen, C-reactive protein (CRP), blood viscosity, genetic epidemiology, diabetes, hypertension.

Continuing activity
Registration and population surveys continue. Cohort studies have been developed from the three surveys and are the only population-based cardiovascular cohort studies in Germany.

Key personnel
PI: Ulrich Keil. Others: Hannelore Löwel, Hans-Werner Hense, Jutta Stieber, Angela Döring, Birgit Filipiak.

Selected publications
Comprehensive list and abstracts available at http://medweb.uni-muenster.de/institute/epi/forschung/index.html

1. Löwel H, Lewis M, Hörmann A, Keil U. Case finding, data quality aspects and comparability of myocardial infarction registers: results of a south German register study. *Journal of Clinical Epidemiology*, 1991, 44:249–260. PMID:1999684.
2. Keil U, Chambless L, Filipiak B, Härtel U. Alcohol and blood pressure and its interaction with smoking and other behavioural variables: results from the MONICA Augsburg Survey 1984/85. *Journal of Hypertension*, 1991, 9:491–498. PMID:1653287.
3. Hense HW, Stender M, Bors W, Keil U. Lack of an association between serum vitamin E and myocardial infarction in a population with high vitamin E levels. *Atherosclerosis*, 1993, 103:21–28. PMID:8280182.
4. Schunkert H, Hense HW, Holmer SR, Stender M, Perz S, Keil U, Lorell BH, Riegger GA. Association between a deletion polymorphism of the angiotensin-converting-enzyme gene and left ventricular hypertrophy. *New England Journal of Medicine*, 1994, 330:1634–1638. PMID:8177269.
5. Koenig W, Sund M, Lowe GDO, Lee AJ, Resch KL, Tunstall-Pedoe H, Keil U, Ernst E. Geographical variations in plasma viscosity and relation to coronary event rates. *Lancet*, 1994, 344:711–714. PMID:7915775.
6. Keil U, Chambless L, Döring A, Filipiak B, Stieber J. The relation of alcohol intake to coronary heart disease and all cause mortality in a beer drinking population. *Epidemiology*, 1997, 8:150–156. PMID:9229206.
7. Keil U, Liese AD, Hense HW, Filipiak B, Döring A, Stieber J, Löwel H. Classical risk factors and their impact on incident non-fatal and fatal myocardial infarction and all-cause mortality in southern Germany. Results from the MONICA Augsburg cohort study 1984–1992. *European Heart Journal*, 1998, 19:1197–1207. PMID:9740341.
8. Hense HW, Filipiak B, Döring A, Stieber J, Liese A, Keil U. Ten-year trends of cardiovascular risk factors in the MONICA Augsburg region in southern Germany: results from the 1984/1985, 1989/1990, and 1994/1995 surveys. *Cardiovascular Disease Prevention*, 1998, 1:318–327. PMID:na.
9. Liese AD, Hense HW, Brenner H, Löwel H, Keil U. Assessing the impact of classical risk factors on myocardial infarction by rate advancement periods. *American Journal of Epidemiology*, 2000, 152:884–888. PMID: 11085401.

Ulrich Keil

#64 Germany-Bremen (GER-BRE, GB)

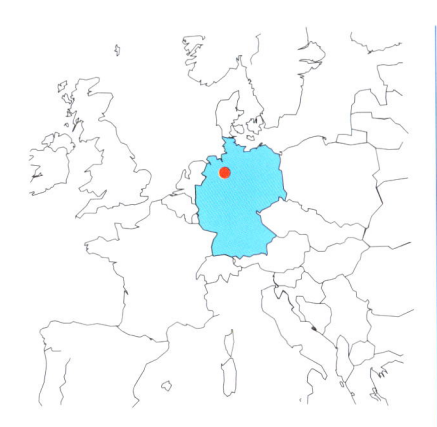

- study of primary prevention in part of the population
- interest in drug utilization
- coronary-event trend and risk-factor populations differ

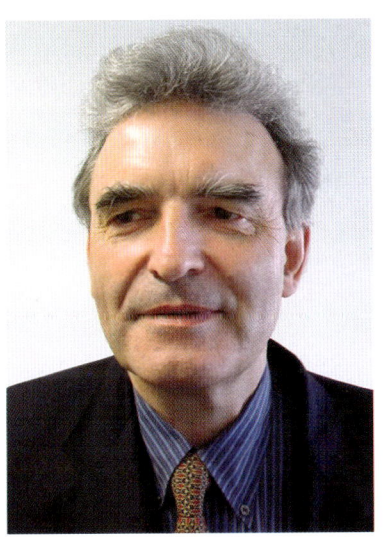

Eberhard Greiser

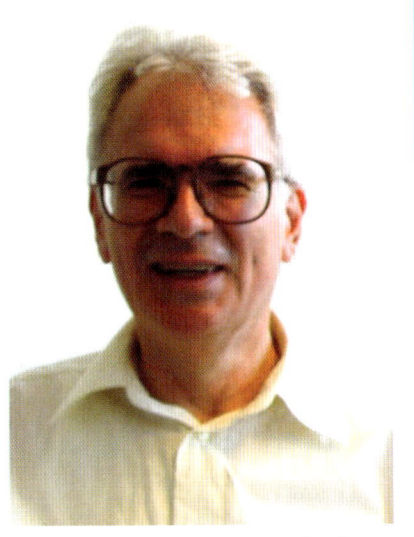

Bert Herman

MCC 24: Bremen
Two Reporting Units, merged for coronary-event registration, (GER-BREb). Risk-factor results in the Monograph and collaborative papers are from one only: North and West Bremen (BREa).

Administrative centre
Bremen Institute for Prevention Research and Social Medicine (BIPS),
Linzer Straße 8-10, D-28359 Bremen, Germany
T +49 421 59596 0; F +49 421 59596 65
Collaborating Centre and Reference Centre for Drug Epidemiology.

Population
Residents aged 25–69 of the city of Bremen in two sub-populations: Bremen North and West (Reporting Unit 1), and Bremen City, South and East (Reporting Unit 2). The area of Bremen North and West, predominantly of blue-collar workers, was contemporaneously one of the intervention regions in the German Cardiovascular Prevention Study. The total population of GER-BREb in 1991 was 552 000.

Funding
1. Bundesanstalt für Arbeit.

Dates
Coronary-event registration and coronary care: 1985–1992. Population surveys: 1984 (Reporting Unit 1 only, BREb), 1988 and 1991/92 (BREa). No stroke registration.

Local research interests
Drug epidemiology. Primary prevention of cardiovascular diseases. Interventions on nutrition and smoking.

Continuing activity
Registration and population surveys have ceased. Analyses with focus on drug utilization continue.

Key personnel
PI: Eberhard Greiser. Co-PI 1986–2000: Bertram Herman. Co-PI 2001: Katrin Janhsen.

Selected publications
Comprehensive list and abstracts available at:
http://www.bips.uni-bremen.de
1. Herman B, Greiser E, Helmert U, Klesse R, Bormann C, Grötschel R. Prevalence of cardiovascular disease risk factors in the City of Bremen—the 1984 Bremen baseline health survey of the German Cardiovascular Prevention Study. *Sozial und Präventivmedizin*, 1987, 32:31–38. PMID:na.
2. Herman B, Helmert U, Greiser E. Factors related to blood lipid levels—the Bremen baseline survey of the German Cardiovascular Prevention Study. *Public Health*, 1988, 102:565–575. PMID:3231696.

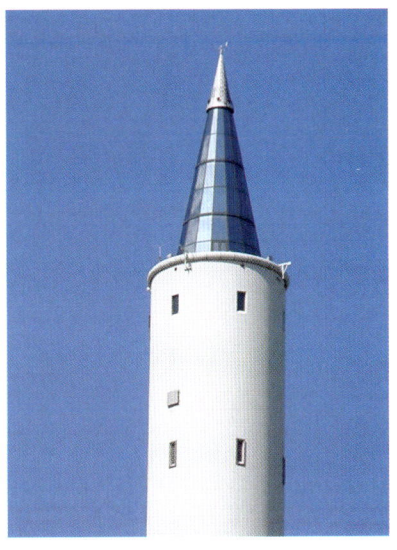

Bremen tower

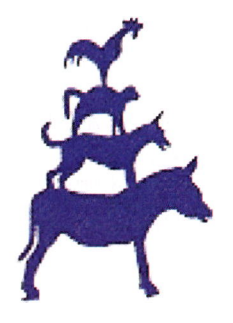

Bremen symbol

3. Herman B, Stüdemann G, Greiser E. Trends in acute myocardial infarction mortality, morbidity and medical care in the city of Bremen: results of a WHO MONICA acute coronary care register, 1985–1988. *Annals of Epidemiology*, 1993, 3 Suppl:62–68. PMID:na.
4. Herman B, Greiser E, Pohlabeln H. A sex difference in short-term survival after initial acute myocardial infarction. The MONICA-Bremen Acute Myocardial Infarction Register, 1985–1990. *European Heart Journal*, 1997, 18:963–970. PMID:9183588.
5. Herman B, Greiser E. Are acute myocardial infarctions becoming smaller? *Journal of Internal Medicine*, 2000, 248:352–354. PMID:11086648.

Eberhard Greiser, Katrin Janhsen

#65 Germany-East Germany (GER-EGE, GE)

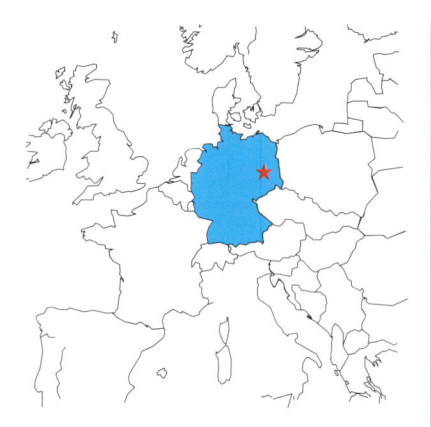

- many Reporting Units scattered over the old East Germany
- majority lost in the early years leaving only 3 at the end
- populations differ for coronary events, coronary care and risk factors
- hosted the Fourth Council of Principal Investigators, Berlin, April 1987

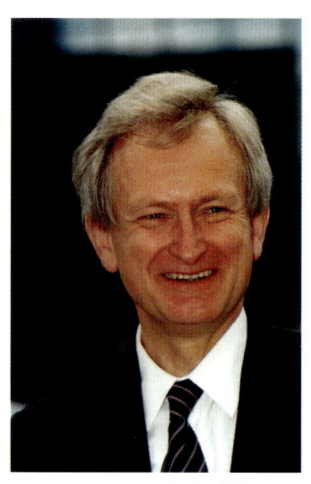

Lothar Heinemann

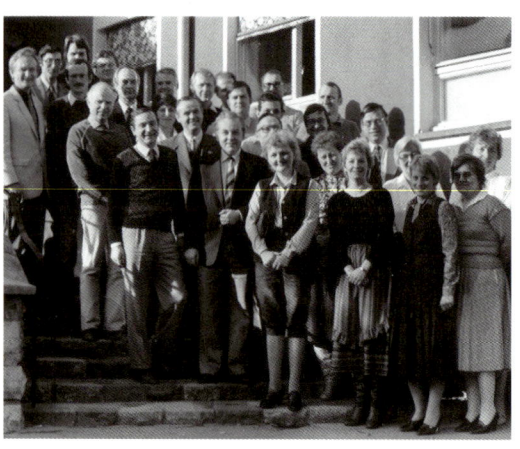

East German MONICA group

MCC 23: MONICA East Germany (previously known as DDR MONICA)

Thirty nine Reporting Units in 1982 became 17 for the MONICA Manual (1990) and fell to three for the main MONICA trends papers and for this Monograph: Erfurt, Chemnitz and Zwickau (EGEa) for coronary-event registration; Chemnitz and Zwickau (EGEb) for risk-factor surveys; Zwickau (EGEd) alone for coronary care. Other Reporting Units contributed to early MONICA Publications through Reporting Unit Aggregates (RUAs) of variable composition named Berlin-Lichtenberg, Cottbus, Halle County, Karl-Marx-Stadt and Rest of DDR MONICA. Detailed analysis of the permutations is beyond the scope of this Monograph but will be available on the MONICA Website.

Administrative centre
Department of Preventive Medicine, Academy of Sciences, Berlin (1982–1990)
after 1990:
ZEG—Centre for Epidemiology & Health Research Berlin,
Invalidenstrasse 115, D-10115 Berlin, Germany
T +49 30 9451 0124; F +49 30 9451 0126
Website: www.zeg-berlin.de

Population
Residents aged 25–74. Of 39 districts in 1982, 22 were excluded before the 1987–89 population survey because of data quality and completeness. After German unification in 1989/90 three Reporting Units (RUs) and the administrative centre continued. The total population of these three in 1991 was 612 000.

Funding
1. Ministry of Health East Germany (GDR). 2. Academy of Sciences Berlin (GDR). 3. Local District Health Departments (GDR). 4. Ministry of Science and Technology (FRG) for continuation of data evaluation (after 1992).

Dates
Coronary-event registration 1984–93: (26, 17, then 3 RUs). Coronary care: 1989–93. Stroke registration—insufficient years for full trend analyses, not included in Monograph (see MONICA Quality assessment of stroke-event registration data). Population surveys: 1982–84, 1988, 1993–94.

Additional description
Health service administrators across East Germany volunteered but found complying with MONICA beyond their resources. Most withdrew, leaving the north unrepresented. German unification involved privatizing healthcare, so East German physicians gave lower priority to MONICA while building their private practices. Funding of MONICA and CINDI (another WHO project) stopped.

Local research interests
Coronary disease and risk-factor differences, social differences and impact of these on life expectancy in East and West Germany.

Key personnel
PIs: Lothar Heinemann and Wolfgang Barth. Coronary-event registration: Ingrid Martin. Stroke registration: Dorothea Eisenblaetter. Psychosocial studies: Michael Weiss. Diet surveys: Chr Thiel. Data management: H Scheadlich, E Claßen.

Surviving RUs: H. Holtz, S. Brasche (Erfurt), S. Böthig (Zwickau), G. Voigt, D Quietsch (Chemnitz).

Selected publications
1. Marti B, Rickenbach M, Keil U, Stieber J, Greiser E, Herman B, Heinemann LAJ, Aßmann A, Schädlich H, Nüssel E, Östor-Lamm E, Gutzwiller F. Variation in coronary risk factor levels of men and women between the German-speaking MONICA centres. *Revue d'Epidémiologie et de Santé Publique*, 1990, 38:479–486. PMID:2082455.
2. Heinemann LAJ, Grabauskas V, Nikitin YP, Rywik SL, Sznajd J. Comparative data on diet from five Eastern Europe communities. *Revue d'Epidémiologie et de Santé Publique*, 1990, 38:525–530. PMID:20822461.
3. Heinemann LAJ, Jones DH. Assessment of physical activity in East Germany. *Annals of Epidemiology*, 1993, 3:86–89. PMID:na.
4. Barth W, Heinemann L. Trends of acute myocardial infarction morbidity and case fatality in East Germany since 1970. *European Heart Journal*, 1994, 15:450–453. PMID:8070469.
5. Eisenblätter D, Heinemann L, Claßen E. Community-based stroke incidence trends from the 1970s through 1980s in East Germany. *Stroke*, 1995, 26:919–923. PMID:7762038.
6. Heinemann LAJ, Barth W, Hoffmeister H. Trend of cardiovascular risk factors in the East German population 1968–1992. *Journal of Clinical Epidemiology*, 1995, 48:787–795. PMID:7769409.
7. Thiel C, Heinemann L. Nutritional behaviour differences in Germany. *Reviews on Environmental Health*, 1996, 11:35–40. PMID:8869524.
8. Barth W, Löwel H, Lewis M, Claßen E, Herman B, Quietzsch D, Greiser E, Keil U, Heinemann LA, Voigt G, Brasche S, Böthig S. Coronary heart disease mortality, morbidity and case fatality in five East and West German cities 1985–1989. *Journal of Clinical Epidemiology*, 1996, 49:1277–1284. PMID:8892496.
9. Heinemann L, Helmert U. Social gradient of cardiovascular disease risk in Germany before/after unification. *Reviews in Environmental Health*, 1996, 11:7–14. PMID:8869521.
10. Heinemann L, Dinkel R, Görtler E. Life expectancy in Germany: possible reasons for the increasing gap between East and West Germany. *Reviews in Environmental Health*, 1996, 11:15–26. PMID:8869522.

Lothar Heinemann

#66 Iceland (ICE-ICE, IC)

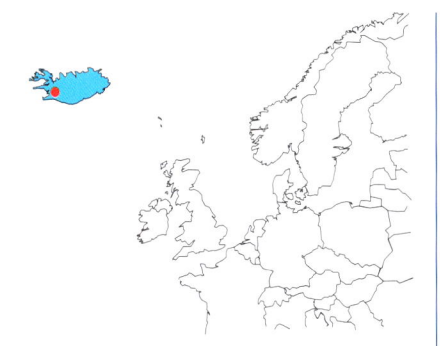

- fourteen years of MONICA coronary-event registration for all Iceland
- declining event rates and large social changes
- coronary-event population and risk-factor populations differ

MCC 28: Iceland
Three Reporting Units: one RUA but varying components. Coronary-event registration from the whole of Iceland (ICEb), population risk-factor data from Reykjavik alone (ICEc).

Administrative centre
The Heart Preventive Clinic of the Icelandic Heart Association—HJARTAVERND, Lágmúla 9, 108-Reykjavík, Iceland
T +354 535 1800; F +354 535 1801

Population
Iceland is the second largest island in Europe, measuring 100 000 square km in area, kissed by the Artic Circle in its far north. Half of the total population of 258 000 (1991) live in Reykjavik, the capital. Industries based on abundant hydro-electric and geothermal power, are replacing fishing and fish exporting as the dominant activity. Hospital inpatient services are paid for through national health insurance.

Funding
1. Icelandic Heart Association. 2. Ministry of Health.

Dates
Coronary-event monitoring: 1981–1994 (fourteen years); age 25–74. Coronary care: 1982–1983, 1990–1992. Population surveys: 1983, 1988/1989, 1993/1994. No stroke registration.

Additional description
The Icelandic Heart Association initiated a population-based cardiovascular cohort study in 1967, the Reykjavík Study, at the Heart Preventive Clinic. This continued until 1997 to measure the prevalence and incidence of various diseases, to detect them in their early stages and to investigate their causes. Related studies continue at the Heart Preventive Clinic which led the MONICA Project in Iceland.

Continuing activity
Coronary-event registration continued from 1995 up to 1998. An additional population survey was carried out in 2001 as well as coronary-care monitoring.

Key personnel
PI 1981–1999: Nikulás Sigfússon. PI 1999–: Uggi Agnarsson. Co–PI: Inga Ingibjörg Guðmundsdóttir. Coronary-event registration and coronary care: Ingibjörg Stefánsdóttir.

Selected publications
1. Sigfússon N. ["Monica"–rannsókn Alðjóða-heilbrigðisstofnunarinnar.] The Monica Project of the World Health Organization. *Hjartavernd*, 1985, 22: 1–2. (Icelandic). PMID:na.
2. Guðmundsdóttir II. [Skráning bráðrar kransæðastíflu. MONICA–rannsókn Hjartaverndar á Íslandi.] Registration of acute myocardial infarction. The MONICA study in Iceland. *Hjartavernd*, 1989, 26: 3–5. (Icelandic). PMID:na.
3. Sigfússon N, Sigvaldason H, Guðmundsdóttir II, Stefánsdóttir I, Steingrímsdóttir L, þorsteinsson þ, Sigurðsson G. [Breytingar á tíðni kransæðastíflu og kransæðadauðsfalla á Íslandi. Tengsl við áhættuðætti og mataræþi.] Changes in fatal and non-fatal myocardial infarction rates in Iceland. Association with risk factors and diet. *Læknabladið (Icelandic Medical Journal)*, 1991, 77:49–58. (Icelandic). PMID:na.
4. Sigfusson N, Sigvaldason H, Steingrimsdottir L, Gudmundsdottir II, Stefansdottir I, Thorsteinsson T, Sigurdsson G. Decline in ischaemic heart disease in Iceland and change in risk-factor levels. *British Medical Journal*, 1991, 302:1371–1375. PMID:2059715.
5. Sigfusson N, Sigvaldason H, Steingrimsdottir L, Gudmundsdottir II, Stefansdottir I, Thorsteinsson T, Sigurdsson G. Recent decline in ischaemic heart disease in Iceland—coincides with a change in risk factors. (Abstract) *European Heart Journal*, 1991, 12:302–302. PMID:na.
6. Agnarsson U, Sigfússon N, Guðmundsdóttir II, Stefánsdóttir I. [Bráð kransæðastífla á Íslandi 1982–1983. Horfur og áhrifaþættir fyrir daga segaleysandi meðferðar.] Acute myocardial infarction in Iceland 1982–1983. Prognosis in the pre-thrombolytic era. *Læknabladið (Icelandic Medical Journal)*, 1996, 82:276–285. (Icelandic, summary in English). PMID:na.
7. Sigfússon N, Guðmundsdóttir II, Stefánsdóttir I, Sigvaldason H. [MONICA rannsóknin á Íslandi 1981–1992.] The MONICA Iceland Study 1981–1992. *Heilbrigdisskýrslur, Fylgirit (Public Health in Iceland)*, 1997, Supplement, no 2. (Icelandic). PMID:na.
8. Salomaa VV, Lundberg V, Agnarsson U, Radisauskas R, Kirchhoff M, Wilhelmsen L, for the MONICA investigators in Nordic countries and Lithuania. Fatalities from myocardial infarction in Nordic Countries and Lithuania. *European Heart Journal*, 1997, 18:91–98. PMID:9049520.

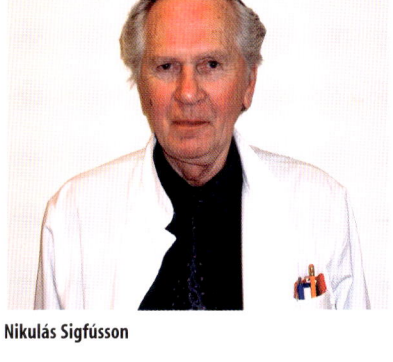

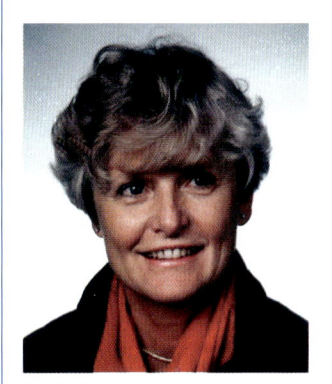

Nikulás Sigfússon

Nikulás Sigfússon

Inga Ingibjörg Gudmundsdóttir

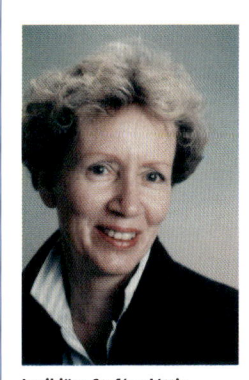

Ingibjörg Stefánsdóttir

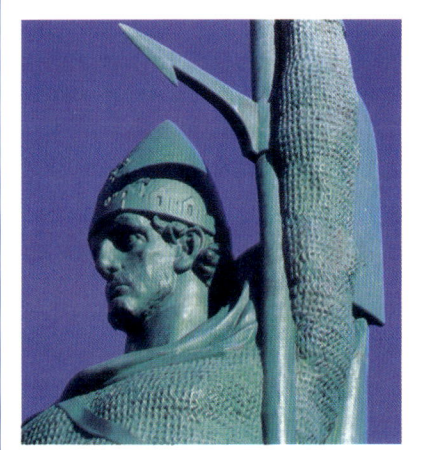

Reykyavik

#67 Italy-Country Coordinating Centre

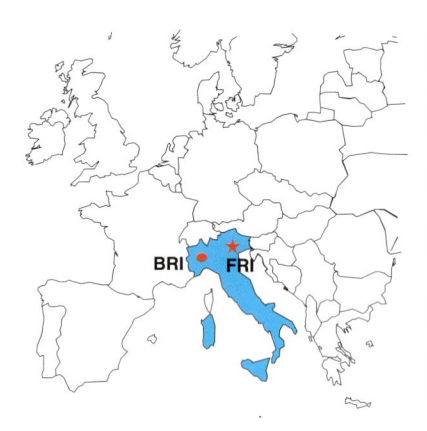

- crucial when MONICA began
- more subtle role at the finish

Administrative centre
Laboratorio di Epidemiologia e Biostatistica
Instituto Superiore di Sanita
Viale Reginea Elena, 299,
00161 Rome, Italy
T +39 06 49902985; F +39 06 49387069

Description
The Italian Coordinating Centre is based in an institute whose involvement in cardiovascular epidemiology goes back to the Seven Countries Study. At the start of MONICA it was active through its then Principal Investigator, Alessandro Menotti, in setting up three MONICA Collaborating Centres in Italy, although that nearest to Rome, Italy-Area Latina lost its funding early and withdrew, see #84 Former MONICA Populations. Alessandro Menotti was also a member of the first MONICA Steering Committee and contributed to the development of the MONICA protocol. Recently, the Coordinating Centre's involvement in MONICA has been less apparent than that of its French equivalent, although its national role in coordinating cardiovascular epidemiology has continued—as demonstrated by its involvement in Italian collaborative publications.

Key personnel
PI: Simona Giampaoli. Former PI: Alessandro Menotti.

Publications
See publications of Italian MCCs.

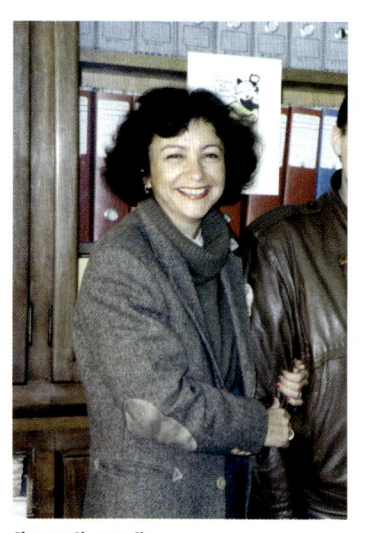

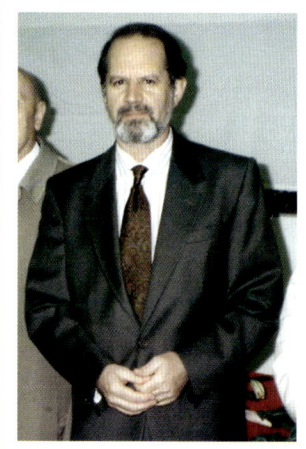

Simona Giampaoli

Simona Giampaoli

Alessandro Menotti

#68 Italy-Brianza (ITA-BRI, IT)

- among the lowest MONICA coronary-event rates
- declining mortality and event rates and case fatality
- studies of socioeconomic differences
- gene-environment interaction from nested case-control studies

MCC 57: Area Brianza
Single Reporting Unit.

Administrative centre
Research Centre for Chronic Degenerative Diseases, Department of Internal Medicine, Department of Prevention and Health Biotechnology, University of Milan-Bicocca, Via Cadore 48, 20052 Monza, Italy
T +39 039 233 3098; F +39 039 365 378

Population
Residents, aged 25–64, of 73 municipalities in Brianza, Lombardy, northern Italy, between Milan and the Swiss border. An urban industrialized population with among the highest average incomes in Italy, it experienced some economic recession in the early 1990s. The total population in 1991 was 850 000.

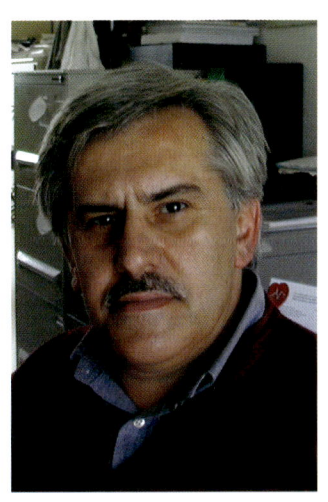

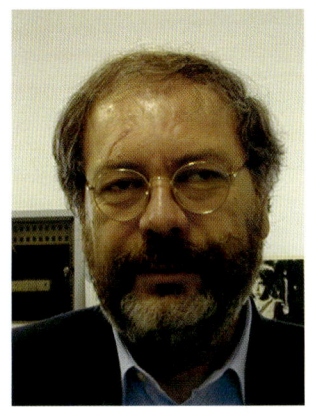

Funding
1. Assessorato alla Sanità della Regione Lombardia. 2. Italian National Research Council.

Dates
Coronary-event registration: 1985–94, (1997–98*). Coronary care: 1986, 1989–94 (1997–98*). Population surveys: 1986/1987, 1989/1990 (1992*) and 1993/4. Stroke-event registration: (1998*). (*) = not in WHO MONICA database.

Additional description
Coronary mortality and event rates for men and women were in the bottom fifth of the MONICA distribution. Declining event rates and case fatality contributed to falling mortality rates but unequally in the two sexes. Attack rates were stable over time if milder events were included, which suggests diminishing severity of disease. Smoking decreased in men, but not in women; blood pressure decreased in both sexes; total cholesterol and BMI (body mass index) increased between the middle and final surveys. Social disparities have been observed in risk factors and in the trends in 28-day case fatality, presumably from pre-hospital factors, as hospital treatment is not biased.

Local research interests
Socio-occupational disparities in coronary disease and its treatment. Simplified methods of registration. Prospective follow-up studies.

Continuing activity
Coronary and stroke-event registration intermittently. Population surveys have ceased. Cohort studies continue using stored material for nested case-control studies.

Key personnel
PIs: Giancarlo Cesana, Marco Ferrario. Population surveys: Roberto Sega. Chief Biochemist: Paolo Mocarelli. Coronary care: Franco Valagussa and Felice Achilli. Data management: Giovanni De Vito. Event registration: Maria Teresa Gussoni.

Selected publications
1. Ferrario M, Sega R, Cesana GC. Lessons from the MONICA Study in Northern Italy. *Journal of Hypertension*, 1991, 9(Suppl 3):S7–S14. PMID:1798004.
2. Cesana GC, Ferrario M, Sega R, Bravi C, Gussoni MT, De Vito G, Valagussa F. [Drop in cardiovascular and coronary mortality in Lombardia, 1969–1987. Evaluation of reliability of the estimates and possible explaining hypothesis.] *Giornale Italiano di Cardiologia*, 1992, 22:293–305. (Italian). PMID:1426772.
3. Ferrario M, Cesana GC, Heiss G, Linn SA, Mocarelli P, Tyroler HA. Demographic and behavioural correlates of high. density lipoprotein cholesterol. An international comparison between northern Italy and the United States. *International Journal of Epidemiology*, 1992, 21:665–675. PMID:1521969.
4. Ferrario M, Cesana GC. [Socioeconomic status and coronary disease: theories, research methods, epidemiological evidence and the results of Italian studies.] *La Medicina del Lavoro*, 1993, 84:18–30. (Italian). PMID:8492732.
5. Cesana GC, De Vito G, Ferrario M, Sega R, Mocarelli P. Trends of smoking habits in Northern Italy (1986–1990) (WHO MONICA Project in Area Brianza). *European Journal of Epidemiology*, 1995, 11:251–258. PMID:7493656.
6. Cesana GC, Ferrario M, De Vito D, Sega R, Grieco A. [Evaluation of the socioeconomic status in epidemiological surveys: hypotheses of research in the Brianza area MONICA project.] *La Medicina del Lavoro*, 1995, 86:16–26. (Italian). PMID:7791660.
7. Achilli F, Valagussa L, Valagussa F, De Vito G, Ferrario M, Cesana G. [Changes in the treatment of cardiac emergencies and their influence on fatalities. Data from the MONICA Project, Brianza Area.] *Giornale Italiano di Cardiologia*, 1997, 27:790–802. (Italian). PMID:9312507.
8. Ferrario M, Sega R, Chatenoud L, Mancia G, Mocarelli P, Crespi P, Cesana GC, for the MONICA- Brianza Research Group. Time trends of major coronary risk factors in a northern Italian population (1986–1994). How remarkable are socio-economic differences in an industrialised southern European population? *International Journal of Epidemiology*, 2001, 30:285–297. PMID:11369728.
9. Ferrario M, Cesana G, Vanuzzo D, Pilotto L, Sega R, Chiodini P, Giampaoli S. Surveillance of ischaemic heart disease: results from the Italian MONICA populations. *International Journal of Epidemiology*, 2001, 30: Suppl 1:S23-S29. PMID:11759847.

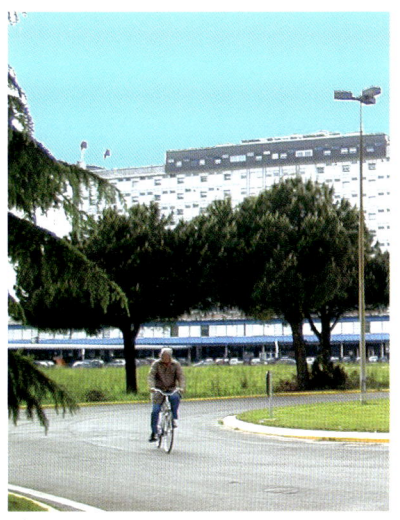

Marco Ferrario, Giancarlo Cesana

#69 Italy-Friuli (ITA-FRI, IF)

- one of the highest cardiovascular disease rates in Italy
- MONICA-Friuli now the model for collecting cardiovascular data in Italy
- hosted 8th Council of Principal Investigators meeting, April 1994

MCC 32: MONICA-Friuli
Five Reporting Units, merged into one RUA.

Administrative centre
Centre for Cardiovascular Disease Prevention,
A.S.S. 4 "Medio Friuli", Agenzia Regionale della Sanità,
Udine, 33100, Italy
E-mail: diego.vanuzzo@ars.sanita.fvg.it
T +39 432 552 456; F +39 432 552 452

Population
Residents aged 25–64 of three provinces of the Friuli-Venezia Giulia region of north-east Italy, bordering Austria and Slovenia. Mountainous near the Alps in the north and flat near the Adriatic sea in the south, the area has a mixed economy and a total population in 1991 of 940 000, including many elderly people. There are three urban centres. Udine with 100 000 people is the largest. Living standards were poor, but are now fairly high. Cardiovascular disease rates are high for Italy. The response rate to surveys was over 75%.

Funding
Regional Health Administration, CVD Registry.

Dates
Coronary and stroke-event registration and coronary care: 1984–1993. Population surveys: 1986, 1989, 1994.

Additional description
Each resident has a unique personal identifier used to track cardiovascular events and deaths through computerized record linkage. Results of the population risk-factor surveys informed regional policies on prevention. Mortality rates have declined in the last decade.

Local research interests
The WHO-CCCCP Martignacco cohort, including haemostatic and homocysteine studies. WHO-CINDI Associate Member. Cardiovascular disease prevention. Event registration. Publication of a disease and risk-factor atlas.

Continuing activity
Follow-up of MONICA survey cohorts with participation in the MORGAM and CUORE projects.

Developing a risk chart of the Italian population. National risk-factor surveillance system (Diego Vanuzzo, Co-Director), using the MONICA protocol, to plot risk-factor distribution and control across Italy. (Initial results can be found at: www.iss.it.)

Key personnel
PI 1995–: Diego Vanuzzo. Former PI–1995: Giorgio Antonio Feruglio. Co-PI: Lorenza Pilotto. Staff: GB Cignacco, G Zanata, M Scarpa, R Marini, M Spanghero, G Zilio.

Selected publications
1. Feruglio GA, Vanuzzo D. [Ischemic heart disease in Italy: dimensions of the problem.] *Giornale Italiano di Cardiologia*, 1989, 19:754–62. (Italian). PMID: 2612821.
2. Prati P, Vanuzzo D, Casaroli M, Di Chiara A, De Biasi F, Feruglio GA, Touboul PJ. Prevalence and determinants of carotid atherosclerosis in a general population. *Stroke*, 1992, 23:1705–11. PMID: 1448818.
3. Grafnetter D, Feruglio GA, Vanuzzo D. [Standardization of the methods of lipid determination according to WHO in the regional project of prevention of cardiovascular diseases in Friuli-Venezia Giulia.] *Giornale Italiano di Cardiologia*, 1996, 26:287–97. (Italian.) PMID: 8690184.
4. Giampaoli S, Vanuzzo D. [Cardiovascular risk factors in Italy: an interpretation with reference to the National Health Plan 1998–2000. Research Group of the Cardiovascular Epidemiologic Observatory.] *Giornale Italiano di Cardiologia*, 1999, 29:1463–71. (Italian). PMID: 10687109.
5. Giampaoli S, Panico S, Meli P, Conti S, Lo Noce C, Pilotto L, Vanuzzo D. [Cardiovascular risk factors in women in menopause.] *Italian Heart Journal*, 2000, 1(Suppl):1180–7. (Italian). PMID: 11140287.
6. Vanuzzo D, Pilotto L, Ambrosio GB, Pyorala K, Lehto S, De Bacquer D, De Backer G, Wood D. Potential for cholesterol lowering in secondary prevention of coronary heart disease in Europe: findings from EUROASPIRE study. European Action on Secondary Prevention through Intervention to Reduce Events. *Atherosclerosis*. 2000, 153:505–17. PMID: 11164441.
7. Giampaoli S, Palmieri L, Dima F, Pilotto L, Vescio MF, Vanuzzo D. [Socioeconomic aspects and cardiovascular risk factors: experience at the Cardiovascular Epidemiologic Observatory.] *Italian Heart Journal*, 2001, 2(Suppl):294–302. (Italian). PMID: 11307787.
8. Giampaoli S, Palmieri L, Pilotto L, Vanuzzo D. Incidence and prevalence of ischemic heart disease in Italy: estimates from the MIAMOD method. *Italian Heart Journal*, 2001, 2:349–55. PPMID: 1139263.

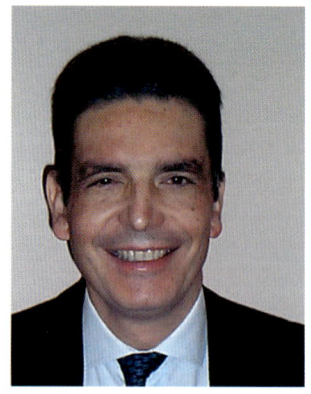

Diego Vanuzzo

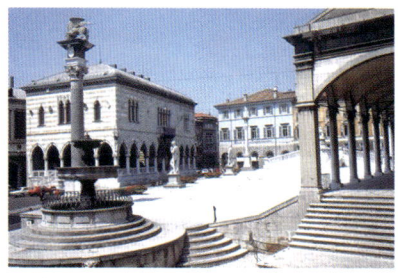

Loggia

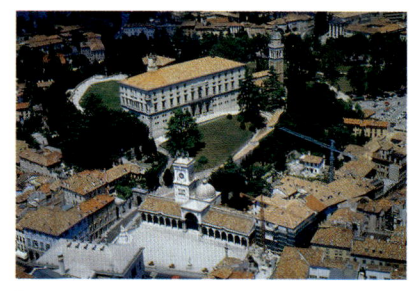

Area

9. Giampaoli S, Palmieri L, Capocaccia R, Pilotto L, Vanuzzo D. Estimating population-based incidence and prevalence of major coronary events. *International Journal of Epidemiology*, 2001, 30 Suppl 1:S5–10. PMID: 11759852.
10. Ferrario M, Cesana G, Vanuzzo D, Pilotto L, Sega R, Chiodini P, Giampaoli S. Surveillance of ischaemic heart disease: results from the Italian MONICA populations. *International Journal of Epidemiology* 2001, 30 Suppl 1:S23–9. PMID: 11759847.

Diego Vanuzzo, Lorenza Pilotto

#70 Lithuania-Kaunas (LTU-KAU, LT)

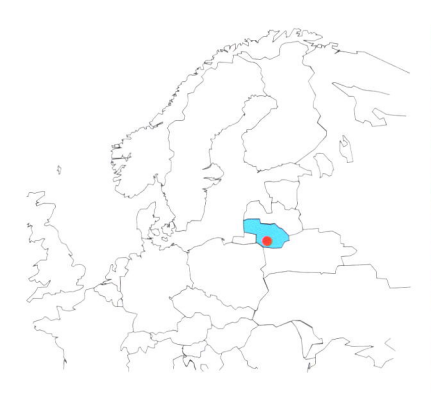

- first study of risk factors in Lithuania that included women
- high cardiovascular mortality in both sexes
- data on disease and risk factors informed national prevention strategies

MCC 45: Kaunas
Single Reporting Unit.

Administrative centre
Institute of Cardiology of the Kaunas University of Medicine,
St Sukileliu 17, Kaunas LT-3007, Lithuania
T +370 7 73 2259; F +370 7 73 2286

Population
Residents aged 25–64 of the city of Kaunas, the second largest city in Lithuania, with a total population in 1991 of 433 000. Kaunas is situated in the centre of Lithuania, at the confluence of the rivers Nemunas and Neris. Its main industries are textiles and food processing. The city has eight universities and schools of higher education, and six hospitals. Mortality rates from the main cardiovascular diseases in Kaunas are similar to those for Lithuania as a whole.

Funding
Ministry of Education and Science.

Dates
Coronary-event registration: 1983–1992. Coronary care: 1987–1992. Stroke-event registration: 1986–1995. Population surveys: 1983/1984, 1987, 1992/1993.

Additional description
Epidemiological studies of heart disease in Kaunas, event registration and population surveys, were started in 1972 as part of the myocardial infarction register and the Kaunas-Rotterdam Intervention study (KRIS) coordinated by WHO. The latter study included only men. In Kaunas the KRIS study still continues as a cohort study. The Kaunas-MONICA study was the first to include both sexes in risk factor surveys, and it also initiated stroke registration. The main results of Kaunas-MONICA have been used to prepare strategies for health promotion and prevention of non-communicable diseases at local and national levels. Since 1994 mortality rates from the main cardiovascular diseases have declined in Lithuania.

Local research interests
Coronary disease, stroke and risk factors in middle-aged men and women. Delivery of care. Diet and vitamins. Trends in cardiovascular diseases and risk factors.

Continuing activity
Cohort studies. Coronary and stroke-event registration. Population surveys, using MONICA standardization.

Key personnel
PI: Juozas Bluzhas. Co-PI population surveys: Stase Domarkiene. Co-PI event registration: Daiva Rastenyte. Biochemist: Lilija Margeviciene. Other staff: Regina Reklaitiene, Abdonas Tamosiunas, Dalia Rasteniene, Regina Grazuleviciene, Ricardas Radisauskas, Zita Petrokiene, Regina Grybauskiene, Kristina Jureniene, Doma Sidlauskiene.

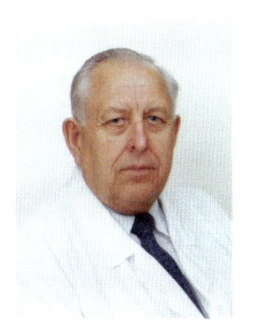

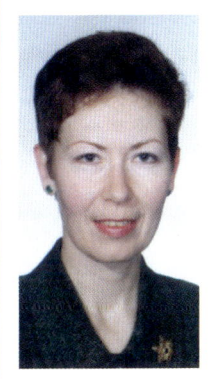

Selected publications
1. Rastenyte D, Salomaa V, Mustaniemi H, Rasteniene D, Grazuleviciene R, Cepaitis Z, Kankaanpaa J, Kuulasmaa K, Torppa J, Bluzhas J, Tuomilehto J. Comparison of trends in ischaemic heart disease between North Karelia, Finland, and Kaunas, Lithuania from 1971 to 1987. *British Heart Journal*, 1992, 68:516–523. PMID: 1467041.
2. Rastenyte D, Cepaitis Z, Sarti C, Bluzhas J, Tuomilehto J. Epidemiology of Stroke in Kaunas, Lithuania: first results from the Kaunas stroke register. *Stroke*, 1995, 26:240–244. PMID:7831695.
3. Domarkiene S. [Ten year trends in the prevalence of the main risk factors of ischaemic heart disease in the Kaunas population aged 35–64 years (the Kaunas MONICA study).] *Medicina*, 1995, 31:61–65. (Lithuanian). PMID:na.
4. Petrokiene Z, Radisauskas R, Jureniene K. Acute coronary care and treatment in Kaunas population during 1987–1993. *Lithuanian Journal of Cardiology*, 1996,1:36–42. PMID:na.
5. Rastenyte D, Tuomilehto J, Sarti C, Cepaitis Z, Bluzhas J. Trends in the incidence and mortality of stroke in Kaunas, Lithuania, 1986–1993. *Cerebrovascular Diseases*, 1996, 6:13–20. PMID:na.
6. Rastenyte D, Tuomilehto J, Sarti C, Cepaitis Z, Bluzhas J. Increasing trends in mortality from cerebral infarction and intracerebral haemorrhage in Kaunas, Lithuania. *Cerebrovascular Diseases*, 1996, 6:216–21. PMID:na.
7. Bluzhas J, Radisauskas R, Rastenyte D, Rasteniene D, Grazuleviciene R, Petrokiene Z. [Morbidity and lethality from ischemic heart disease in the Kaunas population during 1971–1995.] *Medicina*, 1997, 33:20–27. (Lithuanian). PMID:na.
8. Tamosiunas A, Jureniene K, Domarkiene S, Reklaitiene R. Prognostic value of behavioural risk factors for myocardial infarction morbidity and mortality from different causes. *Lithuanian Journal of Cardiology*, 1997, 4:2–6. PMID:na.
9. Domarkiene S, ed. *[Epidemiology and prevention of cardiovascular diseases.]*. Kaunas, 2000, 234 p. (Lithuanian). PMID:na.

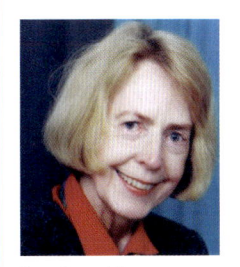

Juozas Bluzhas

Stase Domarkiene

Daiva Rastenyte

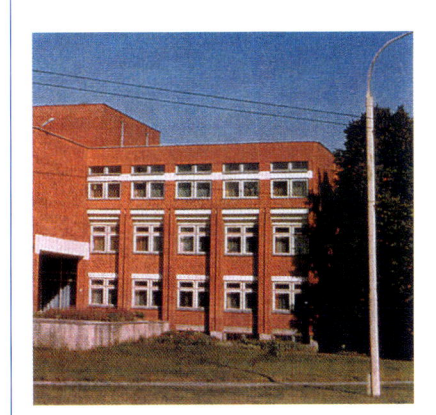

Institute

Juozas Bluzhas, Stase Domarkiene

#71 New Zealand-Auckland (NEZ-AUC, NZ)

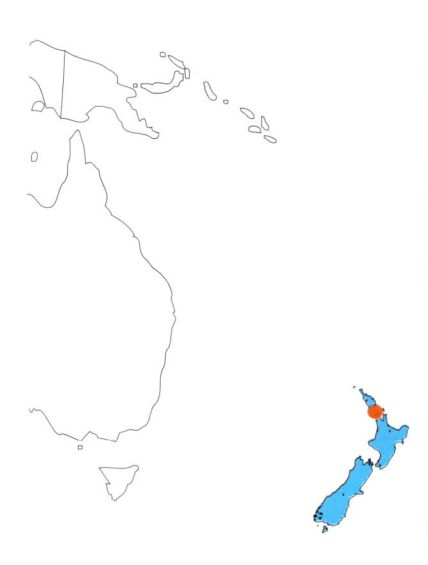

MCC 33: Auckland
Single Reporting Unit.

Administrative centre
Department of Community Health, University of Auckland,
Private Bag 92019, Auckland, New Zealand
T +64 9 373 7599 x6335; F +64 9 373 7503

Population
Residents in the Auckland area aged 35–64. Auckland, with over a quarter of its population, is the largest city in New Zealand, situated towards the north of the North Island on an isthmus with harbours on both east and west coasts. Maori, indigenous to New Zealand, are more likely to live in Auckland than any other city. It is called the Pacific Capital because it has the highest density of Pacific Islanders in the world. The total population in 1991 was 951 000.

Funding
1. Health Research Council of New Zealand. 2. National Heart Foundation of New Zealand.

Dates
Coronary-event registration: 1983–1991(–2)*. Coronary care: 1986, 1989, 1991. Population surveys: 1982, 1993/1994. (A survey was conducted in 1986/7 for a case-control study rather than for MONICA.) (*) = not included in MONICA collaborative publications. No MONICA stroke registration.

Additional description
In 1981 a one-year register of coronary and stroke patients known as ARCOS (Auckland Region Coronary and Stroke Study) was established. This formed the background to the subsequent MONICA study. Auckland participated through its stroke investigator, Ruth Bonita, in MONICA's stroke component, but not through submitting data. Strokes were registered again in 1991 and a 16-year follow-up of the 1981 cases has been completed. Population surveys excluded Maoris as the sampling frame was the general electoral roll and not the Maori only roll. Maori event rates were derived using census data.

Local research interests
Trends in coronary disease. Risk factors, particularly cholesterol. Long-term survival after a coronary event. Coronary disease in Maori and Pacific people.

Continuing activity
Coronary-event registration has ceased. A further stroke register is planned, as is a fourth risk factor survey.

Key personnel
PI: Robert Beaglehole. Co–PI: Rod Jackson. Biostatistician: Alistair Stewart. Co–Investigator: Ruth Bonita

- high coronary-event rates shown to be declining
- improving prognosis in 28-day coronary-event survivors
- decline in blood pressure 1982 to 1993
- studies of disease rates in those of European, Maori and Pacific ethnicity

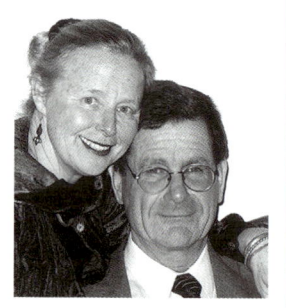

Robert Beaglehole and Ruth Bonita

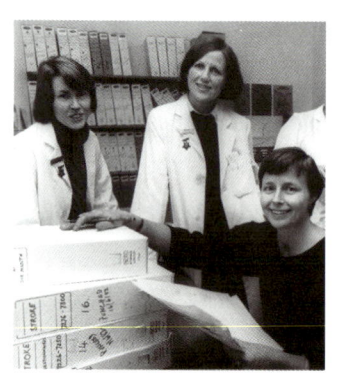

Stroke registration team

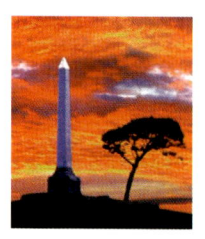

Auckland

Selected publications
1. Beaglehole R. Coronary heart disease trends in Australia and New Zealand. *International Journal of Cardiology*, 1989, 22:1–3. PMID:2784422.
2. Graham P, Jackson R, Beaglehole R, De Boer G. The validity of Maori mortality statistics. *New Zealand Medical Journal*, 1989, 102:124–126. PMID:2927807.
3. Hobbs M, Jamrozik K, Hockey R, Alexander H, Beaglehole R, Dobson A, Heller R, Jackson R, Stewart AW. Mortality from coronary heart disease and incidence of acute myocardial infarction in Auckland, Newcastle and Perth. *Medical Journal of Australia*, 1991, 155:436–442. PMID:1921812.
4. Löwel H, Dobson A, Keil U, Herman B, Hobbs MS, Stewart A, Arstila M, Miettinen H, Mustaniemi H, Tuomilehto J. Coronary heart disease case fatality in four countries: a community study. *Circulation*, 1993, 88:2524–2531. PMID:8252663.
5. Jackson R, Lay Yee R, Priest P, Shaw L, Beaglehole R. Trends in coronary heart disease risk factors in Auckland, 1982–1994. *New Zealand Medical Journal*, 1995, 108:451–454. PMID:8538961.
6. Bell C, Swinburn B, Stewart A, Jackson R, Tukuitonga C, Tipene-Leach D. Ethnic differences and recent trends in coronary heart disease incidence in New Zealand. *New Zealand Medical Journal*, 1996, 109:66–68. PMID:8606820.
7. Trye P, Jackson R, Stewart A, Lay Yee R, Beaglehole R. Trends and determinants of blood pressure in Auckland, New Zealand. 1982–1994. *New Zealand Medical Journal*, 1996, 109:179–181. PMID:8657382.
8. Sonke GS, Beaglehole R, Stewart AW, Jackson R, Stewart FM. Sex differences in case fatality before and after admission to hospital after acute cardiac events: analysis of community-based coronary heart disease register. *British Medical Journal*, 1996, 313:853–855. PMID:8870571.
9. Beaglehole R, Stewart A, Jackson R, Dobson AJ, McElduff P, D'Este K, Heller RF, Jamrozik KD, Hobbs MS, Parsons R, Broadhurst R. Declining rates of coronary heart disease in New Zealand and Australia 1983–1993. *American Journal of Epidemiology*, 1997, 145:707–713. PMID:9125997.
10. Stewart AW, Beaglehole R, Jackson R, Bingley W. Trends in three year survival following acute myocardial infarction, 1983–1992. *European Heart Journal*, 1999, 20:803–807. PMID:10329077.

Alistair Stewart

#72 Poland-Tarnobrzeg Voivodship (POL-TAR, PT)

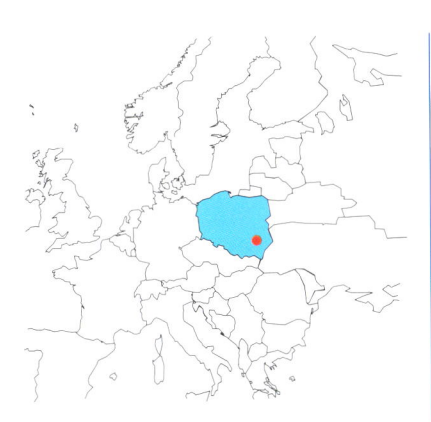

- rural population posed challenges for monitoring
- MONICA monitored rise and fall in cardiovascular deaths
- psychosocial and nutritional factors
- cognitive impairment in old age

MCC 35: POL-MONICA Kraków
Two Reporting Units merged into one RUA.

Administrative centre
Dept of Epidemiology and Population Studies, Institute of Public Health,
Collegium Medicum, Jagiellonian University in Kraków,
St. Grzegórzecka, 31-501 Kraków, Poland
T +48 12 4241360; F +48 12 4217447
Before 1992. Dept of Biochemical Diagnostics and Inpatient Clinic for Metabolic Diseases, Nicolaus Copernicus Medical Academy in Kraków.

Population
Residents aged 25–64 of the south-eastern rural province of Tarnobrzeg Voivodship. There is a steel industry in the south-east, while sulphur industries (now diminished) dominated the centre and north-west. Miners and industrial workers often work smallholdings for agricultural produce as they live in villages and small towns. The total population in 1991 was 609 000.

Funding
1. Ministry of Health. 2. National Committee for Scientific Research contracts: 4 1474 91 1, 4 PO5D 036 08.

Dates
Coronary-event registration: 1984–1993. Coronary care: 1987–93. Population surveys: 1983/84, 1987/88, 1992/93. No stroke registration.

Additional description
Tarnobrzeg Voivodship was chosen for POL-MONICA Krakow to contrast its rural population and health care with that of Warsaw (see POL-MONICA Warsaw). The Project also promoted cardiovascular disease prevention. Additional survey data were used locally and for the Poland and US Collaborative Study on Cardiopulmonary Epidemiology. MONICA monitored risk factors and medical care and trends in coronary heart disease mortality (which increased up to, and decreased after, 1992) during major political, economic and social changes.

Local research interests
Psychosocial and nutritional factors. Cognitive impairment in the elderly. Monitoring secondary prevention.

Continuing activity
Event registration has ceased. Cohort studies until 1998. Population survey in 2001.

Key personnel
PI: Andrzej Pająk. Former PI(–1990: Jan Sznajd. Staff: Ewa Kawalec, Roman Topór-Mądry, Ewa Baczyńska, Aleksander Celiński, Helena Czarnecka, Alicja Hebda, Barbara Idzior-Waluś, Elżbieta Kozek, Marzanna Magdoń, Małgorzata Malczewska-Malec, Maciej Małecki, Adam Markiewicz, Piotr Misiowiec, Ryszard Mizera, Ryszard Morawski, Witold Rostworowski, Iwona Trznadel-Morawska, Urszula Zeman, Andrzej Żarnecki.

Selected publications
1. Pająk A, Broda G, Abernathy JR, Sznajd J, Rywik S, Irving SH, Czarnecka H, Wągrowska H, Thomas RP, Celiński A, et al. Poland-US collaborative study on cardiovascular epidemiology: classification agreement between US National Cholesterol Education Program and European Atherosclerosis Society hyperlipidemia guidelines in selected Polish and US populations. *Atherosclerosis*, 1992, 95:43–50. PMID:1642691.
2. Pająk A. [Myocardial infarction risks and procedures. Longitudinal observational study in 280 000 women and men—POL-MONICA Kraków Project. II. Risk factors and mortality due to ischaemic heart disease in men aged 35–64 years.] *Przegląd Lekarski*, 1996, 53, 707–712. (Polish). PMID:9173437.
3. Pająk A, Jamrozik K, Kawalec E, Topór-Mądry R, Pikoň K, Malczewska-Malec M, Puchalska T. [Myocardial infarction risks and procedures. Longitudinal observational study in 280 000 women and men—POL-MONICA Kraków Project. III. Epidemiology and treatment of myocardial infarction.] *Przegląd Lekarski*, 1996, 53, 767–778. (Polish). PMID:3173437.
4. Pająk A. [Myocardial infarction risks and procedures. Longitudinal observational study in 280 000 women and men—POL-MONICA Kraków Project. IV. Prognosis in non-invasive treatment in myocardial infarction within 28 days from the onset.] *Przegląd Lekarski*, 1996, 53, 779–784. (Polish). PMID:9173438.
5. Pająk A. [Myocardial infarction symptoms and procedures. Longitudinal observation of a study in 280 000 women and men—POL-MONICA Kraków Project. V. Atypical symptoms and prognosis in myocardial infarction.] *Przegląd Lekarski*, 1996, 53, 837–841. (Polish). PMID:9163004.
6. Pająk A, Williams OD, Broda G, Baczyńska E, Rywik S, Davis CE, Kawalec E, Chodkowska E, Irving S, Manolio T. Changes over time in blood lipids and their correlates in Polish rural and urban populations: the Poland-United States Collaborative Study in cardiopulmonary disease epidemiology. *Annals of Epidemiology*, 1997, 7:115–124. PMID:9099399.
7. Pająk A, Broda G, Manolio TA, Kawalec E, Rywik S, Davis CE, Pikoň J, Pytlak A, Thomas RP. Constitutional, biochemical and lifestyle correlates of fibrinogen and factor VII activity in Polish urban and rural populations. *International Journal of Epidemiology*, 1998, 27:953–960. PMID:10024188.
8. Dennis BH, Pająk A, Pardo B, Davis CE, Williams OD, Piotrowski W. Weight gain and its correlates in Poland between 1983 and 1993. *International Journal of Obesity and Related Metabolic Disorders*, 2000, 24:1507–1513. PMID:11126349.

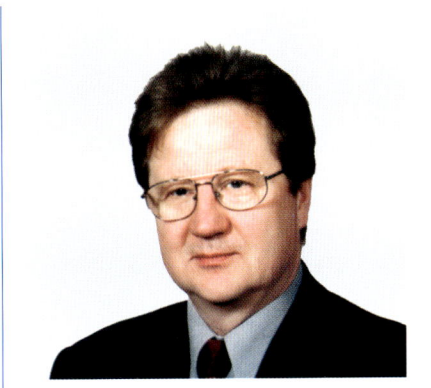

Andrzej Pająk

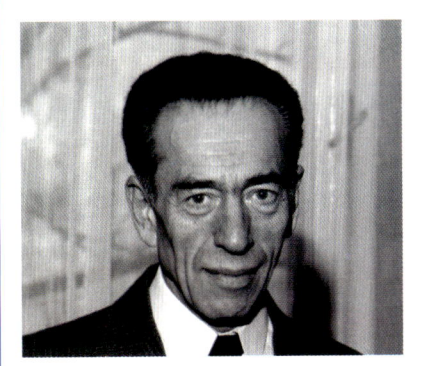

Jan Sznajd (deceased)

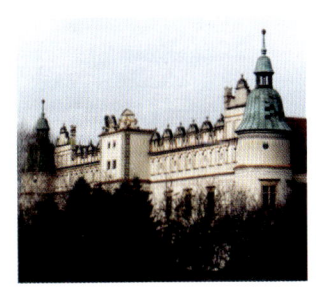

Baranow

Andrzej Pająk, Roman Topór-Mądry

#73 Poland-Warsaw (POL-WAR, PW)

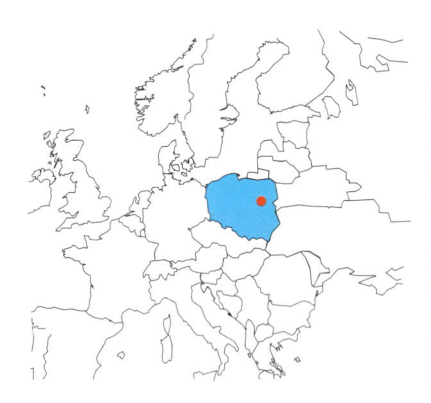

- high initial all-cause mortality, but improving
- high initial case fatality for stroke, but improving
- smoking and blood pressure both high, but not cholesterol
- participated in Poland-United States studies

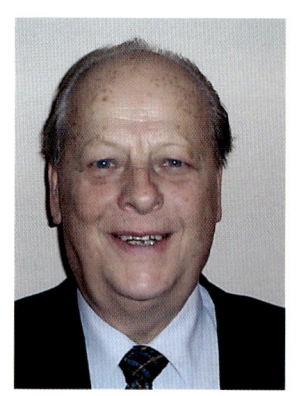

Stefan Rywik

MCC 36: POL-MONICA-Warsaw
Two Reporting Units merged as one Reporting Unit Aggregate (RUA).

Administrative centre
Department of CVD Epidemiology and Prevention,
Stefan Cardinal Wyszyński National Institute of Cardiology,
04-628 Warszawa, Alpejska 42, Poland
T +48 22 815 65 56; F +48 22 613 38 07

Population
Residents aged 25–64 of the two districts of the capital city of Warsaw east of the Vistula. These are partly industrial and partly residential and home to hospitals, banks, governmental offices and universities. Poland's changing economy has affected the living conditions and behaviour of the population. In 1989/90 the free market produced mixed benefits: loss of State social support, high inflation, high unemployment, but greater access to food products previously found only in the western market. Risk-factor profiles have changed. Cardiovascular disease mortality, previously rising, began to decrease from 1991. The total population in 1991 was 494 000.

Funding
1. Government Project: Prevention and Fight against Cardiovascular Disease. 2. State Office Research Grant. 3. Ministry of Health.

Dates
Coronary and stroke-event registration: 1984–1994. Coronary care: 1986–1994. Population surveys: 1984, 1988, 1993.

Additional description
The population surveys included additional factors, including psychosocial factors, nutrition and drug use. Survey, coronary and stroke-registration results were published in data books and used for the Poland-US Collaborative Study.

Local research interests
Cohort study. Correlation of trends in psychosocial factors with mortality trends. Fibrinogen, Factor VII and other haemostatic factors. Nutritional habits of the population and supplementation with vitamins and minerals.

Continuing activity
Registration has ceased. Cohort studies continued until 1998. A new population survey sampling the MONICA population aged 20–74 took place in 2001.

Key personnel
PI: Stefan L. Rywik. Co-PI: Grażyna Broda. Population surveys: Henryka Wągrowska. Event-registration: Maria Polakowska, Aleksandra Pytlak. Biochemist: Ewa Chodkowska. Cooperation with MDC and statistical analyses: Witold Kupść, Walerian Piotrowski, Paweł Kurjata, Danuta Szcześniewska. Nutrition: Elżbieta Sygnowska, Anna Waśkiewicz. Psychosocial: Jerzy Piwoński.

Selected publications
1. Broda G, Rywik S, Kurjata P. Trends in Myocardial Incidence and Fatality in Warsaw Pol-MONICA population from 1984 to 1988. *International Journal of Angiology*, 1995, 4:113–116. PMID:na.
2. Broda G, Davis CE, Pająk A, Williams OD, Rywik S, Baczyńska E, Folsom AR, Szklo M. Poland and United States Collaborative Study on Cardiopulmonary Epidemiology: A Comparison of HDL-cholesterol and its Subfractions in Populations Covered by the United States ARIC Study and the Pol-MONICA Project. Atherosclerosis, *Thrombosis and Vascular Biology*, 1996, 16(2):339–349. PMID:8620351.
3. Waśkiewicz A, Sygnowska E, Broda G, Pardo B. Dietary habits of the Warsaw population observed over 10 years within the framework of the Pol-MONICA Project. *Nutrition, Metabolism and Cardiovascular Diseases*, 1997, 7:425–431. PMID:na.
4. Rywik S, Davis CE, Pająk A, Broda G, Folsom AR, Kawalec E, Williams OD. Poland and US Collaborative Study on cardiovascular epidemiology: Hypertension in the community—prevalence, awareness, treatment and control of hypertension in the Pol-MONICA Project and US ARIC Study. *Annals of Epidemiology*, 1998, 8:3–13. PMID:9465988.
5. Abernathy JR, Rywik S, Pająk A, Thomas RP, Broda G, Kawalec E. Correlates of total and CVD mortality in US and Polish men and women aged 35–64 years. *Cardiovascular Disease Prevention*, 1998, 1:25–31. PMID:na.
6. Rosamond S, Broda G, Kawalec E, Rywik S, Pająk A, Cooper L, Chambless L. Comparison of medical care and survival of hospitalized patients with acute myocardial infarction in Poland and the United States. *American Journal of Cardiology*, 1999, 83:1180–1185. PMID:10215280.
7. Broda G, Davis CE, Pająk A, Rywik S, Irving SH, Kennedy JI, Topór-Mądry R. 10-year trends in cigarette smoking in Polish urban and rural populations in the Pol-MONICA Project. *Cardiovascular Disease Prevention*, 1999, 5:945–954. PMID:na.
8. Pytlak A, Piotrowski W. Prognostic significance of Q-Tc interval for predicting total, cardiac and ischemic heart disease mortality in community-based cohort from Pol-MONICA population. *Annals of Noninvasive Electrocardiology*, 2000, 5:322–329. PMID:na.
9. Broda G. Isolated systolic hypertension is a strong predictor of cardiovascular and all-cause mortality in the middle-aged population: Warsaw Pol-MONICA Follow-up Project. *Journal of Clinical Hypertension* (Greenwich Conn.), 2000, 2, 305–311. PMID:11416666.
10. Rywik SL, Williams OD, Pająk A, Broda G, Davis CE, Kawalec E, Manolio TA, Piotrowski W, Hutchinson R. Incidence and correlates of hypertension in the ARIC Study and the Pol-MONICA project. *Hypertension*, 2000, 18:999–1006. PMID:10953989.

Stefan Rywik

#74 Russia-Moscow (RUS-MOS, RM)

Russia-Moscow Control (RUS-MOC, RC)
Russia-Moscow Intervention (RUS-MOI, RI)

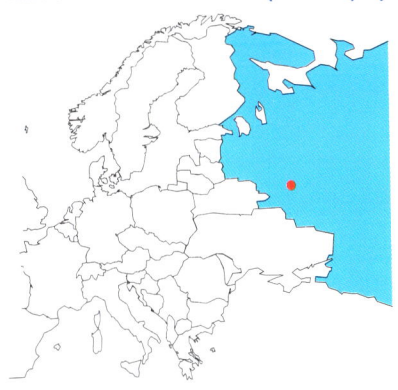

- results from Moscow during a decade of change
- case fatality for coronary events increased
- fall in blood pressure, cholesterol and body mass index (BMI)
- Moscow districts divided into two RUAs
- populations differed for risk-factor and event monitoring

MCC 46: Moscow
Three Reporting Units amalgamated into either two (Russia-Moscow Control, and Russia-Moscow Intervention) or one Reporting Unit Aggregate (Russia-Moscow). In MONICA collaborative analyses RUS-MOS contains all three Reporting Units for coronary care. RUS-MOC covers only the Octyabrsky district. RUS-MOI has two variants: it included the Cheremushkinsky district for coronary events—MOIb, but for risk-factor surveys and stroke covered only the Leninsky district—MOIa.

Administrative centre
State Research Centre for Preventive Medicine,
10 Petroverigsky Lane,
Moscow 101990, Russian Federation
T/F +7 095 925 45 44
E-mail: oganov@online.ru, shalnova@dol.ru

Population
Residents aged 25–64 of the Octyabrsky (RUS-MOC), Leninsky and Cheremushkinsky (RUS-MOI) districts of Moscow. Lifestyle and risk-factor levels typical of megapolis and Russian towns with high mortality and morbidity rates. The total population in 1991 was 214 000 (Moscow-Control) and 601 000 (Moscow-Intervention, MOIb).

Funding
Budget of the Russian Federation.

Dates
Coronary-event registration: 1985–93. Coronary care: 1986, 1989–93. Stroke-event registration: 1985–93. Population surveys: 1984–86, 1988/89*, 1992–95*. (* = middle and final surveys were not carried out in Cheremushkinsky district.)

Additional description
In two districts, Leninsky and Cheremushkinsky, mass redevelopment occurred during the period 1984–1987; many families moved out of this area into new homes elsewhere. This changed the demographic profile of these districts, especially of the smaller Leninsky.

Local Research Interests
Monitoring of main risk factors and mortality in the frame of possible prevention activities at local level.

Continuing activity
Mortality follow-up under development. In 2000–2001 'MONICA-4' took place in the Octyabrsky district, including 424 males and 386 females aged 25–64.

Key personnel*
PI 1997–2001: Georgy Zhukovsky. Former PI 1983–86: Sergei Fedotov. Former PI 1986–97: Tatyana Varlamova. Other staff: A Britov, T Timofeeva, M Osokina, A Alexandri, N Serdyuchenko, V Naumova, N Popova, A Kapustina.
*New team from 2001: PI: Vladimir Konstantinov. Co-PIs: Svetlana Shalnova, Alexander Deev.

Selected publications
1. Volozh OI, Solodkaia ES, Mutso IuKh, Zhukovskii GS, Varlamova TA. [Comparison of the inference of the existence of ischaemic heart disease in epidemiological research with prior polyclinic diagnosis.] *Kardiologiia*, 1985, 25:98–99. (Russian). PMID:3990090.
2. Gorbunov AP, Zhukovskii GS, Nebeiridze DV, Varlamova TA, Oganov RG. [Potential ischaemic heart disease and mortality in the male population 40–59 years old over 6.5 years of observation.] *Kardiologiia*, 1987, 27:39–43. (Russian). PMID:3695111.
3. Varlamova T, Zhukovski G, Chazova L, Britov A. Monitoring of major cardiovascular diseases in Moscow, USSR. *Acta Medica Scandinavica Supplementum*, 1988, 728:73–78. PMID:na
4. Shal'nova SA, Maksimov AB, Kapustina AV, Zhukovskii GS, Varlamova TA. [Prognostic significance of different variants of chest pain in men aged 40–49 years (data of a prospective study).] *Terapevticheskii Arkhiv*, 1988, 60:30–35. (Russian). PMID:3363504.
5. Oganov RG, Zhukovskii GS, Fedin AI, Varlamova TA, Migirov AA. [Morbidity and mortality from stroke among the population of Moscow.] *Terapevticheskii Arkhiv*, 1989, 61:29–32. (Russian). PMID:2595580.
6. Britov A, Varlamova T, Kalinina A, Ostrovskaya T, Konstantinov V, Konstantinov E, Nikulina L, Elisseeva N, Sapozhnikov I. Hypertension studies in the Soviet Union. *Clinical and Experimental Hypertension. Part A, Theory and Practice*, 1989, 11:841–858. PMID:2676258.
7. Britov AN, Zhukovskii GS, Sviderskii VG, Varlamova TA, Liubimova LV, Naumova VV, Deev AD, Spizhovyi VN, Adon'ev BI, Grishenko EA et al. [The results of conducting a programme for the supplementary education of medical workers in the problems of preventing and treating arterial hypertension (a population study).] *Kardiologiia*, 1992, 32:68–73. (Russian). PMID:1487887.

This page was drafted during a break in communication between Moscow and MONICA, but later modified and approved.

**Vladislav Moltchanov,
Hugh Tunstall-Pedoe,
Svetlana Shalnova**

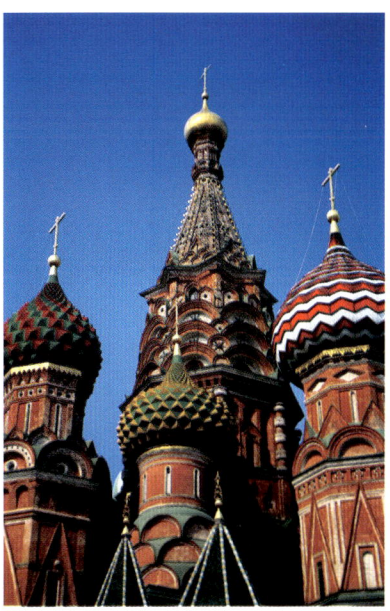

St Basil's Cathedral

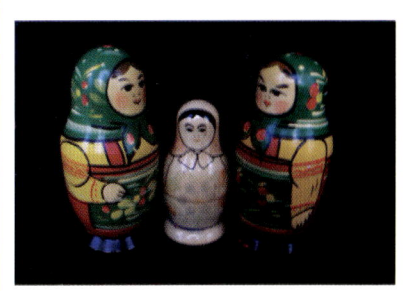

Russian dolls

#75 Russia-Novosibirsk (RUS-NOV, RN)

Russia-Novosibirk Control (RUS-NOC, RO)
Russia-Novosibirk Intervention (RUS-NOI, RT)

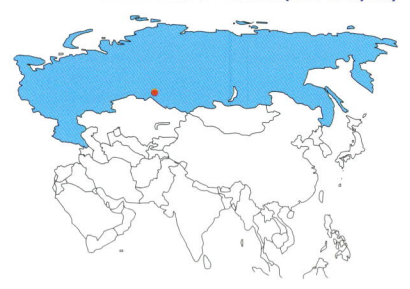

- very high all-causes and cardiovascular mortality
- overall increase in coronary-event rates
- highest stroke event rates in MONICA
- high smoking rates in men and body mass index in women

MCC 47: Siberian MONICA
Three Reporting Units. RUS-NOI covered only the Octyabrsky district. RUS-NOC included both the Kirovsky and Leninsky districts for coronary events and stroke (NOCb), and the baseline survey. For the middle and final risk-factor surveys it covered the Kirowsky district alone—NOCa. All three Reporting Units (districts) are grouped together in RUS-NOV for analyses of coronary care and for Monograph map graphics.

Administrative centre
Institute of Internal Medicine, Siberian Branch of Russian Academy of Medical Science, Vladimirovsky spusk 2a, Novosibirsk 630003, Russian Federation
T +7 38 3229 2048; F +7 38 3222 2821

Population
Residents aged 25–64 of the city of Novosibirsk, central West Siberia, the industrial and scientific centre of Siberia. Coronary heart disease and stroke morbidity and mortality rates are high in men and women. The total population in 1991 was 482 000 (Novosibirsk Control, NOCb) and 160 000 (Novosibirsk Intervention).

Funding
Russian Academy of Medical Science.

Dates
Technical problems affected collaborative analysis of some of the material collected. In collaborative MONICA trend analyses (as distinct from local use) the following dates apply:
RUS-NOC: Coronary-event registration: 1984–1992 (1993 omitted). Coronary care; 1986–1987, 1989–1993. Stroke registration: 1987–1993 (early years and 1994 omitted). Population surveys: 1985/1986, 1988/1989, 1995.
RUS-NOI: Coronary-event registration: 1984–1993. Coronary care: 1986/1987, 1989–1993. Stroke event registration: 1982–1993 (1994 omitted). Population surveys: 1985, 1988, 1994/1995.

Additional description
Population surveys followed the MONICA protocol but with some additional items added. The high cardiovascular mortality in Novosibirsk increased dramatically at the beginning of the 1990s but declined modestly after 1994.

Local research interests
Paradoxical trends of all-cause and cardiovascular diseases mortality in the target population. Comparison of classic with novel risk factors (psychosocial factors, diet, alcohol). Population genetics of cardiovascular diseases.

Continuing activity
Coronary-event registration continues. Stroke-event registration continues in two districts. A repeat population survey of the 45–64 age group was conducted in 1999/2000. Cohort studies continue.

Key personnel
PI: Yuri Nikitin. Other staff: Sofia Malyutina, Valery Gafarov, Valery Feigin, Galina Simonova, Tatyana Vinogradova.

Selected publications
1. Nikitin YP, Shalaurova IY, Serova NV. The validation of serum thiocyanate smoking data in a population survey. *Revue d'Epidémiologie et de Santé Publique*, 1990, 38:469–472. PMID:2082453.
2. Nikitin YP, Mamleeva FR, Efendieva DB. Nutrition and cardiovascular disease in Siberian Residents. *Journal of Progress in Cardiovascular Science*, 1993, I:127–133. PMID:na.
3. Nikitin Y, Malyutina S, Tikhonov A. Lipid spectrum and antioxidant vitamins in urban Siberian population. *Acta Cardiologia*, 1994, 49:400–402. (Conference abstract). PMID: 7976064.
4. Feigin VL, Wiebers DO, Nikitin YP, O'Fallon WM, Whisnant JP. Stroke epidemiology in Novosibirsk, Russia: A population-based study. *Mayo Clinic Proceedings*, 1995, 70:847–852. PMID:7643638.
5. Feigin VL, Wiebers DO, Whisnant YP, O'Fallon WM. Stroke incidence and 30-day case-fatality rates in Novosibirsk, Russia, 1982 through 1992. *Stroke*, 1995, 26:924–929. PMID:7762039.
6. Stegmayr B, Vinogradova T, Malyutina S, Peltonen M, Nikitin Y, Asplund K. Widening gap of stroke between east and west. Eight-year trends in occurrence and risk factors in Russia and Sweden. *Stroke*, 2000, 31: 2–8. PMID:10625707.
7. Gafarov VV. [20 year monitoring of acute cardiovascular disease in the population of a large industrial city in the West Siberia (an Epidemiological Study).] *Terapevticheskii Arkhiv*, 2000, 1:15–21. (Russian. English abstract). PMID:10687199.
8. Nikitin YP, Kazeka LR, Babin VL, Malyutina SK. [Prevalence of Ischemic Heart Disease in Subjects with Hyperinsulinemia (A Population Study).] *Kardiologiia*, 2001, 1:12–16. (Russian. English abstract). PMID:na.
9. Malyutina S, Simonova G, Nikitin YP. The incidence of coronary heart disease and cardiovascular mortality in the urban Siberian population: gender-specific findings from the 10-year cohort study. In: Weidner G. et al, eds. *Heart Disease: Environment, Stress and Gender*, NATO Science Series, 2000, vol.327. ISBN 1 58603 082 5. PMID:na.

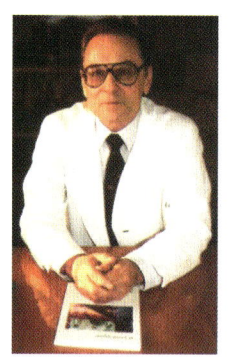

Yuri Nikitin

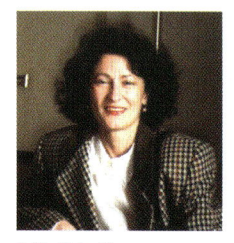

Sofia Malyutina

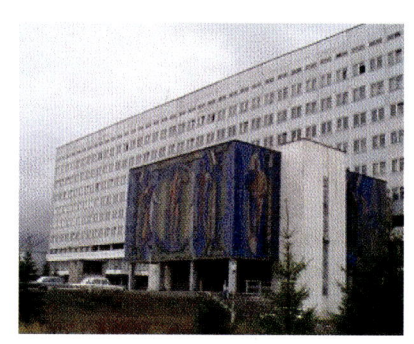

Institute

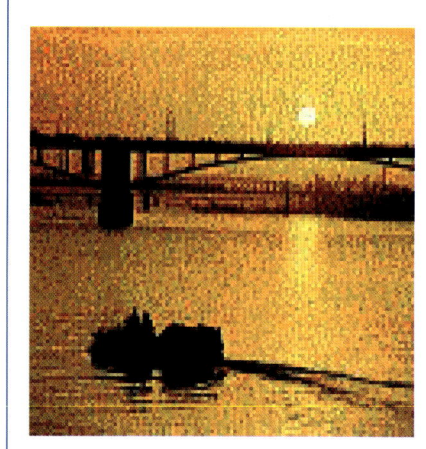

River Ob

Yuri Nikitin, Sofia Malyutina

#76 Spain-Catalonia (SPA-CAT, SP)

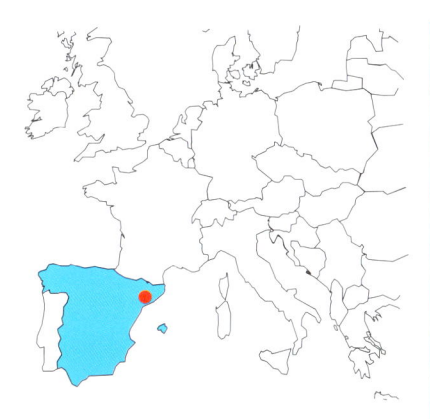

- the only MONICA population in Spain
- Mediterranean population, high smoking, low coronary rates but increasing
- research on coronary disease in women and the elderly
- obesity, diabetes, nutrition, psychosocial factors
- hosted 7th Council of Principal Investigators, August 1992

MCC 39: MONICA-Catalonia
Two areas now counted as one Reporting Unit.

Administrative centre
Programa CRONICAT,
Hospital de la Santa Creu i Sant Pau,
P. Claret 167, Barcelona 08025, Spain
T +34 93 456 3612; F +34 93 433 1572

Population
Residents aged 25–74 of five counties in the metropolitan area of Barcelona, extending from the northern limit of the city towards the Pyrenees. One of the most industrialized areas in Spain, with a minor agricultural sector, it has several hospitals and a university providing a comprehensive health service. Half the population comes from other Spanish regions. High unemployment rates improved during the study period as did socioeconomic development. Response rates for surveys were high. Cardiovascular mortality rates were similar to the Spanish average. The total population in 1991 was 1 119 000.

Funding
1. Institute of Health Studies, Department of Health and Social Security, Generalitat of Catalonia. 2. Manresa Savings Bank. 3. Hospital de la Santa Creu i Sant Pau.

Dates
Coronary-event registration; 1985–94. Coronary care: 1986–87, 1989–94. Population surveys: 1986–88, 1990–92, 1994–96. No stroke registration.

Additional description
Established to evaluate the CRONICAT Programme for the community control of chronic diseases, MONICA-Catalonia originally planned to monitor two areas. However a change of plan led to one single study area. Population surveys included 8990 men and women and additional items. MONICA-Catalonia confirmed the low incidence of coronary heart disease shown in mortality statistics, achieved good quality scores, and is the model for other surveys and registers in Spain. Outside the former 'Eastern bloc' centres of Asia, central and eastern Europe, Catalonia was the only MONICA population to see coronary-event rates increasing—but from a very low level.

Local research interests
Coronary disease and risk factors in women. Obesity, diabetes, nutrition, psychosocial factors. Risk assessment. Delivery of care. Ageing. Epidemiological surveillance methods.

Continuing activity
Registration continued until 1998. Population surveys have ceased. Cohort studies are ongoing.

Key Personnel
PI: Susana Sans. Former Co–PI 1984–93: Ignacio Balaguer-Vintró. Biochemistry: Francesc González Sastre. Former key staff: Lluïsa Balañá, Anna Puigdefàbregas, Guillermo Paluzie.

Selected publications
Comprehensive list available on request
1. Balaguer-Vintró I, Sans S. Coronary heart disease mortality trends and related factors in Spain. *Cardiology*, 1985, 72:97–104. PMID:3872179.
2. Sans S, Balaguer-Vintró I, Fornells J, Borrás J, Méndez E. CRONICAT Programme: review of three years experience in a community chronic diseases prevention programme in Spain. In: Chazov E, Oganov RG, Perova N and V. *Preventive Cardiology*. London: Harwood Academic Publishers, 1985: 481–485. ISBN 3-7186-0338-I.
3. Rodés A, Sans S, Balañá Ll, Paluzie G, Aguilera R, Balaguer-Vintró I. Recruitment methods and differences in early, late and non-respondents in the first MONICA-CATALONIA population survey. *Revue d'Epidémiologie et de Santé Publique*, 1990, 38:447–453. PMID:2082450.
4. Paluzie G, Sans S, Balañá L, Balaguer-Vintro I. Random zero versus standard sphygmomanometer (extended abstract). *Acta Cardiologica*, 1994, 64:327–329. PMID:7976064.
5. Sans S, Kesteloot H, Kromhout D, on behalf of the Task Force. The burden of cardiovascular diseases mortality in Europe. Erratum in: *European Heart Journal*, 1997, 18:1680–1681. *European Heart Journal*, 1997, 18:1231–1248. PMID: 9508543.
6. Sans S. Does change in serum cholesterol of a population influence coronary heart disease mortality? (Editorial). *European Heart Journal*, 1997, 18:540–543. PMID 9129876.
7. Sans S, Puigdefàbregas A, Paluzie G. Acute myocardial infarction is increasing in Spanish men. *European Heart Journal*, 1999, 20 Abstr supl 1:472–472. PMID:10513291.
8. Sans S, Paluzie G, Puigdefàbregas A. Trends of coronary heart disease in Catalonia, 1985–97: MONICA project. *Butlletí Epidemiològic de Catalunya* 2000, XXI (extraordinari 1r trimestre):61–67. (Catalan). ISSN 0211-6340. PMID:na. URL: http://www.gencat.es/sanitat/portal/cat/spbec.htm.
9. Paluzie G, Sans S, Balañá L, Puig T, González-Sastre F, Balaguer-Vintró I. Secular trends in smoking according to educational level between 1986 and 1996: the MONICA Study-Catalonia. *Gaceta Sanitaria*, 2001, 117:303–311. (Spanish, English abstract). PMID:11578559.
10. Sans S, Paluzie G, Balañá L, Puig T, Balaguer-Vintró I. Trends in prevalence, awareness, treatment and control of arterial hypertension between 1986 and 1996: the MONICA-Catalonia study (Erratum in: *Medicina Clínica* (Barc), 2001, 117:731). *Medicina Clínica* (Barc), 2001, 117:246–253. (Spanish, English abstract). PMID:11562326.

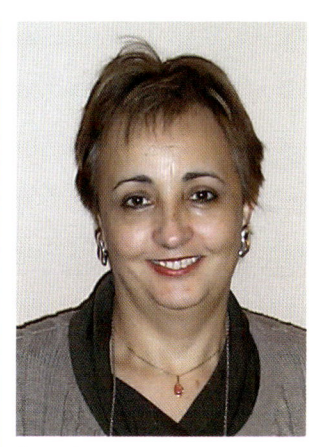

Susana Sans

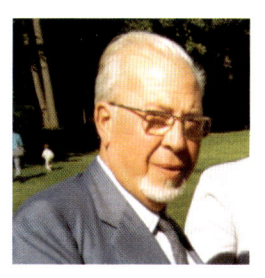

Ignacio Balaguer-Vintró

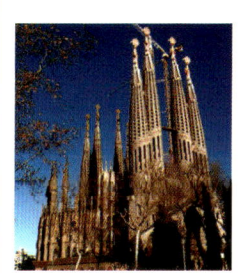

Barcelona

**Susana Sans,
Ignacio Balaguer-Vintró**

#77 Sweden-Gothenburg (SWE-GOT, SG)

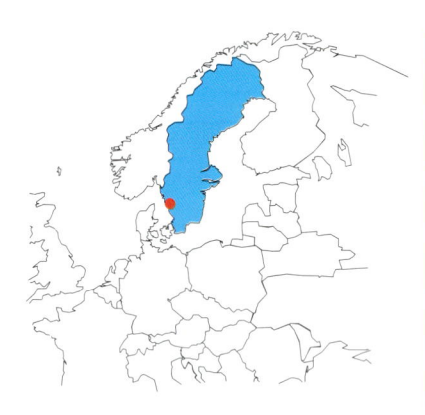

- Gothenburg population has contributed much to cardiovascular epidemiology
- low all-causes mortality, coronary and stroke rates
- changes in event rates in the mid-range
- good improvements in risk factors
- results contrast with those from Northern Sweden

MCC 40:GOT-MONICA
Single Reporting Unit.

Administrative centre
Section of Preventive Cardiology,
Institute of Cardiovascular Diseases, Göteborg University,
Drakegatan 6, SE–41250 Göteborg, Sweden
T +46 31 703 1884; F +46 31 703 1890
The base for coronary and stroke registers and for population surveys was Sahlgrenska University Hospital, Göteborg.

Population
Residents aged 25–64 of the city of Göteborg (Gothenburg), in the south-west of Sweden. It is Sweden's largest port. Industries include car manufacturing, space and information technology and several universities. Immigrants make up 17% of the population. They suffer high unemployment rates. In addition, there are social and health-related differences within the city. The total population in 1991 was 433 000.

Funding
1. Swedish Medical Research Council. 2. Swedish Heart and Lung Foundation. 3. The Inga-Britt and Arne Lundberg Foundation.

Dates
Coronary and stroke-event registration: 1984–1994. Coronary care: 1986–1987 and 1991–1992. Population surveys: 1985/1986, 1990/1991, 1994–1996.

Additional description
Screening of random population samples has been carried out since 1963 on 50-year old men born in 1913, 1923, 1933 and 1943; on men aged 47–55 born in 1915–1925 (excluding 1923). Samples were examined in 1970–1973, 1974–1977 and 1980. Screening was also carried out on women aged 35–64 in 1980 and on women aged 55–84 in 1997. Serum cholesterol, smoking and blood pressure as well as coronary-event rates and mortality have all declined over this period.

Continuing activity
Population screening continues, but registration of events via hospital records is now carried out nationally.

Key personnel
PI: Lars Wilhelmsen. Co-PI: Annika Rosengren. Other staff: Saga Johansson, Per Harmsen (stroke). Statistician: Georg Lappas.

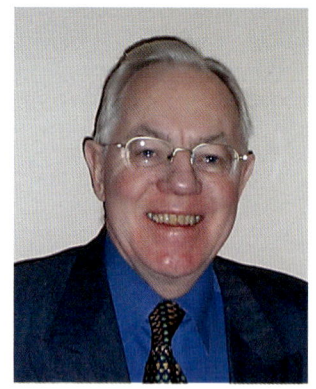

Selected publications
1. Harmsen P, Tsipogianni A, Wilhelmsen L. Stroke incidence rates were unchanged while fatality rates declined, during 1971–1987 in Göteborg, Sweden. *Stroke,* 1992, 23:1410–1415. PMID:1412576.
2. Landin-Wilhelmsen K, Wilhelmsen L, Wilske J, Lappas G, Rosén T, Lindstedt G, Lundberg PA, Bengtsson B-A. Sunlight increases serum 25 (OH) vitamin D concentration, whereas 1,25(OH)2D3 is unaffected. Results from a general population study in Gothenburg, Sweden (the WHO MONICA Project). *European Journal of Clinical Nutrition,* 1995, 49:400–407. PMID:7656883.
3. Wilhelmsen L, Rosengren A, Johansson S, Lappas G. Coronary heart disease attack rate, incidence and mortality 1975–1994 in Göteborg, Sweden. *European Heart Journal,* 1997, 18:572–581. PMID:9129885.
4. Wilhelmsen L, Johansson S, Rosengren A, Wallin I, Dotevall A, Lappas G. Risk factors for cardiovascular disease during 1985–1995 in Göteborg, Sweden. The GOT–MONICA Project. *Journal of Internal Medicine,* 1997, 42:199–211. PMID:9350164.
5. Wilhelmsen L. Cardiovascular monitoring of a city during 30 years, ESC population studies lecture for 1996. *European Heart Journal,* 1997, 18:1220–1230. PMID:9458414.
6. Wilhelmsen L, Rosengren A, Lappas G. Relative importance of improved hospital treatment and primary prevention. Results from 20 years of the Myocardial Infarction Register in Göteborg, Sweden. *Journal of Internal Medicine,* 1999, 245:185–191. PMID: 10081521.
7. Rosengren A, Stegmayr B, Johansson I, Huhtasaari F, Wilhelmsen L. Coronary risk factors, diet and vitamins as possible explanatory factors of the Swedish north-south gradient in coronary disease: a comparison of two MONICA centres. *Journal of Internal Medicine,* 1999, 246:577–586. PMID:10620101.
8. Rosengren A, Eriksson H, Larsson B, Svärdsudd K, Tibblin G, Welin L, Wilhelmsen L. Secular changes in cardiovascular risk factors over 30 years in Swedish men aged 50: the study of men born in 1913, 1923, 1933 and 1943. *Journal of Internal Medicine,* 2000, 247:111–118. PMID:10672138.
9. Dotevall A, Rosengren A, Lappas G, Wilhelmsen L. Does immigration contribute to decreasing CHD incidence? Coronary risk factors among immigrants in Göteborg, Sweden. *Journal of Internal Medicine,* 2000, 247:331–339. PMID:10762449.
10. Manhem K, Dotevall A, Wilhelmsen L, Rosengren A. Social gradients in cardiovascular risk factors and symptoms of Swedish men and women: The Göteborg MONICA study 1995. *Journal of Cardiovascular Risk,* 2000, 7:359–368. PMID:11143766.

Lars Wilhelmsen

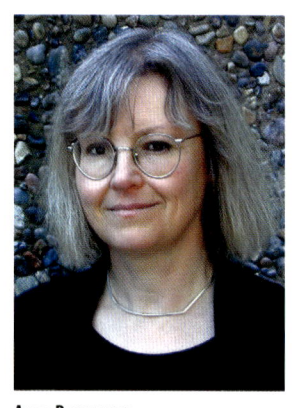

Anna Rosengren

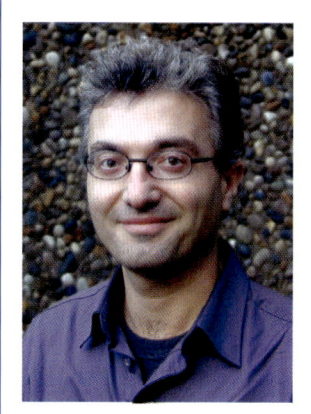

George Lappas

Lars Wilhelmsen

#78 Sweden-Northern Sweden (SWE-NSW, SN)

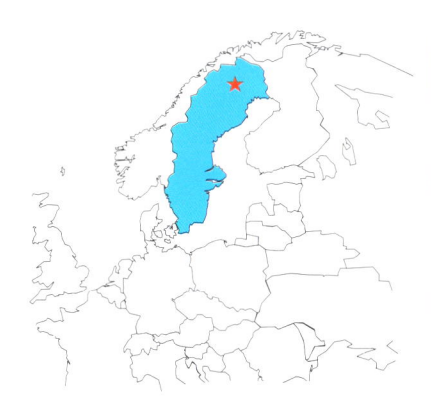

- MONICA crossing the Arctic Circle
- event rates much higher than southern Sweden (see Gothenburg)
- biggest reduction in coronary deaths in men
- highest treatment score for coronary events
- score for risk-factor change in mid-range

MCC 60: Northern Sweden
Two Reporting Units merged into one Reporting Unit Aggregate (RUA).

Administrative centres
MONICA Secretariat, Department of Medicine, University Hospital, SE-901 85 Umea, Sweden and
MONICA Secretariat, Kalix Hospital, SE-952 82 Kalix, Sweden
T +46 90 785 2518 or +46 92 31 3133 ; F +46 90 13 7633
E-mail: Kjell.Asplund@medicin.umu.se and torbjorn.messner@nll.se

Population
Residents aged 25–64 (for coronary events), 25–74 (for strokes and risk-factor surveys) of the Norrbotten and Vasterbotten counties in the north of Sweden. Income and employment in these counties are below average. The people are of south Scandinavian, Saamish and Finnish ethnicity. Skiing, hiking, fishing and hunting during long summer days and winter nights. There are nine acute hospitals. Participation in population surveys was high. The total population in 1991 was 518 000.

Funding
1. Swedish Medical Research Council. 2. Heart and Chest Fund. 3. Vasterbotten and Norrbotten County Councils. 4. King Gustaf V and Queen Victoria's Foundation. 5. Swedish Public Health Institute.

Dates
Coronary-event registration: 1985–1995. Coronary care: 1986–1987, 1989–1995. Stroke-event registration: 1985–94. Population surveys: 1986, 1990, 1994.

Additional description
Excess cholesterol levels fell with the adoption of a pasta-type food culture. Smoking rates extremely low in men but many use smokeless tobacco. The huge decline in male coronary deaths resulted both from declining case fatality and event rates. Coronary-event rates in women and stroke rates were stable. MONICA helped build a biobank of frozen material from 85 000 people with record-linkage for events.

Local research interests
Social and sex differences in risk factors and events. Smokeless tobacco, diabetes and the fibrinolytic system as risk factors. Long-term stroke epidemiology. Gene-environment interactions in cardiovascular disease.

Continuing activity
Coronary and stroke event registration continue with extended coronary age-group. Population survey in 1999 included re-examination of the 1986–94 survey subjects. Use of MONICA data in the GENOS Project (Gene-Environment Interactions in Northern Sweden) and MORGAM collaboration.

Key personnel
PIs 1994–: Kjell Asplund, 2000–: Torbjorn Messner. Former PIs 1984–94: Per-Olov Wester, 1984–2000: Fritz Huhtasaari. Other staff, event-registration and population surveys: Birgitta Stegmayr, Vivan Lundberg, Elsy Jagare-Westerberg, Gunborg Ronnberg, Asa Johansson.

Selected publications
Full list available from the MONICA Secretariat, Umea. Northern Sweden MONICA Project features in Scandinavian Journal of Public Health, 2002, Supplement.

1. Peltonen M, Lundberg V, Huhtasaari F, Asplund K. Marked improvement in survival after acute myocardial infarction in middle-aged men but not in women. The Northern Sweden MONICA Study 1985–1994. *Journal of Internal Medicine*, 2000, 247:579–587. PMID:10809997.
2. Peltonen M, Asplund K, Rosén M. Social patterning of myocardial infarction and stroke in Sweden: incidence and survival. *American Journal of Epidemiology*, 2000, 151:283–292. PMID: n/a.
3. Stegmayr B, Vinogradova T, Malyutina S, Peltonen M, Nikitin Y, Asplund K. Widening gap of stroke between east and west. Eight-year trends in occurrence and risk factors in Russia and Sweden. *Stroke*, 2000, 31:2–8. PMID:10625707.
4. Johansson L, Jansson JH, Boman K, Nilsson TK, Stegmayr B, Hallmans G. Tissue plasminogen activator, plasminogen activator inhibitor-1, and tissue plasminogen activator/plasminogen activator inhibitor-1 complex as risk factors for the development of a first stroke. *Stroke*, 2000, 31: 26–32. PMID:10625711.
5. Ohgren B, Weinehall L, Stegmayr B, Boman K, Hallmans G, Wall S. What else adds to hypertension in predicting stroke? *Journal of Internal Medicine*, 2000, 248:475–82. PMID: 11155140.
6. Rask E, Olsson T, Soderberg S, Andrew R, Livingstone DE, Johnson O, Walker BR. Tissue-specific dysregulation of cortisol metabolism in human obesity. *Journal of Clinical Endocrinology and Metabolism*, 2001, 86:1418–21. PMID: 11238541.
7. Nilsson M, Trehn G, Asplund K. Use of complementary and alternative medicine remedies in Sweden. *Journal of Internal Medicine*, 2001, 250:225–33. PMID: 11555127.
8. Soderberg S, Ahren B, Eliasson M, Dinesen B, Brismar K, Olsson T. Circulating IGF binding protein-1 is inversely associated with leptin in non-obese men and obese postmenopausal women. *European Journal of Endocrinology*, 2001, 144:283–90. PMID: 11248749.
9. Lundberg V, Wikstrom B, Bostrom S, Asplund K. Exploring sex differences in case fatality in acute myocardial infarction or coronary death events in the Northern Sweden MONICA Project. *Journal of Internal Medicine*, 2002, 251:235–44. PMID: 11886483.
10. Persson M, Carlberg B, Mjorndal T, Asplund K, Bohlin J, Lindholm L. 1999 WHO/ISH Guidelines applied to a 1999 MONICA sample from northern Sweden. *Journal of Hypertension*, 2002, 20:29–35. PMID:11791023.

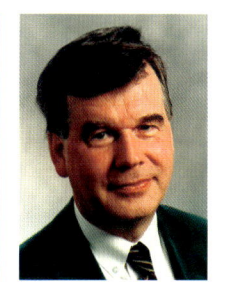

Kjell Asplund

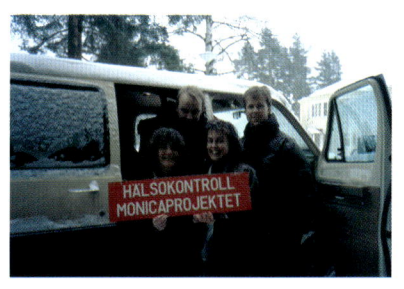

Survey team

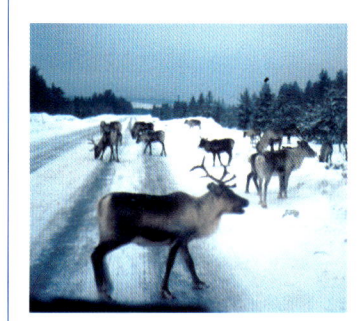

Reindeer on the road

Kjell Asplund

#79 Switzerland (SWI-SWI, SW)

Switzerland-Vaud/Fribourg (SWI-VAF, SV)
Switzerland-Ticino (SWI-TI, ST)

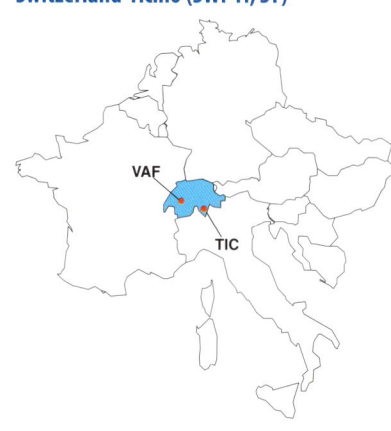

- low event rates despite high total cholesterol levels
- no coronary-event registration in women
- included the 65–74 age group
- hosted 6th Council of Principal Investigators, Lugano, April 1990

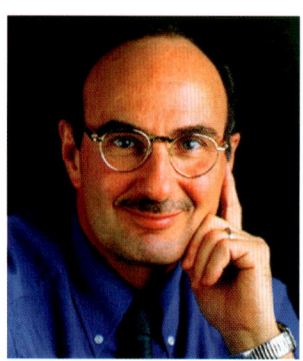

Felix Gutzwiller

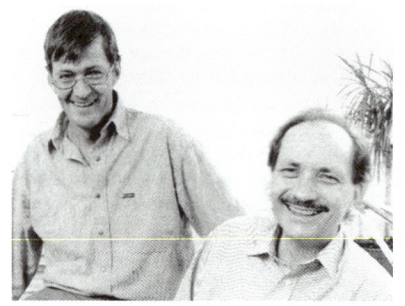

Vincent Wietlisbach and Martin Rickenbach

MCC 50: MONICA Switzerland
Two distinct Reporting Units merged for coronary care.

Administrative centre
Institut universitaire de médecine sociale et préventive,
rue du Bugnon, 17, 1005 Lausanne, Switzerland
T +41 21 314 72 72; F +41 21 314 73 73.

Population
Residents aged 25–74 of the French-speaking cantons of Vaud and Fribourg, and the Italian-speaking canton of Ticino. They are both mixed urban and rural communities but had the lowest and highest mortality from coronary heart disease in Switzerland. Women were excluded from event-registration because projected numbers of female events were considered too low for estimating trends. The total population of Vaud-Fribourg in 1991 was 791 000, and of Ticino was 288 000.

Funding
1. Swiss National Science Foundation (grant numbers 3.856–0.83, 3.938.0.85, 32–9271.87, 32–30110.90). 2. Canton of Vaud. 3. Canton of Ticino.

Dates
Coronary-event registration: 1985–1993*. Coronary care: 1986, 1990, 1992/93*. Population surveys: 1984–86, 1988/89, 1992/93. No stroke registration. *Men only.

Additional description
A community programme for primary prevention of coronary heart disease was launched in Ticino in 1984. The evaluation used the results of the three MONICA population surveys, with Vaud-Fribourg acting as the control comparator region. The surveys inspired opportunistic studies such as a study of the decline in blood lead as the use of unleaded petrol increased; and monitoring of physical activity over a one-week period using a pedometer. MONICA serum is being used extensively as an archive of reference values for Switzerland, for example of serum 25–Hydoxyvitamin D, serum lipoprotein(a), and antibodies to the herpes simplex virus.

Local research interests
Association between blood lipids and obesity. Epidemiological transition (comparison with the Seychelles Heart Study). Diffusion of health technology in coronary care.

Continuing activity
All activities have ceased but coronary-event registration using a coronary-care survey is planned for a one-year period in the near future.

Key personnel
Initiators: Felix Gutzwiller (PI, moved to Zurich in 1988), Gianfranco Domenighetti (Ticino). Co-ordinator 1988–: Fred Paccaud. Medical Officers: Martin Rickenbach (Vaud–Fribourg), Fabrizio Barazzoni (Ticino). Statistician: Vincent Wietlisbach.

Selected publications
1. Rickenbach M, Wietlisbach V, Beretta-Piccoli C, Moccetti T, Gutzwiller F. [Smoking, blood pressure and body weight in the Swiss population. MONICA study 1988–89.] *Schweizerische Medizinische Wochenschrift Supplementum*, 1993, 48:21–28. (German). PMID:8446868.
2. Burnand B, Wietlisbach V, Riesen W, Noseda G, Barazzoni F, Rickenbach M, Gutzwiller F. [Blood lipids in the Swiss population. MONICA study 1988–89.] *Schweizerische Medizinische Wochenschrift Supplementum*, 1993, 48:29–37. (French). PMID:8446869.
3. Sequeira MM, Rickenbach M, Wietlisbach V, Tullen B, Schutz Y. Physical activity assessment using a pedometer and its comparison with a questionnaire in a large population survey. *American Journal of Epidemiology*, 1995, 142:989–999. PMID:7572981.
4. Wietlisbach V, Paccaud F, Rickenbach M, Gutzwiller F. Trends in cardiovascular risk factors (1984–1993) in a Swiss region: results of three population surveys. *Preventive Medicine*, 1997, 26:523–533. PMID:9245675.
5. Bourquin MG, Wietlisbach V, Rickenbach M, Perret F, Paccaud F. Time trends in the treatment of acute myocardial infarction in Switzerland from 1986 to 1993: do they reflect the advances in scientific evidence from clinical trials? *Journal of Clinical Epidemiology*, 1998, 51:723–732. PMID:9731920.
6. Paccaud F, Schlüter-Fasmeyer V, Wietlisbach V, Bovet P. Dyslipidemia and abdominal obesity: an assessment in three general populations. *Journal of Clinical Epidemiology*, 2000, 53:393–400. PMID:10785570.

Vincent Wietlisbach

#80 United Kingdom-Belfast (UNK-BEL, UB)

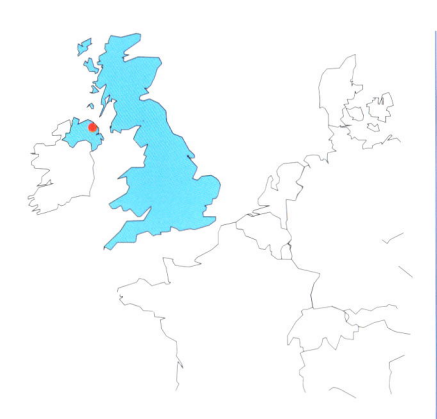

- very high coronary-event rates in both sexes
- less extreme than Glasgow, its neighbour across the sea, but similar
- significant decline in event rates and risk factors
- high scores for treatment of coronary disease

MCC 34: Belfast
Single Reporting Unit.

Administrative centre
Department of Epidemiology and Public Health (formerly Community Medicine), Mulhouse Building, Queen's University Belfast, Grosvenor Road, Belfast, BT12 6BJ, Northern Ireland, United Kingdom
T +44 28 9023 7153; F +44 28 9023 6298
Coordinating centre for the MONICA Optional Study on Haemostatic Factors, and antioxidant studies. Registration centre was in the Royal Victoria Hospital.

Population
Residents aged 25–64 of Belfast city and the Castlereagh, North Down and Ards health districts in Counties Antrim and Down. MONICA covered one-third of the Province's population. Approximately 60% were Belfast city dwellers. Shipbuilding, engineering and textiles are in decline. Dairy farming dominates rural areas. MONICA took place against a backdrop of sectarian strife, now thankfully reduced, in common with a once very high coronary mortality. The total population in 1991 was 477 000.

Funding
1. Medical Research Council (UK). 2. Department of Health and Social Services (NI). 3. Northern Ireland Chest Heart and Stroke Association. 4. British Heart Foundation.

Dates
Coronary-event registration: 1983–1993. Population surveys: 1983/1984, 1986/1987, 1991/1992. Coronary care: 1985, 1988–1993. No stroke registration.

Local research interests
Local studies linked to MONICA included physical activity, diet and homocysteinaemia. Belfast joined up with the three French MONICA centres in the ECTIM Study, a case-control study exploring the genetic basis of myocardial infarction (leader: François Cambien), and the PRIME cohort study of 10 600 Northern Irish and French men (leader: Pierre Ducimetière). The Belfast PI has been active in the administration and coordination of research and secured European Commission funding for MONICA between 1996 and 1999 through a BIOMED 2 grant, as well as funding for the MORGAM study (see below).

Continuing activity
The MORGAM (MOnica Risk Genetics Archiving and Monograph) involves many MONICA and other centres and is coordinated from Belfast. It includes a general risk cohort, a genetic cohort, archiving the MONICA Database, and support for work on this Monograph.

Key personnel
PI: Alun Evans. Others: Malcolm Kerr, Zelda Mathewson, Mary McConville, Evelyn McCrum, Dermot O'Reilly, Susan Cashman.

Selected publications
1. Gey KF, Stahelin HB, Puska P, Evans A. Relationship of plasma level of vitamin C to mortality from ischemic heart disease. *Annals of the New York Academy of Sciences*, 1987, 498:110–123. PMID:3497600.
2. Evans AE, Kerr MM, McCrum EE, McMaster D, McCartney LK, Mallaghan M, Patterson CC. Coronary risk factor prevalence in a high incidence area: results from the Belfast MONICA Project. *Ulster Medical Journal*, 1989, 58:60–68. PMID:2788947.
3. McClean R, McCrum E, Scally G, McMaster D, Patterson C, Evans A. Dietary patterns in the Belfast MONICA Project. *Proceedings of the Nutrition Society*, 1990, 49:297–305. PMID:2236094.
4. Evans AE, Patterson CC, Mathewson Z, McCrum EE, McIlmoyle EL. Incidence, delay and survival in the Belfast MONICA Project coronary event register. *Revue d'Epidémiologie et de Santé Publique*, 1990, 38:419–427. PMID:2082447.
5. Parra HJ, Arveiler D, Evans AE, Cambou JP, Amouyel P, Bingham A, McMaster D, Shaffer P, Douste-Blazy P, Luc G et al. A case-control study of lipoprotein particles in two populations at contrasting risk for coronary heart disease: the ECTIM Study. *Arteriosclerosis and Thrombosis*, 1992, 12:701–707. PMID: 1534257.
6. Cambien F, Poirier O, Lecerf L, Evans A, Cambou JP, Arveiler D, Luc G, Bard JM, Bara L, Ricard S, Tiret L, Amouyel P, Alhenc-Gelas F, Soubrier F. Deletion polymorphism in the gene for angiotensin converting enzyme is a potent risk factor for myocardial infarction. *Nature*, 1992, 359:641–644. PMID:1328889
7. Evans AE, Zhang W, Moreel JF, Bard JM, Ricard S, Poirier O, Tiret L, Fruchart JC, Cambien F. Polymorphisms of the apolipoprotein B and E genes and their relationship to plasma lipid variables in healthy Chinese men. *Human Genetics*, 1993, 92:191–197. PMID: 8370587.
8. Evans AE, Ruidavets JB, McCrum EE, Cambou JP, McClean R, Douste-Blazy P, McMaster D, Bingham A, Patterson CC, Richard JL et al. Autres pays, autres coeurs? Dietary patterns, risk factors and ischaemic heart disease in Belfast and Toulouse. *Quarterly Journal of Medicine*, 1995, 88:469–77. PMID:7633873.
9. Marques-Vidal P, Arveiler D, Evans A, Amouyel P, Ferrières J, Ducimetière P. Different alcohol drinking and blood pressure relationships in France and Northern Ireland: The PRIME Study. *Hypertension*, 2001, 38: 1361–1366.

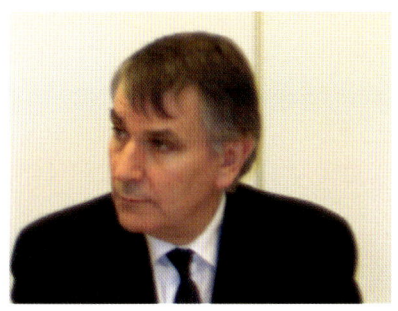

Alun Evans

Alun Evans

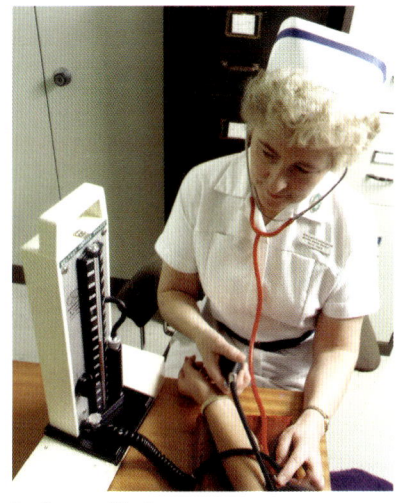

Random-zero blood pressure measurement

#81 United Kingdom-Glasgow (UNK-GLA, UG)

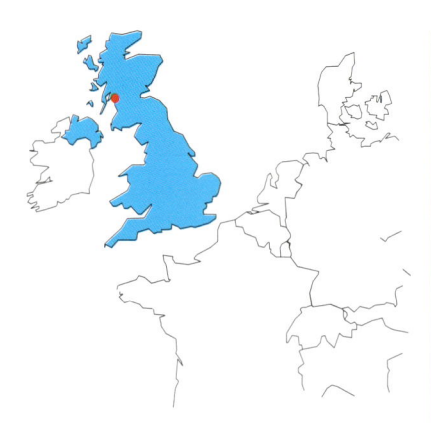

- only MONICA population from mainland Britain
- extreme coronary-event rates, particularly in women
- high scores for risk-factor change and implementing coronary care
- modest change in end-points during study period
- researching sex differences, deprivation, fibrinogen, left ventricular dysfunction, new risk factors

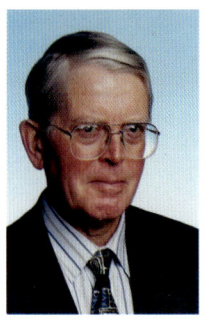

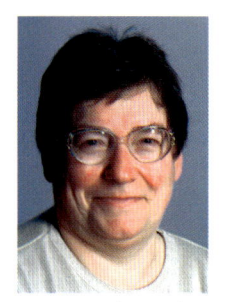

Hugh Tunstall-Pedoe

Caroline Morrison

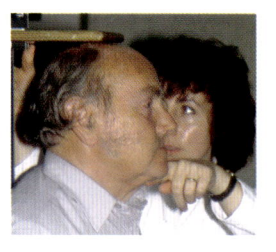

Measuring height

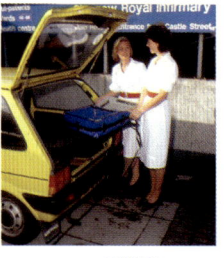

MONICA nurses

MCC 37: Scottish MONICA
Single Reporting Unit.

Administrative centre
Cardiovascular Epidemiology Unit, Dundee University, Ninewells Hospital,
Dundee DD1 9SY, Scotland, United Kingdom
T +44 1382 641 764; F +44 1382 641 095
Website: http://www.dundee.ac.uk/cardioepiunit
MONICA Quality Control Centre for Event Registration.
Registration centre was in Glasgow Royal Infirmary.

Population
Residents aged 25–64 of Glasgow city, north of the River Clyde. Built on former trade and heavy industry, Glasgow's inner city had high levels of deprivation, chronic disease and population decline. Chosen for its exceptional coronary disease mortality in both sexes, survey response rates were below average for Scotland, and MONICA. The total population in 1991 was 392 000.

Funding
1. Chief Scientist Organization of the Scottish Office Department of Health. 2. British Heart Foundation.

Dates
Coronary-event registration and coronary care together: 1985–94 (*–96). Population surveys: 1986, (1989*), 1992, 1995. No stroke registration. (*) = omitted from WHO MONICA database.

Additional description
Originally Scottish MONICA planned to compare two differing populations but the loss of Edinburgh left Glasgow alone to represent Scotland and mainland Britain. The first population survey, with many items added to the MONICA protocol as the Scottish Heart Health Study, visited 25 districts across Scotland recruiting 12 000 men and women in 1984–87. Results of this study of risk factors and lifestyle led to national policies on prevention. World-record disease rates in Glasgow, now in decline, caused national embarrassment—as well as perverse pride. The Dundee Unit was home to the Rapporteur and oversaw quality control work. It was also responsible for editing two MONICA Congress supplements, and this Monograph.

Local research interests
Coronary disease and risk factors in women. Deprivation. Delivery of care. Sudden death and resuscitation. Comparison of classic with new risk factors: fibrinogen, other haemostatic factors, diet and vitamins. Left ventricular dysfunction and heart failure. Helicobacter pylori, Chlamydia pneumoniae.

Continuing activity
Extended ECTIM study, MORGAM (See Belfast page). Registration ceased 1996, no MONICA population surveys after 1995. Cohort studies continue.

Key personnel
PI: Hugh Tunstall-Pedoe. Co-PI 1986–: Caroline Morrison. Former Co-PI (Population Surveys) 1984–90: Cairns Smith. Former Co-PI (Event Registration) 1984–86: Graham Watt. Biochemist 1984–: Roger Tavendale.

Selected publications
Comprehensive list and abstracts available at:
http://www.dundee.ac.uk/cardioepiunit

1. Tunstall-Pedoe H, Smith WCS, Crombie IK, Tavendale R. Coronary risk factor and lifestyle variation across Scotland: results from the Scottish Heart Health Study. *Scottish Medical Journal*, 1989, 34:556–60. PMID:2631202.
2. Smith WCS, Lee AJ, Crombie IK, Tunstall-Pedoe H. Control of blood pressure in Scotland: the rule of halves. *British Medical Journal*, 1990, 300:981–3. PMID:2344507.
3. Lean MEJ, Han TS, Morrison CE. Waist circumference as a measure for indicating the need for weight management. *British Medical Journal*, 1995, 311:158–161. PMID:7613427.
4. Leslie WS, Fitzpatrick B, Morrison CE, Watt GCM, Tunstall-Pedoe H. Out-of-hospital cardiac arrest due to coronary heart disease: a comparison of survival before and after the introduction of defibrillators in ambulances. *Heart*, 1996, 75:195–199. PMID:8673761.
5. Tunstall-Pedoe H, Morrison C, Woodward M, Fitzpatrick B, Watt G. Sex differences in myocardial infarction and coronary deaths in the Scottish MONICA population of Glasgow 1985–91. *Circulation*, 1996, 93:1981–1992. PMID:8640972.
6. Morrison C, Woodward M, Leslie W, Tunstall-Pedoe H. Effect of socio-economic group on incidence of, management of, and survival after myocardial infarction and coronary death: analysis of community coronary event register. *British Medical Journal*, 1997, 314:541–546. PMID:9055711.
7. Tunstall-Pedoe H, Woodward M, Tavendale R, A'Brook R, McCluskey MK. Comparison of the prediction by 27 different factors of coronary heart disease and death in men and women of the Scottish Heart Health Study: cohort study. *British Medical Journal*, 1997, 315:722–729. PMID:9314758.
8. McDonagh TA, Morrison CE, Tunstall-Pedoe H, Ford I, McMurray JJV, Dargie HJ. Symptomatic and asymptomatic left ventricular dysfunction in an urban population. *Lancet*, 1997, 350:829–833, PMID: 9310600.
9. Woodward M, Lowe GD, Rumley A, Tunstall-Pedoe H. Fibrinogen as a risk factor for coronary heart disease and mortality in middle-aged men and women. The Scottish Heart Health Study. *European Heart Journal*, 1998, 19:55–62. PMID:9503176.
10. Wrieden WL, Hannah MK, Bolton-Smith C, Tavendale R, Morrison C, Tunstall-Pedoe H. Plasma vitamin C and food choice in the third Glasgow MONICA population survey. *Journal of Epidemiology and Community Health*, 2000, 54:355–60. PMID:10814656.

Hugh Tunstall-Pedoe,
Caroline Morrison

#82 United States-Stanford (USA-STA, US)

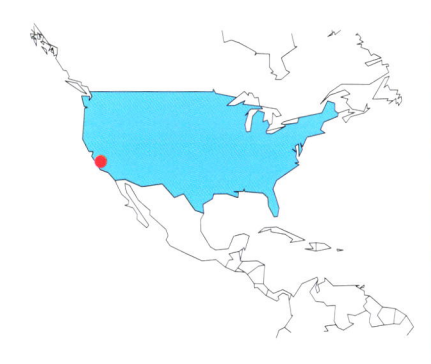

- the only MONICA population from the USA
- derived from monitoring of a community prevention programme
- rapidly falling coronary heart disease mortality but rising revascularization rates
- good risk-factor trends apart from increasing obesity
- researching prevention and control of chronic disease

MCC 43: Stanford
Four geographically separate Reporting Units merged into one Reporting Unit Aggregate (RUA).

Administrative centre
Stanford Center for Research in Disease Prevention,
Stanford University School of Medicine,
1000 Welch Road, Palo Alto, California, 94304-1825 USA
T +1 650 723 6145; F +1 650 725 6906
Website: http://prevention.stanford.edu/

Population
Residents aged 25–64 of four of the Stanford Five-City Project cities, a community cardiovascular disease prevention study. Salinas and Modesto serve agricultural areas with related industries, canning and wine production. Monterey is a coastal city with a declining fishing industry but tourism and military bases. San Luis Obispo hosts a state university. All four were predominantly middle-class but Salinas and Modesto now include large economically-disadvantaged and Mexican-American populations. The total population in 1991 was 380 000.

Funding
National Heart, Lung, and Blood Institute, National Institutes of Health, Public Health Service (HL 21906), 1978–98.

Dates
Coronary-event registration: 1979–1992. Coronary care: 1981–1982, 1985–1986, 1988–1992. Population surveys: 1979/80, 1985/86, 1989/90. No stroke registration for MONICA.

Additional description
The Stanford Five-City Project began in 1978 with two intervention cities (Monterey and Salinas) and three controls (Modesto, San Luis Obispo, and Santa Maria). Population surveys were not conducted in Santa Maria. Community health education took place during 1980–86. Coronary and stroke events were registered to evaluate the interventions. When MONICA was proposed in 1980 the Stanford MCC participated using data from the Five-City Project. The registration procedures predated MONICA so challenging manipulations were needed to provide compatible coronary-event data—not attempted for stroke.

Local research interests
Cardiovascular disease epidemiology and prevention, cancer prevention, behavioural sciences, health communication, exercise, nutrition, lipid disorders, tobacco interventions and control, successful ageing, women's health, social and cultural determinants of health, disease prevention in children and adolescents.

Continuing activity
Registers and population surveys have ended.

Key Personnel
PI: Stephen Fortmann. Other staff: Ann Varady, John Farquhar, William Haskell, Mary Hull, Marilyn Winkleby.

Selected publications
Comprehensive list available at:
http://prevention.stanford.edu/

1. Gillum RF, Fortmann SP, Prineas RJ, Kottke TE. International diagnostic criteria for acute myocardial infarction and acute stroke. *American Heart Journal*, 1984, 108:150–158. PMID:6731265.
2. Farquhar JW, Fortmann SP, Maccoby N, Haskell WL, Williams PT, Flora JA, Taylor CB, Brown BW Jr, Solomon DS, Hulley SB. The Stanford Five-City Project: Design and methods. *American Journal of Epidemiology*, 1985, 122:323–334. PMID:4014215.
3. Fortmann SP, Haskell WL, Williams PT, Varady AN, Hulley SB, Farquhar JW. Community surveillance of cardiovascular diseases in the Stanford Five-City Project: methods and initial experience. *American Journal of Epidemiology*, 1986, 123:656–669. PMID:3953544.
4. Farquhar JW, Fortmann SP, Flora JA, Taylor CB, Haskell WL, Williams PT, Maccoby N, Wood PD. Effects of community-wide education on cardiovascular disease risk factors. The Stanford Five-City Project. *Journal of the American Medical Association*, 1990, 264:359–365. PMID:2362332.
5. Fortmann SP, Winkleby MA, Flora JA, Haskell WL, Taylor CB. Effect of long-term community health education on blood pressure and hypertension control. The Stanford Five-City Project. *American Journal of Epidemiology*, 1990, 132:629–646. PMID:2403104.
6. Taylor CB, Fortmann SP, Flora J, Kayman S, Barrett DC, Jatulis D, Farquhar JW. Effect of long-term community health education on body mass index. The Stanford Five-City Project. *American Journal of Epidemiology*, 1991, 134:235–249. PMID:1877583.
7. Fortmann SP, Taylor CB, Flora JA, Jatulis DE. Changes in adult cigarette smoking prevalence after 5 years of community health education: the Stanford Five-City Project. *American Journal of Epidemiology*, 1993, 137:82–96. PMID:8434576.
8. Fortmann SP, Taylor BC, Flora JA, Winkleby MA. Effect of community health education on plasma cholesterol levels and diet: the Stanford Five-City Project. *American Journal of Epidemiology*, 1993, 137:1039–1055. PMID:8317434.
9. Winkleby MA, Taylor CB, Jatulis D, Fortmann SP. The long-term effects of a cardiovascular disease prevention trial: the Stanford Five-City Project. *American Journal of Public Health*, 1996, 86:1773–1779. PMID:9003136.
10. Fortmann S, Varady A. Effects of a community-wide health education program on cardiovascular disease morbidity and mortality: the Stanford Five-City Project. *American Journal of Epidemiology*, 2000, 152:316–323. PMID:10968376.

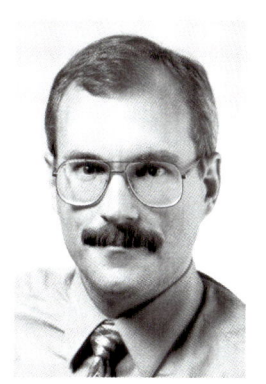

Stephen Fortmann

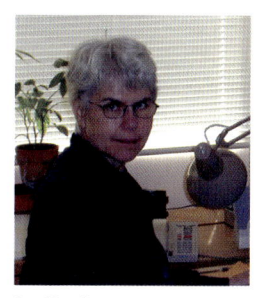

Ann Varady

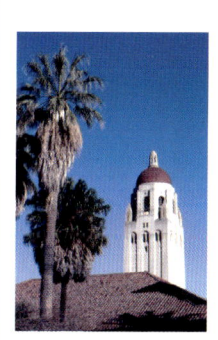

Stanford

Stephen Fortmann

#83 Yugoslavia-Novi Sad (YUG-NOS, YU)

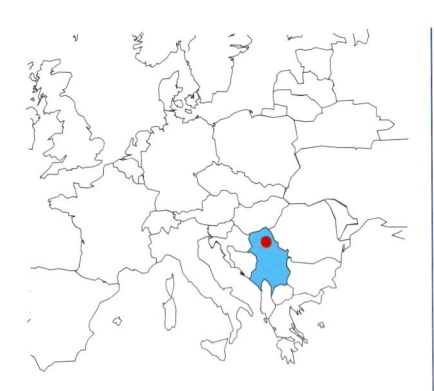

- from the banks of the Danube in Yugoslavia
- greatest increase and highest risk-factor scores in MONICA
- declining event rates reversed into increase
- maintained MONICA collaboration despite war and economic sanctions

MCC 49: Novi Sad
Single Reporting Unit.

Administrative centre
Institute of cardiovascular disease
Institutski put 4
21204 Sremska Kamenica,
Novi Sad, Serbia and Montenegro
T +381 21 612 682; F +381 21 622 059
E-mail: zpotic@eunet.yu

Population
Citizens aged 25–64 of the city of Novi Sad, a multiethnic and multicultural society of some 20 nationalities. Novi Sad, on the river Danube, is the administrative, economic, cultural and educational centre of Vojvodina province. There are several hospitals, a medical centre and a university medical school. Mortality from cardiovascular and cerebrovascular disease is the highest in the country. Response to population surveys was very good. The total population in 1991 was 273 000.

Funding
Regular health insurance fund.

Dates
Coronary and stroke-event registration: 1984–1995. Coronary care: 1987–1995. Population surveys: 1984, 1988/1989, 1994/95.

Additional description
Novi Sad is the only MONICA population in Yugoslavia. The first MONICA survey determined the levels and distribution of major risk factors, contributing to preventive work on coronary and cerebrovascular disease. In the period 1984–1990 morbidity and mortality from coronary and cerebrovascular diseases fell by about 20 percent. Since 1991, with war and economic sanctions, this beneficial trend has reversed and rates have increased continually.

Local research interests
Risk factors in children and young people. Primary prevention. Methodology of monitoring and evaluation; management.

Continuing activity
Event registration. Sample surveys, using the MONICA protocol. Preventive activities.

Key personnel
PI: Milutin Planojevic. Former PI 1984–1986: Djordje Jakovljevic. Other staff: A Svircevic, D Stojsic, T Djapic, M Zikic, P Terzic, Z Solak, V Grujic.

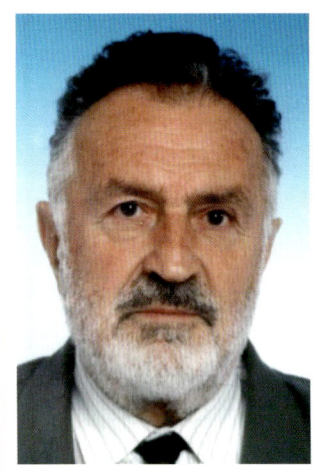

Selected publications
1. Djapic T, Karanov Z. Influence of reduced nutrition on height of systolic and diastolic blood pressure. *Medicinski Pregled*, 1980, 33:369–374. PMID:na.
2. Zikic M. Report of the basic characteristics of the CVD prophylactic program on the territory of Novi Sad community. Abstracts of the 14th World Congress of the Neurology, New Delhi. In: *Neurology – India*, 1989, 37(suppl);102. PMID:na.
3. Zikic M, Knezevic S, Jovanovic M, Slankamenac P. Stroke epidemiology in Novi Sad. *Neurologia Croatica* (Yugoslavia), 1991; 40:171–179. PMID:1932441.
4. Jakovljevic D, Grujic V, Atanackovic D. *Hypertension – text book for general practitioners*, Federal Institute of Public Health, 1995, Belgrade. PMID:na.
5. Planojevic M. The role of the general practitioner in the prevention and control of modern diseases. *Medicinski Pregled*, 1995, 48:231–235. PMID:8524192
6. Radovanovic N, Jakovljevic D. *Quality of life after open heart surgery, a research study*, Institute of Cardiovascular Diseases, Novi Sad, 1997. PMID:na.
7. Dodic B, Planojevic M, Jakovljevic D, Dodic S. [Distribution of the major cardiovascular risk factors in the adult population of Novi Sad.] *Medicinski Pregled*, 1997, 50:53–55. (Serbo-Croat). PMID 9132554.
8. Stojsic D, Benc D, Srdic S, Petrovic M, Tomic N, Stojsic-Milosavljevic A, Panic G, Sakac D. *Treatment of acute coronary syndrome*. Institute of Cardiovascular Diseases, Sremska Kamenica. In press, *Balneoclimatologia*. PMID:na.

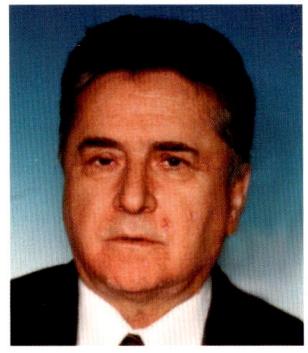

Milutin Planojevic

Djordje Jakovljevic

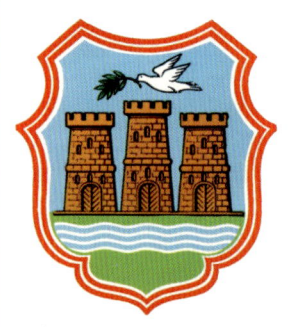

Novi Sad

**Milutin Planojevic,
Djordje Jakovljevic**

#84 Former MONICA Populations

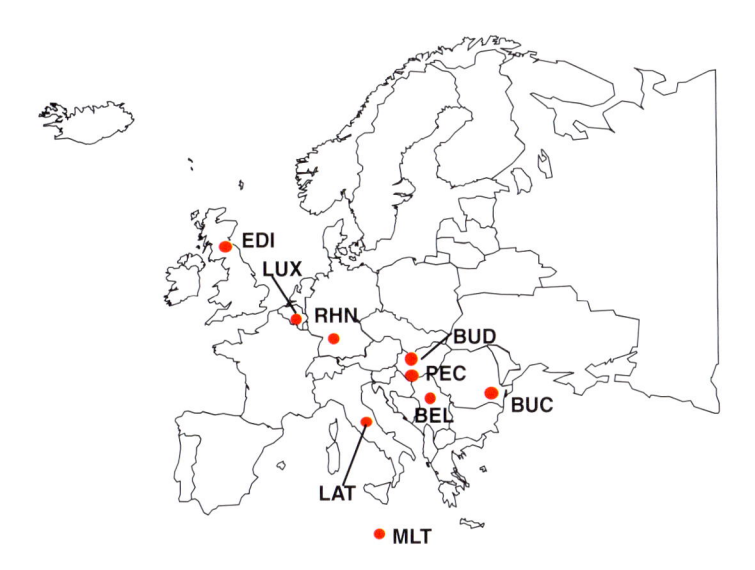

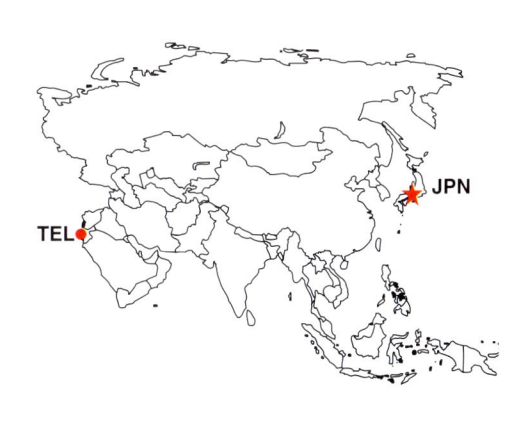

- never started
- stopped early from change in funding or control
- missed deadlines for data transfer
- or transferred data that could not be used

Some MONICA Collaborating Centres did not contribute to collaborative testing of hypotheses on trends because data received in the MONICA Data Centre were too scanty, of inadequate quality, or not received in time to do this. Much time and effort were spent over many years trying to help the MCCs that were experiencing difficulties. Eventually some were encouraged to withdraw, some failed to meet deadlines for data, some discovered major problems with their data which could not be resolved, some failed to obtain continuous funding for the local activities and others simply lost contact, failing to reply to repeated communications. Brief descriptions follow, including what data were registered in the MONICA Data Centre in Helsinki and used in cross-sectional analyses for data books and publications.

Note that comments below on what data were used apply to data that went through the full quality control checks in Helsinki and led to collaborative publications in scientific journals. For some MCCs an accelerated procedure was used for the 1989 *World Health Statistics Annual*, which also included national mortality statistics. Partial data from some of the former MONICA populations, which were not used elsewhere, were used in that publication. (*1*). This applies particularly to routine mortality and demographic data which were collected from the populations before the quality of specific MONICA data was known.

Belgium-Luxembourg (BEL-LUX)
MCC 14: MONICA-Bellux
Luxembourg is the south-east province of Belgium. Rural and forested its low density population is characterized by traditional lifestyles, low socioeconomic status, high mortality and low migration.
PI: M Jeanjean. Inter-University Association for Prevention of Cardiovascular Disease, UCL Brussels.
Routine mortality: 1984–1987. Demographic data: 1981–1994. Coronary-event data: 1985–1991. Coronary care data: none used. Population survey: 1983–1985. No stroke registration.
Problems: after several years of collaboration, data stopped coming to the Data Centre.

Germany-East Germany (GER-EGE)
MCC 23: MONICA East Germany, formerly known as DDR-MONICA
This MCC began with 39 Reporting Units, but managed to survive with only 3, one of which recorded coronary care. The MCC therefore survived and contributed to MONICA. Most of its initial population Reporting Units either did not contribute or did so only to early cross-sectional papers. See #65 *Germany-East Germany*.)

Germany-Rhein-Neckar Region (GER-RHN)
MCC 25: Heidelberg
The region of Baden-Würtenberg is a mixed urban and rural region. It includes the university town of Heidelberg. There is medium industry, the population enjoying high socioeconomic status and average mortality and risk-factor levels.
PI: E Nüssel. *Former Co-PI:* E Östör-Lamm, Dept. of Clinical and Social Medicine, University Medical Clinic, Heidelberg.
Routine mortality: 1983–1989. Demographic data: 1983–1989. Coronary-event data and coronary care data: 1984–1988. Population survey: 1983–1987. Stroke-event data: 1984–1987.
Problems: data stopped coming to the Data Centre following the retirement of Dr Östör-Lamm.

Hungary-Budapest (HUN-BUD), Hungary-Pecs (HUN-PEC)
MCC 27: HUN-MONICA
Budapest: three industrial districts of south Budapest, inhabitants living mainly in blocks of flats with a population of low and middle socioeconomic status.
Pecs: third largest town in Hungary's south-west. The population enjoys above average socioeconomic status. An industrial area dominated by mining. The region was involved in the Healthy Cities and WHO CINDI Projects.
PI: J Duba. National Institute of Cardiology, Budapest.
Routine mortality: 1982–1991. Demographic data: 1982–1992. Coronary-event registration: 1982–1989 (Budapest), 1984–1989 (Pecs). Coronary care data not used. Population surveys: 1982–1984, 1987–1989 (Budapest), 1982–1983, 1987–1988 (Pecs). Stroke-event data: 1983–1989 (Budapest), 1984–1989 (Pecs).
Problems: serious problems were discovered with the quality of initial survey data, and when gaps were discovered in the coverage of coronary and stroke-event registration the combination of problems proved irremediable.

Israel-Tel Aviv (ISR-TEL)
MCC 30: Israel-MONICA
Holom and Bat Jam suburbs of Tel Aviv. The population is mainly middle and lower middle-class with blue-collar workers.
PI: D Brunner. Donolo Institute of Physiological Hygiene, University of Tel Aviv.
Population survey: 1985–1986. No routine mortality, demographic, coronary event, coronary care or stroke-event data used in collaborative analyses.
Problems: non-receipt of data according to MONICA protocol requirements.

Italy-Latina (ITA-LAT)
MCC 31: Area Latina
Province of Latina and neighbouring health units in the region of Lazio, south of Rome. The region was malarious until the 1920s. Eighty

percent of the region is rural. Low incidence area.
PI: G Righetti, Cardiology Dept, SM Goretti Hospital, Latina.
Population survey: 1982–1985. No routine mortality, demographic, coronary-event data, coronary care or stroke-event data used in collaborative analyses.
Problems: early loss of funding led to withdrawal of this population.

Japan (JPN-JPN)
MCC 58: Japan MONICA
Twenty Reporting Units (1985) scattered over Japan.
PI: S Hatano. *Former PI:* I Shigematsu. Japanese Association for Cerebro-Cardiovascular Disease Control.
No Japanese data used in collaborative analyses.
Problems: the MCC's attempt to adapt a large number of different local monitoring studies to the MONICA Project was not successful because of major methodological and structural differences in the study protocols. The very large number of Reporting Units gave the Principal Investigators similar problems to those in East Germany. Loss of this Asian population from MONICA was much regretted.

Malta (MLT-MLT)
MCC 52: Malta
The island of Malta, not including its neighbour Gozo.
PI: Government Chief Medical Officer. *Former Co-PIs:* J Cacciottolo, J Mamo.
Population survey: 1984. No routine mortality, demographic, coronary-event, coronary care or stroke-event data used in collaborative analyses.
Problems: data stopped coming to the Data Centre following the retirement of Dr Cacciottolo.

Romania-Bucharest (ROM-BUC)
MCC 53: Bucharest
Part of Bucharest and possibly a neighbouring rural area.
PIs: C Carp, I Orha. Medical Institute, Fundeni Hospital, Bucharest.
Population survey: 1986–1987. No routine mortality, demographic, coronary-event, coronary care or stroke-event data used in collaborative analyses.
Problem: non-receipt of data according to MONICA protocol requirements, poor definition of study population. Catastrophic earthquake.

United Kingdom-Edinburgh (UNK-EDI)
MCC 38: Scottish MONICA Edinburgh
Edinburgh city, Scotland.
PI: H Tunstall-Pedoe. *Co-PI:* W Symmers.
Population survey: 1986. No data used in collaborative analyses.
Problems: pilot studies showed cold pursuit of coronary cases failed to capture them all, but hot pursuit would need to be prohibitively intensive and expensive because of the rapid movement of cases through the hospitals. Survey data were sent to Helsinki from the 1986 survey but were purged when the MCC was withdrawn. Unlike the survey data from MCCs whose other problems emerged later, Edinburgh's initial survey data were not therefore used in cross-sectional analyses.

Yugoslavia-Belgrade (YUG-BEL)
City of Belgrade.
PI: D Kozarevic. Institute of Chronic Diseases and Gerontology, Belgrade.
No data used in collaborative analyses.
Problems: after an initial pilot period the MCC's parent body was re-organized and decided not to join MONICA.

Reference
1. Anonymous. (Prepared by MONICA Management Centre and MONICA Data Centre with other WHO collaborators.) The WHO MONICA Project. A worldwide monitoring system for cardiovascular diseases: Cardiovascular mortality and risk factors in selected communities. *World Health Statistics Annual*, 1989, 27–149. ISBN 92 4 067890 5. ISSN 0250–3794. MONICA Publication 11.

**Kari Kuulasmaa,
Hugh Tunstall-Pedoe**

MONICA Publications

#85 MONICA Publications List

1. Tuomilehto J, Kuulasmaa K, Torppa J, for the WHO MONICA Project. WHO MONICA Project: geographic variation in mortality from cardiovascular diseases. Baseline data on selected populations, characteristics and cardiovascular mortality. *World Health Statistics Quarterly*, 1987, 40:171–184. PMID: 3617777. MONICA Publication 1.

2. Tunstall-Pedoe H, for the WHO MONICA Project. The World Health Organization MONICA Project (Monitoring Trends and Pająk Determinants in Cardiovascular Disease): a major international collaboration. *Journal of Clinical Epidemiology*, 1988, 41:105–114. PMID: 3335877. MONICA Publication 2.

3. Pająk A, Kuulasmaa K, Tuomilehto J, Ruokokoski E, for the WHO MONICA Project. Geographical variation in the major risk factors of coronary heart disease in men and women aged 35–64 years. *World Health Statistics Quarterly*, 1988, 41:115–140. PMID: 3232405. MONICA Publication 3.

4. Tunstall-Pedoe H. Problems with criteria and quality control in the registration of coronary events in the MONICA study. *Acta Medica Scandinavica Supplementum*, 1988, 728:17–25. PMID: 3202028. MONICA Publication 4.

5. Asplund K, Tuomilehto J, Stegmayr B, Wester PO, Tunstall-Pedoe H. Diagnostic criteria and quality control of the registration of stroke events in the WHO MONICA project. *Acta Medica Scandinavica Supplementum*, 1988, 728:26–39. PMID: 3202029. MONICA Publication 5.

6. Asplund K, Tuomilehto J, Kuulasmaa K, Torppa J, for the WHO MONICA Project. Multinational stroke mortality data at the baseline of the WHO MONICA Project. In: Meyer JS et al., eds. *Cerebral Vascular Disease*, Elsevier Science Publishers, B.V. (Biomedical Division), 1989, 7:167–170. PMID: nil. MONICA Publication 6.

7. Böthig S, for the WHO MONICA Project. WHO MONICA Project: objectives and design. *International Journal of Epidemiology*, 1989, 18(Suppl 1):S29–37. PMID: 2807705. MONICA Publication 7.

8. Tuomilehto J, Kuulasmaa K, for the WHO MONICA Project. WHO MONICA Project: assessing CHD mortality and morbidity. *International Journal of Epidemiology*, 1989, 18(Suppl 1):S38–45. PMID: 2807706. MONICA Publication 8.

9. Keil U, Kuulasmaa K, for WHO MONICA Project. WHO MONICA Project: risk factors. *International Journal of Epidemiology*, 1989, 18(Suppl 1):S46–55. PMID: 2807707. MONICA Publication 9.

10. Tunstall-Pedoe H. Diagnosis, measurement and surveillance of coronary events. *International Journal of Epidemiology*, 1989, 18(3 suppl 1):S169–173. PMID: 2807699. MONICA Publication 10.

11. Anonymous. (Prepared by MONICA Management Centre and MONICA Data Centre with other WHO collaborators.) The WHO MONICA Project. A worldwide monitoring system for cardiovascular diseases: Cardiovascular mortality and risk factors in selected communities. *World Health Statistics Annual*, 1989, 27–149. ISBN 92 4 067890 5. ISSN 0250–3794. MONICA Publication 11.

12. Chambless LE, Dobson AJ, Patterson CC, Raines B. On the use of a logistic risk score in predicting risk of coronary heart disease. *Statistics in Medicine*, 1990, 9:385–396. PMID: 2362977. MONICA Publication 12.

13. Döring A, Pająk A, Ferrario M, Grafnetter D, Kuulasmaa K, for the WHO MONICA Project. Methods of total cholesterol measurement in the baseline survey of the WHO MONICA Project. *Revue d'Epidémiologie et de Santé Publique*, 1990, 38:455–461. PMID: 2082451. MONICA Publication 13.

14. Hense HW, Kuulasmaa K, Zaborskis A, Kupsc W, Tuomilehto J, for the WHO MONICA Project. Quality assessment of blood pressure measurements in epidemiological surveys. The impact of last digit preference and the proportions of identical duplicate measurements. WHO Monica Project. *Revue d'Epidémiologie et de Santé Publique*, 1990, 38:463–468. PMID: 2082452. MONICA Publication 14.

15. Dobson AJ, Kuulasmaa K, Eberle E, Scherer J. Confidence intervals for weighted sums of Poisson parameters. *Statistics in Medicine*, 1991, 10:457–462. PMID: 2028128. MONICA Publication 15.

16. Tunstall-Pedoe H, Kuulasmaa K, Amouyel P, Arveiler D, Rajakangas AM, Pająk A, for the WHO MONICA Project. Myocardial infarction and coronary deaths in the World Health Organization MONICA Project. Registration procedures, event rates, and case-fatality rates in 38 populations from 21 countries in four continents. *Circulation*, 1994, 90:583–612. PMID: 8026046. MONICA Publication 16.

17. Stewart AW, Kuulasmaa K, Beaglehole R, for the WHO MONICA Project. Ecological analysis of the association between mortality and major risk factors of cardiovascular disease. *International Journal of Epidemiology*, 1994, 23:505–516. PMID: 7960374. MONICA Publication 17.

18. Asplund K, Bonita R, Kuulasmaa K, Rajakangas AM, Schädlich H, Suzuki K, Thorvaldsen P, Tuomilehto J, for the WHO MONICA Project. Multinational comparisons of stroke epidemiology. Evaluation of case ascertainment in the WHO MONICA Stroke Study. World Health Organization Monitoring Trends and Determinants in Cardiovascular Disease. *Stroke*, 1995, 26:355–360. PMID: 7886706. MONICA Publication 18.

19. Thorvaldsen P, Asplund K, Kuulasmaa K, Rajakangas AM, Schroll M, for the WHO MONICA Project. Stroke incidence, case fatality, and mortality in the WHO MONICA project. *Stroke*, 1995, 26:361–367. PMID: 7886707. MONICA Publication 19.

20. Hense HW, Koivisto AM, Kuulasmaa K, Zaborskis A, Kupsc W, Tuomilehto J, for the WHO MONICA Project. Assessment of blood pressure measurement quality in the baseline surveys of the WHO MONICA project. *Journal of Human Hypertension*, 1995, 9:935–946. PMID: 8746637. MONICA Publication 20.

21. Asplund K, Rajakangas AM, Kuulasmaa K, Thorvaldsen P, Bonita R, Stegmayr B, Suzuki K, Eisenblätter D, for the WHO MONICA Project. Multinational comparison of diagnostic procedures and management of acute stroke—the WHO MONICA Study. *Cerebrovascular Diseases*, 1996, 6:66–74. PMID: nil. MONICA Publication 21.

22. Dobson A, Filipiak B, Kuulasmaa K, Beaglehole R, Stewart A, Hobbs M, Parsons R, Keil U, Greiser E, Korhonen H, Tuomilehto J. Relations of changes in coronary disease rates and changes in risk factor levels: methodological issues and a practical

example. *American Journal of Epidemiology*, 1996, 143:1025–1034. PMID: 8629609. MONICA Publication 22.

23. Tunstall-Pedoe H. Is acute coronary heart disease different in different countries in the two sexes: lessons from the MONICA Project. *Cardiovascular Risk Factors*, 1996, 6:254–261. PMID: nil. MONICA Publication 23.

24. Salomaa V, Dobson A, Miettinen H, Rajakangas AM, Kuulasmaa K, for the WHO MONICA Project. Mild myocardial infarction—a classification problem in epidemiologic studies. WHO MONICA Project. *Journal of Clinical Epidemiology*, 1997, 50:3–13. PMID: 9048685. MONICA Publication 24.

25. Thorvaldsen P, Kuulasmaa K, Rajakangas AM, Rastenyte D, Sarti C, Wilhelmsen L, for the WHO MONICA Project. Stroke trends in the WHO MONICA project. *Stroke*, 1997, 28:500–506. PMID: 9056602. MONICA Publication 25.

26. Stegmayr B, Asplund K, Kuulasmaa K, Rajakangas AM, Thorvaldsen P, Tuomilehto J, for the WHO MONICA Project. Stroke incidence and mortality correlated to stroke risk factors in the WHO MONICA Project. An ecological study of 18 populations. *Stroke*, 1997, 28:1367–1374. PMID: 9227685. MONICA Publication 26.

27. Molarius A, Seidell JC, Kuulasmaa K, Dobson AJ, Sans S, for the WHO MONICA Project. Smoking and relative body weight: an international perspective from the WHO MONICA Project. *Journal of Epidemiology and Community Health*, 1997, 51:252–260. PMID: 9229053. MONICA Publication 27.

28. Kuulasmaa K, Dobson A, for the WHO MONICA Project. Statistical issues related to following populations rather than individuals over time. *Bulletin of the International Statistical Institute: Proceedings of the 51st Session*, 1997 Aug 18–26, Istanbul, Turkey,Voorburg: International Statistical Institute, 1997, Book 1; 295–298. Also available from URL:http://www.ktl.fi/publications/monica/isi97/isi97.htm. PMID: nil. MONICA Publication 28.

29. Chambless L, Keil U, Dobson A, Mähönen M, Kuulasmaa K, Rajakangas AM, Lowel H, Tunstall-Pedoe H, for the WHO MONICA Project. Population versus clinical view of case fatality from acute coronary heart disease: results from the WHO MONICA Project 1985–1990. *Circulation*, 1997, 96: 3849–3859. PMID: 9403607. MONICA Publication 29.

30. Jackson R, Chambless L, Higgins M, Kuulasmaa K, Wijnberg L, Williams OD, for the WHO MONICA Project and ARIC Study. Gender differences in ischaemic heart disease mortality and risk factors in 46 communities: an ecologic analysis. *Cardiovascular Risk Factors*, 1997, 7:43–54. PMID: nil. MONICA Publication 30.

31. Wolf HK, Tuomilehto J, Kuulasmaa K, Domarkiene S, Cepaitis Z, Molarius A, Sans S, Dobson A, Keil U, Rywik S, for the WHO MONICA Project. Blood pressure levels in the 41 populations of the WHO MONICA Project. *Journal of Human Hypertension*, 1997, 11:733–742. PMID: 9416984. MONICA Publication 31.

32. Dobson AJ, Evans A, Ferrario M, Kuulasmaa KA, Moltchanov VA, Sans S, Tunstall-Pedoe H, Tuomilehto JO, Wedel H, Yarnell J., for the WHO MONICA Project. Changes in estimated coronary risk in the 1980s: data from 38 populations in the WHO MONICA Project. World Health Organization. *Annals of Medicine*, 1998, 30:199–205. PMID: 9667799. MONICA Publication 32.

33. Evans A, Dobson A, Ferrario M, Kuulasmaa K, Moltchanov V, Sans S, Tunstall-Pedoe H, Tuomilehto J, Wedel H, Yarnell J, for the WHO MONICA Project. The WHO MONICA Project: changes in coronary risk in the1980s. Proceedings of the XIth International Symposium on Atherosclerosis, 5–9 October 1997, Paris, France. Elsevier Science. *Atherosclerosis XI*, 1998, 49–55. PMID: nil. MONICA Publication 33.

34. Dobson AJ, Kuulasmaa K, Moltchanov V, Evans A, Fortmann SP, Jamrozik K, Sans S, Tuomilehto J, for the WHO MONICA Project. Changes in cigarette smoking among adults in 35 populations in the mid-1980s. WHO MONICA Project. *Tobacco Control*, 1998, 7:14–21. PMID: 9706749. MONICA Publication 34.

35. Molarius A, Seidell JC, Sans S, Tuomilehto J, Kuulasmaa K, for the WHO MONICA Project. Waist and hip circumferences, and waist-hip ratio in 19 populations of the WHO MONICA Project. *International Journal of Obesity and Related Metabolic Disorders*, 1999, 23:116–125. PMID: 10078844. MONICA Publication 35.

36. Tunstall-Pedoe H, Kuulasmaa K, Mähönen M, Tolonen H, Ruokokoski E, Amouyel P, for the WHO MONICA Project. Contribution of trends in survival and coronary-event rates to changes in coronary heart disease mortality: 10-year results from 37 WHO MONICA project populations. *Lancet*, 1999, 353:1547–1557. PMID: 10334252. MONICA Publication 36.

37. Molarius A, Seidell JC, Sans S, Tuomilehto J, Kuulasmaa K, for the WHO MONICA Project. Varying sensitivity of waist action levels to identify subjects with overweight or obesity in 19 populations of the WHO MONICA Project. *Journal of Clinical Epidemiology*, 1999, 52:1213–1224. PMID: 10580785. MONICA Publication 37.

38. Kuulasmaa K, Tunstall-Pedoe H, Dobson A, Fortmann S, Sans S, Tolonen H, Evans A, Ferrario M, Tuomilehto J, for the WHO MONICA Project. Estimation of contribution of changes in classic risk factors to trends in coronary-event rates across the WHO MONICA Project populations. *Lancet*, 2000, 355:675–687. PMID: 10703799. MONICA Publication 38.

39. Tunstall-Pedoe H, Vanuzzo D, Hobbs M, Mähönen M, Cepaitis Z, Kuulasmaa K, Keil U, for the WHO MONICA Project. Estimation of contribution of changes in coronary care to improving survival, event rates, and coronary heart disease mortality across the WHO MONICA Project populations. *Lancet*, 2000, 355:688–700. PMID: 10703800. MONICA Publication 39.

40. Ingall T, Asplund K, Mähönen M, Bonita R, for the WHO MONICA Project. A multinational comparison of subarachnoid haemorrhage epidemiology in the WHO MONICA stroke study. *Stroke*, 2000, 31:1054–1061. PMID: 10797165. MONICA Publication 40.

41. Molarius A, Seidell JC, Sans S, Tuomilehto J, Kuulasmaa K, for the WHO MONICA Project. Educational level, relative body weight, and changes in their association over 10 years: an international perspective from the WHO MONICA Project. *American Journal of Public Health*, 2000, 90:1260–1268. PMID: 10937007. MONICA Publication 41.

42. Molarius A, Parsons RW, Dobson AJ, Evans A, Fortmann SP, Jamrozik K, Kuulasmaa K, Moltchanov V, Sans S, Tuomilehto J, Puska P, for the WHO MONICA Project. Trends in cigarette smoking in 36 populations from the early 1980s to the mid 1990s: findings from the WHO MONICA Project. *American Journal of Public Health*, 2001, 91:206–212. PMID: 11211628. MONICA Publication 42.

43. Evans A, Tolonen H, Hense HW, Ferrario M, Sans S, Kuulasmaa K, for the WHO MONICA Project. Trends in coronary risk factors in the WHO MONICA Project. *International Journal of Epidemiology*, 2001, 30(Suppl 1):S35–S40. PMID: 11211628. MONICA Publication 43.

44. Kulathinal SB, Kuulasmaa K, Gasbarra D. Estimation of an errors-in-variables regression model when the variances of the measurement errors vary between the observations. *Statistics in Medicine*, 2002,21(8):1089–1101. PMID: 11933035. MONICA Publication 44.

45. Tolonen H, Mähönen M, Asplund K, Rastenyte D, Kuulasmaa K, Vanuzzo D,Tuomilehto J, for the WHO MONICA Project. Do trends in population levels of blood pressure and other cardiovascular risk factors explain trends in stroke event rates? Comparisons of 15 populations in 9 countries within the WHO MONICA Stroke Project. *Stroke*, 2002;33(10): 2367–2375. PMID: 12364723. MONICA Publication 45.

Editor

#86 Abstracts of MONICA Publications

The following 45 publications, which have appeared in print, are those regarded as central to the WHO MONICA Project. They include descriptions of the MONICA methods during the development stage of the project, early cross-sectional results, theoretical, particularly statistical papers from individuals eventually involved in the final analyses, some analyses of sub-sets of data, done to explore methods for the final results, and then major papers on the final collaborative findings. These publications are complemented by a very much larger literature from individual centres, published locally, and described in the pages from individual MONICA Collaborating Centres (MCCs) based on their own populations, see #51–#83.

The publications are numbered to correspond with those on the WHO MONICA Project Website and the Monograph CD-ROM, and also with the references in the text of this Monograph. They are used particularly in section #89 *MONICA Graphics*. The electronic media contain both an additional list and the text of Web publications from MONICA, some of which are appendices to the main published MONICA papers, such as MONICA Publications 38 and 39. They also contain a list of secondary publications such as editorials which appeared in print but have no abstracts.

The way in which the authorship of the papers is cited in some cases does not correspond exactly with what appears in the original papers. MONICA publication policy changed and it took time before the eventual method was agreed of sharing the responsibility between the authors (preparers) of the papers and the WHO MONICA Project, putting names first. The Principal Investigators agreed to make this division of credit retrospective for all MONICA citations, see #41 *Preparation of Manuscripts and Presentations*. When this compromise was agreed on for the authorship of papers, journal editors still sometimes changed citations in the proof of new papers and subsequently had to publish corrections. All those named below as authors were responsible for the papers concerned. However, the original paper might have appeared to give almost all the credit to the WHO MONICA Project and none to the authors, or all to the authors and none to the WHO MONICA Project. Earlier methods of citing MONICA caused serious problems for indexing and citation systems. (For example, although very similar and from the same journal, MONICA Publications 1 and 3 are cited differently by PUBMED, the former as having three named authors and the latter as having no authors. MONICA Publication 24 was attributed by one indexing system to the complete list of MONICA participants, naming the first one named in the appendix of sites and personnel first, although he was not part of the manuscript group named on the front page, and did not feel he deserved it.)

Where there is no attribution "for the WHO MONICA Project" in the authorship of the papers below, this could be for several reasons: the authors concerned were operating as individuals, or invited as individuals addressing a problem of importance to MONICA, not on a remit from the MONICA Steering Committee or as representatives of MONICA, and/or they were not using unpublished MONICA core collaborative data. These papers have been adopted as MONICA publications because they are relevant to the problems that the project as a whole was addressing.

The place of work of the corresponding (usually the first) author has been listed, usually as it appears on the front page of the publication concerned. Sometimes work was done whilst visiting the institution concerned. This listing shows the large number of different institutions involved in the authorship of MONICA Publications. We apologise to the later authors, whose contributions were also important, but it would have taken up too much space to list all the universities and institutions involved in the preparation of all the papers.

Readers involved in major collaborative studies may be interested in the administration of MONICA collaborative publications and authorship. This is discussed elsewhere in this Monograph in #41 *Preparation of Manuscripts and Presentations*, and in the MONICA Manual Part I, Section 2, paragraph 7, Publication Rules. The latter is available from the above MONICA Website and on the Monograph CD-ROM.

Note that the copyrights of abstracts belong to the publishing journal and are published here with permission.

This list of papers is complete as of December 2002. Other papers are in preparation and awaiting publication. Further additions will be listed on the MONICA Website as they appear. MONICA Website: http://www.ktl.fi/monica/

MONICA Publication 1

Tuomilehto J, Kuulasmaa K, Torppa J, for the WHO MONICA Project.
WHO MONICA Project: Geographic variation in mortality from cardiovascular diseases. Baseline data on selected population characteristics and cardiovascular mortality.
World Health Statistics Quarterly, 1987, 40(2):171–184.
MONICA Data Centre, Department of Epidemiology and Health Promotion, National Public Health Institute, Helsinki, Finland

Introduction to paper, no abstract published. Death certificates are the most commonly used source of information for the estimation of the frequency of cardiovascular diseases (CVD) in populations. National mortality statistics have been the major tool used for studying geographic variations in CVD. Such comparisons have suggested that major differences in CVD mortality trends can be found between countries, and that, even national trends can show diverging temporal variations.

To draw conclusions on the incidence and prevalence of CVD from national mortality statistics only is very difficult. Many epidemiologists and statisticians have questioned the accuracy of disease-specific death rates which are obtained from the certification of an underlying cause of death based on the International Classification of Diseases (ICD). The current state of medical knowledge, improper or varying coding practices and insufficient clinical or laboratory data are the main causes of inaccuracies in death certification. The ways in which underlying causes of death are classified in vital statistics offices may also introduce a bias that can contribute to international differences in cause-specific mortality. Another project, specific to geographic comparisons, is that national mortality statistics are produced by pooling data from large populations that may include several heterogeneous sub-populations presenting different mortality experiences.

A great deal of epidemiological research was initiated after the 1950s to explain the risk factors and natural history of CVD. However, neither these studies nor an analysis of national mortality statistics could adequately explain the dynamics of changes in CVD. There was an obvious need for more careful investigation of this disease group which accounts for about 30–50% of all deaths in the middle-aged population of most industrialized countries and is increasing in many countries in the world.

A series of consultations with experts in the field led to the development of a multinational research project, the MONICA Project. This article describes the patterns of CVD mortality by age and sex in the populations which are included in the MONICA Project.

PMID: 3617777.

MONICA Publication 2
Tunstall-Pedoe H, for the WHO MONICA Project.
The World Health Organization MONICA Project (Monitoring Trends and Determinants in Cardiovascular Disease): A major international collaboration.
Journal of Clinical Epidemiology, 1988, 41(2):105–114.

Cardiovascular Epidemiology Unit, Ninewells Hospital and Medical School, Dundee, Scotland

A World Health Organization Working Group has developed a major international collaborative study with the objective of measuring over 10 years, and in many different populations, the trends in, and determinants of, cardiovascular disease. Specifically the programme focuses on trends in event rates for validated fatal and non-fatal coronary heart attacks and strokes, and on trends in cardiovascular risk factors (blood pressure, cigarette smoking and serum cholesterol) in men and women aged 25–64 in the same defined communities. By this means it is hoped to measure changes in cardiovascular mortality and to see how far they are explained on the one hand by changes in incidence mediated by risk factor levels; and on the other by changes in case-fatality rates, related to medical care. Population centres need to be large and numerous; to reliably establish 10-year trends in event rates within a centre 200 or more fatal events in men per year are needed, while for the collaborative study a multiplicity of internally homogeneous centres showing differing trends will provide the best test of the hypotheses. Forty-one MONICA Collaborating Centres, using a standardized protocol, are studying 118 Reporting Units (sub-populations) with a total population aged 25–64 (both sexes) of about 15 million.

PMID: 3335877.

MONICA Publication 3
Pająk A*, Kuulasmaa K, Tuomilehto J, Ruokokoski E, for the WHO MONICA Project.
Geographical variation in the major risk factors of coronary heart disease in men and women aged 35–64 years.
World Health Statistics Quarterly, 1988, 41(3/4):115–140.
*MONICA Data Centre, Department of Epidemiology and Health Promotion, National Public Health Institute, Helsinki, Finland. *School of Public Health, Jagiellonian University, Krakow, Poland*

The WHO MONICA Project is designed to measure the trends in mortality and morbidity from coronary heart disease (CHD) and stroke, and to assess the extent to which they are related to changes in known risk factors in different populations in 27 countries. Risk-factor data are collected from population samples examined in at least two population surveys (one at the beginning of the study and the other at the end). The results of the baseline population surveys are presented. In the populations studied, the proportion of smokers varied between 34–62% among men and 3–52% among women. The population median of systolic blood pressure varied between 121–146 mmHg in men. In women the figures were 118 mmHg and 141 mmHg respectively. In diastolic blood pressure, the variation of median was from 74 mmHg to over 91 mmHg among men and from 72 to 89 mmHg among women. The third major risk factor considered was total cholesterol, with the population median ranging between 4.1 to 6.4 mmol/l among men and 4.2 to 6.3 mmol/l among women. Caution is required when making cross-sectional comparisons between the risk-factor levels as the MONICA Project was not designed for this purpose. Nevertheless, these data do demonstrate clearly the large variety of baseline risk-factor patterns in populations studied in the MONICA Project.

PMID: 3232405.

MONICA Publication 4
Tunstall-Pedoe H.
Problems with criteria and quality control in the registration of coronary events in the MONICA study
Acta Medica Scandinavica Supplementum, 1988, 728:17–25.
MONICA Quality Control Centre for Event Registration, Cardiovascular Epidemiology Unit, Ninewells Hospital and Medical School, Dundee, Scotland, UK

This paper discusses the practical difficulties experienced in registering and coding coronary events. The populations being monitored for fatal and non-fatal coronary events in the World Health Organization MONICA study are too large for surveillance of individuals. Routine medical and medico-legal sources have to be used to identify potential events, which are then coded and categorized according to standard criteria. Methods are dependent on, and have to be adapted to the local system of medical care. Non-fatal cases in hospital are identified and registered either through their admission, 'hot pursuit', or through their discharge, 'cold pursuit'. Each method has its own advantages and disadvantages. Local legal and ethical constraints are also responsible for differences between MONICA Collaborating Centres. Adequacy of investigation of events, and the availability and completeness of medical records are major determinants of the ease and quality of registration. Changes in medical care could cause spurious changes in event rates, and so potential biases need to be monitored and allowed for.

PMID: 3202028.

MONICA Publication 5
Asplund K, Tuomilehto J, Stegmayr B, Wester PO, Tunstall-Pedoe H.
Diagnostic criteria and quality control of the registration of stroke events in the WHO MONICA project.
Acta Medica Scandinavica Supplementum, 1988, 728:26–39.
Department of Medicine, University Hospital, Umea, Sweden

Stroke events are being registered in 27 of the MONICA collaborating centres. Coding of test cases has shown the greatest discrepancies in coding of the type of stroke (different pathoanatomical diagnoses) and of the diagnostic category (whether a definite stroke has occurred or not), as 23% and 14% discrepancies respectively. A check for completeness of stroke registration at the Northern Sweden MONICA Centre showed that more than 91% of the events were retrieved by routine registration procedures. Measures to reduce the discrepancies in coding between centres and to check for completeness of data are suggested. In many centres, the number of stroke events below 65 years of age is too small to permit meaningful analyses. By also including stroke events in the 65 to 74 year age range, the number of fatal events in the Northern Sweden MONICA area increased by 195% and non-fatal events by 149%. Many other MONICA centres have also extended their upper age limit for the registration of stroke events, thus improving the preconditions for statistical evaluations of the long-term changes in stroke incidence.

PMID: 3202029.

MONICA Publication 6
Asplund K, Tuomilehto J, Kuulasmaa K, Torppa J, for the WHO MONICA Project.
Multinational stroke mortality data at the baseline of the WHO MONICA Project.
In: Meyer JS et al, eds. Cerebral Vascular Disease, Elsevier Science Publishers, B.V. (Biomedical Division), 1989, 7:167–170.
Department of Medicine, University Hospital, Umea, Sweden

Introduction since no abstract. In several countries, there has been a dramatic decline in age-specific mortality in cerebrovascular diseases over the last decades. In other populations, the stroke mortality rates have shown a much less impressive decline;in others they have been stable or even increasing. The reasons for these different secular trends are poorly understood.

The main aim of the MONICA Project is to monitor long-term trends in cardiovascular morbidity and mortality in well-defined populations and to assess to what extent these trends are related to changes in established cardiovascular risk factors. The project is initiated and managed by the WHO, and its background, methodology and organization have been described elsewhere.

During a 10-year period, data are collected from official vital statistics, population surveys and prospective uniform registration of acute myocardial infarctions and strokes. In this communication, the baseline age-specific mortality from cerebrovascular disorders in the MONICA populations, as derived from official death statistics, are described.

PMID: not listed.

MONICA Publication 7
Böthig S, for the WHO MONICA Project.
WHO MONICA Project: objectives and design.
International Journal of Epidemiology, 1989, 18(3 Suppl 1):S29–37.
World Health Organization, Cardiovascular Diseases Unit, Geneva, Switzerland

The WHO MONICA Project is a multicentre international collaborative project coordinated by the World Health Organization. Its objective is to measure trends in cardiovascular mortality and morbidity and to assess the extent to which these trends are related to changes in risk factor levels and/or medical care, measured at the same time in defined communities in different countries. Thirty-nine collaborating centres from 26 countries of Europe, North America, and the Western Pacific collaborate in this project, using a standardized protocol and covering a population of approximately 10 million men and women aged 3564. The WHO MONICA Project is directed by the Council of Principal Investigators and a Steering Committee, and it is managed by a Management Centre, Data Centre, Quality Control Centres (for event registration, ECG coding and lipid determinations) and Reference Centres (for optional studies). The MONICA methodology is increasingly used as a measurement tool for cardiovascular and noncommunicable disease prevention and control programmes by centres within and outside the project.

PMID: 2807705.

MONICA Publication 8
Tuomilehto J, Kuulasmaa K, for the WHO MONICA Project.
WHO MONICA Project: assessing CHD mortality and morbidity.
International Journal of Epidemiology, 1989, 18(3 Suppl 1):S38–45.
Department of Epidemiology, National Public Health Institute, Helsinki, Finland

In the WHO MONICA Project mortality and morbidity from acute myocardial infarction is being monitored in 39 Collaborating Centres in 26 countries for a period of 10 years. The myocardial infarction registration procedures have been standardized and suspect coronary events are classified into diagnostic categories according to common criteria. This paper presents ischaemic heart disease mortality figures, based on routine statistics for the study populations and discusses cross-sectional comparability of morbidity data from event registration. Because of differences in availability of data used for diagnostic classification of events (such as autopsy data) the proportions of different diagnostic categories vary from centre to centre. There are, therefore, problems in cross-sectional comparison of morbidity data between the centres. The primary target of event registration in the project is to monitor morbidity changes within centres during the 10-year period. This goal should not be affected by the problems described in this paper.

PMID: 2807706.

MONICA Publication 9

Keil U, Kuulasmaa K, for WHO MONICA Project.
WHO MONICA Project: risk factors.
International Journal of Epidemiology, 1989, 18(3 Suppl 1):S46–55. Erratum appears in Int J Epidemiol, 1990, Sep, 19(3):following 775.
Ruhr-Universität Bochum, Abteilung fur Sozialmedizin und Epidemiologie, Neuherberg, Federal Republic of Germany

The WHO MONICA Project was designed to measure trends and determinants in cardiovascular disease mortality and coronary heart disease and cerebrovascular disease morbidity, and to assess the extent to which these trends are related to changes in known risk factors in 39 collaborative centres in 26 countries. Results of the baseline population surveys are presented. Use of standardized methods allows cross-sectional comparisons to be made of data from the 39 collaborating centres. The proportion of smokers varied between 34 and 62% among men and 3 and 52% among women. The median systolic blood pressure (SBP) values varied from 121 mmHg to 145 mmHg in men and from 117 mmHg to 143 mmHg in women. Median diastolic blood pressure (DBP) values varied from 74 mmHg to 91 mmHg in men and from 72 mmHg to 89 mmHg in women. The prevalence of actual hypertension, defined as SBP and/or DBP greater than 159/94 mmHg, or on antihypertensive medication, varied between 8.4% and 45.3% in men and between 12.6% and 40.5% in women. Median serum total cholesterol values varied from 4.1 mmol/l to 6.4 mmol/l in men and from 4.2 mmol/l to 6.4 mmol/l in women. The results show that there is a large variability in the risk-factor patterns among the MONICA populations. They also indicate that populations with low levels of risk factors are in the minority.

PMID: 2807707.

MONICA Publication 10

Tunstall-Pedoe H.
Diagnosis, measurement and surveillance of coronary events.
International Journal of Epidemiology, 1989, 18(3 suppl 1):S169–173.
Cardiovascular Epidemiology Unit, Ninewells Hospital and Medical School, Dundee, Scotland, UK

Surveillance, monitoring, or registration of coronary heart disease (CHD) in populations large enough to follow trends involve the collection and coding of data provided by routine medical and medico-legal sources. The data may be inadequate, missing from file, or in conflict, but because of the need for completeness, all cases must be used. Registration of a chronic disease in the form of episodes causes some logical problems, as does the need to allocate an underlying cause of death in fatal cases. The problems of extracting and coding the relevant information are discussed with reference to specific items and the results of an international quality control exercise are used to demonstrate how items differ in their consistency of coding. Possible causes of spurious trends are discussed, including inaccurate population data.

PMID: 2807699.

MONICA Publication 11

Anonymous. (Prepared by MONICA Management Centre and MONICA Data Centre with other WHO collaborators.)
The WHO MONICA Project. A worldwide monitoring system for cardiovascular diseases: cardiovascular mortality and risk factors in selected communities.
World Health Statistics Annual, 1989, 27–149.

No abstract in document—introductory paragraphs. Cardiovascular diseases are a major cause of preventable morbidity and premature mortality. They are not diseases of the developed world only, but are increasing and will continue to increase in developing countries as the major communicable diseases come under control.

There is evidence that coronary heart disease, cerebrovascular disease, hypertension, rheumatic fever and rheumatic heart disease are largely preventable. Furthermore, appropriate technology exists for the prevention and control of these diseases.

The main strategies of the WHO Cardiovascular Disease (CVD) Programme are:

— prevention in the population including the development and implementation of national action plans
— primordial prevention and prevention in early life
— integrated cardiovascular disease and non-communicable disease prevention and control measures, since they share common risk factors and common preventive measures.

In order to be able to design proper interventions and to measure their effectiveness, the basic disease pattern of a community has to be established. An appropriate health information system is therefore a necessity for targeted prevention and control programmes.

The WHO MONICA Project (multinational MONItoring of trends and determinants in CArdiovascular disease) was established to clarify the reasons for the differences in mortality trends of coronary heart disease, which in the 1970s were declining in several countries, but constant or rising in many others. The reasons for these differences in mortality trends were not clear since the changes might be caused by a decline in the disease incidence or by better survival of those affected; however, data on morbidity and risk factors were scarce or patchy and were not being collected in a uniform manner. The WHO MONICA Project for monitoring cardiovascular mortality and risk factors in selected countries was the response to this challenge.

PMID: not listed. ISBN 92 4 067890 5. ISSN 0250-3794.

MONICA Publication 12

Chambless LE, Dobson AJ, Patterson CC, Raines B.
On the use of a logistic risk score in predicting risk of coronary heart disease.
Statistics in Medicine, 1990, Apr, 9(4):385–396.
Department of Biostatistics, University of North Carolina, Chapel Hill 27514, USA

Many studies over the last 20 years have used logistic regression to model the relationship between the risk of developing coronary heart disease (CHD) and the levels of risk factors such as high blood pressure, high serum cholesterol, and cigarette smoking. Subsequently, several investigators have proposed the use of some of the published estimated logistic risk functions to predict risk in new populations. Because of great variation in the definition of events, duration of follow-up, population characteristics, definition of risk variables, and selection of other variables in the logistic functions, direct use of such established functions would generally not have validity for the prediction of absolute risk levels. A review of fifteen of these studies indicates on the one hand generally similar results in direction and order of magnitude of effects of the major risk factors, confirming the importance of these risk factors of CHD. On the other hand the reviews indicate sufficient variation to suggest that extrapolation to new populations even to predict relative risk is not justified.

PMID: 2362977.

MONICA Publication 13

Döring A, Pająk A, Ferrario M, Grafnetter D, Kuulasmaa K, for the WHO MONICA Project.
Methods of total cholesterol measurement in the baseline survey of the WHO MONICA Project.
*Revue d'Epidémiologie et de Santé Publique, 1990, 38(5–6):455–461.
Erratum appears in 1991, 39(3):following 317.*
GSF-Medis Institute, München-Neuherberg, Federal Republic of Germany

In the WHO MONICA Project (Monitoring of Trends and Determinants of Cardiovascular Disease) total cholesterol was measured in representative samples from 51 study populations in 26 countries. The biochemical measurements were done locally by the laboratories of collaborating. Differences in measurement procedures among the populations were found in the following factors: fasting status, posture of the subject, tourniquet use, use of serum or plasma, storage conditions, and the analytical method itself. This paper gives an overview of the methods used, and discusses the possible effects of the differences on the comparability of the results. The use of a posture other than that recommended and the use of EDTA (ethylene diaminetetraacetate) plasma are considered to be the most important factors, and were found in nine out of the 51 populations.

PMID: 2082451.

MONICA Publication 14

Hense HW, Kuulasmaa K, Zaborskis A, Kupsc W, Tuomilehto J, for the WHO MONICA Project.
Quality assessment of blood pressure measurements in epidemiological surveys. The impact of last digit preference and the proportions of identical duplicate measurements. WHO Monica Project.
*Revue d'Epidémiologie et de Santé Publique, 1990, 38(5–6):463–468.
Erratum appears in 1991, 39(3):following 317.*
GSF-Medis Institute, Epidemiology Unit, Munich-Neuherberg, Federal Republic of Germany

In the WHO MONICA Project, cardiovascular risk-factor surveys, including measurements of arterial blood pressure (BP), were conducted in more than 50 different populations. In the course of a retrospective BP measurement quality assessment effort, two indicators of 'prejudiced' blood pressure reading, last digit preference and high proportions of identical results in duplicate measurements, are used in addition to other items to evaluate blood pressure measurement quality. We used fictitious blood pressure distributions and applied to them Last Digit Preference scores and Proportions of Identical Duplicate Measurements actually found in the MONICA surveys. The analysis showed that Last Digit Preference affects predominantly the shape of the BP distribution curve, whereas high Proportions of Identical Duplicate Measurements may cause a shift of the entire BP distribution curve. Although the two items are partly interrelated, a clear distinction between them and their effects is advocated.

PMID: 2082452.

MONICA Publication 15

Dobson AJ, Kuulasmaa K, Eberle E, Scherer J.
Confidence intervals for weighted sums of Poisson parameters.
Statistics in Medicine, 1991, Mar, 10(3):457–462.
Department of Statistics, University of Newcastle, New South Wales, Australia

Directly standardized mortality rates are examples of weighted sums of Poisson rate parameters. If the numbers of events are large then normal approximations can be used to calculate confidence intervals, but these are inadequate if the numbers are small. We present a method for obtaining approximate confidence limits for the weighted sum of Poisson parameters as linear functions of the confidence limits for a single Poisson parameter, the unweighted sum. The location and length of the proposed interval depend on the method used to obtain confidence limits for the single parameter. Therefore several methods for obtaining confidence intervals for a single Poisson parameter are compared. For single parameters and for weighted sums of parameters, simulation suggests that the coverage of the proposed intervals is close to the nominal confidence levels. The method is illustrated using data on rates of myocardial infarction obtained as part of the WHO MONICA Project in Augsburg, Federal Republic of Germany.

PMID: 2028128.

MONICA Publication 16

Tunstall-Pedoe H, Kuulasmaa K, Amouyel P, Arveiler D, Rajakangas AM, Pająk A, for the WHO MONICA Project.
Myocardial infarction and coronary deaths in the World Health Organization MONICA Project. Registration procedures, event rates, and case-fatality rates in 38 populations from 21 countries in four continents.
Circulation, 1994, Jul, 90(1):583–612.
Cardiovascular Epidemiology Unit, University of Dundee, Ninewells Hospital, Scotland, UK

Background The WHO MONICA Project is a 10-year study that monitors deaths due to coronary heart disease (CHD), acute myocardial infarction, coronary care, and risk factors in men and women aged 35 to 64 years in defined communities. This analysis of methods and results of coronary-event registration in 1985 through 1987 provides data on the relation between CHD morbidity and mortality.

Methods and Results Fatal and nonfatal coronary events were monitored through population-based registers. Hospital cases were found by pursuing admissions ('hot pursuit') or by retrospective analysis of discharges ('cold pursuit'). Availability of diagnostic data on identified non-fatal myocardial infarction was good. Information on fatal events (deaths occurring within 28 days) was limited and constrained in some populations by problems with access to sources such as death certificates. Age-standardized annual event rates for the main diagnostic group in men aged 35 to 64 covered a 12-fold range from 915 per 100 000 for North Karelia, Finland, to 76 per 100 000 for Beijing, China. For women, rates covered an 8.5-fold range from 256 per 100 000 for Glasgow, UK, to 30 per 100 000 for Catalonia, Spain. Twenty-eight-day case-fatality rates ranged from 37% to 81% for men (average, 48% to 49%), and from 31% to 91% for women (average, 54%). There was no significant correlation across populations for men between coronary-event and case-fatality rates (r = −.04), the percentages of coronary deaths known to have occurred within one hour of onset (r = .08), or the percentages of known first events (r = −.23). Event and case-fatality rates for women correlated strongly with those for men in the same populations (r = .85, r = .80). Case-fatality rates for women were not consistently higher than those for men. For women, there was a significant inverse correlation between event and case-fatality rates (r = −.33, P < .05), suggesting that non-fatal events were being missed where event rates were low. Rankings based on MONICA categories of fatal events placed some middle- and low-mortality populations, such as the French, systematically higher than they would be based on official CHD mortality rates. However, rates for non-fatal myocardial infarction correlated quite well with the official mortality rates for CHD for the same populations. For men (aged 35 to 64 years), approximately 1.5 (at low event rates) to one (at high event rates) episode of hospitalized, non-fatal, definite myocardial infarction was registered for every death due to CHD. The problem in categorizing deaths due to CHD was the large proportion of deaths with no relevant clinical or autopsy information. Unclassifiable deaths averaged 22% across the 38 populations but represented half of all registered deaths in two populations and a third or more of all deaths in 15 populations.

Conclusions The WHO MONICA Project, although designed to study longitudinal trends within populations, provides the opportunity for relating rates of validated CHD deaths to non-fatal myocardial infarction across populations. There are major differences between populations in non-fatal as well as fatal coronary-event rates. They refute suggestions that high CHD mortality rates are associated with high case-fatality rates or a relative excess of sudden deaths. The high proportion of CHD deaths for which no diagnostic information is available is a cause for concern.

PMID: 8026046.

MONICA Publication 17

Stewart AW, Kuulasmaa K, Beaglehole R, for the WHO MONICA Project.
Ecological analysis of the association between mortality and major risk factors of cardiovascular disease.
International Journal of Epidemiology, 1994, 23(3):505–516.
Department of Community Health, University of Auckland, Auckland, New Zealand

Background The WHO Multinational Monitoring of Trends and Determinants in Cardiovascular Disease (MONICA) Project has been established to measure trends in cardiovascular mortality and coronary heart disease and cerebrovascular disease morbidity and to assess the extent to which these trends are related to changes in known risk factors at the same time in defined communities in different countries. This cross-sectional study is based on data from the early part of the Project and assesses the association between mortality and population risk-factor levels.

Methods Thirty-five populations of men and women aged 35–64 years are used in correlation analyses between four mortality measures (deaths from all causes, cardiovascular diseases, ischaemic heart disease and stroke) and three cardiovascular risk factors (regular cigarette smoking, blood pressure and total cholesterol).

Results In male populations all-causes mortality and stroke mortality had more than 39% of their variance explained by the three risk factors but all cardiovascular and ischaemic heart disease mortality had less than 25% of their variance explained. For female populations each mortality measure except ischaemic heart disease mortality had more than 33% of their variance accounted for by the three risk factors. For both the male and female populations each of the mortality measures shows strong associations with high blood pressure but the associations with smoking and high cholesterol are generally weaker and much less consistent.

Conclusions This analysis has shown that accepted cardiovascular mortality risk factors measured cross-sectionally at the population level do not reflect well the variation in mortality between populations.

PMID: 7960374.

MONICA Publication 18

Asplund K, Bonita R, Kuulasmaa K, Rajakangas AM, Schädlich H, Suzuki K, Thorvaldsen P, Tuomilehto J, for the WHO MONICA Project.
Multinational comparisons of stroke epidemiology. Evaluation of case ascertainment in the WHO MONICA Stroke Study. World Health Organization Monitoring Trends and Determinants in Cardiovascular Disease.
Stroke, 1995, Mar, 26(3):355–360. Erratum appears in 1995, Aug, 26(8):1504.
Department of Medicine, University Hospital, Umea, Sweden

Background and Purpose As part of the WHO MONICA Project (World Health Organization Monitoring Trends and Determinants in Cardiovascular Disease), mortality and incidence rates of acute stroke in 14 centres covering 21 populations from 11 countries were compared.

Methods In this report, coverage and quality of the MONICA stroke registers were evaluated for five key indicators using data submitted to the MONICA Data Centre.

Results A low ratio of MONICA stroke register to routine statistics of stroke mortality and a low proportion of non-fatal out-of-hospital events were the most common biases; they indicate that identifications of fatal cases and/or case finding of non-fatal events occurring outside the hospital were inadequate in many MONICA centres. In 10 populations, the data quality analyses suggested that clarification of possible biases would be needed before these populations can be included in a comparative study. Data from the remaining 11 populations meet the data quality standards for multinational comparisons with respect to case ascertainment.

Conclusions These results show that multinational comparisons of stroke incidence involve considerable problems in developing and maintaining appropriate standards of data quality. However, after considerable efforts to ensure quality, comparisons of stroke data within the MONICA Project are possible among a large number of the MONICA populations. Our observations also indicate that results from multinational comparisons of stroke mortality based on routine statistics must be interpreted with caution.

PMID: 7886706.

MONICA Publication 19

Thorvaldsen P, Asplund K, Kuulasmaa K, Rajakangas AM, Schroll M, for the WHO MONICA Project.
Stroke incidence, case fatality, and mortality in the WHO MONICA project. World Health Organization Monitoring Trends and Determinants in Cardiovascular Disease.
Stroke, 1995, Mar, 26(3):361–367. Errata appear in 1995, Aug, 26(8):1504 and 1995, Dec, 26(12):2376.
WHO MONICA Project Annex, Glostrup Population Studies, Glostrup University Hospital, Denmark

Background and Purpose This report compares stroke incidence, case fatality, and mortality rates during the first years of the WHO MONICA Project in 16 European and two Asian populations.

Methods In the stroke component of the WHO MONICA Project, stroke registers were established with uniform and standardized rules for case ascertainment and validation of events.

Results A total of 13 597 stroke events were registered from 1985 to 1987 in a total background population of 2.9 million people aged 35 to 64 years. Age-standardized stroke incidence rates per 100 000 varied from 101 to 285 in men and from 47 to 198 in women. The combined stroke attack rates for first and recurrent events were approximately 20% higher than incidence rates in most populations and varied to the same extent. Stroke incidence rates were very high among the population of Finnish men tested. The incidence of stroke was, in general, higher among populations in eastern than in western Europe. It was also relatively high in the Chinese population studied, particularly among women. The case-fatality rates at 28 days varied from 15% to 49% among men and from 18% to 57% among women. In half of the populations studied, there were only minor differences between official stroke mortality rates and rates measured on the basis of fatal events registered and validated for the WHO MONICA stroke study.

Conclusions The WHO MONICA Project provides a unique opportunity to perform cross-sectional and longitudinal comparisons of stroke epidemiology in many populations. The present data show how large differences in stroke incidence and case-fatality rates contribute to the more than threefold differences in stroke mortality rates among populations.

PMID: 7886707.

MONICA Publication 20
Hense HW, Koivisto AM, Kuulasmaa K, Zaborskis A, Kupsc W, Tuomilehto J, for the WHO MONICA Project.
Assessment of blood pressure measurement quality in the baseline surveys of the WHO MONICA project.
Journal of Human Hypertension, 1995, Dec, 9(12):935–946.
Institute of Epidemiology and Social Medicine, University Munster, Germany

Because of the general unavailability of reference standards, there exist no common procedures to assess the quality of blood pressure measurements in epidemiological population surveys. To approach this problem within the collaborative international WHO MONICA Project, a standardized assessment of BP measurement quality was developed and applied to the forty-seven baseline surveys of that project. The entire assessments were carried out in retrospect, that is, only after each population survey had been completed. The assessment was focused on the procedures of quality assurance and control as reportedly applied in each survey, and on quality indicators which were derived from the recorded blood pressure values of each survey. The definitions of specific quality assessment items were based on the MONICA Project protocol and on sources in the pertinent literature. The available information on quality assurance and control procedures depended solely on self-reports by local survey organizers and on site visits, and was occasionally found to be at variance with the actual blood pressure recordings. Therefore, quality indicators derived from actual blood pressure recordings were far more informative and comparable between surveys. Each survey was rated as optimal, satisfactory, or unsatisfactory with regard to single quality items and these single scores were used jointly to compute a summary score of blood pressure measurement quality for each survey. This summary score indicated that 39 out of 47 MONICA baseline surveys showed optimal or satisfactory BP measurement quality. Limitations and potential for improvement of quality assessments became apparent. We conclude that a standardized assessment of BP measurement quality in epidemiological population surveys seems feasible and propose that quality assessment methods similar to the ones suggested here become a routine part of future epidemiological analyses of blood pressure values and hypertension in populations. This should facilitate valid study comparisons.

PMID: 8746637.

MONICA Publication 21
Asplund K, Rajakangas AM, Kuulasmaa K, Thorvaldsen P, Bonita R, Stegmayr B, Suzuki K, Eisenblätter D, for the WHO MONICA Project.
Multinational comparison of diagnostic procedures and management of acute stroke—the WHO MONICA Study.
Cerebrovascular Diseases, 1996, 6:66–74.
Department of Medicine, University Hospital, Umea, Sweden

Background and Purpose In the stroke component of the WHO MONICA Project, community-based registers of acute stroke have been undertaken in 20 populations in Finland, Sweden, Denmark, Germany, Italy, Yugoslavia, Hungary, Poland, Lithuania, Russia and China. This paper reports on diagnostic procedures and management of acute stroke in these populations.

Methods The MONICA stroke registers apply uniform registration procedures and diagnostic criteria. Data for three years were pooled and used for cross-sectional comparisons. Longitudinal analyses of the use of computerized tomography (CT) scans and autopsy rates were based on all years up to 1990 for which information was available. The total population in the age range investigated (35–64 years) was 3 250 000. Strokes were also recorded for the 65- to 74-year age range in seven of the 20 populations.

Results In all populations, more than three quarters of all 35–64-year-old stroke patients were managed in hospital; in nine populations more than 90% were managed in hospital. The use of CT scans ranged from 0% in Russia to 70–76% in West Germany, Italy, Sweden and two of the Finnish populations. During the mid-1980s, use of CT scan increased rapidly in China (Beijing), Denmark, Finland and Yugoslavia but spread only slowly in Poland, Lithuania and Russia. Autopsy rates varied from 0% in China to 76% in the Hungarian and one of the Russian populations. During the 1980s, autopsy rates were stable in most populations, but declined considerably in Lithuania, Poland and Sweden. Elderly patients (65–74 years) were less often hospitalized in China but this was not the case in European populations. In all populations, CT scan and autopsy were less often performed in older subjects.

Conclusions Large variations exist between countries in the use of diagnostic procedures and the management of acute stroke. Data obtained before the late 1980s permit only very limited multinational epidemiological comparisons of stroke subtypes, but the possibility for making such comparisons is rapidly improving.

PMID: not listed.

MONICA Publication 22

Dobson A, Filipiak B, Kuulasmaa K, Beaglehole R, Stewart A, Hobbs M, Parsons R, Keil U, Greiser E, Korhonen H, Tuomilehto J.
Relations of changes in coronary disease rates and changes in risk factor levels: methodological issues and a practical example.
American Journal of Epidemiology, 1996, May 15, 143(10):1025–1034.
Centre for Clinical Epidemiology and Biostatistics, University of Newcastle, Australia

One of the main hypotheses of the World Health Organization (WHO) MONICA Project is that trends in the major coronary disease risk factors are related to trends in rates of fatal and non-fatal coronary disease events. The units of study are populations rather than individuals. The WHO MONICA Project involves continuous monitoring of all coronary disease events in the populations over a 10-year period and periodic risk-factor surveys in random samples of the same populations. Estimation of associations between average annual changes in mortality and risk-factor levels is illustrated with the use of data from a subset of MONICA centres. Crude estimates of regression coefficients are compared with estimates obtained by weighting for standard errors in both the outcome and explanatory variables. The results show that the strength of association may be either underestimated or overestimated if these errors are not taken into account.

PMID: 8629609.

MONICA Publication 23

Tunstall-Pedoe H.
Is acute coronary heart disease different in different countries in the two sexes: lessons from the MONICA Project.
Cardiovascular Risk Factors, 1996, 6:254–261.
Cardiovascular Epidemiology Unit, University of Dundee, Ninewells Hospital, Dundee, Scotland, UK

The World Health Organization Monitoring Cardiovascular Disease (MONICA) Project involves standardized recording of information on all acute coronary events (coronary deaths and acute myocardial infarction) occurring in men and women <65 in different populations in 21 countries. Although the long-term objective is to measure trends over time, interim analyses from the international study, and from the Scottish MONICA population in Glasgow, have exploited a unique opportunity for comparing acute coronary heart attacks in men and women. Women on average have a higher 28-day case fatality than men, but this is most marked where event rates are low, and not where they are very high, suggesting that a large number of non-fatal episodes in women may not be recognized and reported in low-incidence populations. The international study showed that more women than men had investigations carried out in fatal cases, and the data on survival showed a systematic difference across almost all centres, in that male fatalities occurred earlier than those in women. This has been corroborated in a very detailed comparison from Glasgow, where the case fatality at 28 days was the same in men and women, but more men died outside the hospital early in the attack and more women after admission. Women have a greater number of unconfirmed or possible infarcts compared with men and more subendocardial infarction. A number of other differences are reported from the Glasgow findings. Even given the apparent failure to recognize some attacks in women, there nonetheless seem to be true differences in the way in which coronary attacks behave in the two sexes. However, these differences are few and subtle, and for many, factors are equal. The study of trends during 10 years will show whether differences are widening or narrowing over time.

PMID: not listed.

MONICA Publication 24

Salomaa V, Dobson A, Miettinen H, Rajakangas AM, Kuulasmaa K, for the WHO MONICA Project.
Mild myocardial infarction—a classification problem in epidemiologic studies. WHO MONICA Project.
Journal of Clinical Epidemiology, 1997, Jan, 50(1):3–13.
Department of Epidemiology and Health Promotion, National Public Health Institute, Helsinki, Finland

In studies assessing the trends in coronary events, such as the World Health Organization (WHO) MONICA Project (Multinational MONItoring of Trends and Determinants of CArdiovascular Disease), the main emphasis has been on coronary deaths and non-fatal definite myocardial infarctions (MI). It is, however, possible that the proportion of milder MIs may be increasing because of improvements in treatment and reductions in levels of risk factors. We used the MI register data of the WHO MONICA Project to investigate several definitions for mild non-fatal MIs that would be applicable in various settings and could be used to assess trends in milder coronary events. Of 38 populations participating in the WHO MONICA MI register study, more than half registered a sufficiently wide spectrum of events that it was possible to identify subsets of milder cases. The event rates and case-fatality rates of MI are clearly dependent on the spectrum of non-fatal MIs, which are included. On clinical grounds we propose that the original MONICA category 'non-fatal possible MI' could be divided into two groups: 'non-fatal probable MI' and 'prolonged chest pain'. Non-fatal probable MIs are cases, which in addition to 'typical symptoms' have electrocardiogram (ECG) or enzyme changes suggesting cardiac ischemia, but not severe enough to fulfil the criteria for non-fatal definite MI. In more than half of the MONICA Collaborating Centres, the registration of MI covers these milder events reasonably well. Proportions of non-fatal probable MIs vary less between populations than do proportions of non-fatal possible MIs. Also rates of non-fatal probable MI are somewhat more highly correlated with rates of fatal events and non-fatal definite MI. These findings support the validity of the category of non-fatal probable MI. In each centre the increase in event rates and the decrease in case-fatality due to the inclusion of non-fatal probable MI was larger for women than men. For the WHO MONICA Project and other epidemiological studies the proposed category of non-fatal probable MIs can be used for assessing trends in rates of milder MI.

PMID: 9048685.

MONICA Publication 25

Thorvaldsen P, Kuulasmaa K, Rajakangas AM, Rastenyte D, Sarti C, Wilhelmsen L, for the WHO MONICA Project.
Stroke trends in the WHO MONICA project.
Stroke, 1997, Mar, 28(3):500–506.
Glostrup Population Studies, Glostrup University Hospital, Denmark

Background and Purpose Stroke registers were established as part of the international collaborative World Health Organization Monitoring of Trends and Determinants in Cardiovascular Disease (WHO MONICA) Project in 17 centres in 10 countries. The aim of the present analyses was to estimate and compare temporal stroke trends across the MONICA populations.

Methods All stroke events in defined populations were ascertained and validated according to a common protocol and uniform criteria. Almost 25 000 stroke events in more than 15 million person-years were analysed. Age-standardized rates for fatal stroke and for all stroke events were calculated for whole calendar years for each of the populations. Temporal stroke trends were estimated using annual rates for five to six years.

Results Annual stroke attack rates decreased among men in 13 populations and among women in 15 of the 17 MONICA populations. Stroke mortality rates declined among men in 11 populations and among women in 14 of the populations studied. The estimated trends reached the level of statistical significance at the 5% level in only a small number of populations. The trends in official cerebrovascular death rates were in agreement with those estimated on the basis of MONICA data in the majority of the populations studied.

Conclusions Decreasing stroke mortality and attack rates in a large proportion of populations studied can be interpreted as an indication of declining stroke rates in most of the populations studied. The numbers of populations with statistically significant trends were small, and it is therefore not possible to determine with certainty in which of the populations the changes were real.

PMID: 9056602.

MONICA Publication 26

Stegmayr B, Asplund K, Kuulasmaa K, Rajakangas AM, Thorvaldsen P, Tuomilehto J, for the WHO MONICA Project.
Stroke incidence and mortality correlated to stroke risk factors in the WHO MONICA Project. An ecological study of 18 populations.
Stroke, 1997, Jul, 28(7):1367–1374.
Department of Medicine, University Hospital, Umea, Sweden

Background The aim of the present study was to determine the extent to which the variation in conventional risk factors contributed to the variation in stroke incidence among these populations.

Methods Within the WHO MONICA Project, stroke has been recorded in 18 populations in 11 countries. In population surveys, risk factors for cardiovascular diseases have been examined in the 35 to 64 year age group. Over a 3-year period, 12 224 acute strokes were registered in men and women within the same age range.

Results The highest stroke attack rates were found in Novosibirsk in Siberia, Russia, and Finland, with a more than three-fold higher incidence than in Friuli, Italy. The mean diastolic blood pressure among the populations differed by 15 mmHg between Novosibirsk (highest) and Denmark (lowest). In multiple regression analyses, the presence of conventional cardiovascular risk factors (smoking and elevated blood pressure) explained 21% of the variation in stroke incidence among the population in men and 42% in women. In Finland, in China, and in men in Lithuania, the stroke incidence rates were higher than expected from the population risk factor levels.

Conclusion Prevalence of smoking and elevated blood pressure explains a substantial proportion of the variation of stroke attack rates between populations. However, other risk factors for stroke that were not measured in the present study also contribute considerably to inter-population differences in stroke rates.

PMID: 9227685.

MONICA Publication 27

Molarius A, Seidell JC, Kuulasmaa K, Dobson AJ, Sans S, for the WHO MONICA Project.
Smoking and relative body weight: an international perspective from the WHO MONICA Project.
Journal of Epidemiology and Community Health, 1997, Jun, 51(3):252–260.
MONICA Data Centre, Department of Epidemiology and Health Promotion, National Public Health Institute, Helsinki, Finland

Study Objective To investigate the magnitude and consistency of the associations between smoking and body mass index (BMI) in different populations.

Design A cross-sectional study.

Setting and Participants About 69 000 men and women aged 35–64 years from 42 populations participating in the first WHO MONICA survey in the early and mid-1980s.

Main Results Compared to never smokers, regular smokers had significantly ($p < 0.05$) lower median BMI in 20 (men) and 30 (women) out of 42 populations (range -2.9 to $0.5\,kg/m^2$). There was no population in which smokers had a significantly higher BMI than never smokers. Among men, the association between leanness and smoking was less apparent in populations with relatively low proportions of regular smokers and high proportions of ex-smokers. Ex-smokers had significantly higher BMI than never smokers in 10 of the male populations but in women no consistent pattern was observed. Adjustment for socioeconomic status did not affect these results.

Conclusions Although in most populations the association between smoking and BMI is similar, the magnitude of this association may be affected by the proportions of smokers and ex-smokers in these populations.

PMID: 9229053.

MONICA Publication 28

Kuulasmaa K, Dobson A, for the WHO MONICA Project.
Statistical issues related to following populations rather than individuals over time.
Bulletin of the International Statistical Institute: Proceedings of the 51st Session, 1997, Aug 18–26, Istanbul, Turkey, Voorburg: International Statistical Institute, 1997. Book 1: 295–298.
Also available from
URL:http://www.ktl.fi/publications/monica/isi97/isi97.htm.
MONICA Data Centre, Department of Epidemiology and Health Promotion, National Public Health Institute, Helsinki, Finland

The paper considers the common situation where data on populations have been obtained by measurement of the individuals in a series of independent samples (e.g. risk factors of cardiovascular disease) and by continuous counting of events in individuals of the entire population (e.g. population mortality or incidence), but the risk factors of those getting the events are not known. Methods are described for the estimation of changes in the population mean of the risk factors, estimation of changes in the disease incidence and estimation of the extent to which the observed incidence changes are explained by the observed changes in the risk factors when data are available from a large number of populations. The units of the last analysis are the populations rather than the individuals, but the variances of the variables (i.e. risk factor changes and incidence changes) as well as qualitative information on the quality of the data are available for each population.

PMID: not listed.

MONICA Publication 29

Chambless L, Keil U, Dobson A, Mähönen M, Kuulasmaa K, Rajakangas AM, Lowel H, Tunstall-Pedoe H, for the WHO MONICA Project.
Population versus clinical view of case fatality from acute coronary heart disease: results from the WHO MONICA Project 1985–1990. Multinational MONItoring of Trends and Determinants in CArdiovascular Disease.
Circulation, 1997, Dec 2, 96(11):3849–3859.
Institute of Epidemiology and Social Medicine, University of Münster, Germany

Background The clinical view of case fatality (CF) from acute myocardial infarction (AMI) in those reaching the hospital alive is different from the population view. Registration of both hospitalized AMI cases and out-of-hospital coronary heart disease (CHD) deaths in the WHO MONICA Project allows both views to be reconciled. The WHO MONICA Project provides the largest data set worldwide to explore the relationship between CHD, CF and age, sex, coronary-event rate, and first versus recurrent event.

Methods and Results All 79 669 events of definite AMI or possible coronary death, occurring from 1985 to 90 among 5 725 762 people, 35 to 64 years of age, in 29 MONICA populations are the basis for CF calculations. Age-adjusted CF (percentage of CHD events that were fatal) was calculated across populations, stratified for different time periods, and related to age, sex, and CHD-event rate. Median 28-day population CF was 49% (range, 35% to 60%) in men and 51% (range, 34% to 70%) in women and was higher in women than men in populations in which CHD-event rates were low. Median 28-day CF for hospitalized events was much lower: in men 22% (range, 15% to 36%) and in women 27% (range, 19% to 46%). Among hospitalized events CF was twice as high for recurrent as for first events.

Conclusions Overall 28-day CF is halved for hospitalized events compared with all events, and again nearly halved for hospitalized 24-hour survivors. Because approximately two-thirds of 28-day CHD deaths in men and women occurred before reaching the hospital, opportunities for reducing CF through improved care in the acute event are limited. Major emphasis should be on primary and secondary prevention.

PMID: 9403607.

MONICA Publication 30

Jackson R, Chambless L, Higgins M, Kuulasmaa K, Wijnberg L, Williams OD, for the WHO MONICA Project and ARIC Study.
Gender differences in ischaemic heart disease mortality and risk factors in 46 communities: an ecologic analysis.
Cardiovascular Risk Factors, 1997, 7:43–54.
Department of Community Health, University of Auckland, New Zealand

Internationally, mortality from ischaemic heart disease is consistently higher among men than women although the mortality:gender ratios differ considerably between countries. The objective of this study was to estimate the contribution of gender differences in ischaemic heart disease risk factors to gender differences in ischaemic heart disease mortality between selected communities in different countries.

Methods This cross-sectional study uses communities as the unit of analysis. Gender differences in age-adjusted ischaemic heart disease mortality between communities were correlated with gender differences in the age-adjusted prevalence of five major ischaemic heart disease risk factors [i.e. cigarette smoking, obesity, high blood pressure, high blood total cholesterol and low blood high density lipoprotein cholesterol].

Data came from the World Health Organization coordinated MONICA (Multinational Monitoring of Trends and Determinants in Cardiovascular Disease) Project and the US National Heart Lung and Blood Institute sponsored ARIC (Atherosclerosis Risk in Communities) Study, which have been collecting gender-specific data on ischaemic heart disease risk factors, morbidity and mortality from geographically defined communities in over 25 countries. Data from 46 communities in 24 countries participating in either the MONICA Project or the ARIC Study are included in these analyses. The analyses are restricted to the age group 45 to 64 years.

Results Ischaemic heart disease mortality rates in women were less than half the male rates in all but one community, suggesting that intrinsic biological factors influence gender differences in ischaemic heart disease. There was a more than one-fold variation in gender-specific ischaemic heart disease mortality between communities and a strong positive correlation between male and female ischaemic heart disease mortality across the 46 communities, indicating that environmental or lifestyle factors are also important determinants of gender differences in ischaemic heart disease death rates.

In multiple regression analyses using ischaemic heart disease mortality ratios as the dependant variable, only obesity (partial correlation coefficient: $r = 0.43$, $p = 0.008$) and cigarette smoking ($r = 0.48$, $p = 0.003$) contributed significantly to the model. There were strong correlations between gender ratios in the five risk factors. Approximately 40% of the variation in the gender ratios of ischaemic heart disease mortality across the communities could be explained by differences in the gender ratios of the five risk factors examined.

Conclusions The observed cross-national variation in gender differences in ischaemic heart disease mortality appears to be significantly influenced by gender differences in the standard ischaemic heart disease risk factors, particularly obesity and smoking. However, the strong correlations between the risk-factor gender differences illustrate the potential for substantial confounding in this type of ecological analysis.

PMID: not listed.

MONICA Publication 31
Wolf HK, Tuomilehto J, Kuulasmaa K, Domarkiene S, Cepaitis Z, Molarius A, Sans S, Dobson A, Keil U, Rywik S, for the WHO MONICA Project.
Blood pressure levels in the 41 populations of the WHO MONICA Project.
Journal of Human Hypertension, 1997, Nov, 11(11):733–742.
Department of Physiology and Biophysics, Dalhousie University, Halifax NS, Canada

In the early to mid-1980s, the WHO MONICA Project conducted cardiovascular risk-factor surveys in 41 study populations in 22 countries. Study populations aged 35–64 years comprised 32422 men and 32554 women. Blood pressures (BP) and body mass index (BMI) were measured according to a standard protocol. Participants were asked about antihypertensive medication. In men, the average age-standardized BPs ranged among the populations from 124 to 148 mmHg for systolic (SBP) and from 75 to 93 mmHg for diastolic (DBP). The corresponding values in women were 118 to 145 mmHg for SBP and 74 to 90 mmHg for DBP. In all populations, women had lower SBP than men in the 35–44 age group. However, SBP in women rose more steeply with age so that in 34 of 41 populations women had higher SBP than men in the 55–64 age group. The proportion of participants with untreated major elevation of BP ranged from 4.5% to 33.7% in men and from 1.9% to 22.3% in women. The proportions of participants receiving antihypertensive medication were 4.3–17.7% for men and 6.0–22.0% for women. These proportions were not correlated with the prevalence of untreated hypertensives. Age-adjusted BMI was associated with SBP and accounted for 14% of the SBP variance in men and 32% in women. We found a large difference in SBP among the MONICA study populations and conclude that the results represent a valid estimate of the public health problem posed by elevated BP. We also have shown that almost universally the problem of elevated BP is more prevalent in women than in men, especially in the older age groups.

PMID: 9416984.

MONICA Publication 32
Dobson AJ, Evans A, Ferrario M, Kuulasmaa KA, Moltchanov VA, Sans S, Tunstall-Pedoe H, Tuomilehto JO, Wedel H, Yarnell J, for the WHO MONICA Project.
Changes in estimated coronary risk in the 1980s: data from 38 populations in the WHO MONICA Project. World Health Organization. Monitoring trends and determinants in cardiovascular diseases.
Annals of Medicine, 1998, Apr, 30(2):199–205.
University of Newcastle, Australia

The World Health Organization (WHO) MONICA Project is a 10-year study monitoring trends and determinants of cardiovascular disease in geographically defined populations. Data were collected from over 100 000 randomly selected participants in two risk-factor surveys conducted approximately five years apart in 38 populations using standardized protocols. The net effects of changes in the risk factor levels were estimated using risk scores derived from longitudinal studies in the Nordic countries. The prevalence of cigarette smoking decreased among men in most populations, but the trends for women varied. The prevalence of hypertension declined in two-thirds of the populations. Changes in the prevalence of raised total cholesterol were small but highly correlated between the genders (r = 0.8). The prevalence of obesity increased in three-quarters of the populations for men and in more than half of the populations for women. In almost half of the populations there were statistically significant declines in the estimated coronary risk for both men and women, although for Beijing the risk score increased significantly for both genders. The net effect of the changes in the risk factor levels in the 1980s in most of the study populations of the WHO MONICA Project is that the rates of coronary disease are predicted to decline in the 1990s.

PMID: 9667799.

MONICA Publication 33
Evans A, Dobson A, Ferrario M, Kuulasmaa K, Moltchanov V, Sans S, Tunstall-Pedoe H, Tuomilehto J, Wedel H, Yarnell J, for the WHO MONICA Project.
The WHO MONICA Project: changes in coronary risk in the 1980s.
Proceedings of the XIth International Symposium on Atherosclerosis, 5–9 October 1997, Paris, France. Elsevier Science. Atherosclerosis XI, 1998, 49–55.
The Queen's University of Belfast, Belfast, Northern Ireland, UK

Background The WHO MONICA project is a 10-year study monitoring trends and determinants of cardiovascular disease in geographically defined populations.

Methods and Results Data were collected from randomly selected participants in two risk factor surveys conducted approximately five years apart. The net effects of changes in the risk-factor levels were estimated using risk scores derived from longitudinal studies in the Nordic countries. Prevalence of cigarette smoking decreased among men in most populations, but trends for women varied. Prevalence of hypertension declined in two-thirds of the populations. Changes in prevalence of raised total cholesterol were small. Prevalence of obesity increased in about three-quarters of the populations for both men and women. In almost half the populations there were statistically significant declines in estimated coronary risk for both men and women although for Beijing the risk score increased significantly for both genders.

Conclusions The net effect of changes in risk factor levels in the 1980s in the study populations of the WHO MONICA project is that rates of coronary disease are predicted to decline in the 1990s.

PMID: not listed.

MONICA Publication 34
Dobson AJ, Kuulasmaa K, Moltchanov V, Evans A, Fortmann SP, Jamrozik K, Sans S, Tuomilehto J, for the WHO MONICA Project.
Changes in cigarette smoking among adults in 35 populations in the mid-1980s. WHO MONICA Project.
Tobacco Control, 1998, Spring, 7(1):14–21.
Department of Statistics, University of Newcastle, New South Wales, Australia

Objective To examine changes in the prevalence of cigarette smoking in 35 study populations of the World Health Organization's MONICA Project.

Design Data from two independent, community-based surveys conducted, on average, five years apart.

Setting Geographically defined populations in 21 countries mainly in eastern and western Europe.

Subjects Randomly selected men and women aged 25 to 64 years. Numbers of participants in each study population ranged from 586 to 2817 in each survey.

Main Outcome Measures Changes in proportions of current smokers, ex-smokers, and never-smokers by age and sex using data collected by standardized methods.

Results Among men, smoking prevalence decreased in most populations, by three to four percentage points over five years. In Beijing, however, it increased in all age groups—overall by 11 percentage points. Among women there were increases in smoking in about half the populations. The increases were mainly in the age group 35 to 54 years and often in those populations where smoking prevalence among women has been relatively low.

Conclusions Smoking initiation by middle-aged women in parts of southern and eastern Europe and among men of all ages in Beijing is a matter of concern. The various public health measures that have helped to reduce smoking among men in developed countries should be vigorously extended to these other groups now at growing risk of smoking-related disease.

PMID: 9706749.

MONICA Publication 35

Molarius A, Seidell JC, Sans S, Tuomilehto J, Kuulasmaa K, for the WHO MONICA Project.
Waist and hip circumferences, and waist-hip ratio in 19 populations of the WHO MONICA Project.
International Journal of Obesity and Related Metabolic Disorders, 1999, Feb, 23(2):116–125.
MONICA Data Centre, Department of Epidemiology and Health Promotion, National Public Health Institute, Helsinki, Finland

Objective To assess differences in waist and hip circumferences and waist-to-hip ratio (WHR) measured using a standard protocol among populations with different prevalences of overweight. In addition, to quantify the associations of these anthropometric measures with age and degree of overweight.

Design Cross-sectional study of random population samples.

Subjects More than 32 000 men and women aged 25–64 y from 19 (18 in women) populations participating in the second MONItoring Trends and Determinants in CArdiovascular Disease (MONICA) survey from 1987–1992.

Results Age-standardized mean waist circumference ranges between populations from 83–98 cm in men and from 78–91 cm in women. Mean hip circumference ranged from 94–105 cm and from 97–108 cm in men and women, respectively, and mean WHR from 0.87–0.99 and from 0.76–0.84, respectively. Together, height, body mass index (BMI), age group and population explained about 80% of the variance in waist circumference. BMI was the predominant determinant (77% in men, 75% women). Similar results were obtained for hip circumference. However, height, BMI, age group and population, accounted only for 49% (men) and 30% (women) of the variation in WHR.

Conclusion Considerable variation in waist and hip circumferences and WHR were observed among the study populations. Waist circumference and WHR, both of which are used as indicators of abdominal obesity, seem to measure different aspects of the human body: waist circumference reflects mainly the degree of overweight whereas WHR does not.

PMID: 10078844.

MONICA Publication 36

Tunstall-Pedoe H, Kuulasmaa K, Mähönen M, Tolonen H, Ruokokoski E, Amouyel P, for the WHO MONICA Project.
Contribution of trends in survival and coronary-event rates to changes in coronary heart disease mortality: 10-year results from 37 WHO MONICA Project populations. Monitoring trends and determinants in cardiovascular disease.
Lancet, 1999, May 8, 353(9164):1547–1557.
Cardiovascular Epidemiology Unit (MONICA Quality Control Centre for Event Registration), University of Dundee, Ninewells Hospital and Medical School, Dundee, UK

Background The WHO MONICA (Monitoring Trends and Determinants in Cardiovascular Disease) Project monitored, from the early 1980s, trends over 10 years in coronary heart disease (CHD) across 37 populations in 21 countries. We aimed to validate trends in mortality, partitioning responsibility between changing coronary-event rates and changing survival.

Methods Registers identified non-fatal definite myocardial infarction and definite, possible, or unclassifiable coronary deaths in men and women aged 35–64 years, followed up for 28 days in or out of hospital. We calculated rates from population denominators to estimate trends in age-standardized rates and case fatality (percentage of 28-day fatalities = [100- survival percentage]).

Findings During 371 population-years, 166 000 events were registered. Official CHD mortality rates, based on death certification, fell (annual changes: men −4.0% [range −10.8 to 3.2]; women −4.0% [−12.7 to 3.0]). By MONICA criteria, CHD mortality rates were higher, but fell less (−2.7% [−8.0 to 4.2] and −2.1% [−8.5 to 4.1]). Changes in non-fatal rates were smaller (−2.1%, [−6.9 to 2.8] and −0.8% [−9.8 to 6.8]). MONICA coronary-event rates (fatal and non-fatal combined) fell more (−2.1% [−6.5 to 2.8] and −1.4% [−6.7 to 2.8]) than case fatality (−0.6% [−4.2 to 3.1] and −0.8% [−4.8 to 2.9]). Contribution to changing CHD mortality varied, but in populations in which mortality decreased, coronary-event rates contributed two-thirds and case fatality one-third.

Interpretation Over the decade studied, the 37 populations in the WHO MONICA Project showed substantial contributions from changes in survival, but the major determinant of decline in CHD mortality is whatever drives changing coronary-event rates.

PMID: 10334252.

MONICA Publication 37

Molarius A, Seidell JC, Sans S, Tuomilehto J, Kuulasmaa K, for the WHO MONICA Project.
Varying sensitivity of waist action levels to identify subjects with overweight or obesity in 19 populations of the WHO MONICA Project.
Journal of Clinical Epidemiology, 1999, Dec, 52(12):1213–1224.
MONICA Data Centre, Department of Epidemiology and Health Promotion, National Public Health Institute, Helsinki, Finland

It has been suggested in the literature that cut-off points based on waist circumference (waist action levels) should replace cut-off points based on body mass index (BMI) and waist-to-hip ratio in identifying subjects with overweight or obesity. In this article, we examine the sensitivity and specificity of the cut-off points when applied to 19 populations with widely different prevalences of overweight. Our design was a cross-sectional study based on random population samples. A total of 32 978 subjects aged 25–64 years from 19 male and 18 female populations participating in the second MONICA survey from 1987 to 1992 were included in this study. We found that at waist action level 1 (waist circumference > or = 94 cm in men and > or = 80 cm in women), sensitivity varied between 40% and 80% in men and between 51% and 86% in women between populations when compared with the cut-off points based on BMI (> or = 25 kg/m2) and waist-to-hip ratio (> or = 0.95 for men, > or = 0.80 for women). Specificity was high (> or = 90%) in all populations. At waist action level 2 (waist circumference > or = 102 cm and > or = 88 cm in men and women, respectively, BMI > or = 30 kg/m2), sensitivity varied from 22% to 64% in men and from 26% to 67% in women, whereas specificity was >95% in all populations. Sensitivity was in general lowest in populations in which overweight was relatively uncommon, whereas it was highest in populations with relatively high prevalence of overweight. We propose that cut-off points based on waist circumference as a replacement for cut-off points based on BMI and waist-to-hip ratio should be viewed with caution. Based on the proposed waist action levels, very few people would unnecessarily be advised to have weight management, but a varying proportion of those who would need it might be missed. The optimal screening cut-off points for waist circumference may be population specific.

PMID: 10580785.

MONICA Publication 38

Kuulasmaa K, Tunstall-Pedoe H, Dobson A, Fortmann S, Sans S, Tolonen H, Evans A, Ferrario M, Tuomilehto J, for the WHO MONICA Project.
Estimation of contribution of changes in classic risk factors to trends in coronary-event rates across the WHO MONICA Project populations.
Lancet, 2000, Feb 26, 355(9205):675–687.
Department of Epidemiology and Health Promotion, National Public Health Institute (KTL), Helsinki, Finland

Background From the mid-1980s to mid-1990s, the WHO MONICA Project monitored coronary events and classic risk factors for coronary heart disease (CHD) in 38 populations from 21 countries. We assessed the extent to which changes in these risk factors explain the variation in the trends in coronary-event rates across the populations.

Methods In men and women aged 35–64 years, non-fatal myocardial infarction and coronary deaths were registered continuously to assess trends in rates of coronary events. We carried out population surveys to estimate trends in risk factors. Trends in event rates were regressed on trends in risk score and in individual risk factors.

Findings Smoking rates decreased in most male populations but trends were mixed in women; mean blood pressures and cholesterol concentrations decreased, body mass index increased, and overall risk scores and coronary-event rates decreased. The model of trends in 10-year coronary-event rates against risk scores and single risk factors showed a poor fit, but this was improved with a 4-year time lag for coronary events. The explanatory power of the analyses was limited by imprecision of the estimates and homogeneity of trends in the study populations.

Interpretation Changes in the classic risk factors seem to partly explain the variation in population trends in CHD. Residual variance is attributable to difficulties in measurement and analysis, including time lag, and to factors that were not included, such as medical interventions. The results support prevention policies based on the classic risk factors but suggest potential for prevention beyond these.

PMID: 10703799.

MONICA Publication 39

Tunstall-Pedoe H, Vanuzzo D, Hobbs M, Mähönen M, Cepaitis Z, Kuulasmaa K, Keil U, for the WHO MONICA Project.
Estimation of contribution of changes in coronary care to improving survival, event rates, and coronary heart disease mortality across the WHO MONICA Project populations.
Lancet, 2000 Feb 26, 355(9205):688–700.
Cardiovascular Epidemiology Unit, (MONICA Quality Control Centre for Event Registration), University of Dundee, Ninewells Hospital and Medical School, Dundee, UK

Background The revolution in coronary care in the mid-1980s to mid-1990s corresponded with monitoring of coronary heart disease (CHD) in 31 populations of the WHO MONICA Project. We studied the impact of this revolution on coronary end-points.

Methods Case fatality, coronary-event rates, and CHD mortality were monitored in men and women aged 35–64 years in two separate 3–4-year periods. In each period, we recorded percentage use of eight treatments: coronary-artery reperfusion before, thrombolytics during, and beta-blockers, antiplatelet drugs, and angiotensin-converting-enzyme (ACE) inhibitors before and during non-fatal myocardial infarction. Values were averaged to produce treatment scores. We correlated changes across populations, and regressed changes in coronary end-points on changes in treatment scores.

Findings Treatment changes correlated positively with each other but inversely with change in coronary end-points. By regression, for the common average treatment change of 20, case fatality fell by 19% (95% CI 12–26) in men and 16% (5–27) in women; coronary-event rates fell by 25% (16–35) and 23% (7–39); and CHD mortality rates fell by 42% (31–53) and 34% (17–50). The regression model explained an estimated 61% and 41% of variance for men and women in trends for case fatality, 52% and 30% for coronary-event rates, and 72% and 56% for CHD mortality.

Interpretation Changes in coronary care and secondary prevention were strongly linked with declining coronary end-points. Scores and benefits followed a geographical east-to-west gradient. The apparent effects of the treatment might be exaggerated by other changes in economically successful populations, so their specificity needs further assessment.

Comment in: *Lancet*, 2000, Feb 26, 355(9205):668–9.

PMID: 10703800.

MONICA Publication 40

Ingall T, Asplund K, Mähönen M, Bonita R, for the WHO MONICA Project
A multinational comparison of subarachnoid haemorrhage epidemiology in the WHO MONICA stroke study.
Stroke, 2000, May, 31(5):1054–1061.
Department of Neurology, Mayo Clinic, Scottsdale, Arizona, USA

Background and Purpose By official, mostly unvalidated statistics, mortality from subarachnoid haemorrhage (SAH) show large variations between countries. Using uniform criteria for case ascertainment and diagnosis, a multinational comparison of attack rates and case fatality rates of SAH has been performed within the framework of the WHO MONICA Project.

Methods In 25- to 64-year-old men and women, a total of 3368 SAH events were recorded during 35.9 million person-years of observation in 11 populations in Europe and China. Strict MONICA criteria were used for case ascertainment and diagnosis of stroke subtype. Case fatality was based on follow-up at 28 days after onset.

Results Age-adjusted average annual SAH attack rates varied 10-fold among the 11 populations studied, from 2.0 (95% CI 1.6 to 2.4) per 100 000 population per year in China-Beijing to 22.5 (95% CI 20.9 to 24.1) per 100 000 population per year in Finland. No consistent pattern was observed in the sex ratio of attack rates in the different populations. The overall 28-day case fatality rate was 42%, with 2-fold differences in age-adjusted rates between populations but little difference between men and women. Case fatality rates were consistently higher in eastern than in western Europe.

Conclusions Using a uniform methodology, the WHO MONICA Project has shown very large variations in attack rates of SAH across 11 populations in Europe and China. The generally accepted view that women have a higher risk of SAH than men does not apply to all populations. Marked differences in outcomes of SAH add to the wide gap in the burden of stroke between east and west Europe.

PMID: 10797165.

MONICA Publication 41
Molarius A, Seidell JC, Sans S, Tuomilehto J, Kuulasmaa K, for the WHO MONICA Project.
Educational level, relative body weight, and changes in their association over 10 years: an international perspective from the WHO MONICA Project.
American Journal of Public Health, 2000, Aug, 90(8):1260–1268.
MONICA Data Centre, Department of Epidemiology and Health Promotion, National Public Health Institute, Helsinki, Finland

Objectives This study assessed the consistency and magnitude of the association between educational level and relative body weight in populations with widely different prevalences of overweight and investigated possible changes in the association over 10 years.

Methods Differences in age-adjusted mean body mass index (BMI) between the highest and the lowest tertiles of years of schooling were calculated for 26 populations in the initial and final surveys of the World Health Organization (WHO) MONICA (Monitoring Trends and Determinants in Cardiovascular Disease) Project. The data are derived from random population samples, including more than 42 000 men and women aged 35 to 64 years in the initial survey (1979–1989) and almost 35 000 in the final survey (1989–1996).

Results For women, almost all populations showed a statistically significant inverse association between educational level and BMI; the difference between the highest and the lowest educational tertiles ranged from −3.3 to 0.4 kg/m2. For men, the difference ranged from −1.5 to 2.2 kg/m2. In about two-thirds of the populations, the differences in BMI between the educational levels increased over the 10-year period.

Conclusion Lower education was associated with higher BMI in about half of the male and in almost all of the female populations, and the differences in relative body weight between educational levels increased over the study period. Thus, socioeconomic inequality in health consequences of obesity may increase in many countries.

PMID: 10937007.

MONICA Publication 42
Molarius A, Parsons RW, Dobson AJ, Evans A, Fortmann SP, Jamrozik K, Kuulasmaa K, Moltchanov V, Sans S, Tuomilehto J, Puska P, for the WHO MONICA Project.
Trends in cigarette smoking in 36 populations from the early 1980s to the mid 1990s: findings from the WHO MONICA Project.
American Journal of Public Health, 2001, 91(2):206–212.
MONICA Data Centre, Department of Epidemiology and Health Promotion, National Public Health Institute, Helsinki, Finland

Objectives This report analyses cigarette smoking over 10 years in populations in the World Health Organization (WHO) MONICA Project (to monitor trends and determinants of cardiovascular disease).

Methods Over 300 000 randomly selected subjects aged 25 to 64 years participated in surveys conducted in geographically defined populations.

Results For men, smoking prevalence decreased by more than 5% in 16 of the 36 study populations, remained static in most others, but increased in Beijing. Where prevalence decreased, this was largely due to higher proportions of never smokers in the younger age groups rather than to smokers quitting. Among women, smoking prevalence increased by more than 5% in six populations and decreased by more than 5% in nine populations. For women, smoking tended to increase in populations with low prevalence and decrease in populations with higher prevalence; for men, the reverse pattern was observed.

Conclusions These data illustrate the evolution of the smoking epidemic in populations and provide the basis for targeted public health interventions to support the WHO priority for tobacco control.

PMID: 11211628.

MONICA Publication 43
Evans A, Tolonen H, Hense HW, Ferrario M, Sans S, Kuulasmaa K, for the WHO MONICA Project.
Trends in coronary risk factors in the WHO MONICA Project.
International Journal of Epidemiology, 2001, 30(Suppl 1):S35–S40.
Department of Epidemiology and Public Health, The Queen's University of Belfast, Mulhouse Building, Belfast BT12 6BJ, Northern Ireland, UK

Background The World Health Organization (WHO) MONICA Project was established to determine how trends in event rates for coronary heart disease (CHD) and, optionally, stroke were related to trends in classic coronary risk factors. Risk factors were therefore monitored over 10 years across 38 populations from 21 countries in four continents (overall period covered: 1979–1996).

Methods A standard protocol was applied across participating centres, in at least two, and usually three, independent surveys conducted on random samples of the study populations, well separated within the 10-year study period.

Results Smoking rates decreased in most male populations (35–64 years) but in females the majority showed increases. Systolic blood pressure showed decreasing trends in the majority of centres in both sexes. Mean levels of cholesterol generally showed downward trends, which, although the changes were small, had large effects on risk. There was a trend of increasing body mass index (BMI) with half the female populations and two-thirds of the male populations showing a significant increase.

Conclusions It is feasible to monitor the classic CHD risk factors in diverse populations through repeated surveys over a decade. In general, the risk factor trends are downwards in most populations but in particular, an increase in smoking in women in many populations and increasing BMI, especially in men, are worrying findings with significant public health implications.

PMID: 11759849.

MONICA Publication 44

Kulathinal SB, Kuulasmaa K, Gasbarra D.
Estimation of an errors-in-variables regression model when the variances of the measurement errors vary between the observations.
Statistics in Medicine, 2002, Apr 30, 21(8):1089–1101.
Department of Epidemiology and Health Promotion, National Public Health Institute, Mannerheimintie 166, 00300 Helsinki, Finland

It is common in the analysis of aggregate data in epidemiology that the variances of the aggregate observations are available. The analysis of such data leads to a measurement error situation, where the known variances of the measurement errors vary between the observations. Assuming multivariate normal distribution for the 'true' observations and normal distributions for the measurement errors, we derive a simple EM algorithm for obtaining maximum likelihood estimates of the parameters of the multivariate normal distributions. The results also facilitate the estimation of regression parameters between the variables as well as the 'true' values of the observations. The approach is applied to re-estimate recent results of the WHO MONICA Project on cardiovascular disease and its risk factors, where the original estimation of the regression coefficients did not adjust for the regression attenuation caused by the measurement errors.

PMID: 11933035.

MONICA Publication 45

Tolonen H, Mähönen M, Asplund K, Rastenyte D, Kuulasmaa K, Vanuzzo D, Tuomilehto J, for the WHO MONICA Project.
Do trends in population levels of blood pressure and other cardiovascular risk factors explain trends in stroke event rates? Comparisons of 15 populations in 9 countries within the WHO MONICA Stroke Project.
Stroke, 2002;33(10):2367–2375.
Department of Epidemiology and Health Promotion, National Public Health Institute, Mannerheimintie 166, 00300 Helsinki, Finland

Background and Purpose Previous studies have indicated a reasonably strong relationship between secular trends in classic cardiovascular risk factors and stroke incidence within single population. To what extent variations in stroke trends between populations can be attributed to differences in classic cardiovascular risk factor trends is unknown.

Methods In the World Health Organization Monitoring of Trends and Determinants in Cardiovascular Disease (WHO MONICA) Project, repeated population surveys of cardiovascular risk factors and continuous monitoring of stroke events have been conducted in 35- to 64-year-old people over a 7- to 13-year period in 15 populations in 9 countries. Stroke trends were compared with trends in individual risk factors and their combinations. A 3- to 4-year time lag between changes in risk factors and change in stroke rates was considered.

Results Population-level trends in systolic blood pressure showed a strong association with stroke trends in women but there was no association in men. In women, 38% of the variation in stroke event trends was explained by changes in systolic blood pressure when the 3 to 4-year time lag was taken into account. Combining trends in systolic blood pressure, daily cigarette smoking, serum cholesterol, and body mass index into a risk score explained only a small fraction of the variation in stroke event trends.

Conclusions In this study, it appears that variations in stroke trends between populations can be explained only in part by changes in classic cardiovascular risk factors. The associations between risk factor trends and stroke trends are stronger for women than for men.

PMID: 12364723.

#87 MONICA Publications on the World Wide Web

1. WHO MONICA Project. MONICA Manual. (1998–1999). Available from URL: http://www.ktl.fi/publications/monica/manual/index.htm, URN:*NBN:fi-fe19981146*. MONICA Web Publication 1.
2. Mähönen M, Tolonen H, Kuulasmaa K, Tunstall-Pedoe H, Amouyel P, for the WHO MONICA Project. Quality assessment of coronary event registration data in the WHO MONICA Project. (January 1999). Available from URL: http://www.ktl.fi/publications/monica/coreqa/coreqa.htm, URN:NBN:*fi-fe19991072*. MONICA Web Publication 2.
3. Moltchanov V, Kuulasmaa K, Torppa J, for the WHO MONICA Project. Quality assessment of demographic data in the WHO MONICA Project. (April 1999). Available from URL: http://www.ktl.fi/publications/monica/demoqa/demoqa.htm, URN:*NBN:fi-fe19991073*. MONICA Web Publication 3.
4. Mähönen M, Cepaitis Z, Kuulasmaa K, for the WHO MONICA Project. Quality assessment of acute coronary care data in the WHO MONICA Project. (February 1999). Available from URL: http://www.ktl.fi/publications/monica/accqa/accqa.htm, URN:*NBN:fi-fe19991081*. MONICA Web Publication 4.
5. Mähönen M, Tolonen H, Kuulasmaa K, for the WHO MONICA Project. Quality assessment of stroke event registration data in the WHO MONICA Project. (November 1998). Available from URL: http://www.ktl.fi/publications/monica/strokeqa/strokeqa.htm, URN:*NBN:fi-fe19991080*. MONICA Web Publication 5.
6. Kuulasmaa K, Tolonen H, Ferrario M, Ruokokoski E, for the WHO MONICA Project. Age, date of examination and survey periods in the MONICA surveys. (May 1998). Available from URL: http://www.ktl.fi/publications/monica/age/ageqa.htm, URN:*NBN:fi-fe19991075*. MONICA Web Publication 6.
7. Wolf HK, Kuulasmaa K, Tolonen H, Ruokokoski E, for the WHO MONICA Project. Participation rates, quality of sampling frames and sampling fractions in the MONICA Surveys. (September 1998). Available from URL: http://www.ktl.fi/publications/monica/nonres/nonres.htm, URN:*NBN:fi-fe19991076*. MONICA Web Publication 7.
8. Molarius A, Kuulasmaa K, Evans A, McCrum E, Tolonen H, for the WHO MONICA Project. Quality assessment of data on smoking behaviour in the WHO MONICA Project. (February 1999). Available from URL: http://www.ktl.fi/publications/monica/smoking/qa30.htm, URN:*NBN:fi-fe19991077*. MONICA Web Publication 8.
9. Kuulasmaa K, Hense HW, Tolonen H, for the WHO MONICA Project. Quality assessment of data on blood pressure in the WHO MONICA Project. (May 1998). Available from URL: http://www.ktl.fi/publications/monica/bp/bpqa.htm, URN:*NBN:fi-fe19991082*. MONICA Web Publication 9.
10. Ferrario M, Kuulasmaa K, Grafnetter D, Moltchanov V, for the WHO MONICA Project. Quality assessment of total cholesterol measurements in the WHO MONICA Project. (April 1999). Available from URL: http://www.ktl.fi/publications/monica/tchol/tcholqa.htm, URN:*NBN:fi-fe19991083*. MONICA Web Publication 10.
11. Marques-Vidal P, Ferrario M, Kuulasmaa K, Grafnetter D, Moltchanov V, for the WHO MONICA Project. Quality assessment of data on HDL cholesterol in the WHO MONICA Project. (June 1999). Available from URL: http://www.ktl.fi/publications/monica/hdl/hdlqa.htm, URN:*NBN:fi-fe19991137*. MONICA Web Publication 11.
12. Molarius A, Kuulasmaa K, Sans S, for the WHO MONICA Project. Quality assessment of weight and height measurements in the WHO MONICA Project. (May 1998). Available from URL: http://www.ktl.fi/publications/monica/bmi/bmiqa20.htm, URN:*NBN:fi-fe19991079*. MONICA Web Publication 12.
13. Molarius A, Sans S, Kuulasmaa K, for the WHO MONICA Project. Quality assessment of data on waist and hip circumferences in the WHO MONICA Project. (October 1998). Available from URL: http://www.ktl.fi/publications/monica/waisthip/waisthipqa.htm, URN:*NBN:fi-fe19991091*. MONICA Web Publication 13.
14. Molarius A, Kuulasmaa K, Moltchanov V, Ferrario M, for the WHO MONICA Project. Quality assessment of data on marital status and educational achievement in the WHO MONICA Project. (December 1998). Available from URL: http://www.ktl.fi/publications/monica/educ/educqa.htm, URN:*NBN:fi-fe19991078*. MONICA Web Publication 14.
15. Molarius A, Tuomilehto J, Kuulasmaa K, for the WHO MONICA Project. Quality assessment of data on hypertension control in the WHO MONICA Project. (October 1998). Available from URL: http://www.ktl.fi/publications/monica/hyperten/hbpdrug.htm, URN:*NBN:fi-fe19991084*. MONICA Web Publication 15.
16. Tolonen H, Ferrario M, Minoja M, for the WHO MONICA Project. Quality assessment of data on awareness and treatment of high cholesterol in the WHO MONICA Project. (June 1999). Available from URL: http://www.ktl.fi/publications/monica/hich/hchdrug.htm, URN:*NBN:fi-fe19991130*. MONICA Web Publication 16.
17. Tolonen H, Kuulasmaa K, for the WHO MONICA Project. Quality assessment of data on use of aspirin in the WHO MONICA Project. (June 1999). Available from URL: http://www.ktl.fi/publications/monica/aspirin/aspirinqa.htm, URN:*NBN:fi-fe19991129*. MONICA Web Publication 17.

18. Lundberg V, Tolonen H, Kuulasmaa K, for the WHO MONICA Project. Quality assessment of data on menopausal status and hormones in the WHO MONICA Project. (June 1999). Available from URL: http://www.ktl.fi/publications/monica/womenqa/womenqa.htm, URN:*NBN:fi-fe19991131*. MONICA Web Publication 18.

19. Molarius A, Seidell JC, Sans S, Tuomilehto J, Kuulasmaa K, for the WHO MONICA Project. Varying sensitivity of waist action levels to identify subjects with overweight or obesity in 19 populations of the WHO MONICA Project—tables and figures for waist action level 1. (December 1999). Available from URL: http://www.ktl.fi/publications/monica/waction/waction.htm, URN:*NBN:fi-fe19991138*. MONICA Web Publication 19.

20. Kuulasmaa K, Dobson A, Tunstall-Pedoe H, Fortmann S, Sans S, Tolonen H, Evans A, Ferrario M, Tuomilehto J, for the WHO MONICA Project. Estimation of contribution of changes in classical risk factors to trends in coronary-event rates across the WHO MONICA Project populations: methodological appendix to a paper published in the *Lancet*. (February 2000). Available from URL: http://www.ktl.fi/publications/monica/earwig/appendix.htm, URN:*NBN:fi-fe19991356*. MONICA Web Publication 20.

21. Vanuzzo D, Pilotto L, Pilotto L, Mähönen M, Hobbs M, for the WHO MONICA Project. Pharmacological treatment during AMI and in secondary prevention: the scientific evidence. (February 2000). Available from URL: http://www.ktl.fi/publications/monica/carpfish/appenda/evidence.htm, URN:*NBN:fi-fe976567*. MONICA Web Publication 21.

22. Hobbs M, Mähönen M, Jamrozik K, for the WHO MONICA Project. Constructing an evidence-based treatment score for relating changes in treatment to changes in mortality, coronary events and case fatality in the WHO MONICA Project. (February 2000). Available from URL: http://www.ktl.fi/publications/monica/carpfish/appendb/wts.htm, URN:*NBN:fi-fe976568*. MONICA Web Publication 22.

23. Tunstall-Pedoe H, Mähönen M, Cepaitis Z, Kuulasmaa K, Vanuzzo D, Hobbs M, Keil U, for the WHO MONICA Project. Derivation of an acute coronary care quality score for the WHO MONICA Project. (February 2000). Available from URL: http://www.ktl.fi/publications/monica/carpfish/appendc/accqscore.htm, URN:*NBN:fi-fe976569*. MONICA Web Publication 23.

24. Mähönen M, Tunstall-Pedoe H, Rajakangas AM, Cepaitis Z, Kuulasmaa K, Dobson A, Keil U, for the WHO MONICA Project. Definitions of case fatality for coronary events in the WHO MONICA Project. (February 2000). Available from URL: http://www.ktl.fi/publications/monica/carpfish/appendd/cfdef.htm URN:*NBN:fi-fe976570*. MONICA Web Publication 24.

25. Mähönen M, Tolonen H, Kuulasmaa K, for the WHO MONICA Project. MONICA Coronary event registration data book 1980–1995. (October 2000). Available from URL: http://www.ktl.fi/publications/monica/coredb/coredb.htm, URN:*NBN:fi-fe20001204*. MONICA Web Publication 25.

26. Mähönen M, Tolonen H, Kuulasmaa K, for the WHO MONICA Project. MONICA stroke event registration data book 1982–1995. (October 2000). Available from URL: http://www.ktl.fi/publications/monica/strokedb/strokedb.htm, URN:*NBN:fi-fe20001205*. MONICA Web Publication 26.

27. Tolonen H, Kuulasmaa K, Ruokokoski E, for the WHO MONICA Project. MONICA population survey data book. (October 2000). Available from URL: http://www.ktl.fi/publications/monica/surveydb/title.htm, URN:*NBN:fi-fe20001206*. MONICA Web Publication 27.

28. Mähönen M, Asplund K, Tolonen H, Kuulasmaa K, for the WHO MONICA Project. Stroke event trend quality score for the WHO MONICA Project. (November 2001). Available from URL: http://www.ktl.fi/publications/monica/strokescore/score.htm, URN:*NBN:fi-fe20011554*. MONICA Web Publication 28.

29. Mähönen M, Cepaitis Z, Kuulasmaa K, for the WHO MONICA Project. MONICA acute coronary care data book 1981–1995. (December 2001). Available from URL: http://www.ktl.fi/publications/monica/accdb/accdb.htm, URN:*NBN:fi-fe20011304*. MONICA Web Publication 29.

30. Tolonen H, Kuulasmaa K, Asplund K, Mähönen M, for the WHO MONICA Project. Do trends in population levels of blood pressure and other cardiovascular risk factors explain trends in stroke event rates?—methodological appendix. to a paper published in *Stroke*. (August 2002). Available from URL: http://www.ktl.fi/publications/monica/strokeah1/appendix.htm URN:*NBN:fi-fe20021258*. MONICA Web Publication 30.

#88 MONICA Memos

'(a)' or 'Add' after a memo number initially meant follow-up circulation of additional material or a correction. Memos were circulated very widely. Those restricted and confidential to MONICA investigators were later labelled 'A' after the number, while 'E' means that the memo was distributed primarily by e-mail and/or through the World Wide Web. Scanned images of most of the MONICA Memos are to be found in the scanned document archive on the second CD-ROM attached to this Monograph. Exceptions are copies of unpublished papers still considered confidential in December 2002.

Number	Date	Title
1	21.02.83	Serum banks
2	22.02.83	Quality assurance of monitoring of diseases
3	15.03.83	Codes and 'optional' studies
4	30.03.83	MONICA substudies—Environmental risk factors for cancer
5	30.03.83	Analysis of expired air carbon monoxide concentration
6	27.04.83	Validation of smoking trends with plasma/serum thiocyanate
6(a)	17.05.83	The determination of thiocyanate in blood serum
7	10.05.83	MONICA Steering Committee
8	31.05.83	MONICA Steering Committee (report of MSC Meeting Helsinki, 9–10 February 1983; amendments to MONICA Protocol)
9	31.05.83	MONICA ECG Coding and Standardization
10	31.05.83	Socioeconomic and behavioural factors (Section 14 of MONICA Protocol)
11	06.06.83	Monitoring administrative data of health services
12	06.06.83	Annual progress report
13	22.07.83	Physical activity surveys
13a	06.09.83	Indices of physical activity
14	10.08.83	Drug monitoring in MONICA
15	12.08.83	MONICA local manuals
16	15.09.83	Drug monitoring in MONICA
17	27.09.83	Meeting of MONICA Principal Investigators (timing, manuals, test case histories, population descriptions)
18	04.10.83	Sample case histories for test coding
19	04.10.83	Local MONICA manuals (checklist, choice of ICD codes to be selected for screening from hospital discharge records)
20	20.10.83	Specimen case histories (sudden death)
21	26.10.83	Minutes of Second MONICA Steering Committee, Liège, Belgium, 8–9 September 1983
22	10.11.83	Monitoring of radical scavenging vitamins in MONICA
23	09.12.83	Includes: list of MONICA centres, information on Meeting of PIs 1984, possible myocardial infarction, manuals, coding, pooling records
24	16.01.84	MONICA data management
25	16.01.84	Draft pooling record—acute coronary care
26	18.01.84	Classification of drugs in the MONICA Project
27	06.02.84	Recommendation for research on the surveillance of the dietary habits of the population with regard to CHD
28	12.03.84	MONICA optional study on vitamins and CHD
29	02.04.84	MONICA data management
30	11.05.84	Report of the MONICA PIs meeting, Geneva, 28 February–1 March 1984
31	21.05.84	ECGs for coding with MONICA criteria
31 Add 1	05.02.87	1985 ECG Test Set—explanatory letter
32	14.05.84	Model codes for case histories
33	23.05.84	MONICA data management
34	15.08.84	Surveillance of population dietary habits with regard to cardiovascular diseases
35	10.12.84	Official MONICA Project appendix listing MONICA sites and key personnel
36	19.12.84	Minutes of MONICA SC/6 and SC/7 and report of US-CCSP liaison meeting
37	25.01.85	Stability of lipids in frozen sera—a report to the MONICA Project
38	25.01.85	MONICA Quality Control Centre for ECG coding, Budapest, 1984 activity report
39	08.02.85	Reporting Units
40	25.02.85	Derivation of MONICA diagnostic categories
41	08.03.85	Electrocardiographic coding for MONICA—A diagnostic algorithm and test code sequences
42	08.03.85	Confidentiality of MONICA data
43	25.03.85	MONICA Annual Reports
44	06.05.85	Test case histories 1985 series
45	15.05.85	Monitoring of other chronic diseases within the MONICA Project
46	07.06.85	Plan for MONICA data collection documents
47	07.06.85	Dr Chambless' report of his visit to the MDC in April 1985
48	27.06.85	Coding exercise on test case histories, second series (coronary events, acute coronary care and stroke events)
49	28.06.85	Description of data collection procedures for the MONICA Project (draft)
50	06.07.85	Sample selection description (including questionnaire)
50 Add 1	31.10.85	Responses received to MNM 50
51	09.07.85	Descriptive presentation of data from the WHO MONICA Project (survey data and event registration data)

Number	Date	Title
52	26.07.85	Organization and management of the WHO MONICA Project
53	06.08.85	MONICA Collaborating Centres and Reporting Units
54	07.08.85	Transfer of demographic and mortality data
55	12.08.85	MONICA Annual Reports (up to June 1985)
56	16.08.85	Annual Hospital Enzyme Use Reporting Form
56 Add 1	18.08.85	Set of Forms
57	02.12.85	Revised Coronary Event and Acute Coronary Care Record Formats and Specific Instructions
58	27.02.86	Reports on MONICA Meeting of Principal Investigators and MONICA Steering Committee, Helsinki and Porvoo, August 1985
59	15.04.86	Report on Test Case Histories 1985 Series—Coronary Events
60	27.09.85	Autopsy Studies
61	18.12.85	MONICA Collaborating Centres and Reporting Units
62	25.01.86	MONICA Optional Studies Report
63	06.02.86	Transfer of Event Registration and Population Survey Data to the MONICA Data Centre
64	07.02.86	Annual Hospital Enzyme Use Reports
65	06.03.86	Quality Control of ECG Measurements
65 Add 1	07.04.86	Minnesota Code Learning Packets and Answer Sheets (no longer available)
66	14.03.86	Test Case Histories (Coronary Events) 1986 series
66 Add 1	22.07.86	Compliance Report on Test Case Histories (Coronary Events), 1986 Series
67	04.07.86	Electrocardiographic Coding for the MONICA Project
68	20.03.86	Site Visit Procedures
69	21.04.86	Standard Population for the MONICA Project
70	21.04.86	Berlin PIs Meeting, 6–11 April 1987
71	21.04.86	2nd International MONICA Congress, August 1987
71 Corr 1	04.07.86	2nd International MONICA Congress, August 1987
72	23.05.86	Electrocardiogram Test Set
73	29.05.86	Dr Heinemann's visit to IARC, May 1986
74	04.07.86	MONICA Diagnostic Algorithm—Coronary Events
75	19.06.86	Annual Reports 1985/86
76	04.07.86	Revised Population Survey Data Transfer Formats
77	04.07.86	Draft Edit Specifications for Coronary-Events Data
78	17.07.86	MONICA Data Collection Forms
79	28.07.86	Revised Stroke Event Data Transfer Formats
79 Corr 1	25.09.86	Revised Stroke Event Data Transfer Formats—enclosing revised page 17/18
80	25.09.86	Report of MONICA Steering Committee 10
81	05.09.86	Analysis of expired air carbon monoxide concentration
82	02.09.86	MONICA Collaborative Publication
83	17.09.86	MONICA Optional Studies on Physical Activity
84	17.09.86	Quality Control Activities in the MONICA project
85	03.10.86	Material Shipment from the MCCs to the MDC and the Use of Problem Communication Forms
86	03.10.86	Preparation of Magnetic Tapes
87	10.12.86	Annual Reports 1985/1986
88	15.12.86	Stroke Case Histories for Coding
88 Corr 1	19.02.87	Stroke Case Histories for Coding—test case history form stroke events (Form M)
89	18.12.86	Monitoring of Medical Care in MONICA
90	22.01.87	Results of 1986 Coronary-Event Coding Exercise
91	23.01.87	MONICA Manual (explanatory letter)
92	12.02.87	Optional Study Meeting on Physical Activity, 8 April 1987
93	22.02.87	ECG Coding Seminar, Budapest, 30 March–3 April 1987
94	05.03.87	Results of the 1986 ECG Test Coding
95	09.03.87	Evaluation of Quality Control
96	11.03.87	Optional Study Meeting—EURONUT-MONICA: Surveillance of Dietary Habits of the Population with regard to Cardiovascular Diseases
97	22.03.87	Management Reports to MONICA Council of Principal Investigators
98	23.03.87	MONICA Optional Study Meetings, Berlin, 8 April 1987
99	24.06.87	New Genetic Risk Factors for Coronary Heart Disease: Proposal for a Case Control and Family Study
100	02.08.87	MONICA physical activity questionnaire
101	12.02.88	MONICA Key Sites and Personnel—request for update
102	31.07.87	1986/87 MONICA Annual Reports
103	04.08.87	WHO Lipid Reference Programme—Attempt to Standardize Dry Chemistry Cholesterol Method
104	14.08.87	Coronary-Event Data and Population Survey Data Edit Specifications
105	28.08.87	1987 Test Set of Electrocardiograms for Standardized Coding
105 Add	02.10.87	1987 Test Set of Electrocardiograms for Standardized Coding
106	09.09.87	Call for research workers to assist MDC in analysis and preparation of data reports
107	28.10.87	Changes in administrative structure of the MONICA Data Centre
108	28.10.87	Minutes of the 4th Council of Principal Investigators, Berlin, GDR, 9–11 April 1987
109	–.–.–	Not issued

Number	Date	Title
110	28.10.87	Test Case Histories—Coronary Events 1987 series
111	28.10.87	Acute Coronary Care
112	12.11.87	Confidential Distribution of MONICA Memos
113A	23.11.87	Copies of Transparencies presented at the 2nd MONICA Congress, Helsinki, 14–15 August 1987
114	23.11.87	Data checking system for the MONICA data
115	04.12.87	Optional Study: Physical Activity
116	11.12.87	Use of electronic mail
117	17.12.87	Coronary and stroke procedure questionnaire
118	–.–.–	Not issued
119	11.01.88	Call for stroke case histories
120	11.02.88	Possible study of heart disease and risk factors in migrants
121	15.02.88	5th MONICA PIs' meeting, Augsburg, 1988—accommodation request form.
122	03.03.88	Draft Agenda for Augsburg PIs' meeting 1-3 October 1988
123	03.03.88	Information to authors and for Principal Investigators on the preparation of the Acta Medica Scandinavica
124A	28.03.88	Draft manuscript on collaborative MONICA Risk-Factor Data to be published in the World Health Statistics Quarterly, September 1988
125	11.03.88	Cumulative list of MONICA publications
126	11.03.88	New mortality statistics reporting forms
127	15.04.88	MONICA Optional Study on the Surveillance of Dietary Habits
128	11.05.88	Optional Study of Physical Activity: (Questionnaire of Dr K. Powell)
129	19.05.88	Assessment of Medical Care in MONICA: Availability of Routinely Collected Hospital Data. (Questionnaire of Professor M. Hobbs)
130	06.06.88	5th Council of MONICA Principal Investigators, Augsburg, FRG—finalized programme
131	15.06.88	MONICA Optional Study on Physical Activity—meeting to be held on 1 October in Augsburg
132A	04.07.88	Draft Baseline Population Survey Data Book
133	01.08.88	MONICA Council of Principal Investigators—Travel to Augsburg from Munich and Frankfurt Airports
134	01.08.88	MONICA Optional Study on Genetics
135	01.08.88	MONICA Council of Principal Investigators 1988: Workshop on Internal Quality Control—Survey
136	10.08.88	Meeting of MONICA Principal Investigators, Augsburg: Workshop on Coding of Stroke Events (Item 9b of Agenda)
137	10.08.88	Meeting of MONICA Principal Investigators, Augsburg: Proposal for Monitoring of Medical Care in MONICA
138	–.–.–	Not issued
139	–.–.–	Not issued
140	10.08.88	New Questions for the Core Data Transfer Format: Population Survey Data
141	12.08.88	Status of Acute Coronary Care Data Transfer to MDC
142	30.08.88	MONICA Council of Principal Investigators: Optional Study Meeting on Nutrition
143	31.08.88	MONICA Council of Principal Investigators: Discussion Paper for Monitoring of Medical Care in MONICA
144	19.09.88	Management Reports to the MONICA Council of Principal Investigators
145A	20.09.88	Corrections for Draft Baseline Population Survey Data Book
146	20.09.88	Proposed revision of MONICA Manual Section 3
147	12.10.88	New telephone numbers and postal code at the MONICA Data Centre
148A	26.10.88	Assessing Trends in Coronary Heart Disease Mortality and Morbidity: The MONICA Project
149	14.11.88	Issues relating to the monitoring of Stroke
150A	05.12.88	MONICA Articles for clearance
151	05.12.88	MONICA Publications: WHSQ and Congress Proceedings
152	05.12.88	Study of Heart Disease and Risk Factors in Migrants: Results of Survey
153	16.01.89	3rd MONICA Congress Nice 15–16 September 1989
154(i)	18.01.89	1988 ECG Test Set (i) 25 mm/sec
154(ii)	18.01.89	1988 ECG Test Set (ii) 50 mm/sec
155	06.02.89	Physical Activity Optional Study—Visit of Dr Carl Casperson to Europe
156	25.02.89	MONICA Annual Reports 1987–88
157	25.02.89	MONICA Manual Version 2—Preliminary Order Form
158	17.03.89	Changes to telephone, telex and telefax numbers at the MDC
159	01.05.89	1989 Stroke Case Histories for Coding
160	01.05.89	1989 Coronary-Event Case Histories for Coding
160 Add	14.06.89	Coronary case histories for coding—Form L
161A	04.12.89	Methods of total cholesterol measurements in the baseline survey
162A	13.06.89	Quality Assessment of Blood Pressure Measurements in the First Surveys of the WHO MONICA Project
163	11.07.89	Suggested Revision to MONICA Manual Section 3: Additional Survey Questions
164A	13.07.89	World Health Statistics Annual 1989
165	28.07.89	Third MONICA Congress, Nice, 15–16 September 1989: Programme

Number	Date	Title
166	28.09.89	MONICA Presentations in Nice, September 1989
167	28.09.89	Instructions for the preparation of publications after the 3rd MONICA Congress
168	22.09.89	MONICA Data Centre—new telephone and telefax numbers
169	18.10.89	6th Council of MONICA Principal Investigators, Lugano, Switzerland, 26 April—2 May 1990—preliminary information, draft agenda and accommodation reservation form
169 Add	03.11.89	6th Council of MONICA Principal Investigators—hotel categories and prices
170	24.10.89	Assessment of Medical Care in MONICA: Annual Structural Medical Care Assessment
171	31.10.89	Vacancy for an Epidemiologist in the MONICA Data Centre
172	29.11.89	Proposed Teleconference following the MONICA Council of Principal Investigators in Lugano
173A	11.02.90	Coronary Event Registration Quality Assessment Report
174	13.02.90	WHO MONICA presentations at the Regional European Meeting of the International Epidemiological Association, "Epidemiological Evaluation of the Strategy Health for All", Granada, Spain, 14–16 February 1990.
175A	14.02.90	Quality Assessment of Total Cholesterol Measurements in the first surveys of the MONICA Project
176A	12.03.90	Quality Assessment of Smoking Data in the first surveys of the WHO MONICA Project
177	15.02.90	Eligibility of MCCs for publication of Coronary-Event Data
178A	16.02.90	MONICA Baseline Population Survey Data Book
179A	02.03.90	MONICA Coronary Event Registration Data Book—1980–86
179A(Add)	02.03.90	Annex II to Coronary Event Registration Data Book: Distribution limited to MSC, SAG, and those who prepared the document. MCCs to receive their own data direct from MDC.
180	08.03.90	Update: Satellite Teleconference on Cardiovascular Diseases
181	09.03.90	Third MONICA Survey
182	14.03.90	MONICA Publications Priorities
183A	15.03.90	Ecological Analysis of the Relationship between Mortality Data and Major Risk Factors of Cardiovascular Disease: paper for clearance
184	19.03.90	Report of the 5th Meeting of MONICA Principal Investigators, Augsburg, FRG, 3–5 October 1988
185	22.03.90	Atherosclerosis in Selected European Regions (ASER Project)—Outline of a study proposed by MONICA-France.
186	06.04.90	Schedules of MONICA Meetings, Lugano, 26 April–2 May 1990
187A	05.04.90	Quality Assessment of Blood Pressure Measurements in Epidemiologic Surveys
188	06.04.90	WHO MONICA Project: 1990 Mid-term Review
189	06.04.90	Global MONICA Network
190	25.06.90	Advocacy of CVD Prevention
191	03.08.90	Questionnaire on Global MONICA Network
192	06.12.90	Timing of the 3rd MONICA Survey
193	07.12.90	MONICA Population Survey Data Component
194	12.12.90	MONICA Optional Study of Haemostatic Factors and CHD
195	14.12.90	MONICA Publications Plan and Priorities
196	11.12.90	Proposed Training Video for the 3rd Survey
197	01.03.91	Report of the 6th Meeting of Principal Investigators, Lugano, Switzerland, 30 April–2 May 1990
198	14.03.91	Proceedings 3rd MONICA Congress—RESP Contents List
198 Add 1	29.04.91	Erratum to above
199(i)	18.04.91	1991 Test Set of Electrocardiograms for Standardized Coding: 25 mm/sec paper speed
199(ii)	18.04.91	1991 Test Set of Electrocardiograms for Standardized Coding: 50 mm/sec paper speed
200	22.04.91	7th Council of MONICA Principal Investigators, Barcelona, 1992
201	01.05.91	MONICA Data Centre—new telephone and telefax numbers
202A	11.10.92	Draft report—HDL-Cholesterol (HDL-CH)
203	14.10.91	Health Services Reporting Forms
204	16.10.91	Schedule of meetings for remaining years of MONICA
205	12.11.91	Stroke Case Histories for Coding, 1991
206	15.11.91	Coronary Case Histories for Coding, 1991
205/6 Add	12.02.92	Coronary Case Histories for Coding 1991, electronic transfer
207	17.01.92	7th Council of MONICA Principal Investigators, Barcelona, Spain, 24–29 August 1992
208	20.01.92	Atherosclerosis in Selected Regions: The ASER Project
209A	30.01.92	Quality Assessment of Smoking Data in the First Survey of the WHO MONICA Project
210A	30.01.92	Assessment of Blood Pressure Measurement in the Baseline Surveys of the WHO MONICA Project
211A	03.02.92	Stroke Event Registration Quality Report

Number	Date	Title
212A	03.02.92	Draft Stroke Event Registration Data Book 1982–1987
213	06.02.92	Presentation of MONICA Coronary Events in Amsterdam in August 1991
214	04.05.92	MONICA Manual, Part III, Section 1—Population Survey Data Component: Revision, March 1992
215	06.05.92	MONICA Manual, Part V, Section 1—Data Transfer to the MONICA Data Centre: Revision, March 1992
216	08.05.92	Medical Services Reporting Forms—UA, UB, UC, UD
217A	22.05.92	Quality of Stroke Subtype Data in the MONICA Stroke Event Registration
218A	24.06.92	Interim Report: Blood Pressure Measurement Quality in the Second Surveys of the MONICA Project
219A	03.07.92	Coronary-Event Registration—Documents for MONICA Principal Investigators' meeting, Barcelona, August 1992
220A	03.07.92	Workshop on Health Services in MONICA Populations—Documents for MONICA Principal Investigators' Meeting, Barcelona, August 1992
221A	14.07.92	Workshop on Population Surveys (Documents for 7th Council of MONICA Principal Investigators, Barcelona, 24–29 August 1992)
222A	14.07.92	Workshop on Stroke—Documents for 7th Council of MONICA Principal Investigators, Barcelona, 24–29 August 1992
223	14.07.92	Workshop on Methodological Issues-Documents for 7th Council of MONICA Principal Investigators, Barcelona, 24–29 August 1992
224	14.07.92	Schedules of MONICA Meetings, Barcelona, 24–29 August 1992
225	24.07.92	Errors in MONICA Risk-Factor Slides
226	23.07.92	Studies in the Elderly
227A	16.09.92	Assessment of the Quality of Demographic Data in the WHO MONICA Project
228	30.09.92	Management Report of the MONICA Quality Control Centre for Event Registration, Dundee and Reports on Test Case History Exercises 1991–1992
229	26.10.92	Interrelationship between Arterial Blood Pressure and Serum Lipids Across Populations
230	23.10.92	Membership, Working Group on Epidemiology and Prevention, European Society of Cardiology
231	06.11.92	MONICA Participation at IEA Conference, Sydney, Australia, 26–29 September 1993
232A	16.11.92	Action List from the 7th Council of MONICA Principal Investigators, and Minutes of 24th MONICA Steering Committee
233	23.11.92	MONICA Collaborative Publications
234	11.12.92	Preliminary information concerning the organization of a Training Seminar on 3rd MONICA Survey Methods
235	14.12.92	Call for Investigators to analyse the MONICA 2nd Survey data
236	18.12.92	Instruction Manual of MONICA Quality Control Summary Report
237	29.12.92	MONICA Core Data Edit Specifications
238A	26.02.93	Minutes of MONICA Steering Committee Telephone Conferences of 15 October and 16 December 1992
239	14.05.93	Report on the Training Seminar on 3rd MONICA Survey Methods, Gargnano, Italy, 7–12 March 1993
240A	17.05.93	Minutes of MONICA Steering Committee Telephone Conferences of 11 February and 4 March 1993
241A	26.05.93	Abstracts of MONICA presentations
242A	25.06.93	Acute coronary care data (covering letter)
242A(a)	28.06.93	Acute coronary care data—Quality Assessment Report
242A(b)	28.06.93	Acute coronary care data—Quality Assessment Report for longitudinal data
242A(c)	28.06.93	Draft data book for cross-sectional comparisons of data on acute coronary care
242A(d)	28.06.93	Draft data book for preliminary longitudinal analyses on acute coronary care
243	16.07.93	Updating of MONICA Manual appendices
244	23.07.93	MONICA publication rules
245	26.07.93	8th Council of MONICA Principal Investigators, Udine, Italy, week of 18 April 1994
246A	23.08.93	Myocardial infarction and coronary deaths in the World Health Organization MONICA Project: Registration procedures, event rates and case fatality in 38 populations from 21 countries in 4 continents
247A	16.09.93	Quality assessment of smoking data in the 2nd survey
248A	160.9.93	Age and date of examination in the first and second survey
249	03.12.93	8th Meeting of MONICA principal investigators Udine, Italy 18–22 April 1994
250(ii)	03.12.93	1993 test set of electrogardiograms for standardized coding 50 mm/sec paper speed
250(i)	03.12.93	1993 test set of electrogardiograms for standardized coding 25 mm/sec paper speed
251	06.12.93	Presentation of slides at 3rd International Conference on Preventive Cardiology, Oslo, 27 June–1 July 1993
252A	17.12.93	Quality assessment of HDL-cholesterol measurements in the first surveys of the WHO MONICA Project

Number	Date	Title
253A	17.01.94	Quality assessment of data on marital status and educational achievement in the first survey of the MONICA Project
254A	26.01.94	Minutes of MONICA Steering Committee Telephone Conferences 33–38
255	11.02.94	8th Council of MONICA principal Investigators, Udine, Italy, 18–23 April 1994
256	11.02.94	Local arrangements for 8th council of MONICA principal investigators Udine, Italy, 18–23 April 1994
257A	24.02.94	Quality assessment of coronary event data for 1980–1990
258A	01.03.94	Stroke incidence, mortality, and case-fatality in the WHO MONICA Project
259A	01.03.94	Participation rate and the quality of sampling frame in the first and second risk-factor surveys of the WHO MONICA project
260A	01.03.94	Second Population Survey Data Book
261	04.03.94	MONICA streamlined publication plan
262	04.03.94	MONICA Data Centre—new telephone and telefax numbers
263A	07.03.94	Gender differences in IHD mortality and risk factors in 43 communities: an ecological analysis
264	24.03.94	Working documents for CPI-8
265A	16.03.94	Coronary case histories for coding 1994
266	21.03.94	Minutes of 25th MONICA Steering Committee, 15–17 June 1993
267	21.03.94	The WHO MONICA publications plan for centrally generated publications
268A	28.03.94	Minutes of MONICA Steering Committee telephone conferences 39–40
269	5.04.94	Draft strategic plan for MONICA; Section 3.5 Constraints and Solutions
270	28.04.94	Report of the 7th Meeting of MONICA Principal Investigators Barcelona, Catalonia, Spain, 24–29 August 1992
271	02.05.94	A study of baseline risk factors for coronary heart disease: results of population screening in a developing country
272	05.05.94	List of MONICA Memos
273	20.05.94	Abbreviations of MONICA population names
274	30.05.94	ARIC Study and NHLBI activities
275	02.06.94	MONICA Annual Reports 1993–1994
276A	20.06.94	Coronary Event Registration Data Book 1980–90
277A	23.06.94	Quality assessment of stroke event data for 1982–1990
278	24.06.94	Reports of workshops and optional studies at the 8th Council of MONICA Principal Investigators, Udine, Italy, 19–23 April 1994
279(A)	24.08.94	Presentation of slides in the conference on epidemiology and prevention of stroke, Umeå, Sweden 29–31 May 1994
280A	06.09.94	Article on diagnostic procedures and management of stroke
281A	20.10.94	Minutes of MONICA Steering Committee telephone conferences 41–43
282	01.11.94	MONICA publications policy (MONICA Manual Part I, section 2)
283A	21.11.94	Xth International Symposium on Atherosclerosis, Montreal 9–14th October 1994: slides and abstract of presentation on risk factor trends
284A	12.01.95	Quality assessment of weight and height measurements in the first and second MONICA survey
285A	27.01.95	Smoking Questionnaire: Professor Constance Nathanson
286	17.02.95	Coronary event registration quality control—reminder
287A	10.05.95	Non-fatal possible myocardial infarction—a classification problem in epidemiological studies
288A	06.05.95	Minutes of MONICA Steering Committee Telephone Conferences 44–48
289A	15.05.95	Submission to the European Commission for funding for the MONICA project
290A	22.05.95	Stroke publication
291A	05.06.95	Assessment of blood pressure measurement quality in the baseline surveys of the WHO MONICA Project
292A	25.08.95	Changes in cigarette smoking among adults in 35 populations during the 1980s
293	12.10.95	MONICA and the Internet
294A	03.11.95	Smoking and relative body weight: An international perspective from the WHO MONICA project
295(a)	10.11.95	"Life after MONICA"
295(b)	10.11.95	"Life after MONICA"
296A	12.02.96	Draft stroke event registration data book 1982–90
297A	15.02.96	Quality assessment of blood pressure measurements in the 1st and 2nd MONICA surveys
298A	04.04.96	Cigarette smoking and official mortality release of data to MCC 11: Newcastle
299A	26.04.96	Quality assessment of total cholesterol measurements in the first and middle surveys of the WHO MONICA Project
300A	03.05.96	Quality assessment of data on waist and hip circumference in the second survey
301A	10.05.96	Quality assessment of data on marital status and educational achievement in the second survey of the WHO MONICA project
302A	24.05.96	Assessment of the quality of demographic data in the WHO MONICA project
303	25.06.96	Standardization of total cholesterol determinations in MONICA

Number	Date	Title
304A	03.06.96	Quality assessment of the data on hypertension control in the first and second population surveys of the WHO MONICA Project
305	01.07.96	CVDs and alcohol consumption
306	01.07.96	MONICA in Internet
307A	01.07.96	Internal MONICA pages on the World Wide Web
308A	26.08.96	Stroke trends in the WHO MONICA Project
309	30.08.96	9th Council of MONICA Principal Investigators
310A	10.09.96	Future of MONICA data base
311	16.09.96	MONICA Data Centre: new telephone and telefax numbers
312	16.09.96	Life after MONICA
313A	02.10.96	Presentation of slides at the 18th Congress of the European Society of Cardiology, Birmingham, 25–29 August 1996
314	14.11.96	Manuscript groups for papers on ten-year trends
315	18.11.96	Stroke incidence and mortality correlated to stroke risk factors in the WHO MONICA Project: an ecological study of 18 populations
316	26.11.96	9th Council of MONICA Principal Investigators, Milan, 28 September–1 October 1997
317A	02.12.96	Smoking Cross-Sectional Paper—Second Survey: Release of data to MCC 34: Belfast MONICA
318	20.12.96	Updated list of MONICA Collaborating Centres
319A	14.01.97	Large blood pressure differences are found between the populations of the WHO MONICA Project
320A	24.01.97	Draft manuscript of Changes in Estimated Coronary Risk in 1980s: Data from 38 populations in the WHO MONICA Project
321A	14.02.97	Population versus clinical view of case fatality from acute coronary heart disease: results from the WHO MONICA Project 1985–1990.
322A	28.02.97	Subtypes of stroke: international comparisons possible? Observations in 13 populations in the WHO MONICA Project
323A	17.03.97	Quality assessment of HDL-cholesterol measurements in the first and middle surveys of the WHO MONICA Project
324A	26.03.97	Age, date of examination and survey periods in the MONICA surveys
325A	04.04.97	Quality assessment of data on smoking behaviour in the WHO MONICA Project
326A	23.05.97	Quality assessment of weight and height measurements in the WHO MONICA Project
327A	10.06.97	Quality assessment of data on blood pressure in the WHO MONICA Project
328A	27.06.97	Participation rates, quality of sampling frames and sampling fractions in the MONICA surveys
329A	17.06.97	Quality assessment of data on marital status and educational achievement in the WHO MONICA Project
330	17.07.97	9th Council of MONICA Principal Investigators, draft programme
331	17.07.97	9th Council of MONICA Principal Investigators, future governance of MONICA
332	17.07.97	9th Council of MONICA Principal Investigators, certificates of good service
333A	17.07.97	9th Council of MONICA Principal Investigators, future of the MONICA data base
334A	25.07.97	MONICA Steering Committee telephone conferences 58–66: action lists
335A	28.08.97	Quality assessment of data on hypertension control in the WHO MONICA Project
336A	25.08.97	MONICA publications plan (memo includes only about half of the publication plan)
336 Add	17.09.97	MONICA publications plan
337	25.08.97	MONICA publications and internal reports
338A	01.09.97	Quality assessment of coronary event registration data in the WHO MONICA Project
339A	03.09.97	Coronary event registration data book 1980–1995
340A	12.09.97	Quality assessment of stroke event registration data in the WHO MONICA Project
341A	12.09.97	WHO MONICA Project. Stroke event registration data book 1982–1995
342A	04.09.97	2nd application to BIOMED
343	09.09.97	Proposal to modify publication rules (MONICA Manual I.2.7)
344A	19.09.97	Quality assessment of acute coronary care data in the WHO MONICA Project
345A	19.09.97	WHO MONICA Project. Acute coronary care data book: 1981–1995
346A	16.09.97	Second meeting of EARWIG one: MONICA main results manuscript group
347A	29.09.97	Waist and hip circumferences and waist-hip ratio in 19 populations of the WHO MONICA Project
348	07.10.97	MONICA Annual Reports: 1996–1997
349	29.10.97	Global prevention and control of cardiovascular diseases: resolution adopted at CPI9
350	21.11.97	Stroke monitoring
351	21.11.97	Addresses of MONICA Collaborating Centres

Number	Date	Title
352A	08.12.97	Subarachnoid haemorrhage in MONICA Release of stroke data to MCC 60: Northern Sweden/STRAG
353A	18.12.97	MONICA sessions at the 4th International Conference on Preventive Cardiology, Montreal, Canada, 29 June–3 July 1997
354	20.01.98	For information, new telephone numbers of MDC
355A	06.02.98	Myocardial infarction and coronary deaths in the WHO MONICA Project 1985–90: How trends in male and female incidence, population case-fatality and mortality relate across 40 populations
356A	05.03.98	Quality assessment of data on waist and hip circumferences in the WHO MONICA Project
357A	29.04.98	Varying sensitivity of waist action levels to identify subjects with overweight or obesity in 19 populations of the WHO MONICA Project
358A	29.04.98	MONICA Manual Part I, Section 2: Organization and Management of the WHO MONICA Project
359A	17.07.98	Quality assessment of demographic data in the WHO MONICA Project
360A	27.07.98	MONICA symposium at the European Society of Cardiology Working Group on Epidemiology and Prevention Scientific Meeting, Shannon, Ireland, 14–17 May 1998.
361A	27.07.98	MONICA events at the European Congress of Cardiology, Vienna, Austria, 22–26 August 1998
362A	20.08.98	Quality assessment of total cholesterol measurements in the WHO MONICA Project
363A	02.11.98	Relationship between abdominal obesity and dyslipidemia in various populations. Release of data to MCC50: Switzerland
364A	23.11.98	Endorsement of changes to MONICA Manual
365	18.12.98	Newsletter
366A	12.01.99	Educational level and relative body weight, and changes in their association over 10 years—an international perspective from the WHO MONICA Project
367A	12.01.99	Quality assessment of data on menopausal status and hormones in the WHO MONICA Project
368A	12.01.99	Quality assessment of data on awareness and treatment of high cholesterol in the WHO MONICA Project
369A	12.01.99	Variation between populations in the management of myocardial infarction: what the WHO MONICA Project showed in 1989
370A	18.01.99	Quality assessment of data on use of aspirin in the WHO MONICA Project
371A	26.01.99	Election of members of MCCs to the MONICA Steering Committee: Proposed modification of procedures for counting postal votes
372A	27.01.99	Call for nominations for new MSC Member
373	16.02.99	MONICA at IEA XV Scientific Meeting
374A	01.03.99	Quality assessment of data on HDL-cholesterol in the WHO MONICA Project
375A	15.03.99	How trends in survival and coronary-event rates contribute to changing coronary heart disease mortality: ten-year results from 37 WHO MONICA Project populations
375A Add1	25.03.99	How trends in survival and coronary-event rates contribute to changing coronary heart disease mortality: ten-year results from 37 WHO MONICA Project populations
376A	16.03.99	Trends in cigarette smoking in 36 populations from the early 1980s to the mid 1990s: findings from the WHO MONICA Project
377	21.04.99	Result of MONICA Steering Committee Elections—1999
378	27.05.99	MONICA Workshops at IEA satellite symposium in Rome, 6–7 September 1999
379A	06.09.99	Sampling frames and response rates for heart disease risk-factor surveys: the experience of the WHO MONICA Project
380A	16.09.99	WHO MONICA Project Monograph
381A	27.09.99	A multinational comparison of subarachnoid haemorrhage epidemiology in the WHO MONICA stroke study
382A	03.11.99	Major MONICA manuscripts for approval as soon as possible: MONICA first and second hypotheses
383A	20.12.99	Total serum cholesterol in relation to age, body mass index and gender: a multinational comparison
384A	15.02.00	The global burden of coronary heart disease and stroke: release of MONICA data to the MMC for inclusion in the World Health Report 2000
385	24.03.00	Au revoir—Auf wiedersehen!
386E	15.12.00	MONICA Memoranda revived
387E	15.12.00	MONICA Monograph (Updated Proposal)
388E	29.08.01	Manuscripts on 10-year trends in stroke for approval for publication
389E	30.08.01	MONICA posters at the ESC XXIII Congress
390E	16.11.01	Manuscript on current smoking and the risk of non-fatal myocardial infarction for approval for publication
391E	07.02.02	MONICA manuscripts for approval for publication
392E	19.03.02	Postponement of elections of MSC members

Number	Date	Title
393E	16.04.02	MONICA Monograph and Multimedia Sourcebook
394E	07.05.02	Future Management of the MONICA Project
395E	07.05.02	MONICA Monograph about to go to the WHO Editor
396E	10.06.02	Manuscript on trends in the management of myocardial infarction for approval for publication
397E	22.08.02	Manuscript on trends in stroke and coronary heart disease for approval for publication
398E	09.10.02	Call for nominations for members for the MSC for a five years period
399E	06.11.02	Postal ballot for the election of a new MSC
400E	04.12.02	Results of MONICA Steering Committee elections-2002
401E	10.12.02	Manuscript on the relationship between total cholesterol, age and body mass index for approval for publication

MONICA Graphics

Prepared by Hanna Tolonen (Helsinki) and Hugh Tunstall-Pedoe (Dundee)
Commentary and notes by Hugh Tunstall-Pedoe

#89 MONICA Graphics

Introduction

The analysis of the final results of the WHO MONICA Project involved the creation of large numbers of complex tables. These were eventually reduced to six or so for each of the MONICA Publications. Each table needed to encompass between 15 and 38 populations, to show the results for men and women, and to include different factors and end-points. Their preparation involved a formidable amount of work. This was matched by the challenge, first to the editorial staff of the journals and the reviewers, and then to the readers of the papers when they eventually appeared. Understanding a two-by-two table is a problem for many readers. MONICA tables commonly had 20 or more columns and 40 rows.

While the manuscripts were being prepared for publication, preliminary results were being communicated to cardiology, stroke, epidemiology, and public health conferences. Complex tables cannot be projected onto a screen. MONICA needed to summarize its findings graphically, in a way that made sense within a few seconds to a professional audience.

By trial and error we developed a MONICA style. Over a number of years a portfolio of slides was created, shown at international meetings, and distributed to MONICA investigators for local use. Publication of MONICA results in scientific journals might be thought to have made these slide images redundant. Readers of scientific papers tend to be more interested in the conclusions than in the data. But the WHO MONICA Project has an incomparable collection of data, of interest to many investigators beyond those concerned with the testing of the MONICA hypotheses. There was a danger that MONICA graphics summarizing the data would be lost to the wider audience in cardiovascular disease and public health. Even this professional audience preferred graphics to tables, wanted to see them, and to be able to study them in their own time.

The following graphics are therefore a key product of the MONICA collaboration, and one of the reasons for producing this Monograph. No other study has produced standardized data of such range and value. The graphics should encourage those looking at them in this book to go on to do some or all of a number of things: explore the MONICA Publications (*2*) study the MONICA Quality assessment reports (*1*), look at the MONICA Data Books; check the MONICA Website (*1*), and even analyse the sample Data Base on the CD-ROM.

Developed originally for transient presentation, the slides have been reviewed and revised meticulously before appearing here in print. In addition, a number of the graphics that follow have been prepared specifically for this Monograph.

Three slide formats are of particular interest in the history of presenting MONICA collaborative results. One is the presentation of trends, exemplified for example by G15 or by G38, a MONICA standard. The second is their simplified rendering into 'traffic-light' symbols in the spot-maps such as G24, G25 and G39—too simple for publication in scientific journals, but of great educational value. The third illustrates how results of major publications can be simplified into single images such as G23 and G31. These are examples of the formidable challenge of making research results understandable to a wide readership. They illustrate how complex epidemiological findings can be summarized simply through an understanding of mathematical relationships, even though this final format was achieved only after considerable labour and numerous false starts.

1. See Monograph CD-ROM or MONICA Website http://www.ktl.fi/monica/.
2. Full references and summaries of MONICA Publications appear in #85/86.

Populations, data collection and official mortality

1. To qualify for the final testing of the MONICA hypotheses populations needed to provide approximately ten years of 'core data', that is data on trends in coronary-event rates, trends in cardiovascular risk factors and trends in coronary care. For testing the stroke hypotheses, data on trends in stroke rates were needed. These data were sent to the MONICA Data Centre in Helsinki, where they underwent formal quality assessment before they were used. See #7 *MONICA Data Centre (MDC)*, #12 *Quality Assurance*, MONICA Manual Part I, Section 1 (*1*).

2. Populations are known in the WHO MONICA Project as Reporting Unit Aggregates, abbreviated to RUAs. Each is identified in this Monograph and in the later MONICA Publications (*2*) by a seven-character code. The first three characters are the national country code, followed by a hyphen, and then the three-character population code. Characteristics of each population are described in #51–#83. See MONICA Manual Part I, Appendix 2 (*1*), also *Appendix*.

3. Populations from former MONICA Collaborating Centres (see *Glossary*), provided material for the early parts of the study, but are not shown in maps G1 and G2. Either the quantity or the quality of their data were inadequate to contribute to the analysis of 10-year trends, and therefore to hypothesis testing. These populations are listed in #84. Some of their data were processed in the MONICA Data Centre and appear in MONICA Quality assessment reports (*1*), MONICA Data Books (*1*), and in early MONICA Publications of cross-sectional data, or of five-year trends, such as 1, 2, 3, 10, 15 (*2*).

4. There were changes over time in the number of countries involved in the WHO MONICA Project. Some withdrew, some joined together (two Germanies), and some separated (republics of the former Soviet Union). The final total was 21.

5. There are 35 MONICA population RUAs shown in maps G1 and G2, seven outside Europe and 28 within. The number of RUAs used varied between analyses, some using more than 35 and some fewer:

    a. The first major analysis on 10-year trends in coronary-event rates, case fatality and mortality rates, for MONICA Publication 36 (*2*), used 37 RUAs. The two Russian cities shown here, Russia-Moscow, RUS-MOS, see #74, and Russia-Novosibirsk, RUS-NOV, see #75, were each split into 'intervention' and 'control' population RUAs.

    b. The largest number of RUAs was used in testing the First MONICA Hypothesis, also known as the risk-factor hypothesis, see #2 *MONICA Hypotheses and Study Design* for MONICA Publication 38 (*2*). In addition to the 37 RUAs used in the coronary-event paper, Germany-Augsburg, GER-AUG, see #63, was split into 'urban' and 'rural' RUAs, making 38.

    c. In testing the Second MONICA Hypothesis on coronary care, see #2, for MONICA Publication 39 (*2*), the 35 population RUAs shown in G1 and G2 were all used, but only after amalgamating the two from Belgium into one, the two from Switzerland into one, and three from Finland into one, leaving 31 separate RUAs.

    d. The two Swiss populations provided information on core data items in men, but only on risk factors in women. Therefore there are fewer population RUAs for women, compared with men, in many of the following graphics. Exceptions are risk-factor graphics G36–G56 (Swiss men and women both represented) and stroke graphics G26–G35 (neither).

    e. Fifteen RUAs from ten countries provided data for testing the stroke hypotheses. They are identified in #26 *Registration of Stroke Events*, and G9. In addition GER-EGE, see #65, provided data over six years.

6. The MONICA Protocol specified that all data components should be measured in the same defined populations. See MONICA Manual Part I, Section 1 (*1*). For local technical reasons, described in the relevant MONICA Quality assessment reports, this did not always happen. Variants of the same population, where the RUAs may overlap, are shown in Data Books by suffixes a, b, c, for example AUS-PERa, AUS-PERb. Overlapping but different RUAs explain why the graphics occasionally differ from MONICA Publications for a particular RUA. See *Appendix* where the RUAs used in each graphic are defined in terms of their constituent MONICA reporting units. (Other discrepancies from the early MONICA Publications result from different age standardization. See #39 *Age Standardization*.)

1. See Monograph CD-ROM or MONICA Website http://www.ktl.fi/monica/.
2. Full references and summaries of MONICA Publications appear in #85/86.

G1 Populations outside Europe used in testing the MONICA hypotheses

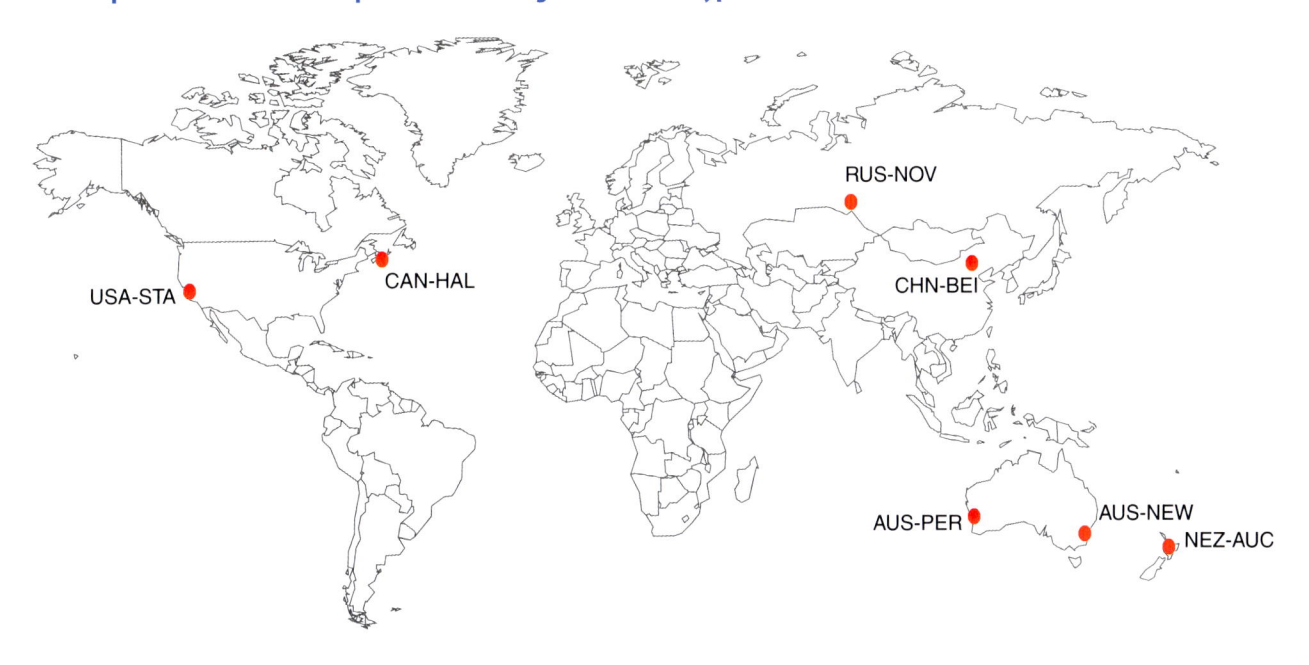

G2 European populations used in testing the MONICA hypotheses

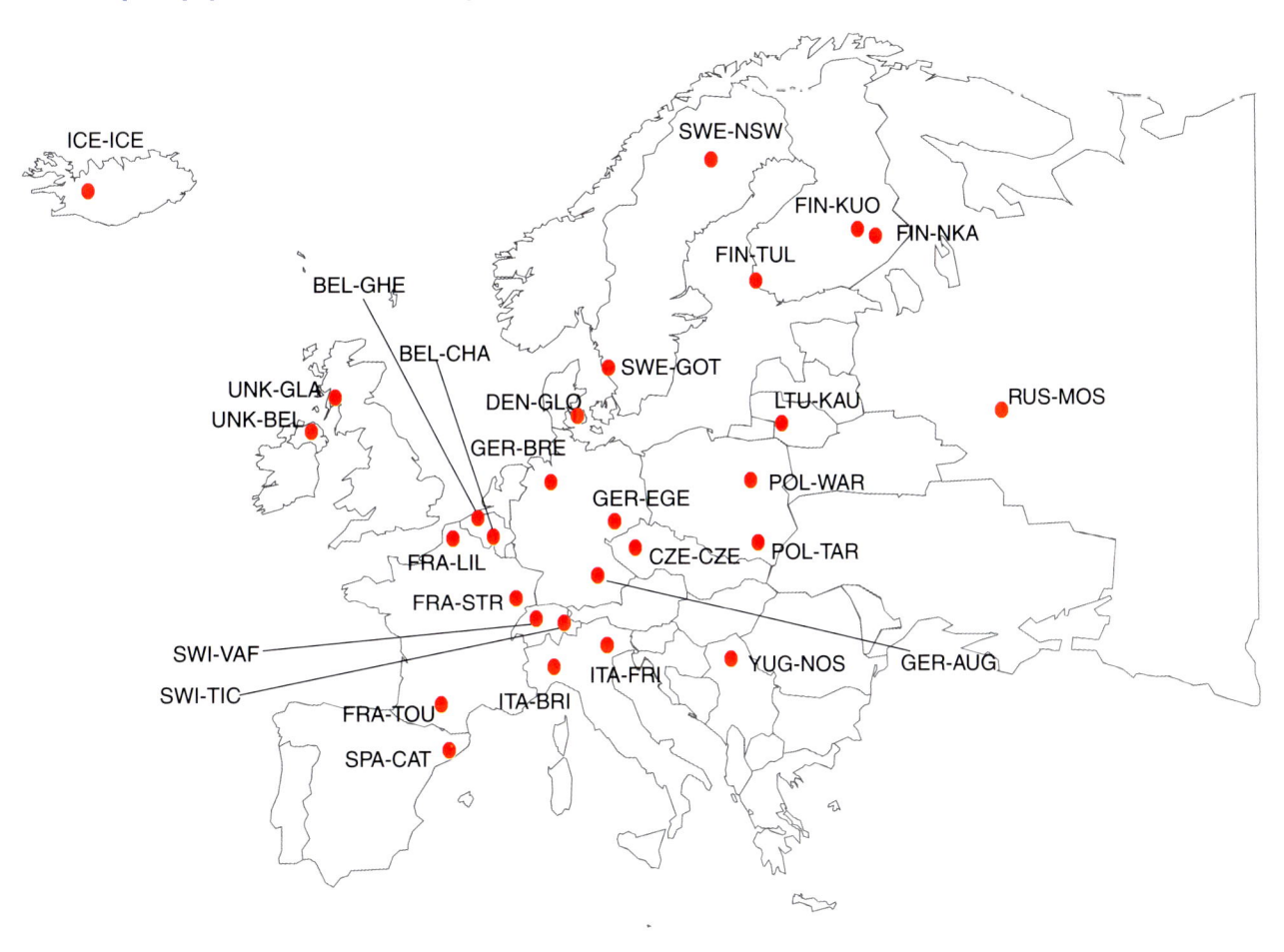

POPULATIONS, DATA COLLECTION AND OFFICIAL MORTALITY

1. These charts incorporate the official, routine, death certificate data, obtained directly from local or national statistical sources. MONICA registration procedures for validation and diagnostic classification of coronary and stroke events have not been applied. Population denominators are the same as those used in calculating MONICA event rates, as are the methods of age standardization. Discrepancies between these results and those for coronary and stroke mortality after MONICA validation therefore result from different numerators, not differences in denominators or in age standardization. See #16 *Routine Mortality Data*, #37 *Event Rates, Case Fatality and Trends*, #39 *Age Standardization*, MONICA Quality assessment of demographic data (*1*).

2. According to basic international coding rules, even if there are several causes, or a sequence of causes of death written on a death certificate, each death is assigned a single 'underlying' cause. Deaths or death rates from single causes can be added up therefore to give the total number of deaths or death rates from all causes (that is, from any cause).

3. CHD is coronary heart disease, also known as IHD, or ischaemic heart disease. See *Glossary*.

4. Stroke is also known as cerebrovascular disease. See *Glossary*.

5. Other CVD are cardiovascular diseases (that is diseases of the heart and circulatory system—arteries, veins and lymphatics) other than coronary heart disease and cerebrovascular disease.

6. Non-CVD are all other causes of death, such as infections, cancer, respiratory disease, injury and poisoning, to name a few.

7. The three years specified for each graph varied by population. They are the starting and stopping years for coronary-event registration in the population concerned, shown graphically in G8.

8. Results, as in many of the following graphs, are age-standardized for the 35–64 age group, using the world standard population. See #39 *Age Standardization*.

9. Note that the scale maximum for women on the x-axis is only half of that for men.

10. The bar charts allow comparison of mortality rates between populations and between the sexes. Comparison of G4 with G3 shows changes in mortality rates and in consequent population ranking over time.

11. Some of these mortality data were used in the early MONICA Publications 1, 6, 10, 16 (*2*).

1. **See Monograph CD-ROM or MONICA Website http://www.ktl.fi/monica/.**
2. **Full references and summaries of MONICA Publications appear in #85/86.**

G3 Death rates from various causes: first three years of coronary-event registration

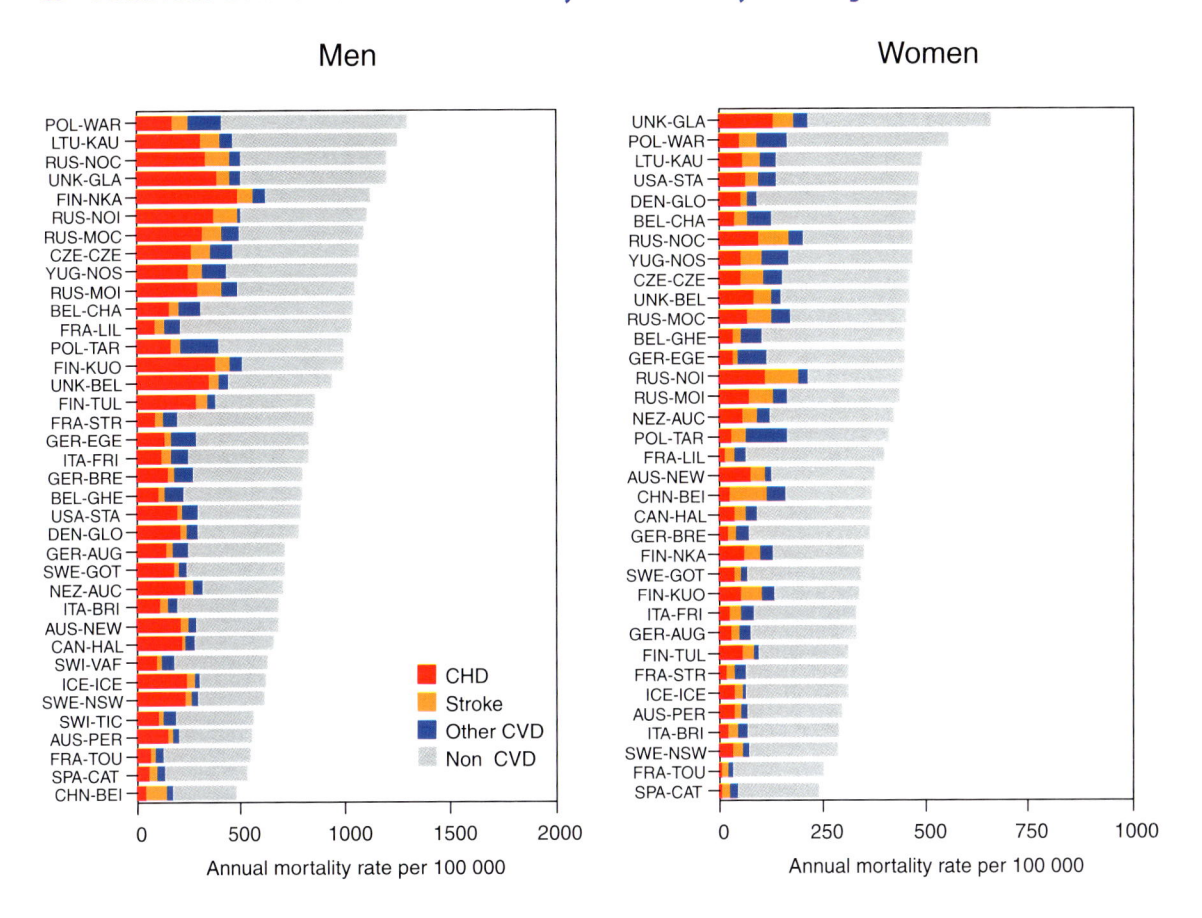

Men

Women

G4 Death rates from various causes: final three years of coronary-event registration

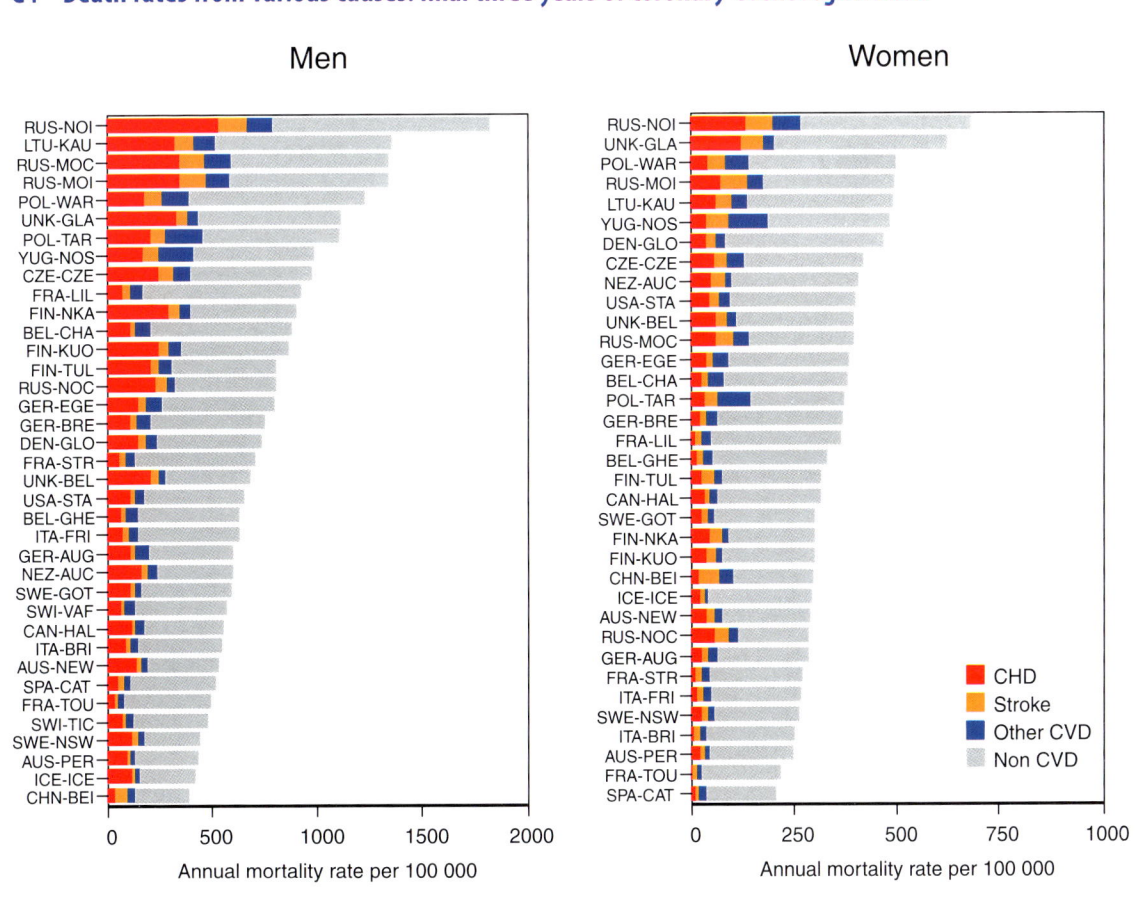

Men

Women

POPULATIONS, DATA COLLECTION AND OFFICIAL MORTALITY

1. As in graphs G3 and G4 the official, unvalidated cause of death is used. Here the denominator is all the deaths in that sex. Demographic data on population numbers are not essential for the calculation of what is called proportional mortality. However in this case the calculation was made using mortality rates.

2. The disease groups are described for G3 and G4 (previous page), as is age standardization.

3. There is more than two-to-one variation in the proportion of all deaths attributable to cardiovascular disease in different populations. The proportion is generally higher in men than women. The sex difference is smaller than the difference within one sex between different populations.

4. There is variation also in the proportion of all cardiovascular deaths attributable to coronary heart disease, stroke and other cardiovascular diseases. A geographical pattern is apparent.

5. The distribution of proportions of deaths from different causes is not changing greatly over time.

6. Proportional mortality analyses such as these have not featured in MONICA Publications.

G5 Ranking of populations by proportion of all deaths from cardiovascular causes: first three years of coronary-event registration

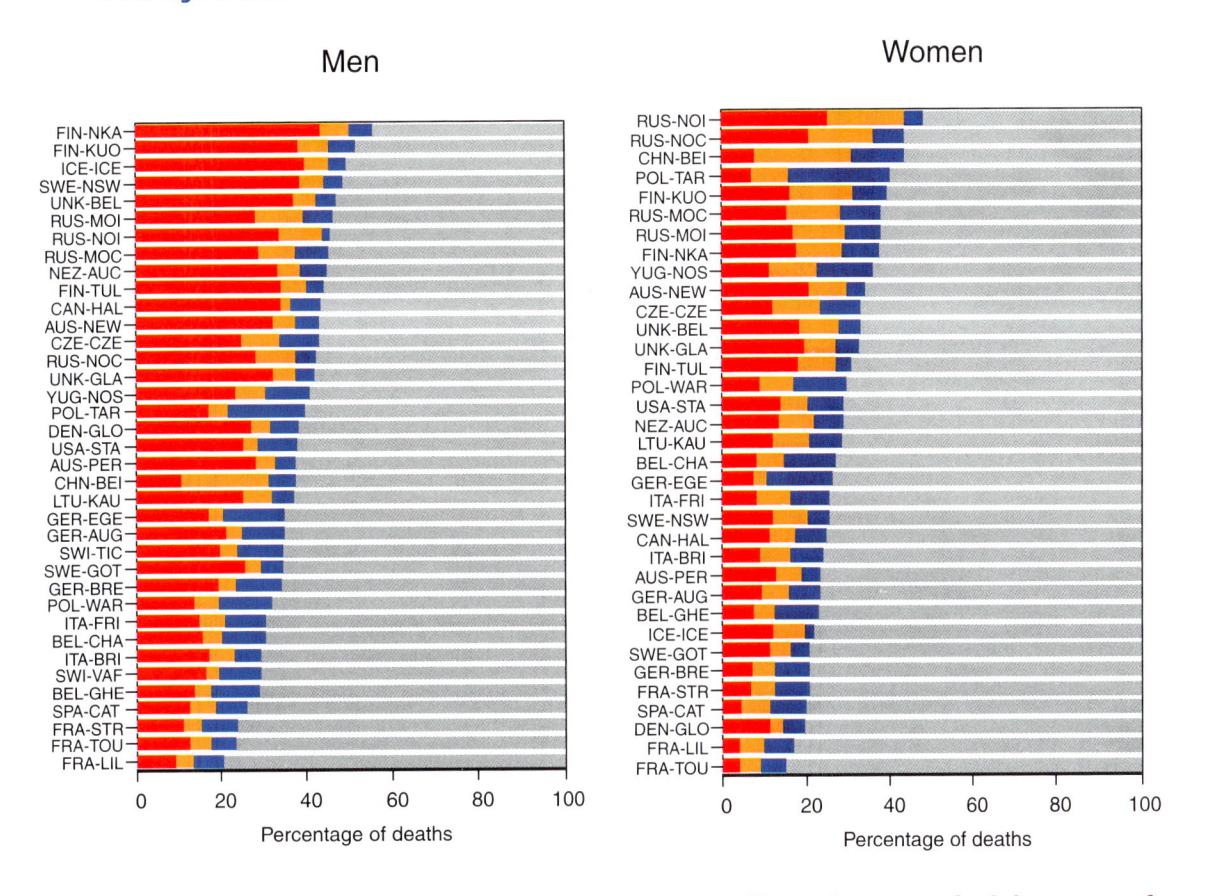

G6 Ranking of populations by proportion of all deaths from cardiovascular causes: final three years of coronary-event registration

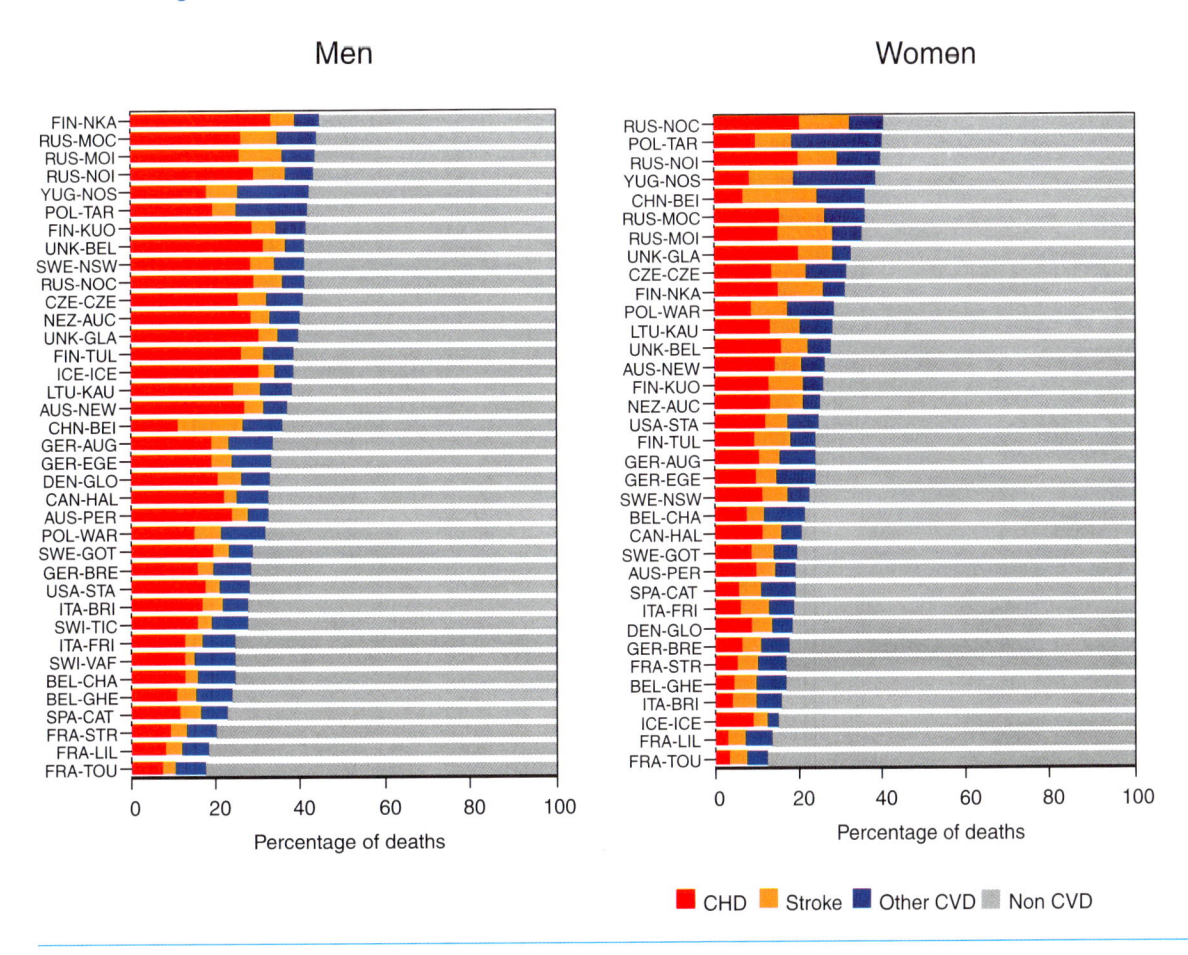

■ CHD ■ Stroke ■ Other CVD ■ Non CVD

POPULATIONS, DATA COLLECTION AND OFFICIAL MORTALITY

G7

1. 'Hot pursuit' (red dots in G7) is the identification of potential cases of non-fatal myocardial infarction from their admission to hospital. 'Cold pursuit' (blue dots in G7) is identification from documents, particularly paper or computer listings produced on discharge from hospital. See #20 *Registration of Coronary Events, Hot and Cold Pursuit*, and MONICA Manual Part IV, Section 1 (*1*), MONICA Publications 4, 10, 16 (*2*). Despite concern about comparability at the time, the method of identifying cases for registration did not appear to show any systematic geographical pattern, or to have a systematic effect on results. G7 shows that different MONICA Collaborating Centres (MCCs) within one country, responsible for neighbouring RUAs, often employed different methods for identifying cases. In some population RUAs a combination or intermediate methods were used—sometimes these changed over time.

G8

2. Years chosen for coronary-event registration were those in which data were available and passed the quality assessments of the MONICA Data Centre. See MONICA Quality assessment of coronary event registration data (*1*). The years shown in G8 define the initial and final years used for graphs G3–G6, and for many later graphs. All 38 of the population RUAs from MONICA Publication 38 (*2*) are included.

3. Starting and stopping dates varied between populations. Twenty-two of the 38 main MONICA hypothesis-testing population RUAs began by 1 January 1984; all 38 monitored coronary events together for the seven years 1 January 1985–31 December 1991; all but two, Denmark-Glostrup, DEN-GLO, see #57, and New Zealand-Auckland, NEZ-AUC, see #71, continued past the end of 1992, and just nine more stopped at the end of 1993. Twenty-seven of the 38 therefore registered coronary events for the same nine years, 1985–1993 inclusive.

4. The 'lagged' registration period, shown in red in G8, was used when testing the First MONICA Hypothesis on coronary risk factors, see #2 *MONICA Hypotheses and Study Design*. Trends in coronary-event rates were calculated twice: firstly over the full period (blue plus red bars) without any time difference from the measurement of trends in risk factors, and secondly after a delayed onset of several years. See G70, G72 and MONICA Publication 38 (*2*).

1. See Monograph CD-ROM or MONICA Website http://www.ktl.fi/monica/.
2. Full references and summaries of MONICA Publications appear in #85/86.

G7 Populations using different methods of identifying non-fatal cases for coronary-event registration

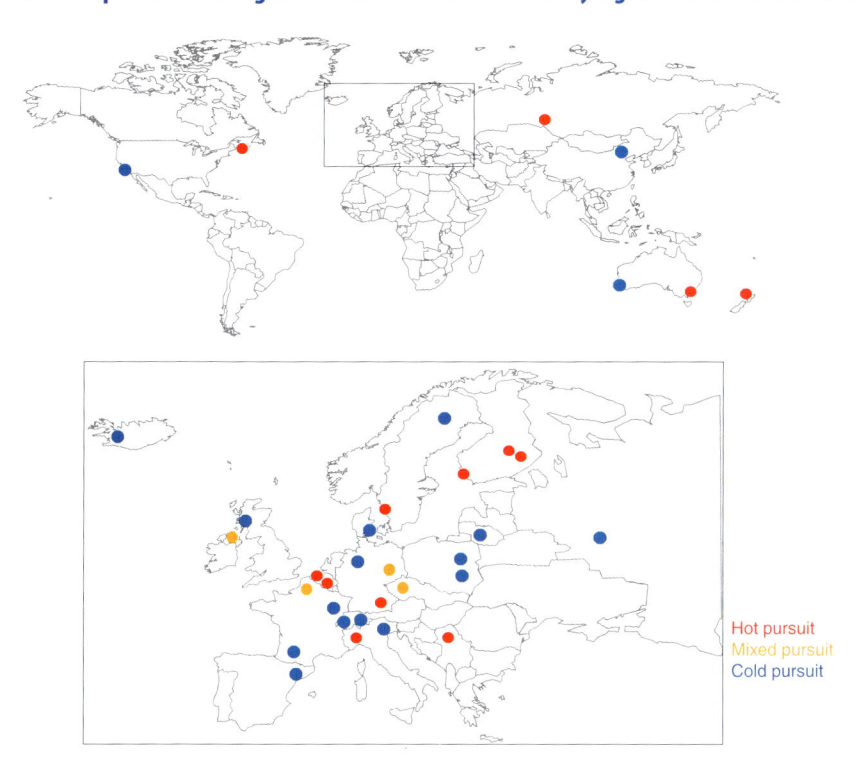

Hot pursuit
Mixed pursuit
Cold pursuit

G8 Years of coronary-event registration in different populations

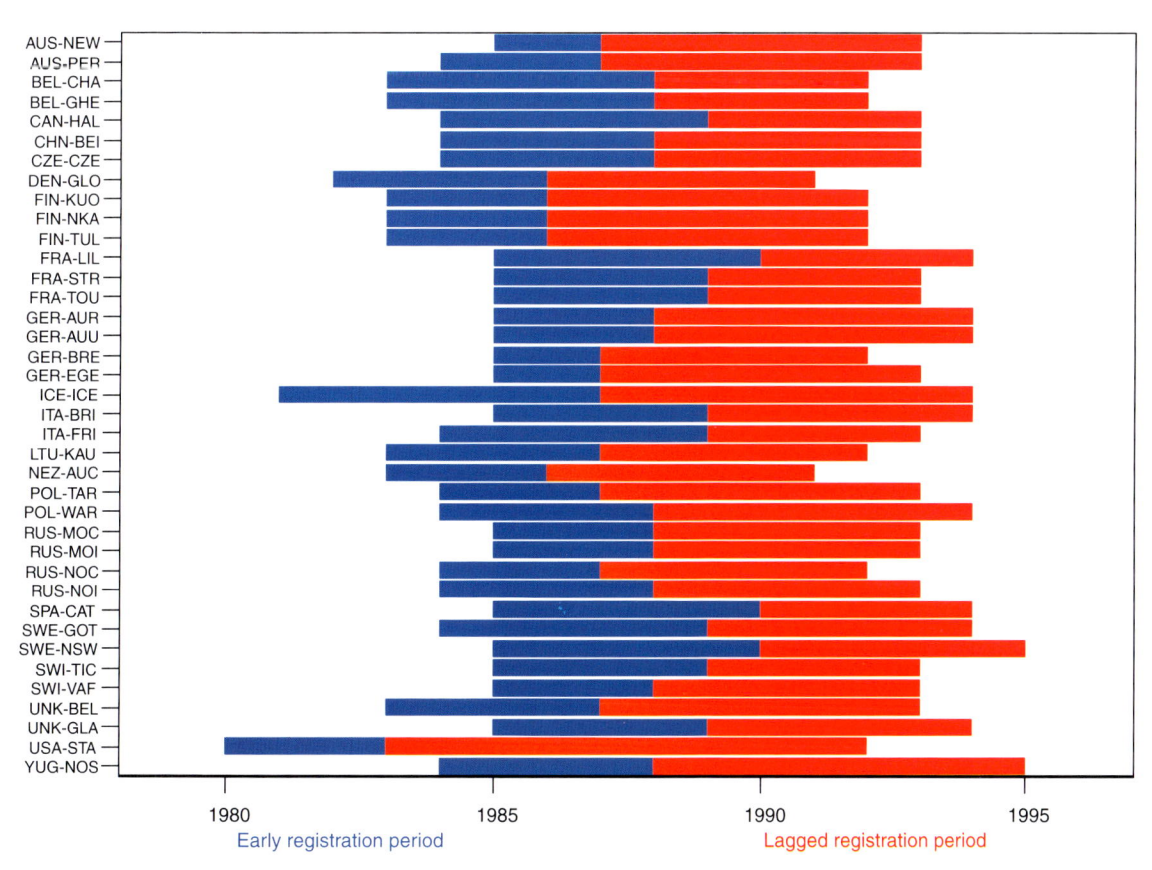

Early registration period   Lagged registration period

POPULATIONS, DATA COLLECTION AND OFFICIAL MORTALITY

G9

1. The 38 MONICA population RUAs in which long-term coronary-event registration took place have been described previously. Equivalent stroke registration took place in 15 RUAs. Years chosen for analysing stroke events were those in which data were available, and passed the MONICA quality control checks for stroke. These years were not necessarily the same years as those in which registration of coronary events took place in the same population RUAs although they could be. Equally, the years were not always the same in related populations. Compare G8 and G9. There are differences in G9 between the three Finnish centres, see #58, and between the two RUAs from Russia-Novosibirsk, see #75. In addition to the 15 populations used to test the MONICA stroke hypotheses, others registered stroke for shorter periods, contributing to early cross-sectional analyses and papers on stroke methods. See MONICA Quality assessment of stroke event registration data (*1*), Germany-East Germany, #65 *GER-EGE*, #84 *Former MONICA Populations*.

2. The 'lagged' registration period was used in testing the First Hypothesis for stroke. See note 4 on previous page referring to G8, G74 and G76. See MONICA Publication 45.

3. Although MONICA was set up to monitor both coronary disease and stroke, monitoring of the latter could not be made obligatory. There were formidable problems in setting up long-term coronary-event registration and conducting repeated population risk-factor surveys before embarking on stroke. Reasons why approximately half of the MONICA Collaborating Centres did not register stroke as well as coronary events included the following:
   - A primarily cardiac focus resulting in lack of interest in stroke.
   - Insufficient resources and manpower to set up a second registration system.
   - Doubts whether numbers of strokes below age 65 would be sufficient to establish local trends, coupled with reluctance to include older age groups. (Half the stroke registers did do so.)
   - Finally in the early 1980s there was concern that registration of non-fatal stroke events would be incomplete in populations where they might be managed away from large hospitals in domiciliary practice. Now modern management of stroke has made referral to hospital a routine.

   MONICA stroke registers tended to reflect local enthusiasm by neurologists or those concerned with diseases of the elderly, as well as epidemiologists. Coronary registers were attractive to cardiologists.

G10

4. To participate in testing the coronary and stroke risk-factor hypotheses, MCCs had to establish trends in risk factors in their population RUAs by mounting an initial and a final population risk-factor survey. A middle survey was recommended but optional.

5. Surveys were not initiated at the same time in different populations. Some lasted only a few months. There was less chance of their occurring simultaneously across populations than was true for coronary or stroke-event registration. That was longer-term.

6. Because risk-factor levels may fluctuate according to the season of the year, investigators were encouraged to standardize the calendar months in which their risk-factor surveys were replicated. This was not always possible through delays in funding, initiating and completing the surveys. See MONICA Quality assessment of age, date of examination and survey periods (*1*).

7. Ideally, the first population surveys in each RUA would have preceded or been simultaneous with the start of event registration. It was not generally feasible to start both registration and population risk-factor surveys together. Coronary and stroke-event registration often started before population risk-factor monitoring. This was because event registration was more problematic. It took longer to pilot and then get up and running smoothly, so attention was focused on that before initiating the population risk-factor surveys. Compare G10, with G8, and G9.

1. See Monograph CD-ROM or MONICA Website http://www.ktl.fi//monica/.

G9 Years of stroke registration in different populations

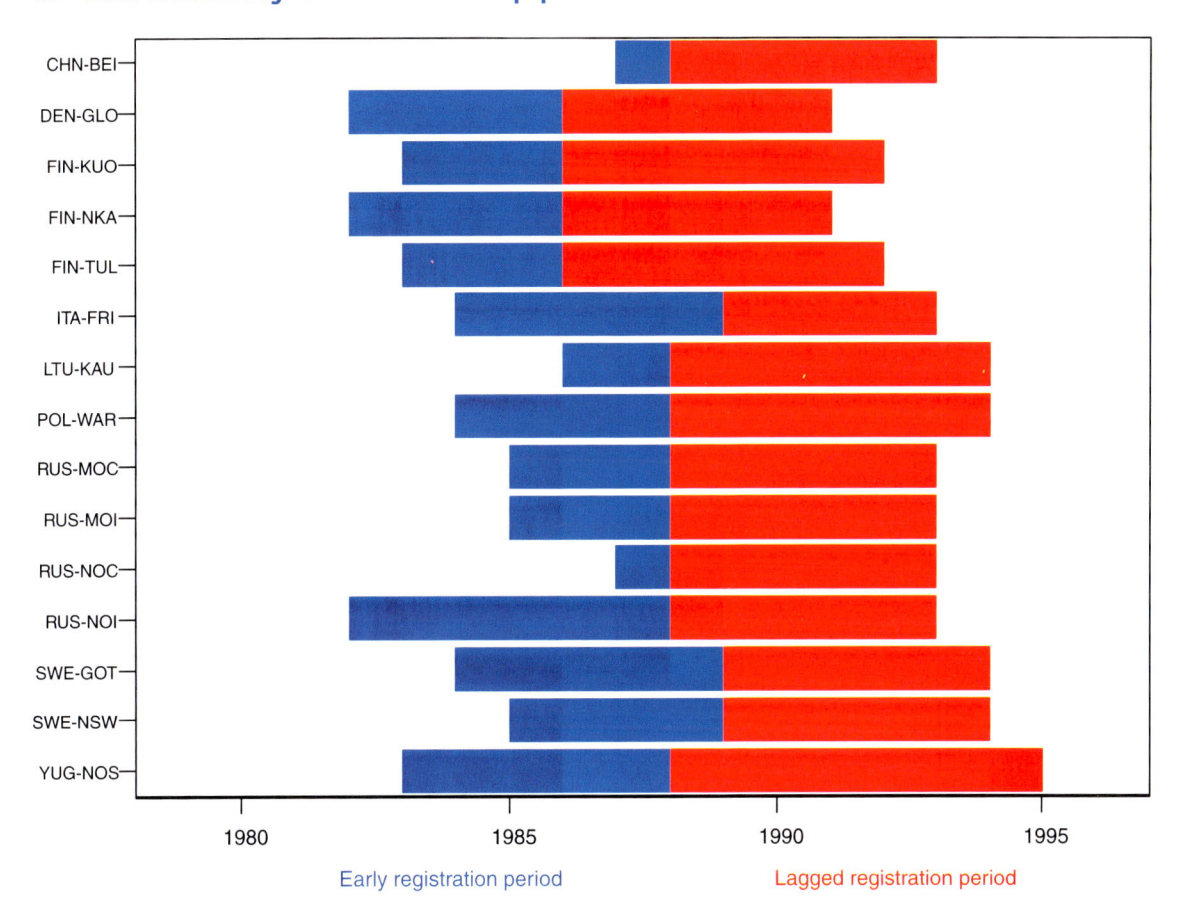

Early registration period — Lagged registration period

G10 Timing of risk-factor surveys in different populations

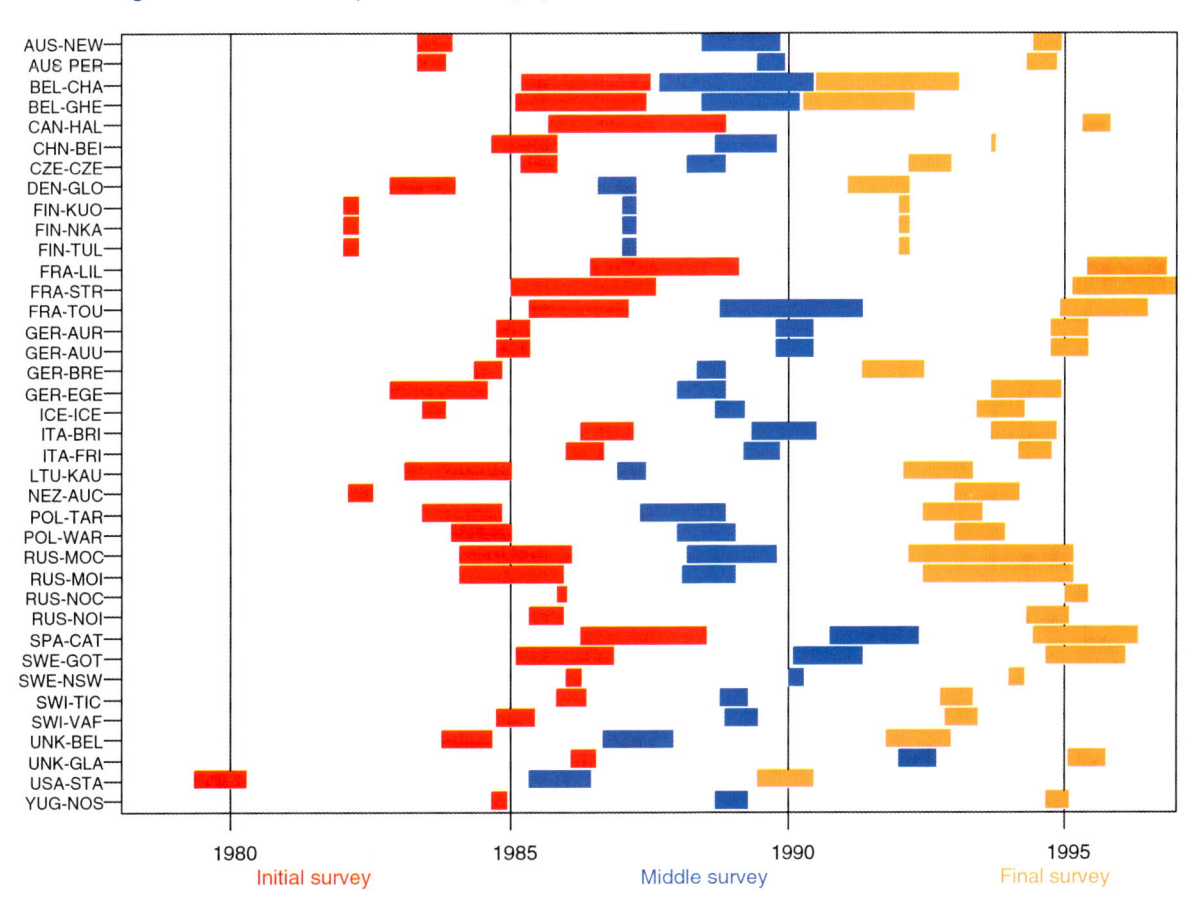

Initial survey — Middle survey — Final survey

POPULATIONS, DATA COLLECTION AND OFFICIAL MORTALITY

1. Coronary-care recording was more limited in duration in most population RUAs than coronary-event registration, particularly in the early years of the MONICA Project. However, some MCCs monitored both data components in their RUAs from start to finish. See #24 *Acute Coronary Care*, MONICA Quality assessment of acute coronary care data (*1*), MONICA Data Book of coronary care (*1*).

2. To test the coronary-care hypothesis, differences in coronary care and rates of coronary end-points were measured across two separate time periods. See G57–G68 and G77, MONICA Publication 39 (*2*).

3. This graph therefore depicts only the defined time periods used in testing that hypothesis, and not the total amount of coronary-care data available. For the same reason G11 shows only part of the coronary-event period of registration.

4. The MONICA collaboration did not require simultaneous recording of coronary care across the MONICA populations. However, comparison of G11 with G10 shows greater uniformity in timing across populations for coronary care than there was for the population risk-factor surveys.

5. The lapse of time between the first and second period differed in different populations. The improvements in treatment between the two periods in different populations (See G57–G68) are specific to those periods and the variable distance between them, as are the associated changes in coronary-event rates. Differences in treatment and in event rates in the same population RUA can be considered together because they are matched for time difference. If either the changes in treatments or the changes in end-point rates are compared across population RUAs, the lack of standardization of the time differences might lead to wrong conclusions.

1. See Monograph CD-ROM or MONICA Website http://www.ktl.fi/monica/.
2. Full references and summaries of MONICA Publications appear in #85/86.

G11 Periods used for testing the MONICA coronary-care (treatment or second) hypothesis

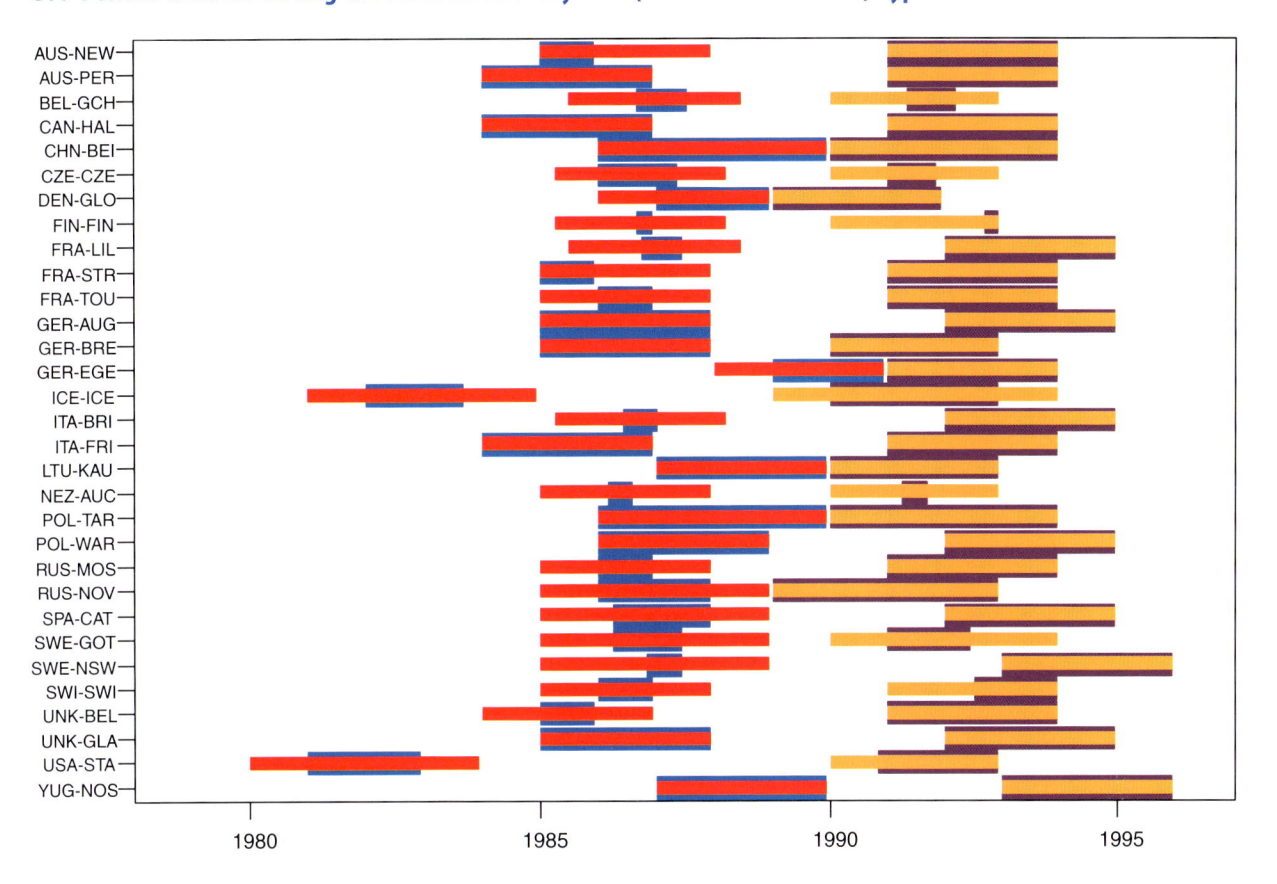

First coronary event registration period
First coronary care recording period

Second coronary event registration period
Second coronary care recording period

Coronary events: incidence, case fatality and mortality rates

1. The specific calendar years included in the two three-year periods differed by population. They were identified previously in G8.

2. Event rates are calculated using registration data for events, and demographic data for population denominators. See #17 *Demographic Data*, #37 *Event Rates, Case Fatality, and Trends*, MONICA Quality assessment of demographic data (*1*), MONICA Quality assessment of coronary-event registration data (*1*), MONICA Data Book of coronary events (*1*).

3. Results are age-standardized for the 35–64 age group, using the world standard population. See #39 *Age Standardization*.

4. Coronary events are defined using MONICA diagnostic criteria. In this case definition 1 is used, incorporating definite non-fatal myocardial infarction and definite, possible and unclassifiable (previously called 'insufficient data') coronary deaths. Non-fatal possible myocardial infarction is excluded from this definition. See #23 *Diagnosing Myocardial Infarction and Coronary Death*, MONICA Manual Part IV, Section 1 (*1*), and MONICA Publication 16 (*2*).

5. Note that the scale maximum for women on the x-axis is half of that for men.

6. Confidence intervals, an indicator of precision, are not shown. Rates are averaged over three years, involving large numbers of events in most populations. Estimates of rates should therefore be reasonably precise. See the MONICA Data Book of coronary events, table 6 (*1*), for numbers.

7. These figures illustrate the five-to-one and ten-to-one variation in event rates between populations of the same sex, and the four to one ratio between coronary-event rates in men and women. Comparison of G13 with G12 shows the changes of coronary-event rates over time and resulting change in population RUA rankings.

1. See Monograph CD-ROM or MONICA Website http://www.ktl.fi/monica/.
2. Full references and summaries of MONICA Publications appear in #85/86.

G12 Coronary-event rates: first three years of registration

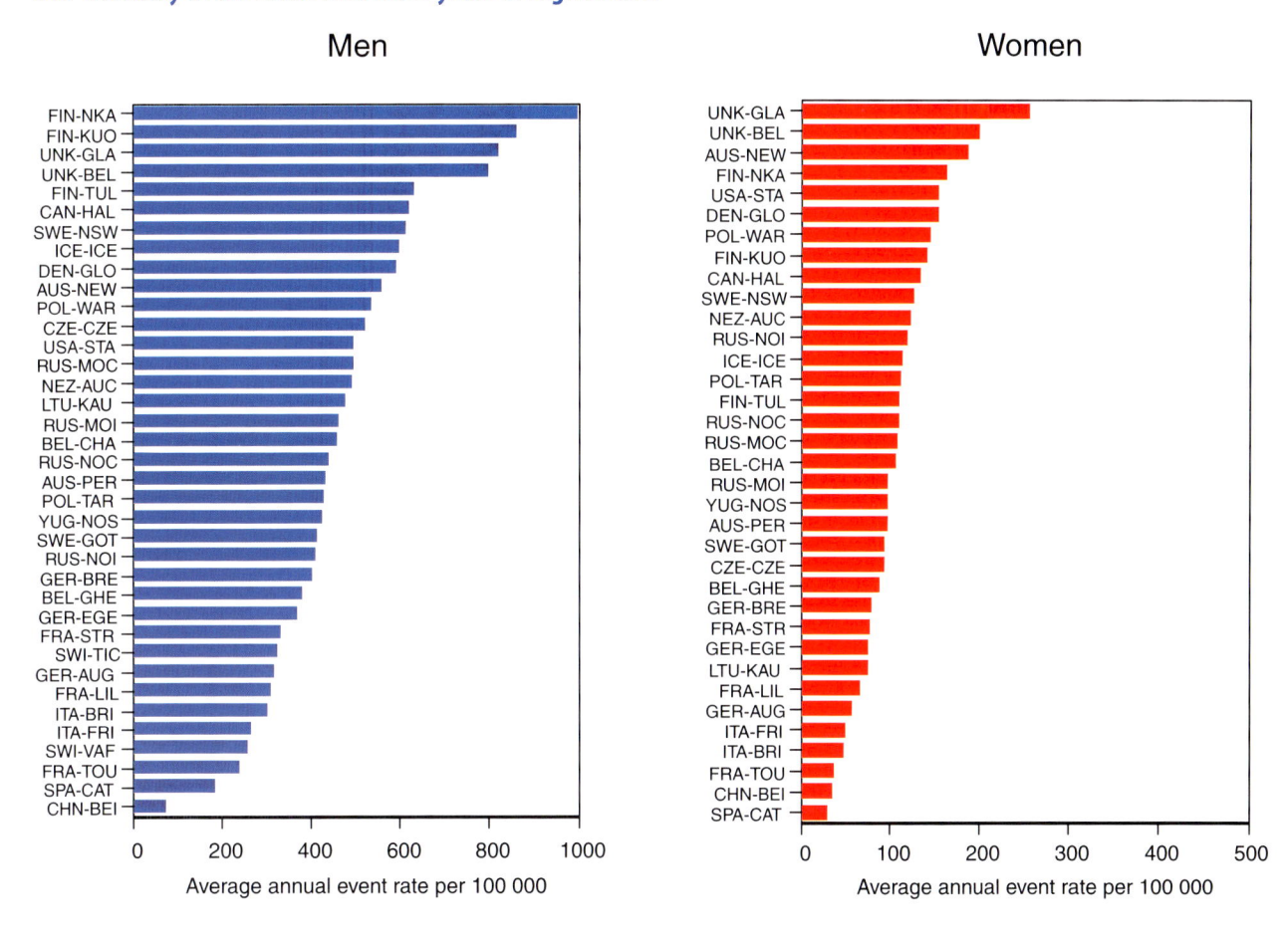

Men

Women

Average annual event rate per 100 000

G13 Coronary-event rates: final three years of registration

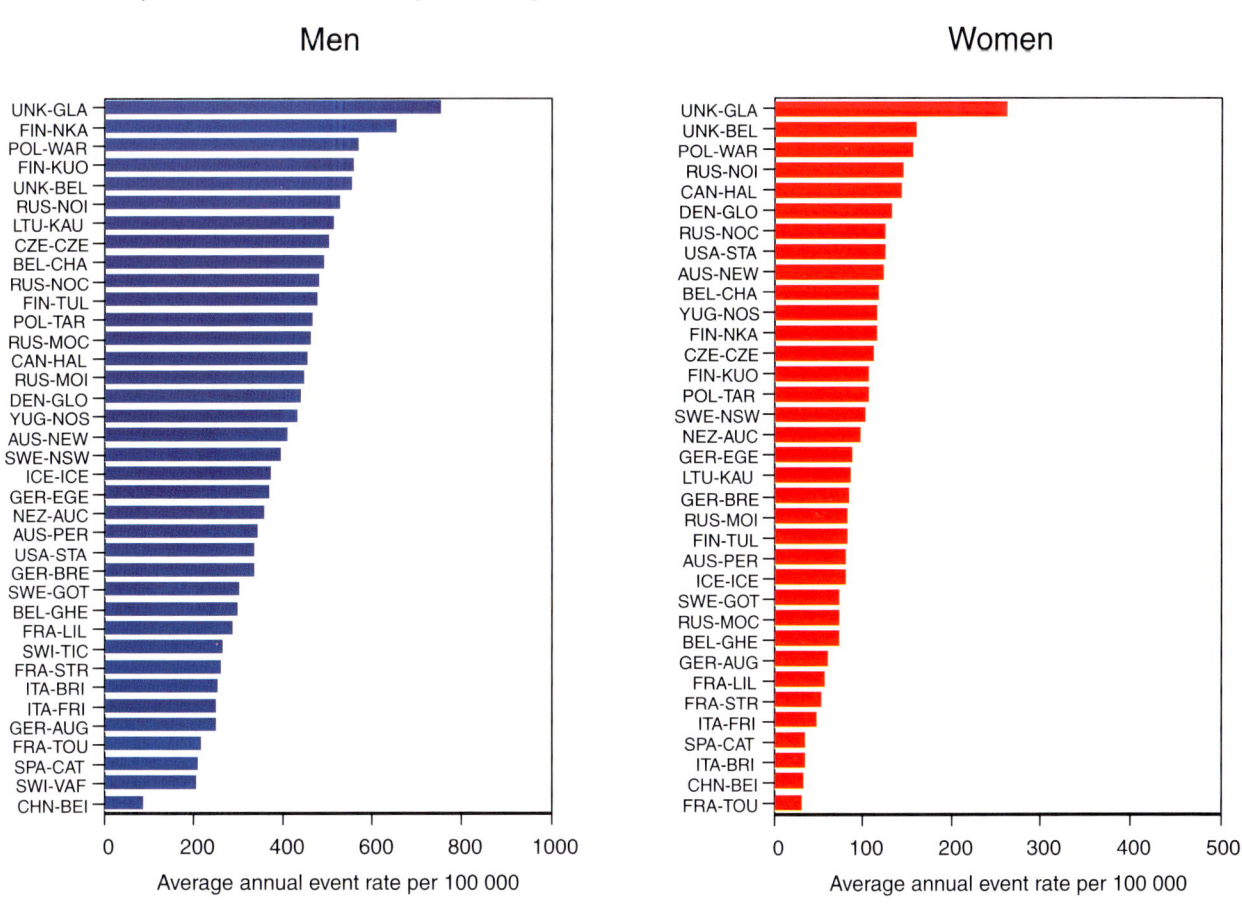

Men

Women

Average annual event rate per 100 000

CORONARY EVENTS: INCIDENCE, CASE FATALITY AND MORTALITY RATES

G14

1. For calculating the trends in population coronary-event rates in MONICA we use a statistical model that assumes that each trend is log-linear in pattern, and that expresses the result as annual percentage change. See #37 *Event Rates, Case Fatality, and Trends*. Graph G14 shows annual event rates before any statistical modelling has been done. Although largely unreadable it is there because it illustrates the problems in the raw data before the statistical model is used. There are large year-on-year fluctuations. Trends in event rates in specific populations may not appear linear, but J-, or U-shaped. A large absolute difference where rates are high will be equivalent, in percentage terms, to a smaller one in different population RUAs where the underlying rate is low.

2. G14 does show a general pattern of decline, but also what is happening at the extremes. Results for Finland-North Karelia, FIN-NKA, see #58, in men and United Kingdom-Glasgow, UNK-GLA, see #81, in women are notable at the top end of the distribution. China-Beijing, CHN-BEI, see #55, in men and Spain-Catalonia, SPA-CAT, see #76, in women have the lowest rates. Yearly numbers of coronary events, and coronary-event rates are published in the MONICA Data Book of coronary events, table 6 (*1*) from which this graph is derived.

3. Note in G14 the difference in scale maximum on the y-axis between men and women. It is almost four-to-one.

G15

4. G15 is derived from the same set of data as G14, but after calculation of trends. See #37 *Event Rates, Case Fatality and Trends*. It is partly coincidental and not inevitable that the extreme values are held by almost the same population RUAs in men in G14 and G15 (Finland-North Karelia, FIN-NKA and China Beijing, CHN-BEI). G14 is plotted for rates, low to high, and G15 for trends in rates, decreasing to increasing. The same pattern is not seen in women, where there is no association between extremes in rates and extremes in trends.

5. Horizontal bars in G15 show the 95% confidence intervals around the estimated annual trend. The smaller the length of the bars the more precise the estimated trend. If the bars fail to cross the zero line the estimated trend is considered to deviate significantly from zero. This graph follows a standard model used for presenting estimated trends in the MONICA results. Declining trends are shown to the left of the zero line, and increasing trends to the right.

6. Confidence intervals are wider for women than for men because there were fewer events. Greater relative year-on-year fluctuations, through the random variation resulting from smaller numbers, are seen well in G14 when the two sexes are compared. This resulted in less precise estimates of trends in women in G15 than in men. Wide confidence intervals are also found where the trend appears to deviate from log-linear.

7. Both G14 and G15 show that the tendency in the majority of MONICA population RUAs is towards a decline in coronary-event rates. In this majority in G15 the estimated annual trend is to the left of the zero line. In men the ratio is four-fifths declining versus one-fifth increasing. In women it is nearer to two-thirds declining to one-third increasing. See the same data presented also in G23, G24 and G25.

8. G15 was previously published in MONICA Publication 36 (*2*). It was important in establishing that there were differing trends in coronary-event rates (rates when non-fatal and fatal coronary events were combined), in the different MONICA population RUAs around the world. The data previously available for multinational comparisons were from routine death certification.

1. See Monograph CD-ROM or MONICA Website http://www.ktl.fi/monica/.
2. Full references and summaries of MONICA Publications appear in #85/86.

G14 Coronary-event rates by calendar year of registration

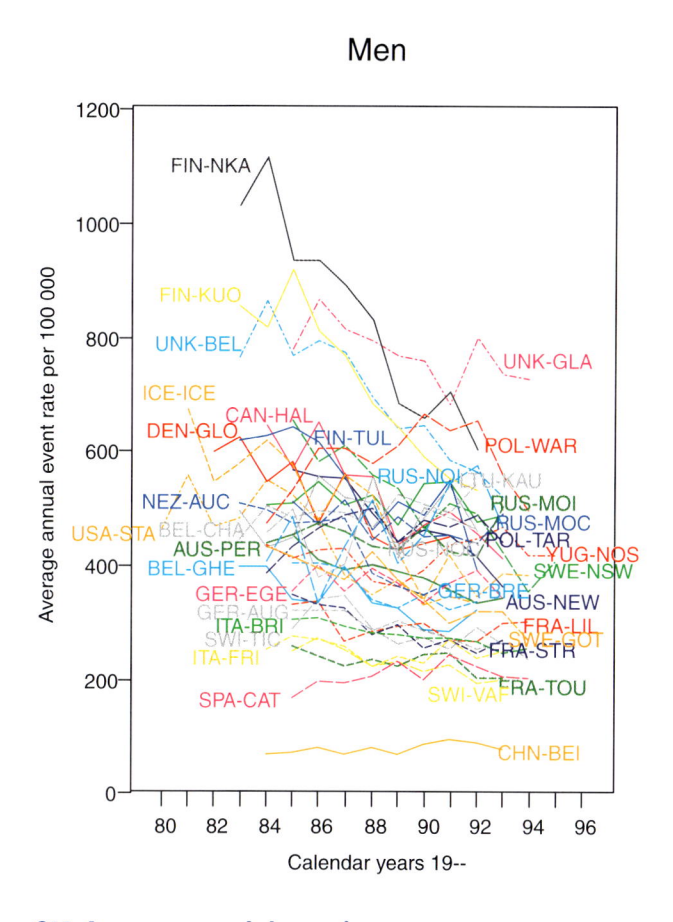

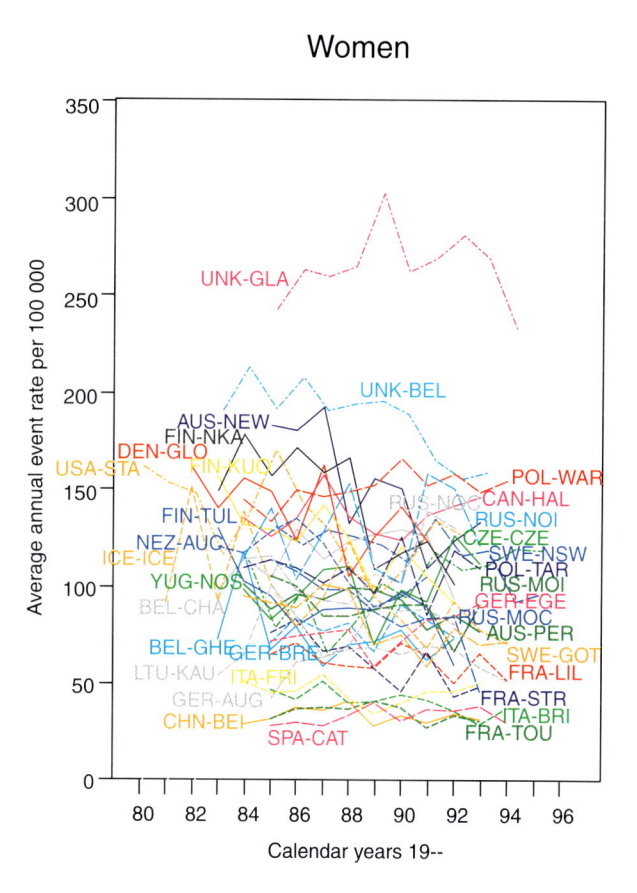

G15 Average annual change in coronary-event rates

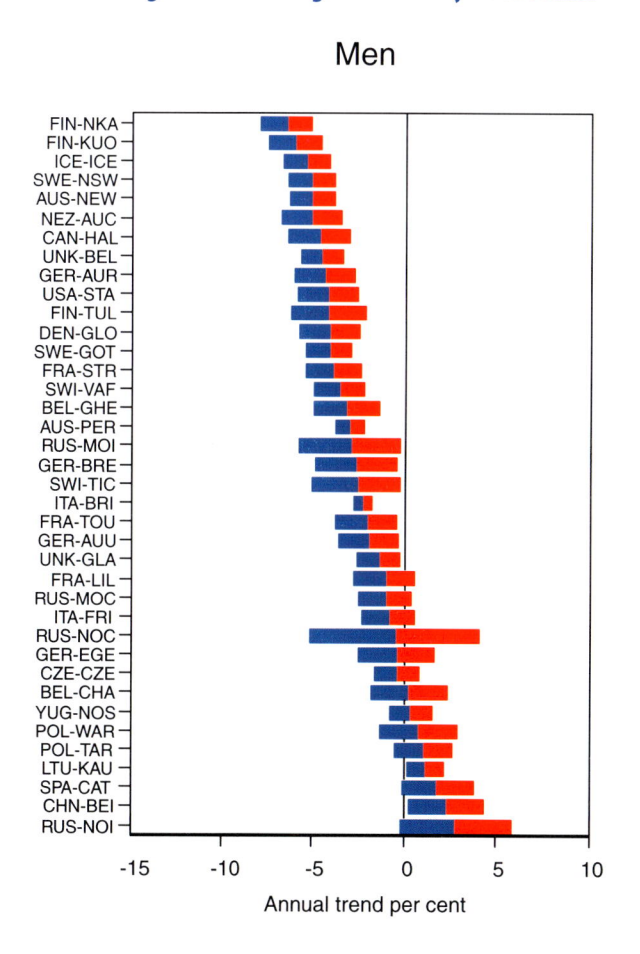

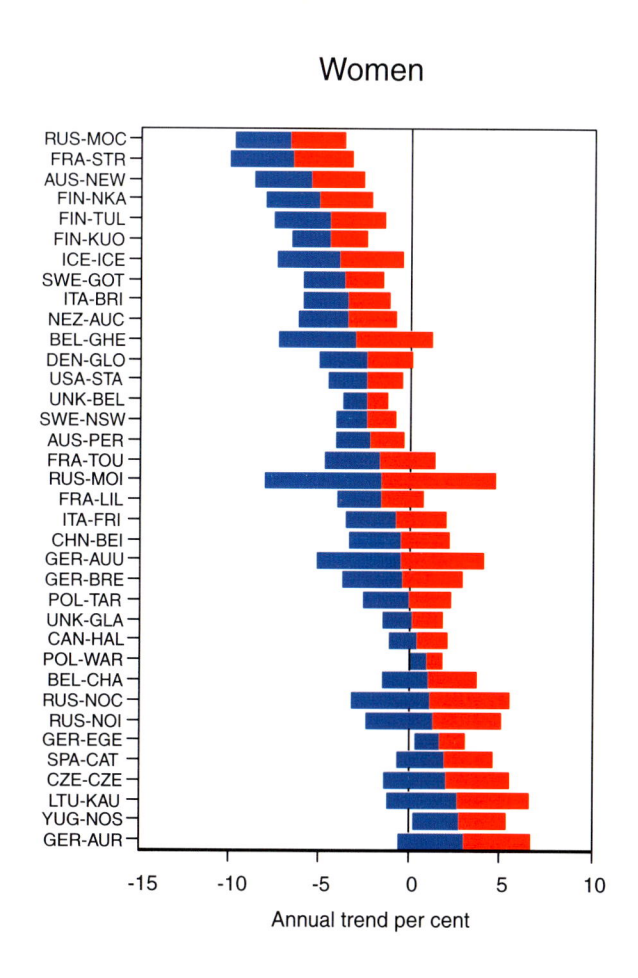

CORONARY EVENTS: INCIDENCE, CASE FATALITY AND MORTALITY RATES

Notes in italics are repeated to help random browsers—systematic readers should ignore them

1. *The specific calendar years included in the two three-year periods differed by population. They were identified in G8.*

2. Case fatality is the proportion of events ending fatally within 28 days from the onset of the attack. See #37 *Event Rates, Case Fatality, and Trends*.

3. The denominator is all events so the scale is the same for men and women. Case fatality does not involve population demographic data.

4. Results are age-standardized for the 35–64 age group, using the MONICA weightings for case fatality. See #39 *Age Standardization*.

5. *The case fatality here is for coronary events defined using MONICA diagnostic criteria, definition 1. Definition 1 incorporates definite non-fatal myocardial infarction and definite, possible and unclassifiable (previously called 'insufficient data') coronary deaths. Non-fatal possible myocardial infarction is excluded from this definition. See #23 Diagnosing Myocardial Infarction and Coronary Death, MONICA Manual Part IV, Section 1 (1), and MONICA Publication 16 (2).*

6. Case fatality here is higher than that in published clinical case series of myocardial infarction. Results include all coronary deaths, two-thirds or more of which occur before admission to hospital. Clinical case series usually start with diagnosed patients' admission to hospital and exclude coronary deaths in patients admitted for other conditions. That is why the case fatality is much lower. Follow-up may cease at hospital discharge or at three weeks rather than the 28 days in MONICA, but that has a smaller impact on case fatality than that from exclusion of pre-hospital sudden deaths. See MONICA Publications 16, 29 (*2*).

7. The complement of case fatality, survival, should relate to treatment. Fatality and survival also reflect the relative success of the MONICA registers in finding and confirming putative fatal and non-fatal coronary cases. This problem is discussed in MONICA Publications 16, 29, 36 (*2*).

8. High case fatality, as in Poland-Tarnobrzeg Voivodship, POL-TAR, see #72, reflects delays and difficulties in obtaining diagnostic confirmation of non-fatal events, to make them definite myocardial infarction. Without early electrocardiographic or serological confirmation, all potential definite non-fatal cases are classified as possibles, and excluded from the case mix for MONICA definition 1. See #23 *Diagnosing Myocardial Infarction and Coronary Death*, MONICA Manual Part IV, Section 1 (*1*), and MONICA Publication 16 (*2*).

9. *Confidence intervals, an indicator of precision, are not shown. Rates are averaged over three years, involving large numbers of events in most population. Estimates of case fatality should therefore be reasonably precise. See MONICA Data Book of coronary events, table 6 (1) for the numbers.*

10. These figures illustrate the variation between populations, and between the two sexes, and changes in ranking over time. On average, case fatality was slightly higher in women than in men. Differences were usually small, and were absent in some populations with high coronary-event rates in both sexes. This question is examined in MONICA Publications 16, 29, 36 (*2*). MONICA Publication 16 showed that high case fatality in women, but not in men, correlated with low population event rates. The authors suggested that this might result from a lower level of suspicion, recognition and ascertainment of myocardial infarction in women patients with non-fatal infarction compared to that in men. MONICA Publication 39 (*2*) discussed trends in case fatality in relation to changes in treatment, examining the Second MONICA Hypothesis. Graphs G16 and G17 show some suggestive geographical polarization between populations with low and high case fatality.

1. See Monograph CD-ROM or MONICA Website http://www.ktl.fi/monica/.
2. Full references and summaries of MONICA Publications appear in #85/86.

G16 Case fatality for coronary events: first three years of registration

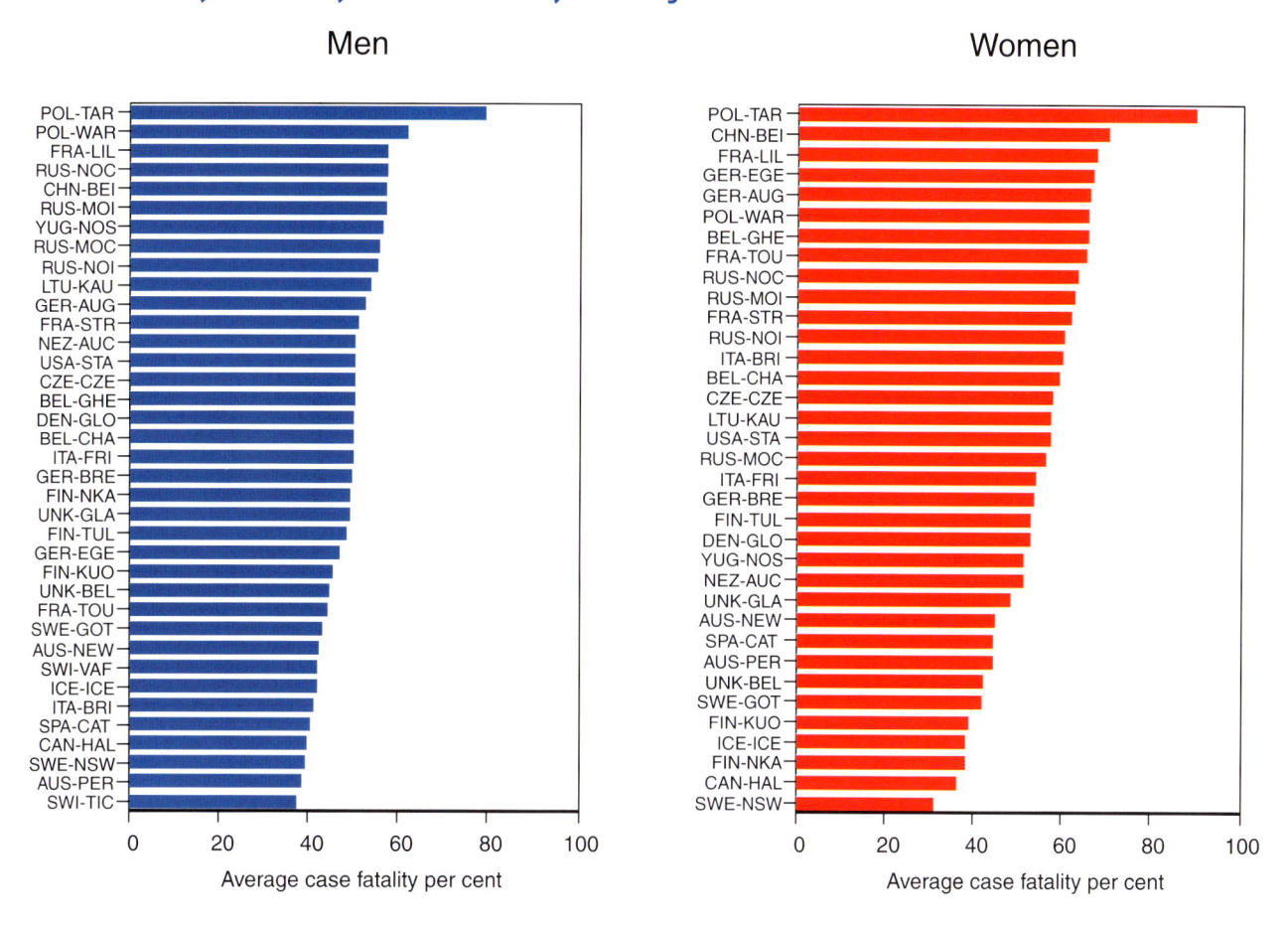

Men / Women

G17 Case fatality for coronary events: final three years of registration

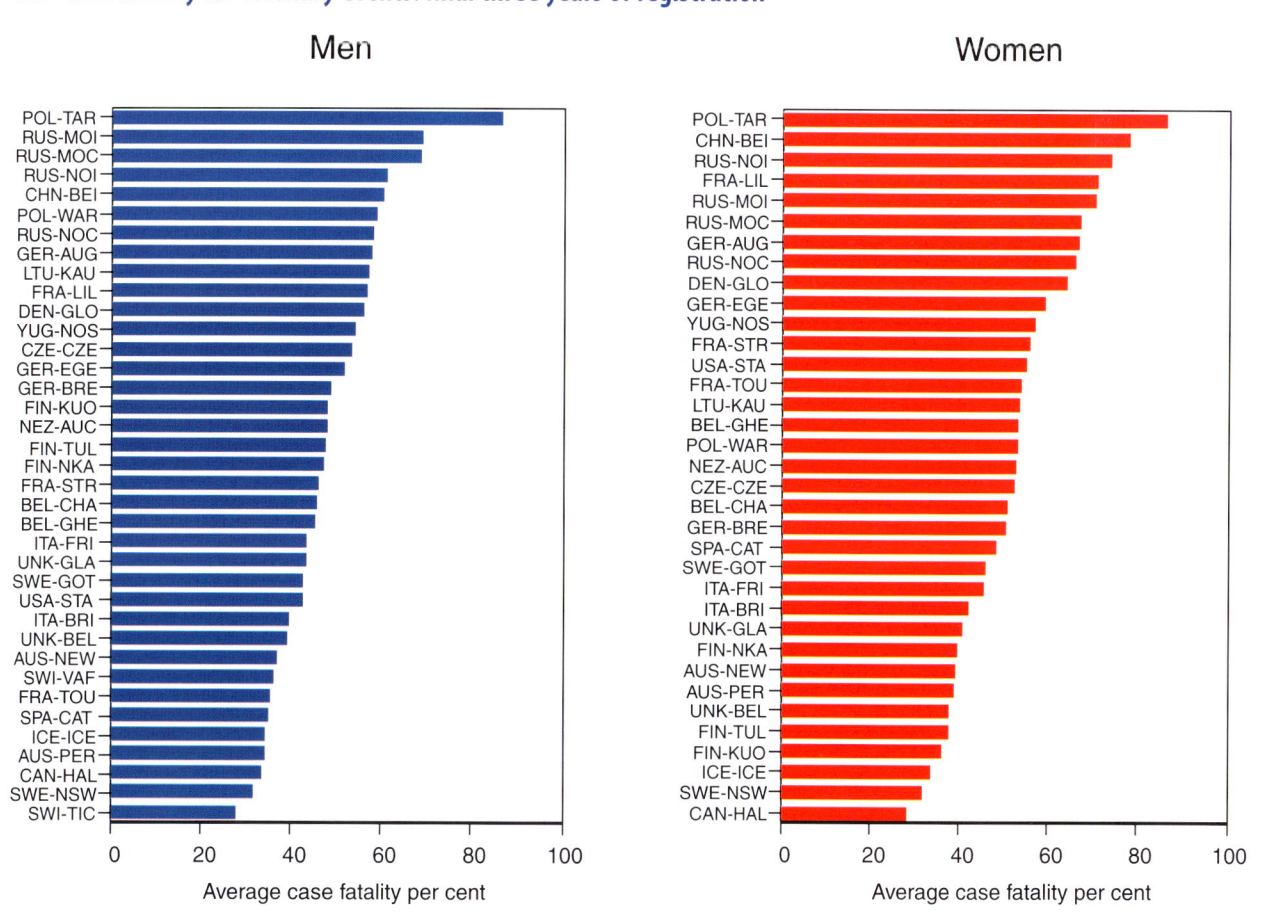

Men / Women

CORONARY EVENTS: INCIDENCE, CASE FATALITY AND MORTALITY RATES

Notes in italics are repeated to help random browsers—systematic readers should ignore them

G18

1. Calculation of trends is explained in #37 *Event Rates, Case Fatality and Trends*. The units of change in case fatality are potentially confusing because its basic unit is per cent, so that a percentage decline can be interpreted as absolute or relative. (Similarly potential confusion arises later for changes in cigarette smokers (see G37).) Because of an important mathematical relationship (see later, G23) the trend shown here is the relative trend. Case fatality averages about 50% overall. If it declined from 50% to 49% the relative decline would be about 2%, as shown in G18, but the absolute change would be 1%.

2. *Horizontal bars in G18 show the 95% confidence intervals around the estimated annual trend. The smaller the length of the bars the more precise the estimated trend. If the bars fail to cross the zero line the estimated trend is considered to deviate significantly from zero. Declining trends are shown to the left of the zero line, and increasing trends to the right.*

3. *Confidence intervals are wider for women than for men because there were fewer events. Greater year-on-year fluctuations through the random variation resulting from smaller numbers resulted in less precise estimates of trends. Wide confidence intervals are also found where the trend appears to deviate from log-linear.*

4. G18 shows that case fatality is tending downwards in most populations in MONICA, although the estimated trend in many individual results fails to differ significantly from zero. The crossover point in the graph for men is slightly lower down than that in the graph for women, but in both there is close to two-thirds of populations with an estimated decline and one-third with an increase. This graph has been published previously in MONICA Publication 36 (*2*).

G19

5. G19 contrasts the results of comparing mortality rates, calculated from two sources: firstly from numbers of MONICA coronary heart disease (CHD) deaths validated through registration, and secondly from numbers of coronary deaths reported by routine official sources. See #16 *Routine Mortality Data*. The same population denominators were used to calculate both event rates. There are substantial discrepancies in some populations but not all, suggesting both potential under-reporting and over-reporting of coronary deaths. A dilemma posed by the discrepancy is whether to include as coronary deaths those that MONICA found unclassifiable—deaths with no available diagnostic information (originally labelled 'insufficient data'). These accounted for 22% of potential coronary deaths overall, and over 40% in some populations. This graph uses MONICA case definition 1, including unclassifiable deaths. MONICA definition 2, which excludes them, gives a different result. The answer may be somewhere between. See #23 *Diagnosing Myocardial Infarction and Coronary Death*, MONICA Manual Part IV, Section 1 (*1*), MONICA Publications 16 (*2*) (which examines this issue in detail) and 36 (*2*).

6. In G19 the scale maximum for men and women is different on the x-axis, that for men being three-and-a-half times greater than for women. Discrepancies between MONICA and official CHD mortality rates in women are proportionately greater than those in men.

7. G19 gives an impression of what is happening across populations, but is less easy to read for single populations. The grey line joining the red and blue marks indicates the extent of the discrepancy. Basic information on which G19 is based is found in the MONICA Data Book of coronary events, table 11 (*1*). Five year cross-sectional data were published in MONICA Publication 16 (*2*).

1. **See Monograph CD-ROM or MONICA Website http://www.ktl.fi/monica/.**
2. **Full references and summaries of MONICA Publications appear in #85/86.**

G18 Average annual change in case fatality

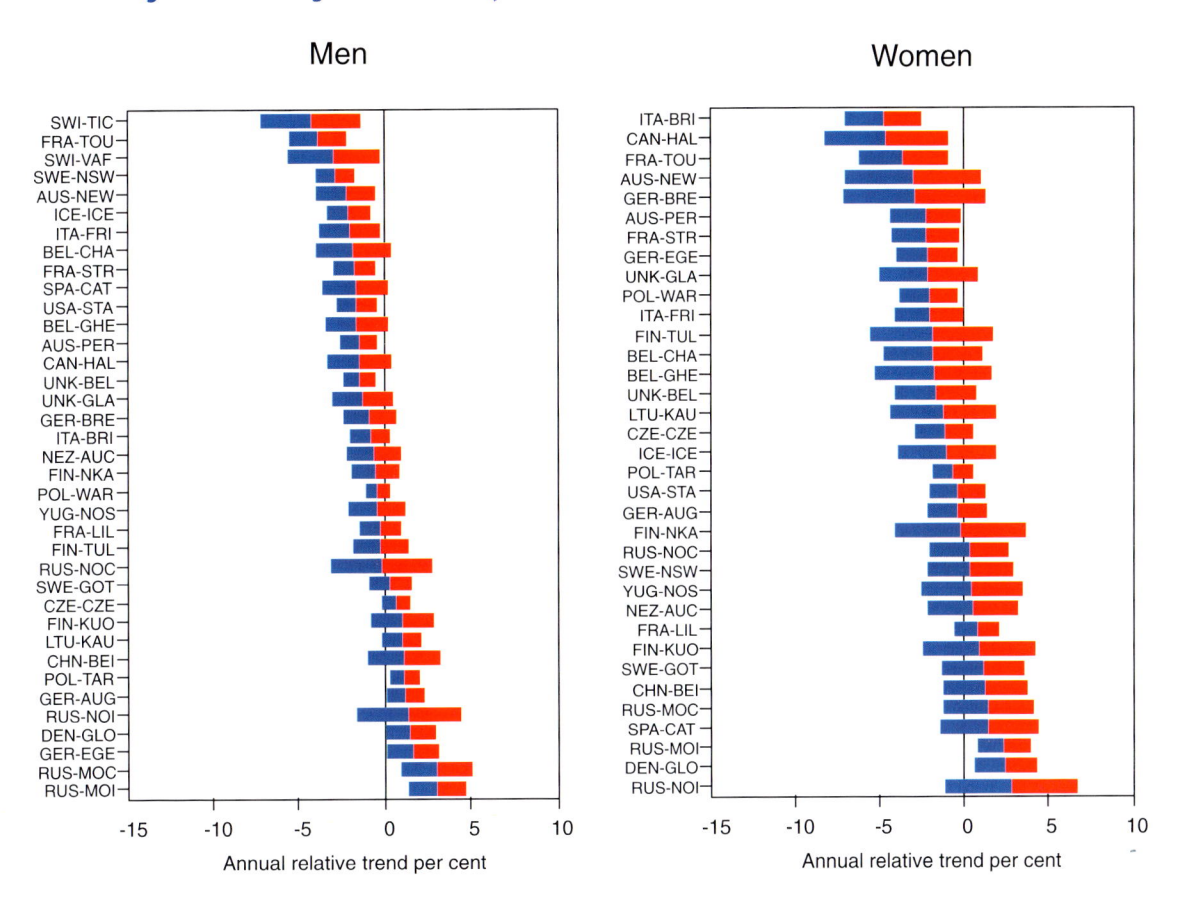

Men

Women

Annual relative trend per cent

G19 Populations ranked by ten-year average MONICA coronary heart disease (CHD) mortality rates showing official unvalidated rates

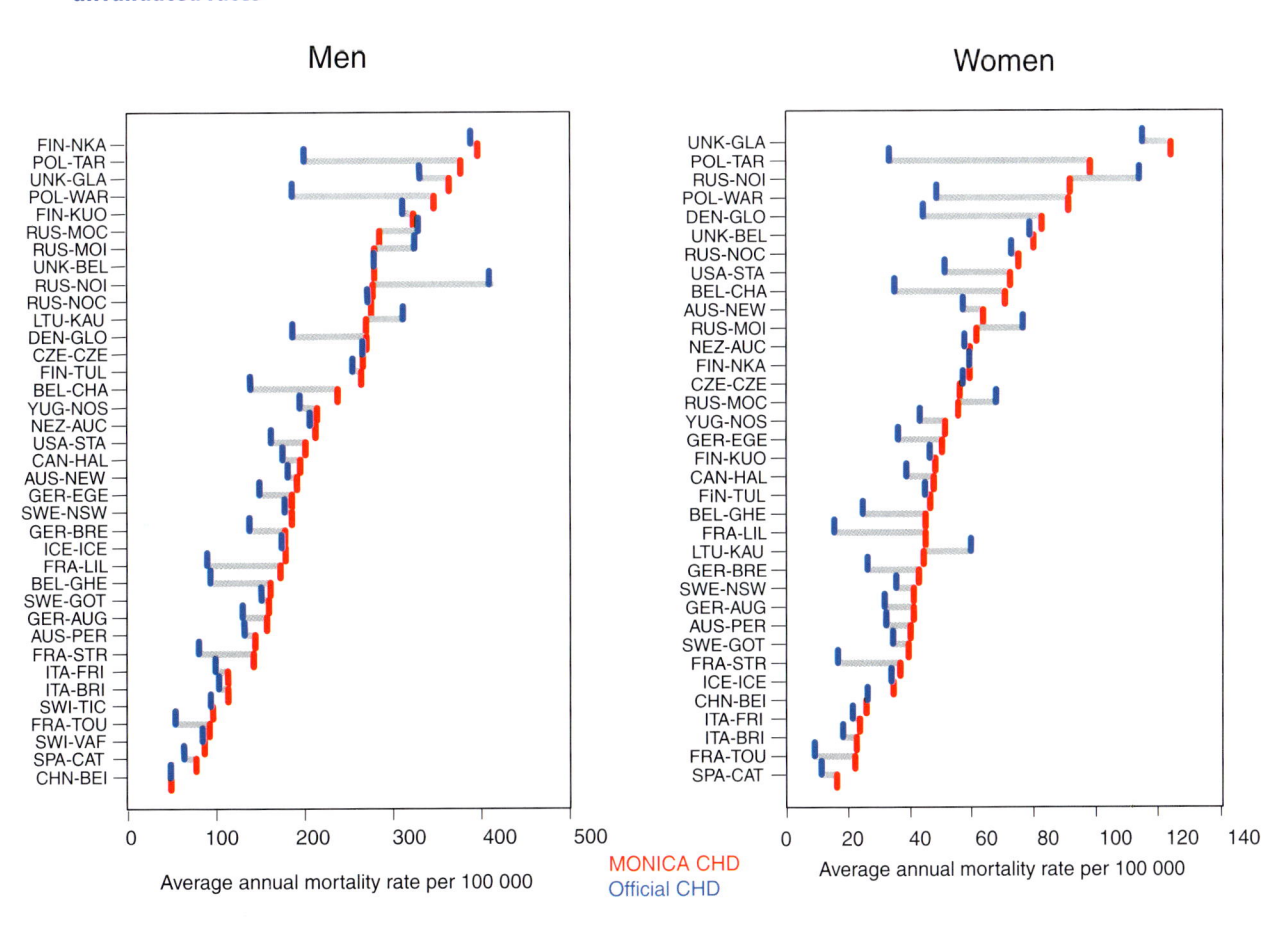

Men

Women

MONICA CHD
Official CHD

Average annual mortality rate per 100 000

CORONARY EVENTS: INCIDENCE, CASE FATALITY AND MORTALITY RATES

Notes in italics are repeated to help random browsers—systematic readers should ignore them

G20

1. *Calculation of trends is explained in #37 Event Rates, Case Fatality, and Trends.*

2. G20 follows on from G19 (see earlier commentary), showing trends over time in the same data components. The original data are found in table 11 of the MONICA Data Book of coronary events (*1*).

3. In men, trends in MONICA CHD mortality rates are often more modest than those in the official mortality rates. However, there is better agreement between the estimated *trends* in official and MONICA CHD mortality rates in G20 in men, than there is for the *mortality rates themselves* in G19.

4. There is relatively less agreement between the two mortality trends in women than there is in men.

5. There are several explanations for the discrepancies, not all implying that MONICA is right. Was registration of events uniformly complete over time? Did the proportion of unclassifiable coronary deaths change over time (see notes for G19)? Did the medico-legal practice in sudden death change, for example for postmortem examination? See MONICA Quality assessment of coronary event registration data table 8 (*1*), MONICA Data Book of coronary events table 5 (*1*), for further information.

6. G20 answers one of the original MONICA questions. When MONICA was planned during the late 1970s and early 1980s there were still many eminent pathologists and cardiologists who denied that mortality rates for coronary heart disease were changing. They claimed that the reported declines were spurious and resulted from changing fashions and inaccuracies in death certification. MONICA discovered numerous problems and discrepancies in death certification, but confirmed that mortality rates from cardiovascular disease were indeed changing.

G21

7. A recurrent concern in MONICA analyses is whether extreme results, or indeed the general pattern of results, could be unduly influenced by variations in the quality of data. Quality assessment was rigorous, the results are explicit, are published on the Web, and are taken into consideration in the major analyses. See MONICA Quality assessment of coronary event registration data (*1*) MONICA Qality assessment of demographic data (*1*).

8. In G21 the relation between trends in coronary endpoints, and the quality score allocated to each population for its coronary-event data is not random. The weak relation that is there is shown on formal calculation not to be strong enough to suggest that study results were significantly compromised or confounded by known variation in data quality. See MONICA Quality assessment of coronary event registration data, Appendix 5—Coronary events trends quality scores (*1*), MONICA Publication 36 (*2*).

1. **See Monograph CD-ROM or MONICA Website http://www.ktl.fi/monica/.**
2. **Full references and summaries of MONICA Publications appear in #85/86.**

G20 Populations ranked by average annual change in MONICA CHD mortality rates, showing unvalidated (from routine mortality reporting) trend equivalents

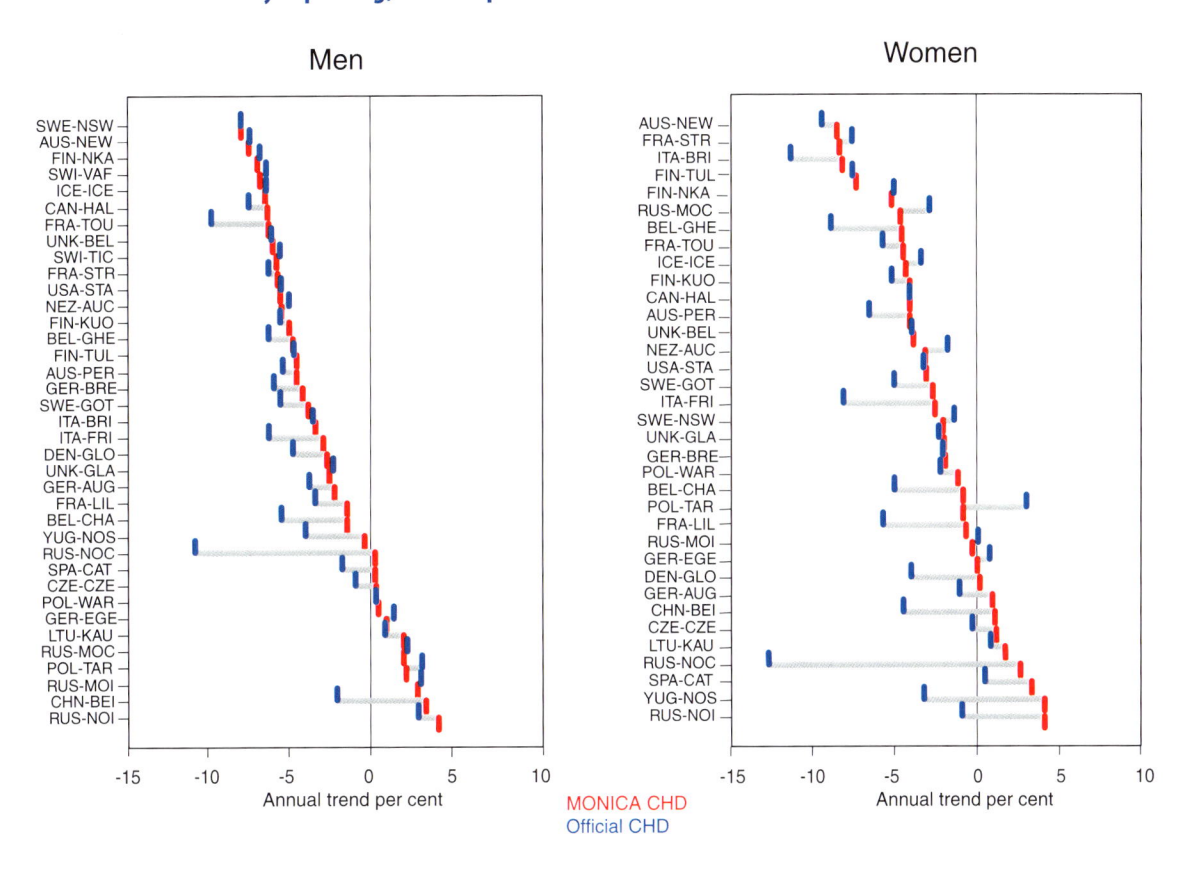

MONICA CHD
Official CHD

G21 Change in coronary end-points, by population, against coronary-event quality score

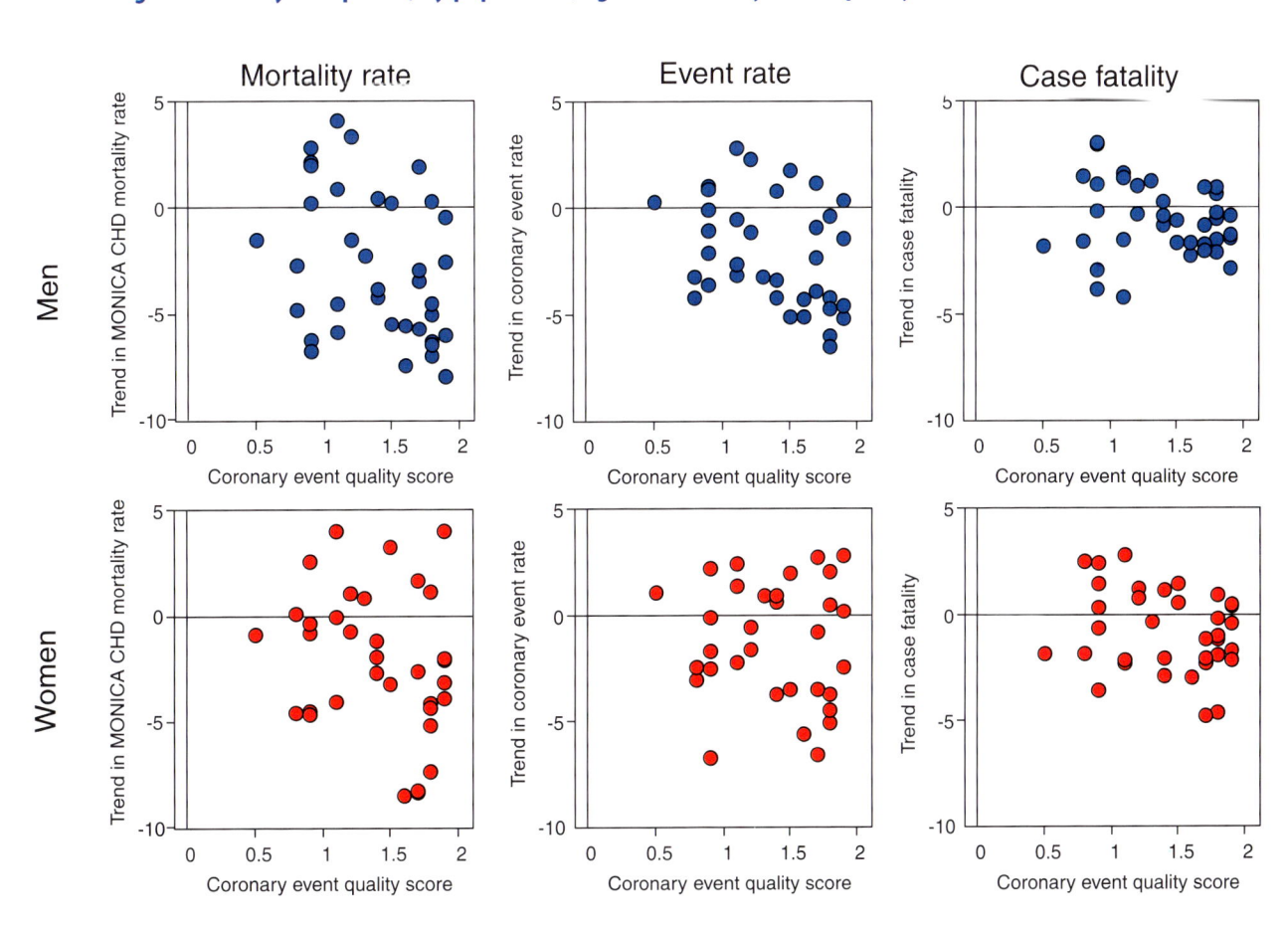

CORONARY EVENTS: INCIDENCE, CASE FATALITY AND MORTALITY RATES

Notes in italics are repeated to help random browsers—systematic readers should ignore them

G22

1. *Calculation of trends is explained in #37 Event rates, Case Fatality, and Trends.*

2. *Horizontal bars in G22 show the 95% confidence intervals around the estimated annual trend. The smaller the length of the bars the more precise the estimated trend. If the bars fail to cross the zero line the estimated trend is considered to deviate significantly from zero. Declining trends are shown to the left of the zero line, and increasing trends to the right.*

3. *Confidence intervals are wider for women than for men because there were fewer events. Greater year-on-year fluctuations through the random variation resulting from smaller numbers resulted in less precise estimates of trends. Wide confidence intervals are also found where the trend appears to deviate from log-linear.*

4. G22 shows that MONICA CHD mortality rates are decreasing in most populations in MONICA, although many individual trends do not deviate significantly from zero. The proportion of populations in which there is an increasing trend, about one-third, is similar in the two sexes.

G23

5. It can be shown mathematically that changes in MONICA CHD mortality rates are the sum of change in coronary-event rates and relative change in case fatality. G23 plots the ranking of change in CHD mortality rates (already shown in G22 with confidence intervals) but this time as the sum of the two contributing components. See #37 *Event Rates, Case Fatality, and Trends*. The overall pattern is for trends in coronary-event rates to explain about two-thirds of the change in CHD mortality rates. Change in case fatality (which is the complement of survival) explains the remaining third.

6. G23 was published in the first major MONICA collaborative paper of final results, MONICA Publication 36 (*2*). G23 shows a key finding of the MONICA Project—that during the mid-1980s to mid-1990s, the decline in mortality rates from coronary disease in MONICA populations resulted more from a falling incidence of disease than from better survival in those affected, although improvement in the latter was significant. Other studies have produced contradictory results, but none of them matched the number of populations and years involved in MONICA.

2. **Full references and summaries of MONICA Publications appear in #85/86.**

G22 Average annual change in MONICA coronary heart disease (CHD) mortality rates

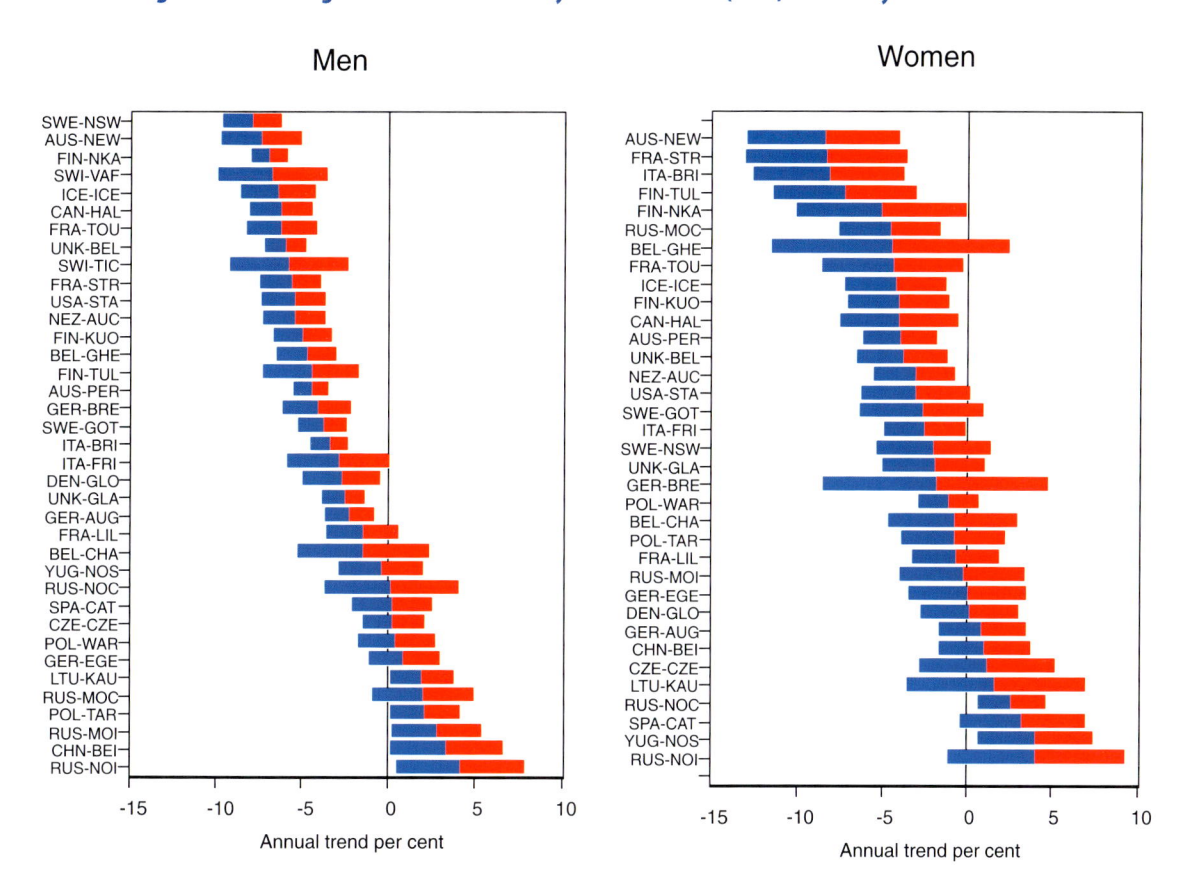

G23 Changes in MONICA coronary heart disease (CHD) mortality rates divided between changes in coronary-event rates and changes in case fatality

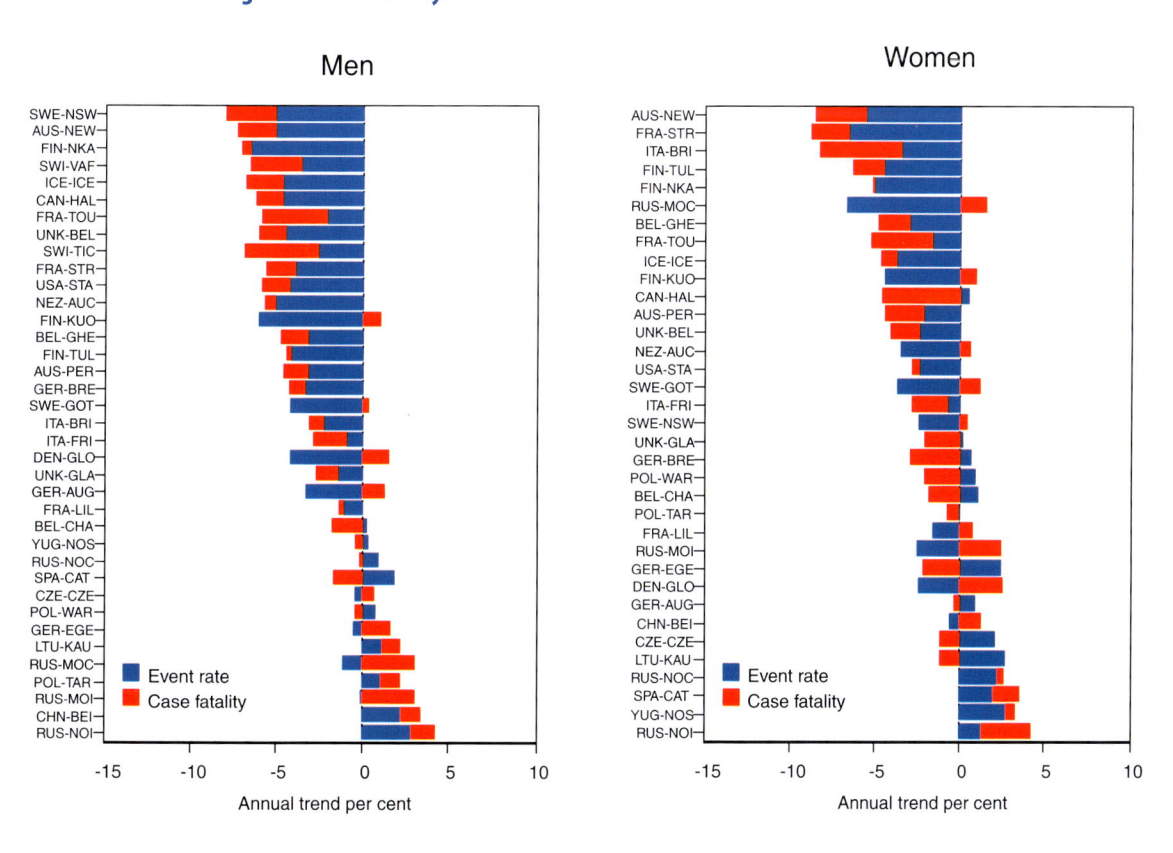

CORONARY EVENTS: INCIDENCE, CASE FATALITY AND MORTALITY RATES

1. G24 and G25 summarize the results shown for trends in mortality in G22, for trends in coronary-event rates in G15, and for trends in case fatality in G18. The Russia-Moscow (RUS-MOS, MOC/MOI, #74) and Russia-Novosibirsk (RUS-NOV, NOC/NOI, #75) populations were split in the previous graphs, but here they feature as single RUAs, with single spots.

2. A blue spot indicates a population RUA whose estimated trend and confidence intervals for that endpoint are to the left of the zero line in the relevant graph indicating a significant decline.

3. Red spots indicate population RUAs whose estimated trends and confidence intervals are to the right of the zero line, showing significant increases.

4. Black spots indicate populations where confidence intervals straddle the zero line, so that trends are not significantly different from zero, even though the trend estimate itself may be to one side of it, as is usually the case.

5. There are more black spots in women, G25, than in men, G24, because estimated trends are less precise, with greater confidence intervals, even though the estimated trends themselves are often as large as those in men.

6. The European and world maps suggest clustering of populations with similar trends in coronary endpoints, shown by the distribution of spots of the same colour.

G24 Spot maps of changes in coronary end-points in men

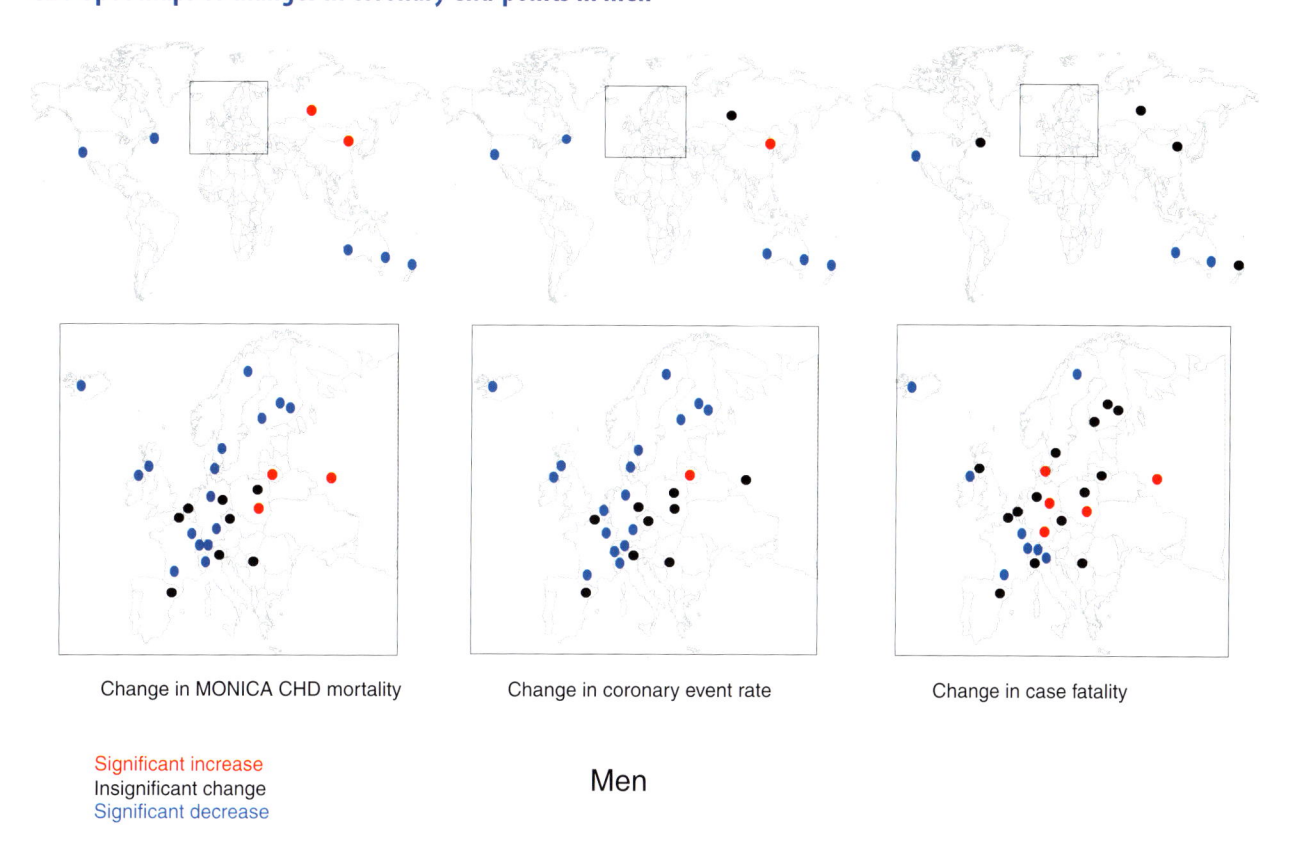

| Change in MONICA CHD mortality | Change in coronary event rate | Change in case fatality |

Significant increase
Insignificant change
Significant decrease

Men

G25 Spot maps of changes in coronary end-points in women

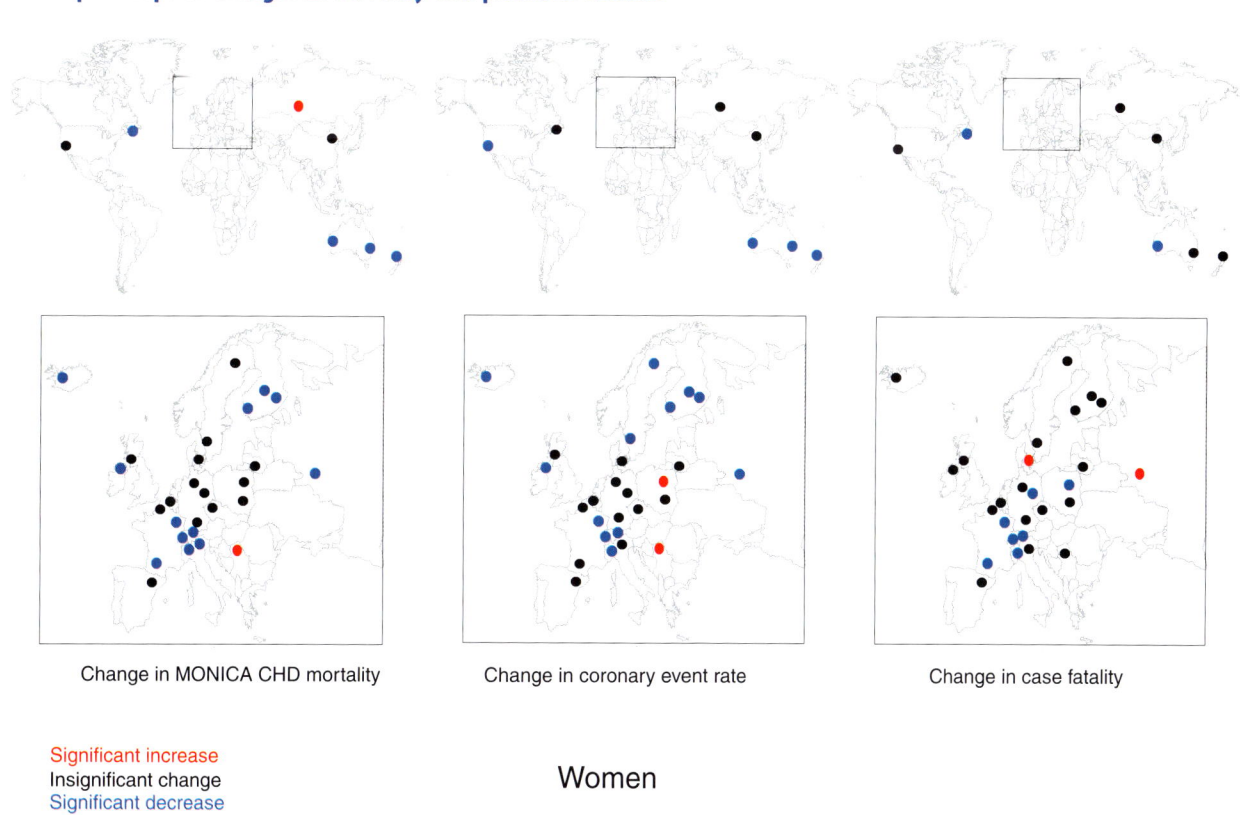

| Change in MONICA CHD mortality | Change in coronary event rate | Change in case fatality |

Significant increase
Insignificant change
Significant decrease

Women

CORONARY EVENTS: INCIDENCE, CASE FATALITY AND MORTALITY RATES

Strokes: incidence, case fatality and mortality rates

1. The specific calendar years included in the two three-year periods differed by population. They were identified in G9, and were not necessarily the same as those used for coronary-event registration.

2. Event rates are calculated using registration data for events, and demographic data for population denominators. See #17 *Demographic Data*, #37 *Event Rates, Case Fatality, and Trends*, MONICA Quality assessment of demographic data (*1*), MONICA Quality assessment of stroke registration data (*1*), MONICA Data Book of stroke events (*1*).

3. Results are age-standardized for the 35–64 age group, using the world standard population. See #39 *Age Standardization*.

4. Strokes are defined using MONICA diagnostic criteria. The criterion for stroke itself is the clinical presentation: symptoms, signs and clinical examination. Stroke does not have simple confirmatory tests equivalent to the electrocardiogram and cardiac enzyme tests used to define definite myocardial infarction, but there was increasing use of imaging techniques over the registration period, which were used to identify what sort of stroke had occurred. The cerebrovascular disease in stroke can be haemorrhage from an artery (subarachnoid haemorrhage, or intracerebal haemorrhage) or ischaemia from atheromatous arterial thrombosis leading to infarction or death of part of the brain (atherothrombotic cerebral infarction). See #26 and #27 *Registration of Stroke Events, Diagnosis of Stroke*, MONICA Manual Part IV, Section 2 (*1*), MONICA Publications 5, 18, 19, 21. (*2*).

G26

5. The x-axes of the graphs for stroke-event rates in G26 show the same maximum readings for men and women as their rates are not as different as those previously described for coronary-event rates. Comparison with the values in G12 and G13 shows that these stroke rates are intermediate between the coronary-event rates in men and women.

6. Confidence intervals, an index of precision, are not shown. Rates are averaged over three years. They are less precise than those for coronary events in men and more similar to those in women. See MONICA Data Book of stroke events, table 5.1 (*1*) for numbers of events from which these rates are derived.

7. These figures show: a four-fold variation in rates across populations in men and six-fold variation in women; on average higher event rates in men than women within populations; the changes in population event rates over time; and the effects of these changes on the population rankings.

G27

8. The lower graph, G27 is unreadable for some populations but deliberately inserted to show what the annual trend data look like before summarizing them statistically in terms of log-linear trends, shown in G29. (See the discussion for G14.) G27 gives an overall picture of the trends over time. Among the year-on-year fluctuations some populations seem to show a decline in rates but others little change. Yearly numbers and rates are available in the MONICA Data Book of stroke events, table 5.1 (*1*), from which this graph is derived.

1. **See Monograph CD-ROM or MONICA Website http://www.ktl.fi/monica/.**
2. **Full references and summaries of MONICA Publications appear in #85/86.**

G26 Overall stroke rates: first three years and final three years of registration

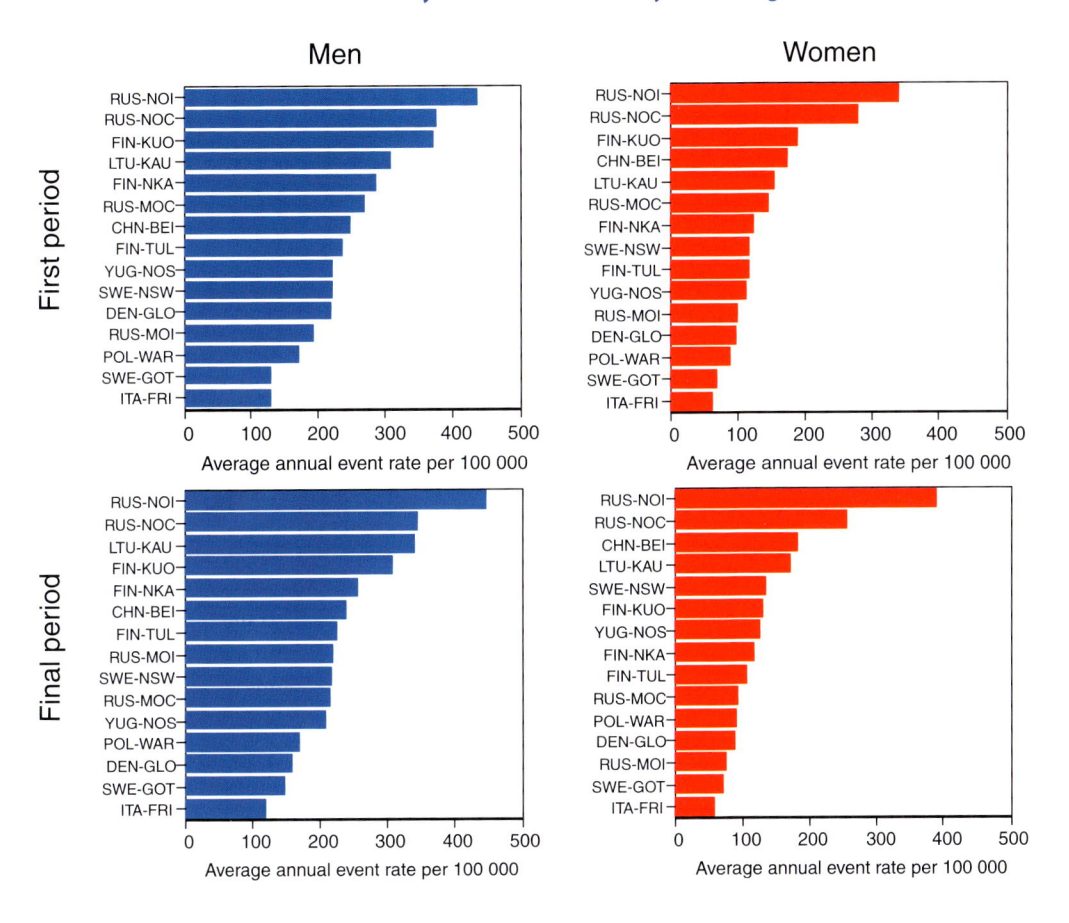

G27 Overall stroke rates by calendar year of registration

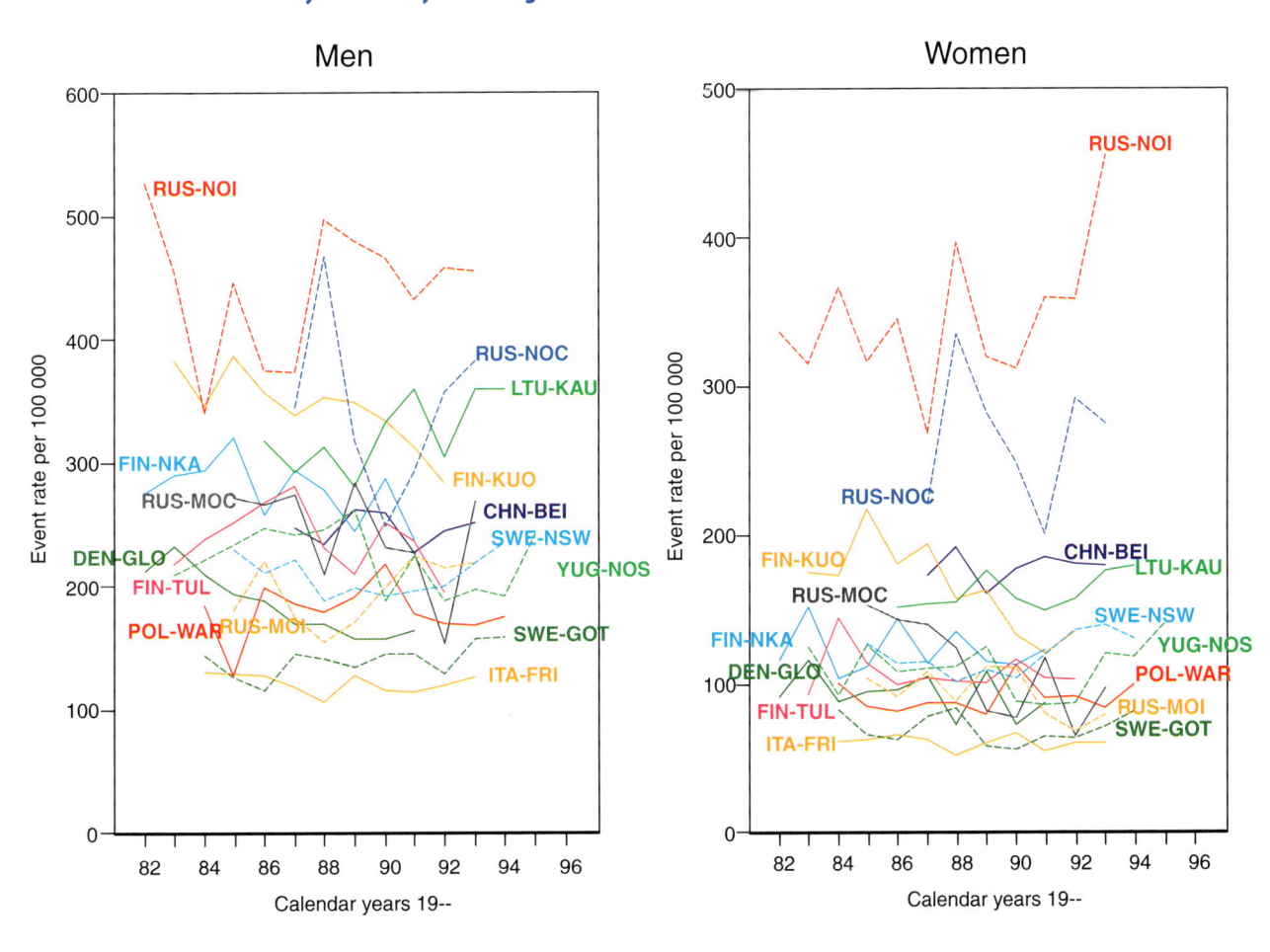

STROKES: INCIDENCE, CASE FATALITY AND MORTALITY RATES

G28

1. *The calendar years involved in each three-year period differed by population, and are identified in G9. They are not necessarily the same as those used in registration of coronary events.*

2. Case fatality is the proportion of events ending fatally within 28 days from onset. See #37 *Event Rates, Case Fatality and Trends,* MONICA Manual Part IV, Section 2 (*1*), MONICA Data Book of stroke events, table 8.1 (*1*), MONICA Publication 19 (*2*).

3. The denominator is all events and the scale is therefore the same for men and women. Case fatality does not involve population demographic data.

4. *Results are age-standardized for the 34–64 age group, using the weightings for case fatality in MONICA. See #39 Age Standardization.*

5. *The case fatality shown is for strokes defined using MONICA diagnostic criteria. See #26 and #27 Registration of Stroke Events, Diagnosis of Stroke, MONICA Publication 5 (2).*

6. Case fatality shown here may be higher than that derived from hospitalized stroke cases. Results include all stroke deaths. Some of these (particularly cerebral haemorrhage) may occur rapidly before admission to hospital, although this is less common than it is for coronary deaths. Clinical case series may start with admission to hospital, and follow-up may cease at hospital discharge, rather than the 28 days used here.

7. The complement of case fatality, survival, should relate to acute management of stroke. Differences in case fatality probably also reflect variations between populations in the distribution of stroke subtypes (haemorrhagic versus ischaemic strokes) and variations in stroke severity at onset. Case-mix also reflects the relative success of the MONICA registers in finding both fatal strokes and non-fatal stroke cases of all degrees of severity. This problem of case ascertainment of fatal versus non-fatal cases is probably greater in the delineation of specific stroke subtypes. (See G35, subarachnoid haemorrhage.)

8. Confidence intervals, an index of precision, are not given. Rates are averaged over three years. See MONICA Data Book of stroke events tables 5.1, 8.1 (*1*) for numbers. As in coronary events, the case fatality appears higher in women than in men. Within each sex there is a nearly four-fold variation across population RUAs in case fatality without any apparent modal values. (Compare with G16 and G17.) G28 illustrates the variation between populations, and between the two sexes, changes in case fatality over time and the resulting change in population rankings. There is some apparent geographical clustering of results.

G29

9. Horizontal bars in G29 show the 95% confidence intervals around estimated annual trends. The smaller the length of the bars, the more precise the estimated trend. If the bars fail to cross the zero line, the estimated trends are considered to deviate significantly from zero. Declining trends are shown to the left of the zero line, and increasing trends to the right.

10. Confidence intervals are similar for men and women because the number of events is similar. Examination of the year-on-year trend for Russia-Novosibirsk Control, RUS-NOC, see #75, in G27 helps to explain lack of precision in the estimated trend in G29.

11. G29 shows that incidence rates of stroke events are tending to decrease in around half the populations but some of the remainder show an increasing trend. The trends in case fatality show a fairly similar pattern. With a few exceptions estimated trends in individual populations are not large enough to be statistically significant, as they are small in relation to the width of the confidence interval. See MONICA Publications 19, 25, 45 (*2*), MONICA Data Book of stroke events table 5.1 (*1*). MONICA Publications on stroke, incorporating these results, were in preparation at the same time as this Monograph. (Note that some of the RUAs used in these differ slightly from those in this Monograph, so the results may disagree on particular populations—see note 6 on G1, G2.)

1. **See Monograph CD-ROM or MONICA Website http://www.ktl.fi/monica/.**
2. **Full references and summaries of MONICA Publications appear in #85/86.**

G28 Stroke case fatality: first three and final three years of registration

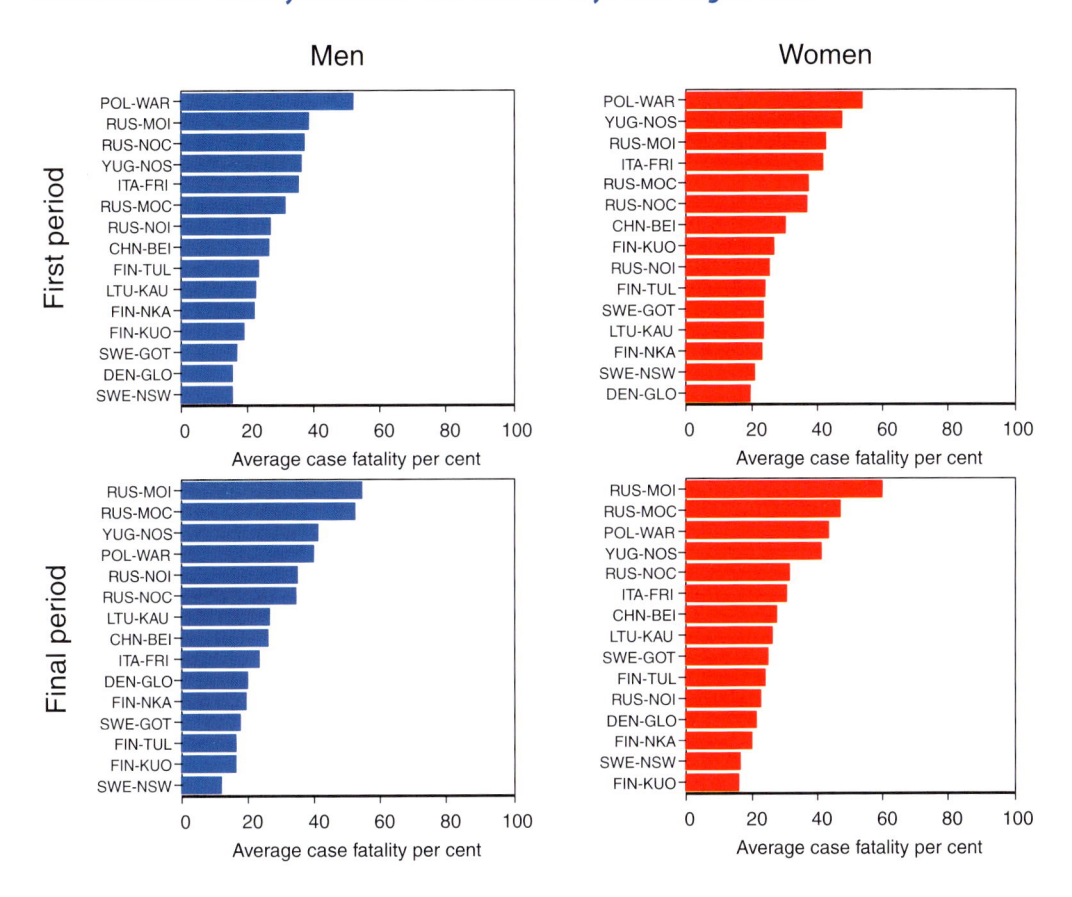

G29 Average annual change in stroke-event rates and in case fatality

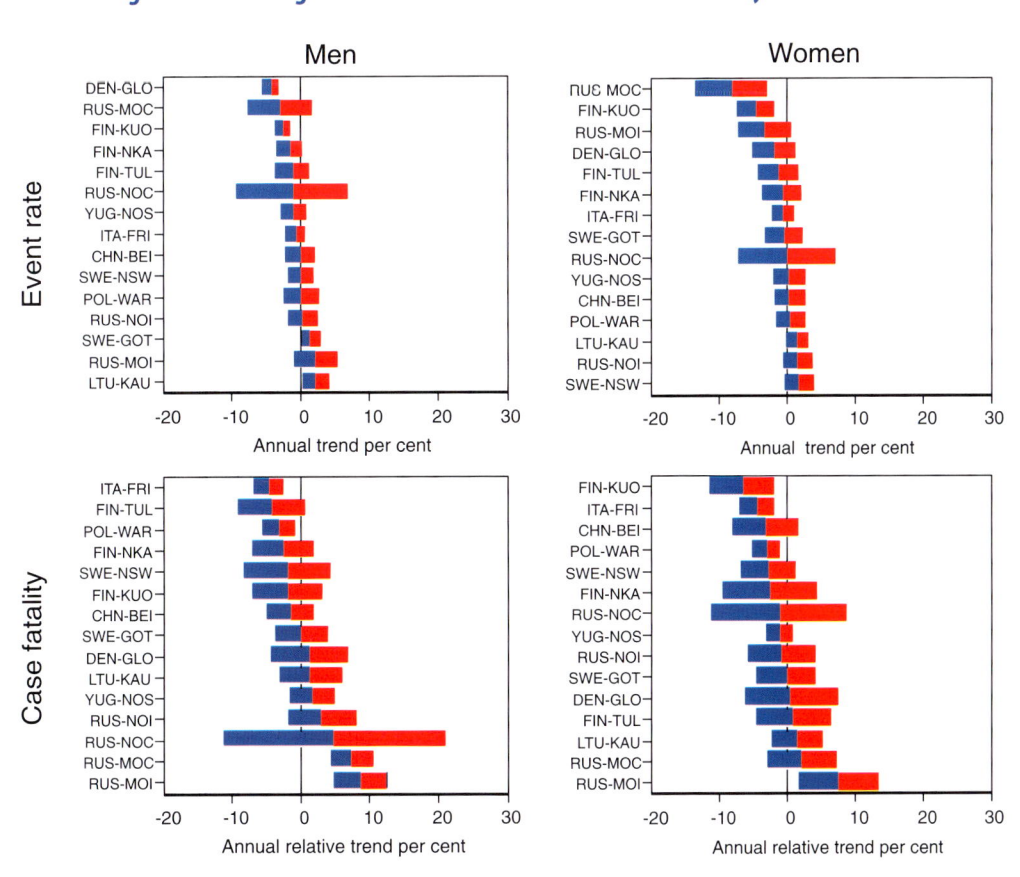

STROKES: INCIDENCE, CASE FATALITY AND MORTALITY RATES

Notes in italics are repeated to help random browsers—systematic readers should ignore them

G30

1. *The calendar years involved in each three-year period differed by population, and are identified in G9. Mortality rates are those for definite and unclassifiable strokes, excluding cases classified as not stroke. See #26 and #27 Registration of Stroke Events, Diagnosis of Stroke, #37 Event Rates, Case Fatality and Trends, MONICA Manual Part IV, Section 2 (1), MONICA Quality assessment of stroke registration data (1), MONICA Data Book of stroke events, table 7.1 (1).*

2. *Results are age-standardized for the 35–64 age group, using the world standard population. See #39 Age Standardization.*

3. Mortality rates in G30 show a four-to-one variation in both men and women, and higher mortality rates in men within each population RUA. There is a geographical gradient in stroke mortality from western and northern Europe towards the east.

4. MONICA stroke data involve fewer RUAs and fewer events, taking both sexes together, than do coronary events, along with different diagnostic and case-finding challenges. In contrast with the findings for coronary events discrepancies between the official and MONICA-validated stroke mortality rates occurred in only a small number of RUAs so we have not included stroke graphs equivalent to G19 and G20. The material for constructing such graphs is found in MONICA Quality assessment of stroke registration data, tables 7 and 8 (1).

G31

5. *Calculation of trends is explained in #37 Event Rates, Case Fatality and Trends. Horizontal bars in the mortality rate plots of G31 show the 95% confidence intervals around the estimated annual trend. The smaller the length of the bars, the more precise the estimated trend. If the bars fail to cross the zero line, the estimated trend is considered to deviate significantly from zero. Declining trends are shown to the left of the zero line and increasing trends to the right.*

6. The upper graph in G31 shows the change in stroke mortality rates. The tendency is towards a decline in the majority of populations in both sexes, but there is a cluster of populations in eastern Europe with increasing mortality.

7. It can be shown mathematically that changes in stroke mortality rates are the sum of changes in stroke-event rates and relative changes in case fatality. The lower graphs in G31 plot the ranking of change in stroke mortality (already shown in G31 with confidence intervals), but this time as the sum of the two contributing components. G31 suggests that change in case fatality is the major contributor to changing mortality rates from stroke, particularly when they are increasing, with a lesser contribution from decline in stroke-event rates.

8. These results contrast with those for coronary events (G22 and G23), which originated with the analyses for MONICA Publication 36 (2). Equivalent MONICA Publications for stroke were in preparation at the same time as this Monograph (1). (Note that some of the RUAs used in these differ slightly from those in this Monograph, so the results may disagree on particular populations. See note 6 on G1, G2.) It was the decline in event rates that accounted for two-thirds of the decline in mortality from coronary heart disease. See G23. The confidence intervals in G29 and G31 are wide in relation to the estimated trends, particularly those for case fatality. Calculation of the relative contribution of trends in event rates, and in case fatality, to declining stroke mortality rates may be more subject to random error or 'noise' than is the case for coronary events.

1. **See Monograph CD-ROM or MONICA Website http://www.ktl.fi/monica/.**
2. **Full references and summaries of MONICA Publications appear in #85/86.**

G30 Stroke mortality rates: first three years and final three years of registration

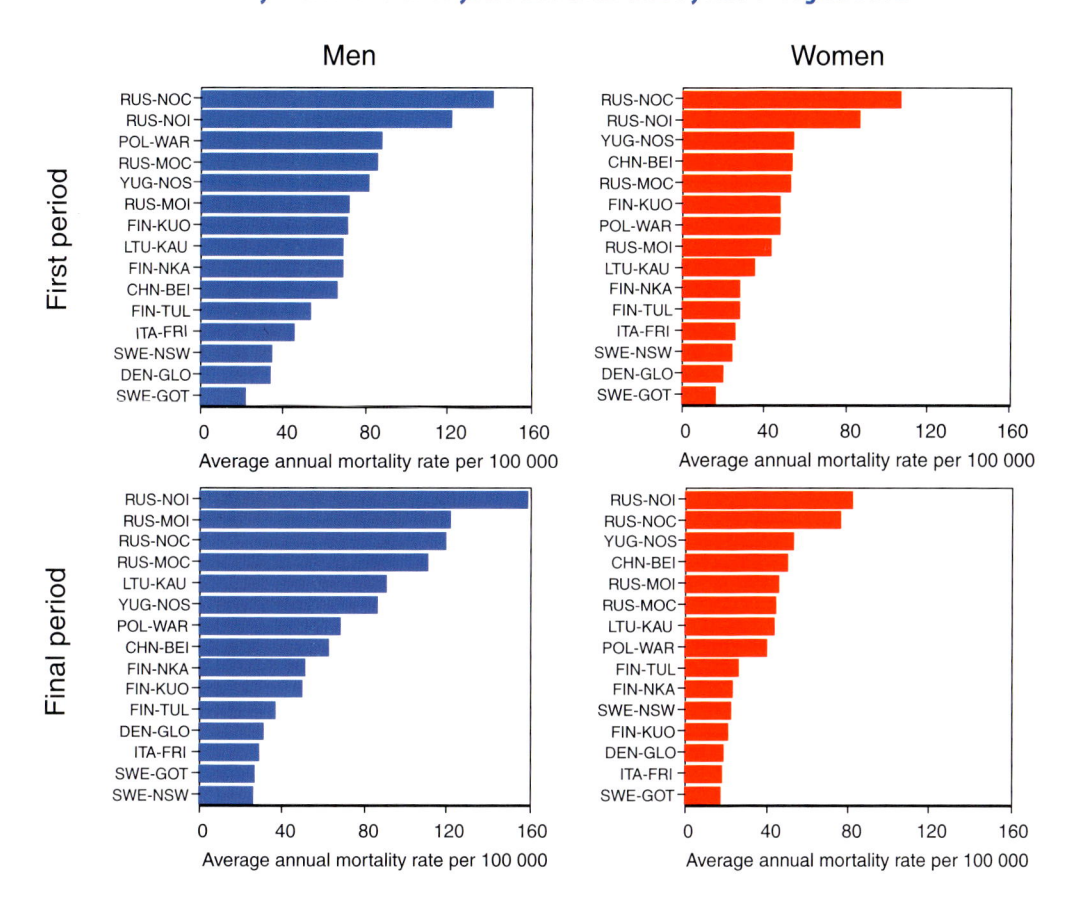

G31 Changes in stroke mortality rates divided between changes in stroke-event rates and changes in case fatality

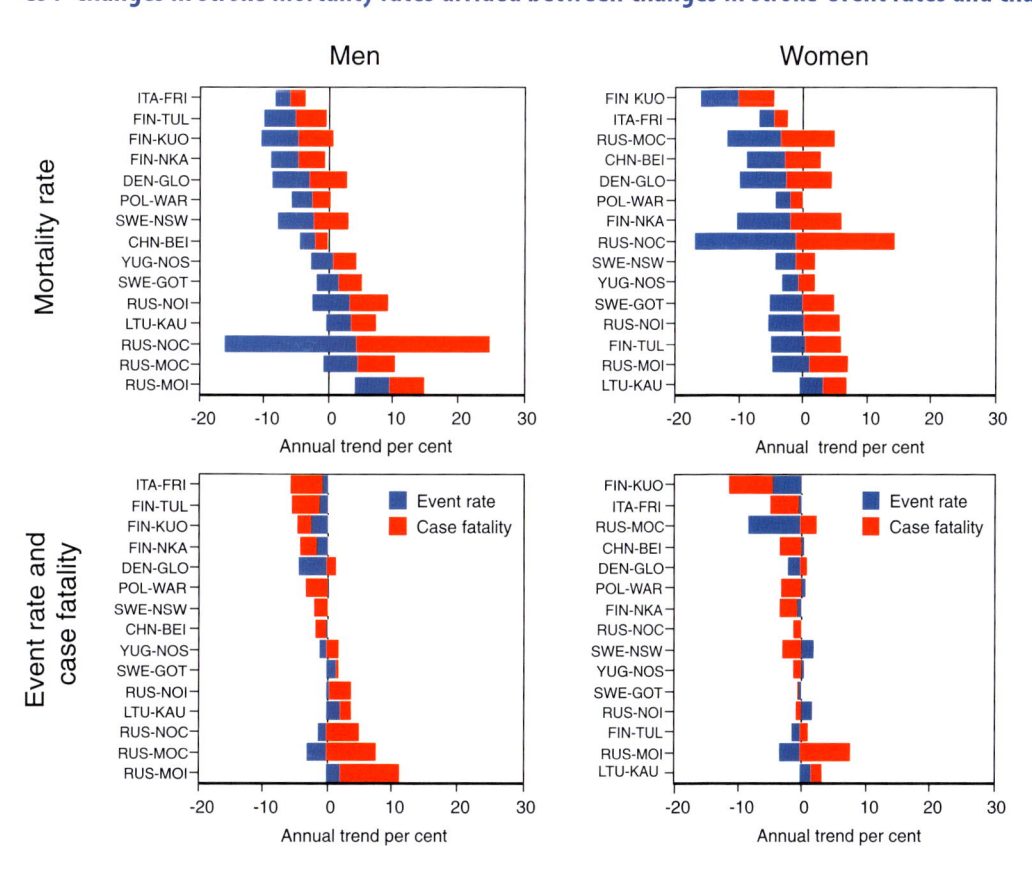

STROKES: INCIDENCE, CASE FATALITY AND MORTALITY RATES

1. The six spot maps, in G32 and G33 are derived directly from the data already shown on trends in stroke-event rates and on trends in case fatality in G29, and on trends in mortality rates in G31. However, the two Moscow population RUAs, and two Novosibirsk RUAs, are combined to produce one RUA for each city in these maps.

2. Blue spots indicate populations whose estimated trend for that end-point and its confidence intervals are to the left of the zero line in G29 or G31 indicating a significant decline.

3. Red spots indicate populations whose estimated trend for that end-point and its confidence intervals are to the right of the zero line in G29 or G31 indicating a significant increase.

4. Black spots indicate populations where confidence intervals straddle the zero line, so the estimated trend does not deviate significantly from zero, even though the trend estimate may be to one side of it, as is usually the case.

5. Fifty-six of the seventy-eight spots in G32 and G33 are black, so most individual estimates of trends failed to deviate significantly from zero. In most populations the number of stroke events being recorded each year in the below 65-year age group was modest in relation to the trends that were being investigated. Stroke numbers were smaller than those for coronary events in men, for which the original MONICA power calculations had been done. Some MONICA centres extended their age-range for stroke to 74, instead of 64, increasing the number of registrations and making analysis of trends more precise. This happened in 8 of the 15 RUAs. Results are not shown here. See MONICA Quality assessment for stroke event registration data (*1*) and MONICA Data Book of stroke events (*1*).

6. Perhaps because there were fewer stroke populations than there were for coronary events and less precision in estimating trends, geographical clustering of the coloured spots seems less obvious. Contrast G32, G33 with G24, G25. There is more of a geographical pattern to be seen in G29 and G31 if tendencies to increasing and decreasing trends are considered. For consistency with other spot maps in this Monograph, G32 and G33 feature only results that reach statistical significance.

1. **See Monograph CD-ROM or MONICA Website http://www.ktl.fi/monica/.**
2. **Full references and summaries of MONICA Publications appear in #85/86.**

G32 Spot maps of changes in stroke end-points in men

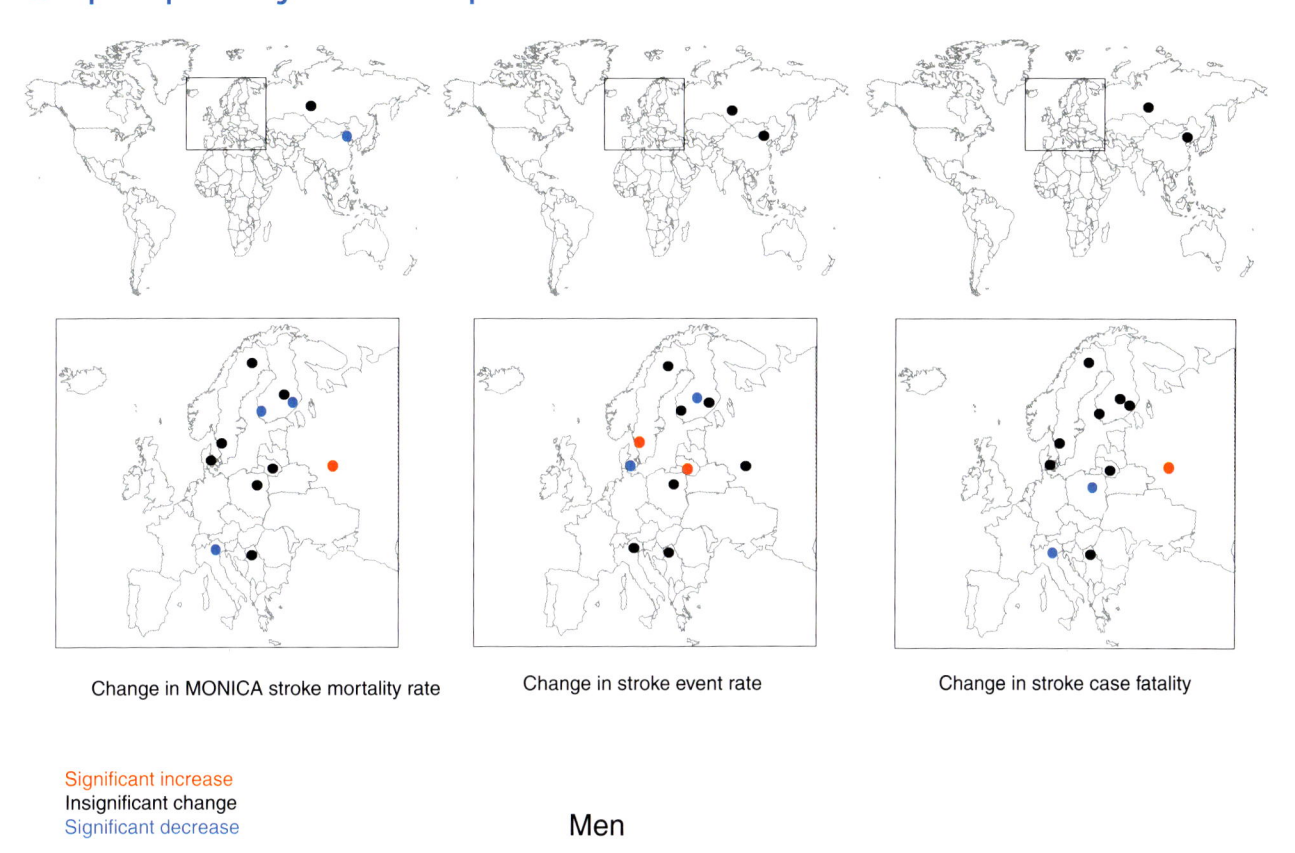

Change in MONICA stroke mortality rate

Change in stroke event rate

Change in stroke case fatality

Significant increase
Insignificant change
Significant decrease

Men

G33 Spot maps of changes in stroke end-points in women

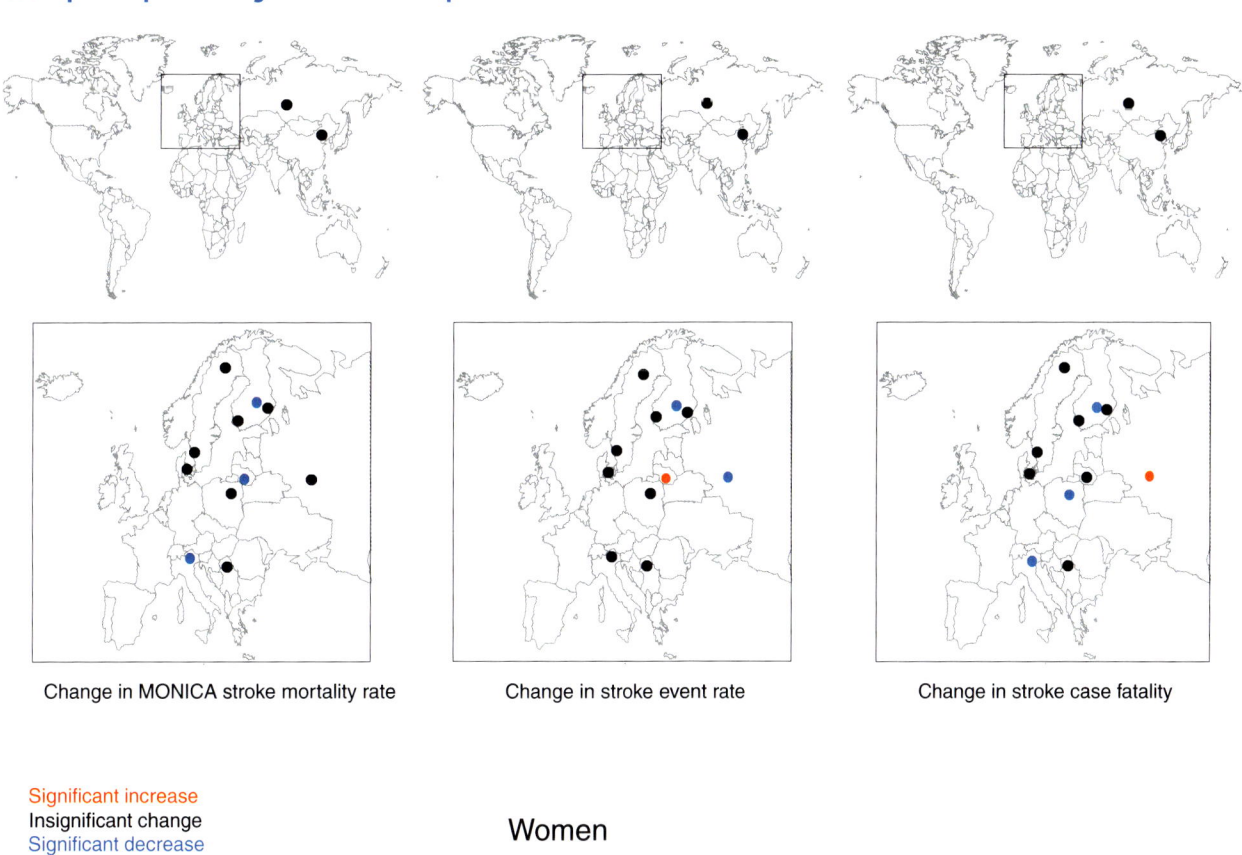

Change in MONICA stroke mortality rate

Change in stroke event rate

Change in stroke case fatality

Significant increase
Insignificant change
Significant decrease

Women

STROKES: INCIDENCE, CASE FATALITY AND MORTALITY RATES

G34

1. A recurrent concern in MONICA analyses is whether extreme results, or indeed the general pattern of results, could be influenced by variations in the quality of data. Quality assessment was rigorous. The results are explicit, are published, and are taken into consideration in the major analyses. See MONICA Quality assessment of stroke event registration data (*1*), MONICA Quality assessment of demographic data (*1*).

2. In G34 the relation between the stroke end-points, and the quality score allocated to each population for its stroke data, may not be random. Patterns are not consistent across the sexes. Any weak relation that there is can be shown in formal calculations not to be strong enough to suggest that study results are being seriously compromised or confounded by the quality of items that have been measured.

3. The document explaining the derivation of the stroke-event quality score is published on the MONICA Website as Stroke Event Trend Quality Score for the WHO MONICA Project (*1*).

G35

4. Subarachnoid haemorrhage is a specific variety of stroke in which there is bleeding into the cerebro-spinal fluid from a congenital weakness in a middle-sized artery at the base of the brain. Confirmation depends upon specific diagnostic tests. Subarachnoid haemorrhage has a younger age-distribution than other subtypes of stroke. It is very commonly considered for neurosurgical treatment to prevent recurrence. See #26 and #27 *Registration of Stroke Events, Diagnosis of Stroke*, MONICA Manual Part IV, Section 2 (*1*), MONICA Data Book of stroke events tables 4.3, 4.4 (*1*), MONICA Publication 40 (*2*).

5. Numbers of cases are small compared with stroke overall. Unlike other graphs in this Monograph, results in G35 are averaged over the whole registration period for the population concerned. Despite this, the estimated rates are small (approximately 10% of overall stroke rates) and cannot be very precise.

6. With the need for greater investigational and diagnostic involvement, some stroke registers had greater problems than others in satisfying MONICA criteria for reliably identifying fatal and non-fatal stroke subtypes such as subarachnoid haemorrhage. Problems of data quality have led to results from fewer population RUAs featuring in G35 than for the other overall stroke results.

7. Since autopsy is not performed in China, the low case fatality there may be from failure to identify all fatal cases of subarachnoid haemorrhage. Through relatively small numbers, some of the other results will have limited precision. Despite these limitations, this is a unique set of data on international variation in frequency and outcome of subarachnoid haemorrhage. See MONICA Publication 40 (*2*) whose subject is subarachnoid haemorrhage in MONICA. In that paper the choice of population RUAs is slightly different from that in G35. Some RUAs shown in the latter have been amalgamated but the paper included data from the limited period of stroke registration in Germany-East Germany, GER-EGE, see #65.

1. **See Monograph CD-ROM or MONICA Website http://www.ktl.fi/monica/.**
2. **Full references and summaries of MONICA Publications appear in #85/86.**

G34 Change in stroke end-points, by population, against stroke-event quality scores

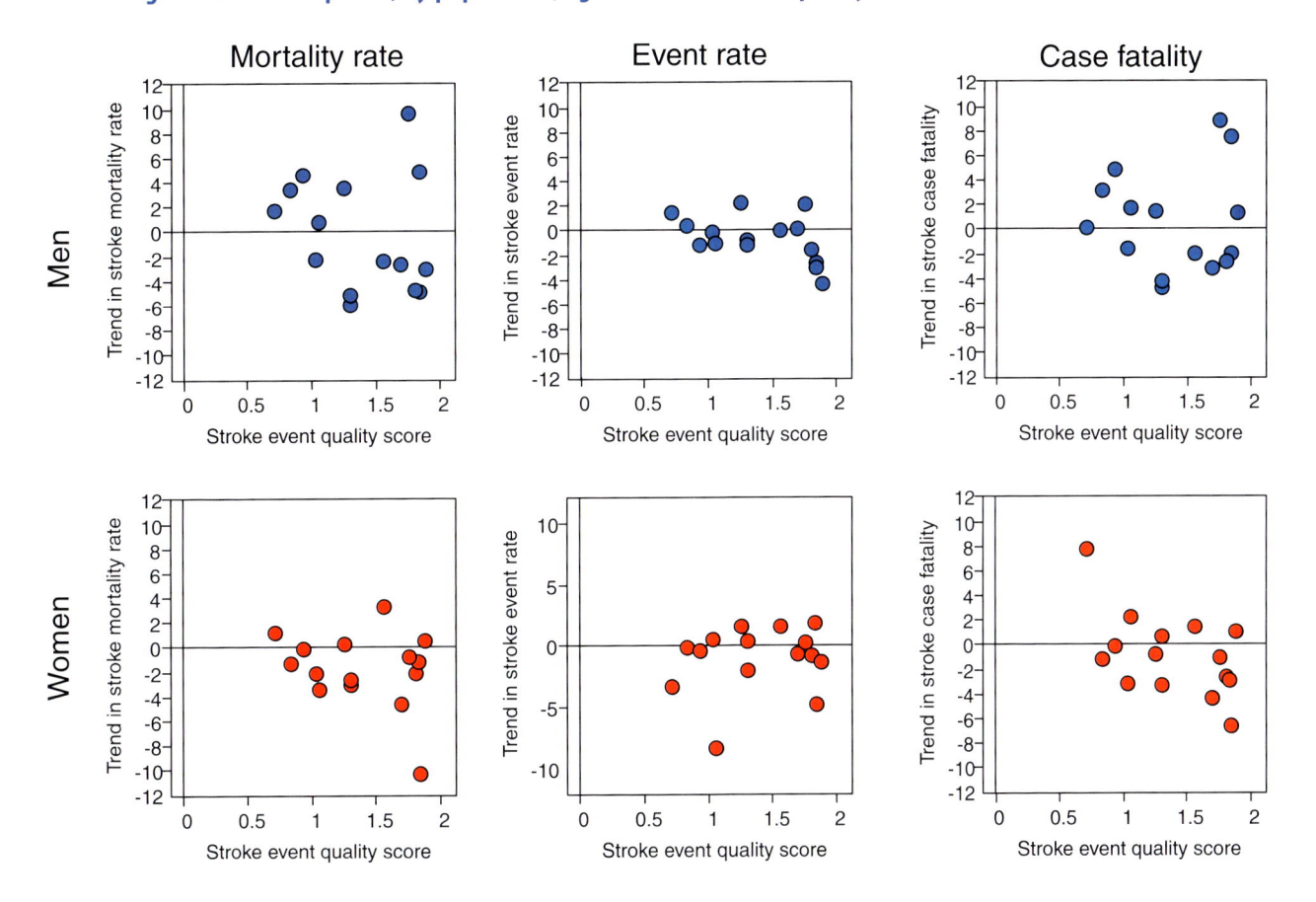

G35 Event rates and case fatality: subarachnoid haemorrhage

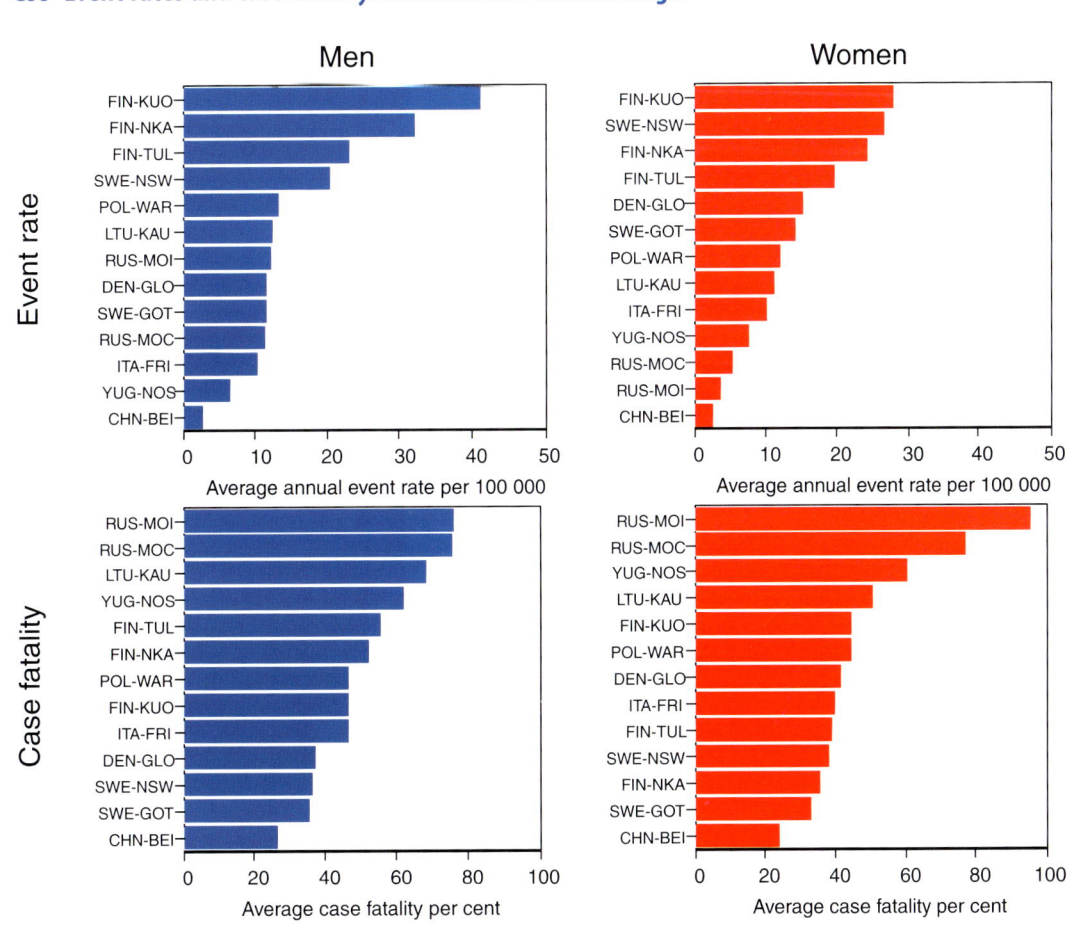

STROKES: INCIDENCE, CASE FATALITY AND MORTALITY RATES

Risk factors: daily cigarette smoking

1. The timing of the initial and final surveys differed by population. These surveys were usually eight to ten years apart but the interval could be as little as six years. The calendar years and months varied. See G10 and MONICA Quality assessment of age, date of examination and survey periods (*1*).

2. Results are shown as the estimated prevalence, or percentage, of daily cigarette smokers in the 34–65 age group. The results are age-standardized to minimize any effect of differing age structures on the apparent findings. See #38 *Population Prevalence and Trends*, #39 *Age Standardization*, #31 *Smoking*.

3. The graphs characterize men and women over a thirty-year age band in each survey for each population with a single value, but levels and trends vary with age. Age-specific data are available in the MONICA Data Book of population surveys, table 6.4.3 (*1*), and early results in MONICA Publication 11 (*2*).

4. Survey results could be influenced by failure to participate by some of those selected for the survey. The issue is complex, as different methods of recruitment and sampling were used in different populations. There is more than one definition of response rates. See #28 *Sampling*, #29 *Recruitment and Response Rates*, MONICA Quality assessment of participation rates, sampling frames and fractions (*1*).

5. A daily cigarette smoker was someone who usually smoked at least one cigarette a day. Comparisons of smoking prevalence between populations are not as simple as they may appear. In addition to the hard core of daily cigarette smokers, easy to categorize, there are variable numbers of additional smokers who are less easy to classify, such as weekend or social smokers, pipe and cigar smokers. These groups create problems in standardizing the assessment of the prevalence of smoking. See #31 *Smoking*, MONICA Quality assessment of data on smoking (*1*), MONICA Manual Part III, Section 1 (*1*).

6. Smoking is the only classical risk factor ascertained by questionnaire. Because of the potential for concealment of smoking by 'deceivers' biochemical validation was attempted in MONICA using serum thiocyanate. See MONICA Manual Part III, Section 3 (*1*). This was found to be neither sensitive nor specific, and it was abandoned. Some centres measured expired-air-carbon-monoxide and/or serum cotinine on all or some of their participants. However it is questionnaire results that are used in these analyses. See MONICA Quality assessment of data on smoking (*1*).

7. The scales for men and women are the same. Smoking prevalence was generally higher in men than in women in the same population, with a few exceptions such as United Kingdom-Glasgow, UNK-GLA, see #81, where findings in the two sexes were similar. Some populations showed a large disparity in their ranking for men and women. This is true of the two Russia-Novosibirsk populations in the initial survey, RUS-NOC, RUS-NOI, see #75, and China-Beijing, CHN-BEI, see #55, in the final survey.

8. Data for these graphs are found in the MONICA Data Book of population surveys, table 6.4.3 (*1*). The Data book and the MONICA Quality assessment of data on smoking (*1*) contain tables describing items of smoking behaviour not shown here, such as the prevalence of never smokers and former or ex-smokers, numbers of cigarettes smoked, and frequency of other varieties of tobacco smoking. See the MONICA Data Book of population surveys, tables 6.4.2–6.4.6 (*1*).

1. **See Monograph CD-ROM or MONICA Website http://www.ktl.fi/monica/.**
2. **Full references and summaries of MONICA Publications appear in #85/86.**

G36 Prevalence of daily cigarette smokers in the initial risk-factor survey

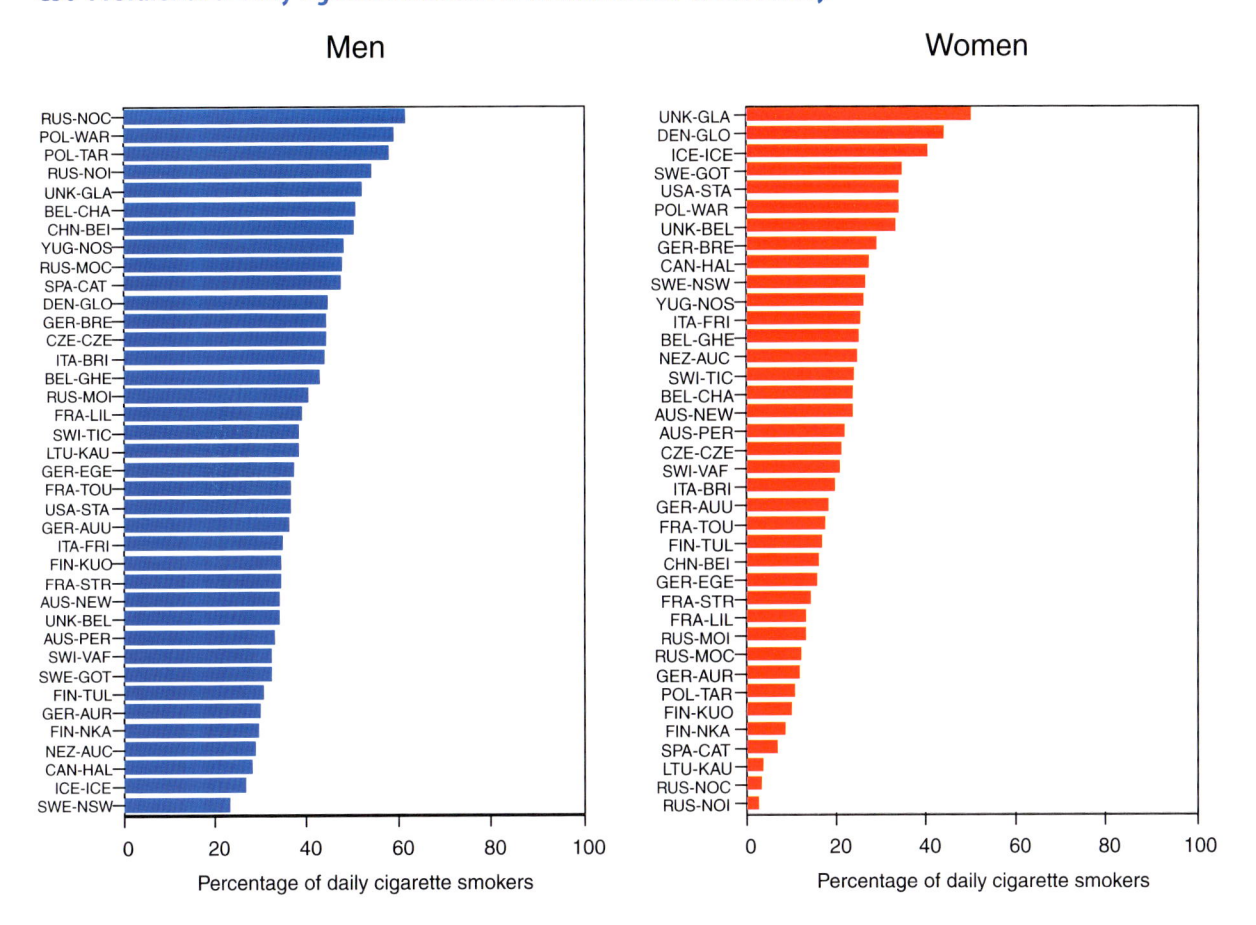

G37 Prevalence of daily cigarette smokers in the final risk-factor survey

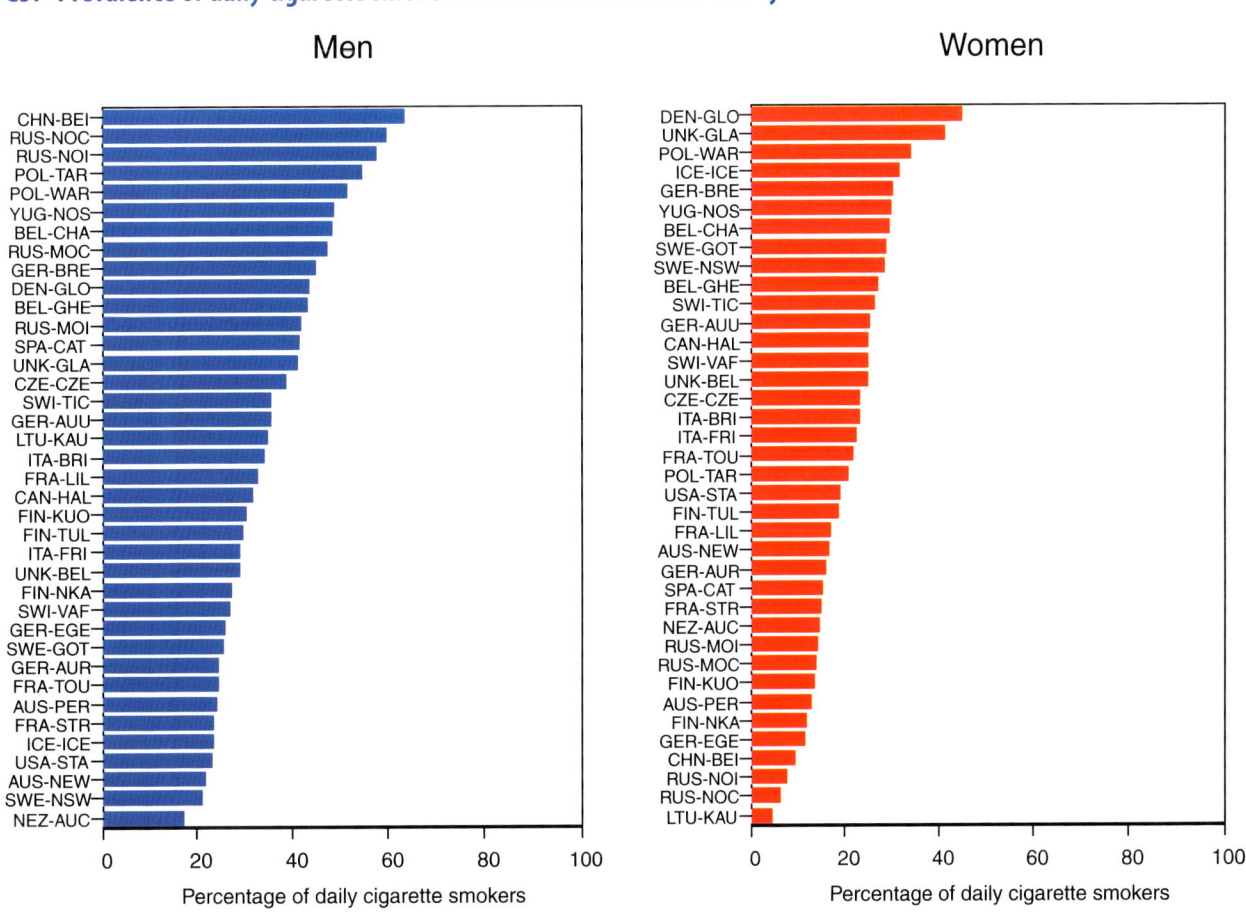

RISK FACTORS: DAILY CIGARETTE SMOKING

G38

1. Calculation of trends is explained in #38 *Population Prevalence and Trends*.

2. The initial and final surveys did not take place exactly ten years apart. G38 incorporates corrections to standardize the differences, as if they were being measured across ten years.

3. Horizontal bars in G38 show the 95% confidence intervals around the estimated 10-year trend. The smaller the length of the bars the more precise the estimated trend. If the bars fail to cross the zero line the estimated trend is considered to deviate significantly from zero. Declining trends are shown to the left of the zero line, and increasing trends to the right.

4. Confidence intervals are similar for men and women; the population surveys sampled them in similar numbers.

5. G38 shows different trends in smoking between men and women in the different populations. The majority of male populations show a decrease in smoking, so that the tendency is to the left of zero in 32 populations and towards an increase, right of the zero line in five. In women, it is a minority of populations that show a decrease in smoking. Twelve are to the left of zero and 25 are to the right. Results varied in different age groups. What is shown here is an age-standardized summary statistic. Age-specific data are available in the MONICA Data Book of population surveys, table 6.4.4 (*1*).

G39

6. G39 is a spot map showing the geographical distribution of the results shown in G38. Half or more of the confidence intervals in G38 include zero. The populations concerned are marked by black spots. Those with a significant decrease in smoking levels are shown with blue spots, while a significant increase is shown with a red spot.

7. G39 shows little difference between the sexes outside Europe. Within Europe however, there are no male populations showing a significant increase in smoking and many show a significant decrease. In women increases and decreases are almost evenly balanced.

8. It is unlikely that smoking data of poor quality had a significant effect on overall MONICA results. G56 (see later) shows acceptable quality scores for most populations and little correlation in the scatter plot between quality scores of the smoking data and the apparent trends in smoking. See MONICA Quality assessment of data on smoking (*1*).

9. Trends in cigarette smoking in the MONICA populations are the subject of MONICA Publications 34 and 42 (*2*); early cross-sectional data are found in MONICA Publication 11 (*2*).

1. See Monograph CD-ROM or MONICA Website http://www.ktl.fi/monica/.
2. **Full references and summaries of MONICA Publications appear in #85/86.**

G38 Ten-year change in prevalence of daily cigarettes smokers

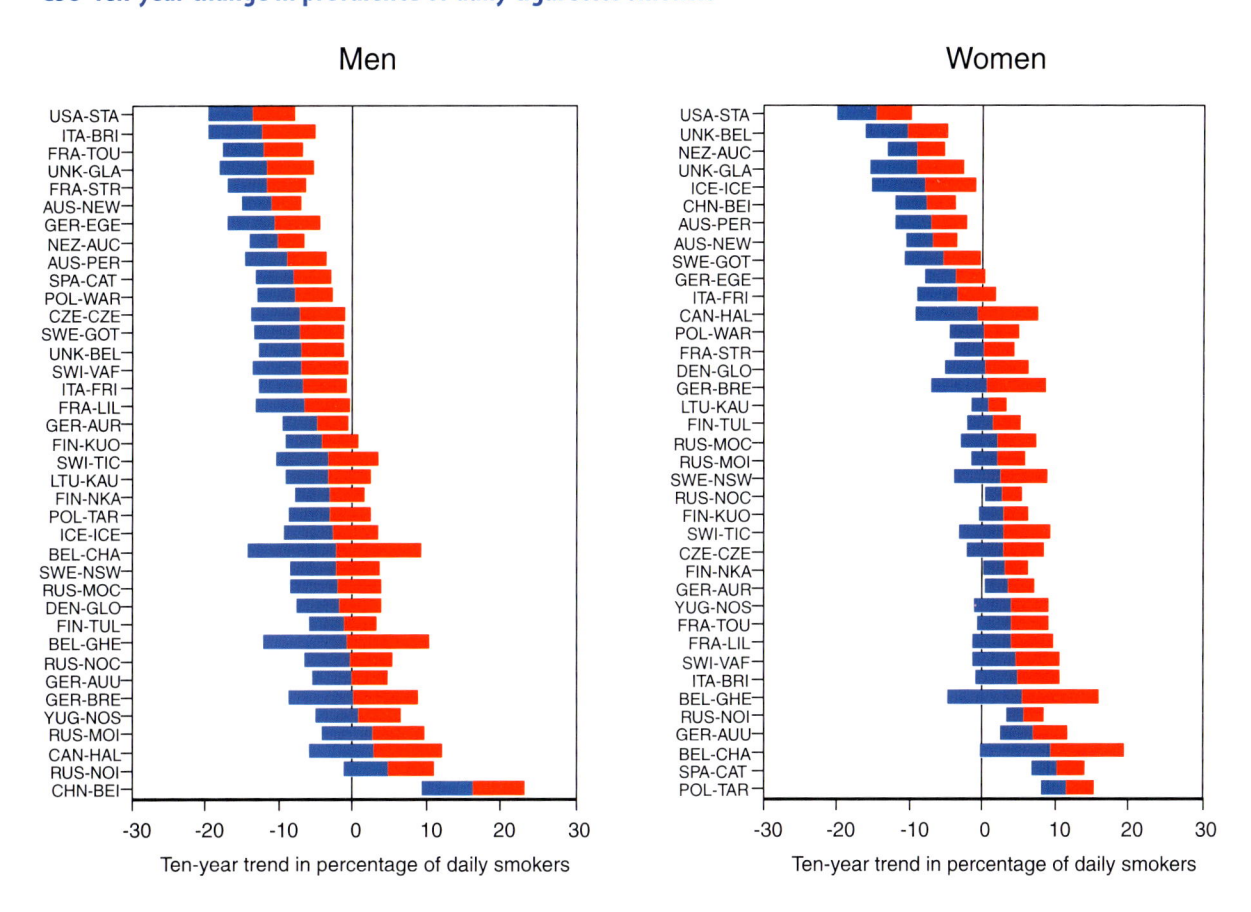

Men | Women

Ten-year trend in percentage of daily smokers

G39 Spot maps of population changes in prevalence of daily cigarette smoking

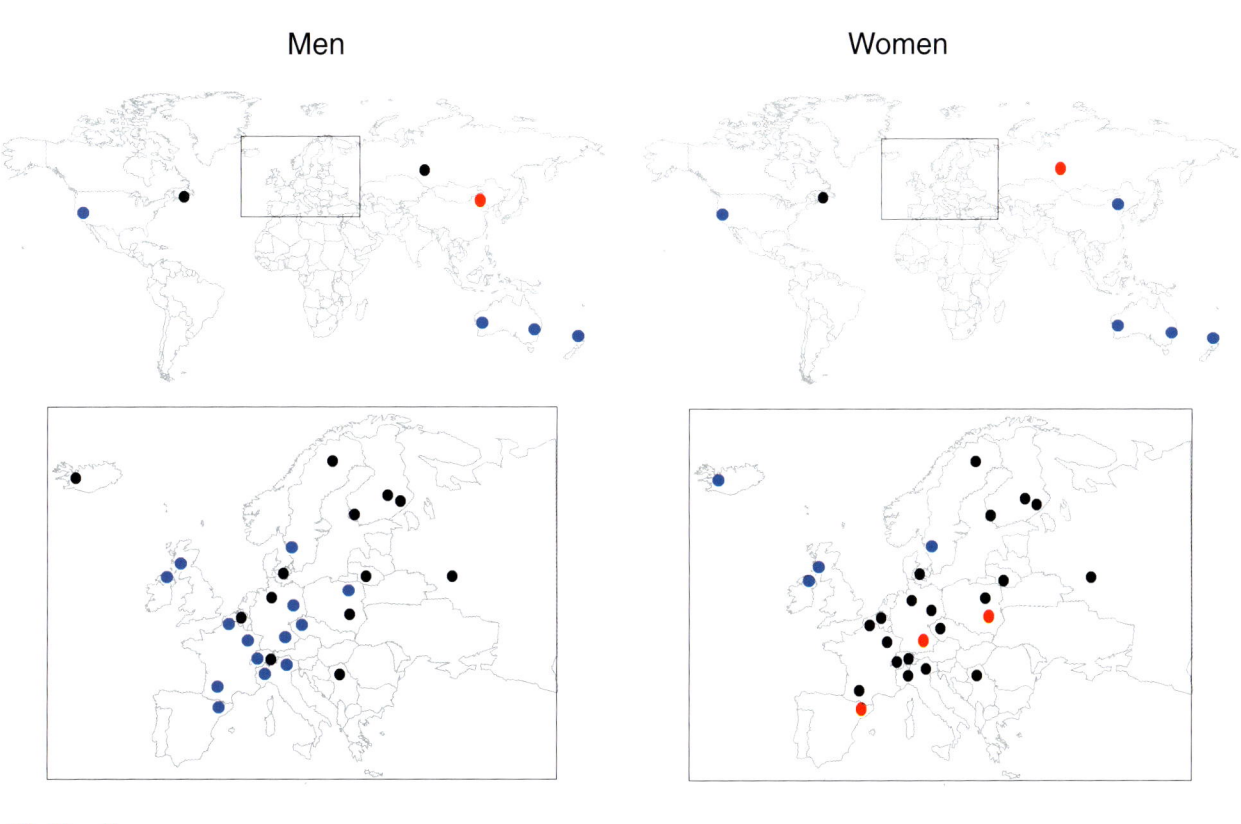

Men | Women

Significant increase
Insignificant change
Significant decrease

RISK FACTORS: DAILY CIGARETTE SMOKING

Risk factors: systolic blood pressure

Notes in italics are repeated to help random browsers—systematic readers should ignore them

1. *The timing of the initial and final surveys differed by population. These surveys were usually eight to ten years apart but the interval could be as little as six years. The calendar years and months varied. See G10 and MONICA Quality assessment of age, date of examination and survey periods (1).*

2. Results are shown as the mean systolic blood pressure in millimetres of mercury, mmHg, for the 35–64 age group. *The results are age-standardized to minimize any effect of differing age structures on the apparent findings. See #38 Population Prevalence and Trends, #39 Age Standardization.*

3. *The graphs characterize men and women over a thirty-year age band in each survey for each population with a single value, but levels and trends vary with age.* Age-specific data are published in the MONICA Data Book of population surveys, table 6.1.2 (*1*), and early results in MONICA Publication 11 (*2*).

4. *Survey results could be influenced by failure to participate by some of those selected for the survey. The issue is complex. Different methods of recruitment and sampling were used in different populations. There is more than one definition of response rates. See #28 Sampling, #29 Recruitment and Response Rates, MONICA Quality assessment of participation rates, sampling frames and fractions (1).*

5. To convert to and from SI Units: 100 mmHg = 13.3 kilopascal (kPa); 10 kPa = 75 mmHg.

6. In a reading such as 156/82, the systolic blood pressure is the first, higher reading—156, and the second lower one—82, is the diastolic blood pressure. It was formerly believed that the diastolic blood pressure was of greater medical significance, and it was the target of medical intervention. Measurement of the systolic blood pressure is easier to standardize; it is now considered to be of equal or greater significance than diastolic blood pressure as a risk factor predicting cardiovascular disease; and it is increasingly the target of treatment. See #32 Blood pressure.

7. In the MONICA population surveys blood pressure was measured twice with the subject at rest, and the average of the two readings was used. See MONICA Manual Part III, Section 1 (*1*), MONICA Quality assessment of data on blood pressure (*1*).

8. Real differences in average blood pressure in populations over time and space are important to epidemiologists, but they could be spuriously created by bad measurement techniques. Readings are ephemeral and cannot be stored for re-measurement like blood specimens. Some centres used simple mercury sphygmomanometers and others more complex 'random-zero' mercury sphygmomanometers, designed to reduce observer bias. Extensive training, quality control and monitoring of performance were done to encourage standardized recording. See #32 *Blood Pressure*, MONICA Quality assessment of data on blood pressure (*1*). MONICA Publications 11, 14, 20, 31 (*2*).

9. The scale for men and women is the same, as is the range across populations of average systolic blood pressure. The latter varied by about 25 mmHg in the initial survey, and rather less in the final survey, where pressures appear more uniform. Rankings appear similar in the two sexes.

10. These graphs are based on the MONICA Data Book of population surveys, table 6.1.2 (*1*). The Data Book contains information on many more blood pressure items, such as diastolic blood pressure, blood pressure categories, and identification and treatment of hypertension in different populations. See MONICA Quality assessment of data on hypertension control (*1*), MONICA Data Book of population surveys, tables 6.1.2–6.1.6 (*1*).

11. The Data book also contains age-specific data (as did MONICA Publication 11) (*2*). These show that in many populations the blood pressure in women aged 35–44 is lower than that in men of the same age, but at 55–64 it is higher. The age-standardized readings shown here conceal this difference in age-gradients.

1. **See Monograph CD-ROM or MONICA Website http://www.ktl.fi/monica/.**
2. **Full references and summaries of MONICA Publications appear in #85/86.**

G40 Average systolic blood pressure in the initial risk-factor survey

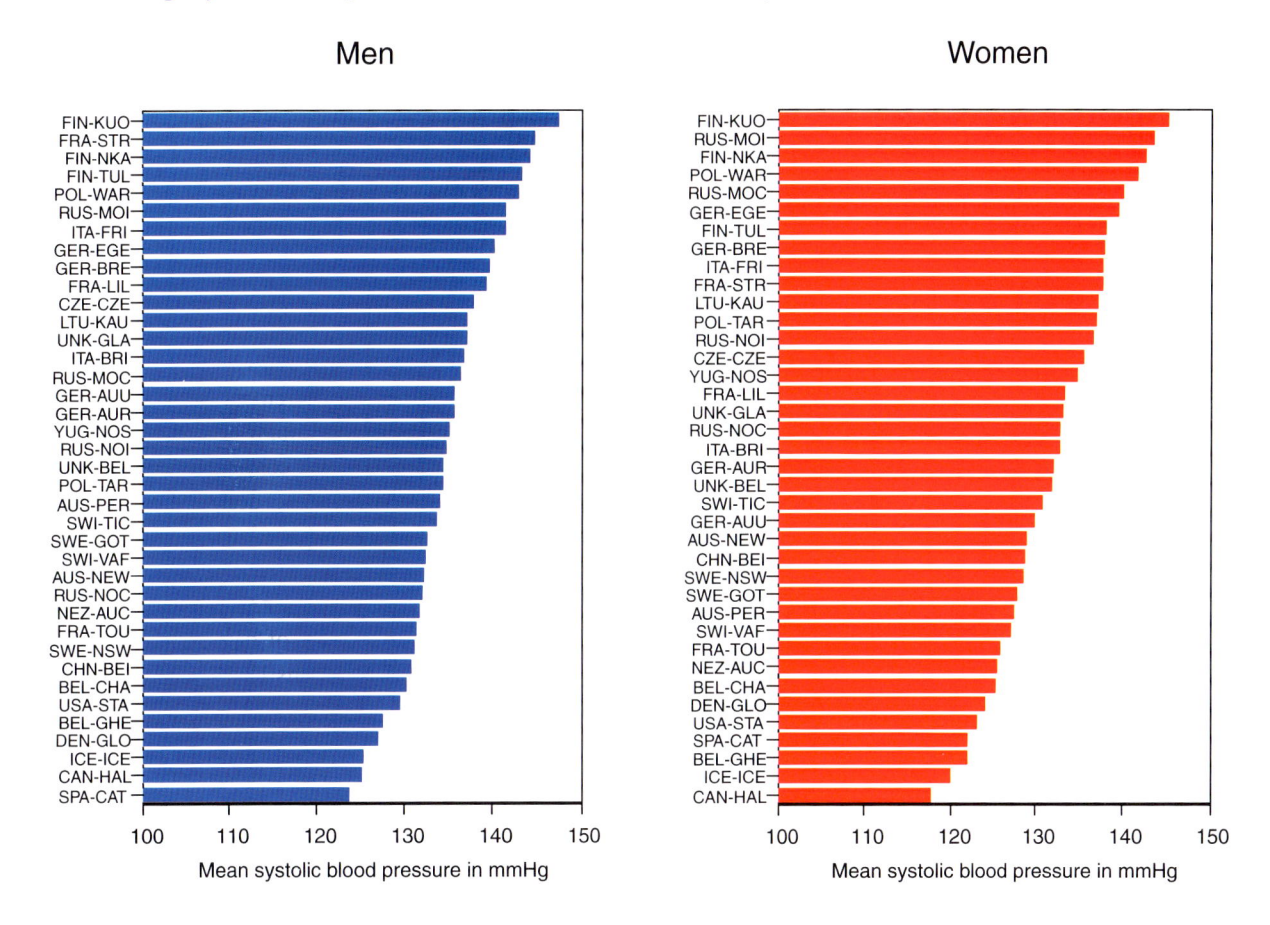

G41 Average systolic blood pressure in the final risk-factor survey

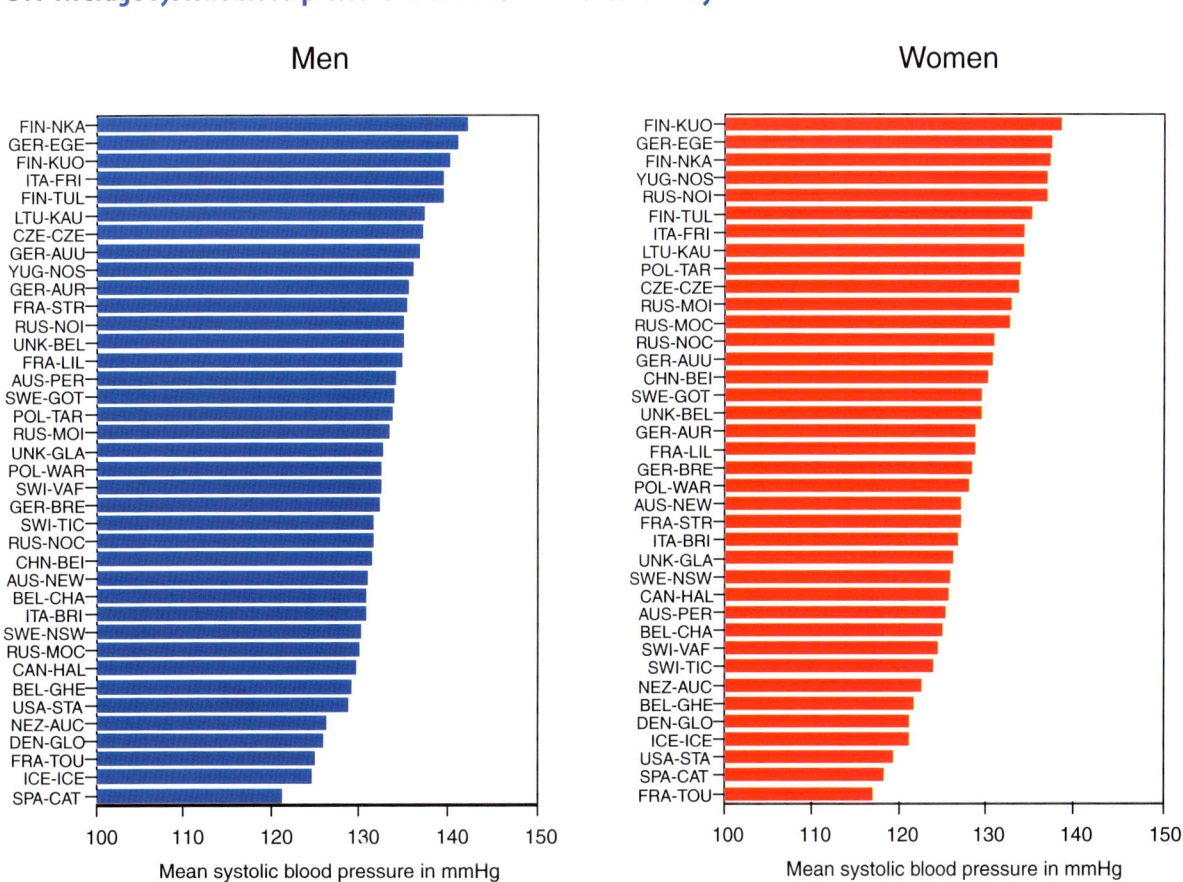

Notes in italics are repeated to help random browsers—systematic readers should ignore them

G42

1. *Calculation of trends is explained in #38 Population Prevalence and Trends.*

2. *The initial and final surveys did not take place exactly ten years apart, but this graph incorporates corrections to standardize the differences, as if they were being measured across ten years.*

3. *Horizontal bars in G42 show the 95% confidence intervals around the estimated 10-year trend. The smaller the length of the bars the more precise the estimated trend. If the bars fail to cross the zero line the estimated trend is considered to deviate significantly from zero. Declining trends are shown to the left of the zero line, increasing trends to the right.*

4. *Confidence intervals are similar for men and women; the population surveys sampled them in similar numbers.*

5. *To convert to and from SI Units: 100 mmHg = 13.3 kiloPascal (kPa); 10 kPa = 75 mmHg.*

6. G42 shows similar trends in systolic blood pressure in men and women in the various populations. The majority of male populations show decreasing trends. Two-thirds of the populations show a decreasing trend, to the left of zero. The trend is increasing, to the right of zero in 12. In women, more populations show a decrease. Only seven have an estimated increasing trend. Age-specific data are available in the MONICA Data Book of population surveys (*1*).

G43

7. G43 is a spot map showing the geographical distribution of the results shown in G42. Many of the confidence intervals in G42 include zero, particularly in men. *The populations concerned are marked with black spots. Those with a significant decrease in systolic blood pressure are shown with blue spots, while those with a significant increase are marked with red spots.*

8. Only one population, Canada-Halifax, CAN-HAL, see #54, had a significant increase in mean systolic blood pressure in both men and women. It had the second lowest average systolic blood pressure in men in the initial population survey, and the lowest average in women. In the final survey CAN-HAL readings had increased but still remained low.

9. It is unlikely that blood pressure data of poor quality had a significant effect on overall MONICA results: G56 (see later) shows that most population RUAs had acceptable blood pressure quality scores and that these did not appear to relate strongly to trends in blood pressure. Ensuring continued high quality readings in the field is difficult however, and it is not possible to carry out external quality control or to archive material. Automatic machines may, in the future, remove some but not all, of the causes of variability and bias in blood pressure measurement. In the mid-1980s to mid-1990s they were not sufficiently tested and standardized for reliability and comparability to be recommended for the MONICA population surveys. Investigators were expected to replicate the same standard methods when repeating their population surveys.

10. See the MONICA Data Book of population surveys, tables 6.1.2–6.1.6 (*1*) for blood pressure items. MONICA Publications 14, 20, 31 (*2*) are on data quality and blood pressure levels, while MONICA Publication 11 (*2*) provided early cross-sectional data. For further information, see #32 *Blood Pressure*, MONICA Quality assessment of data on blood pressure (*1*), MONICA Quality assessment of data on hypertension control (*1*). Further publications will be listed on the MONICA Website (*1*) as they appear.

1. **See Monograph CD-ROM or MONICA Website http://www.ktl.fi/monica/.**
2. **Full references and summaries of MONICA Publications appear in #85/86.**

G42 Ten-year change in average systolic blood pressure

Men

Women

Ten-year trend in systolic blood pressure in mmHg

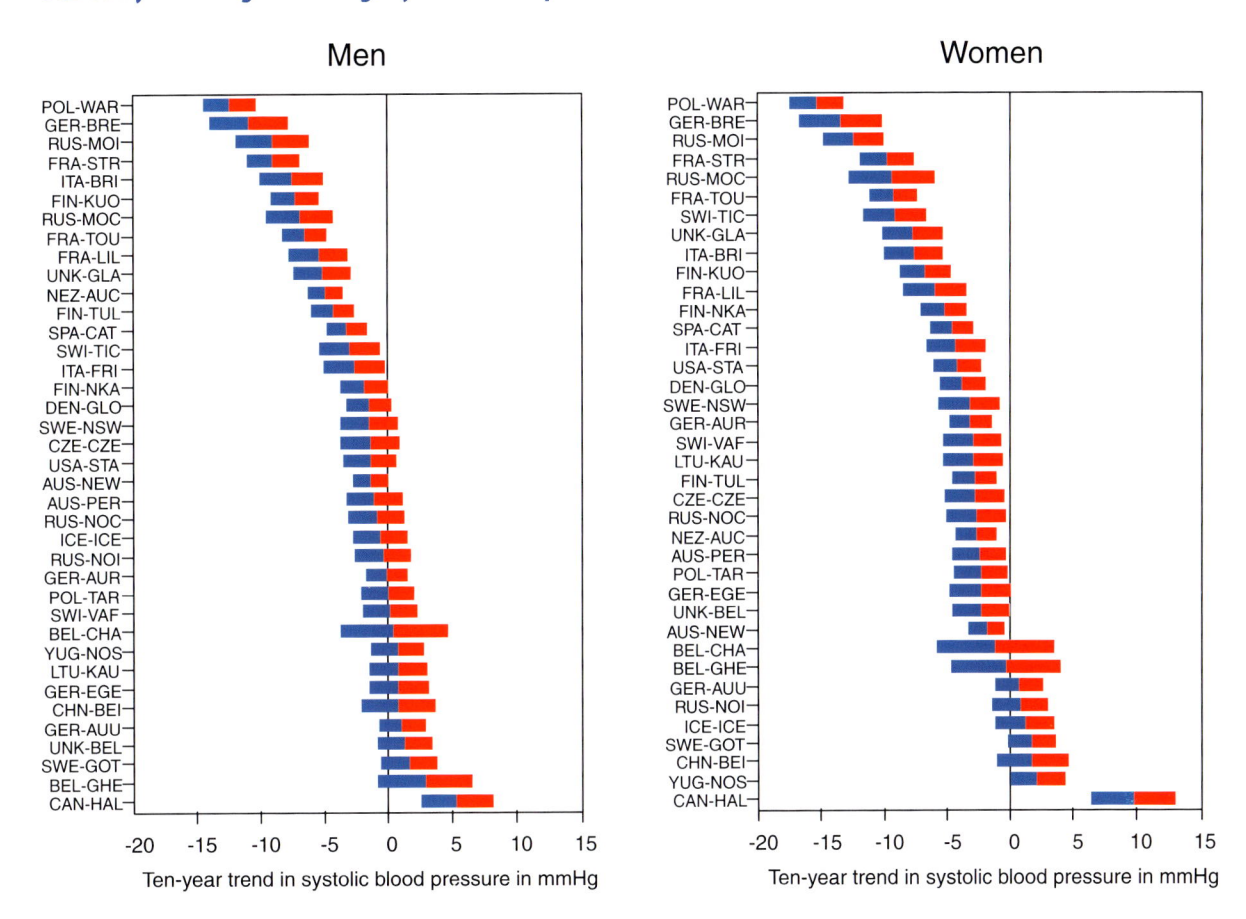

G43 Spot maps of population changes in average systolic blood pressure

Men

Women

Significant increase
Insignificant change
Significant decrease

RISK FACTORS: SYSTOLIC BLOOD PRESSURE

201

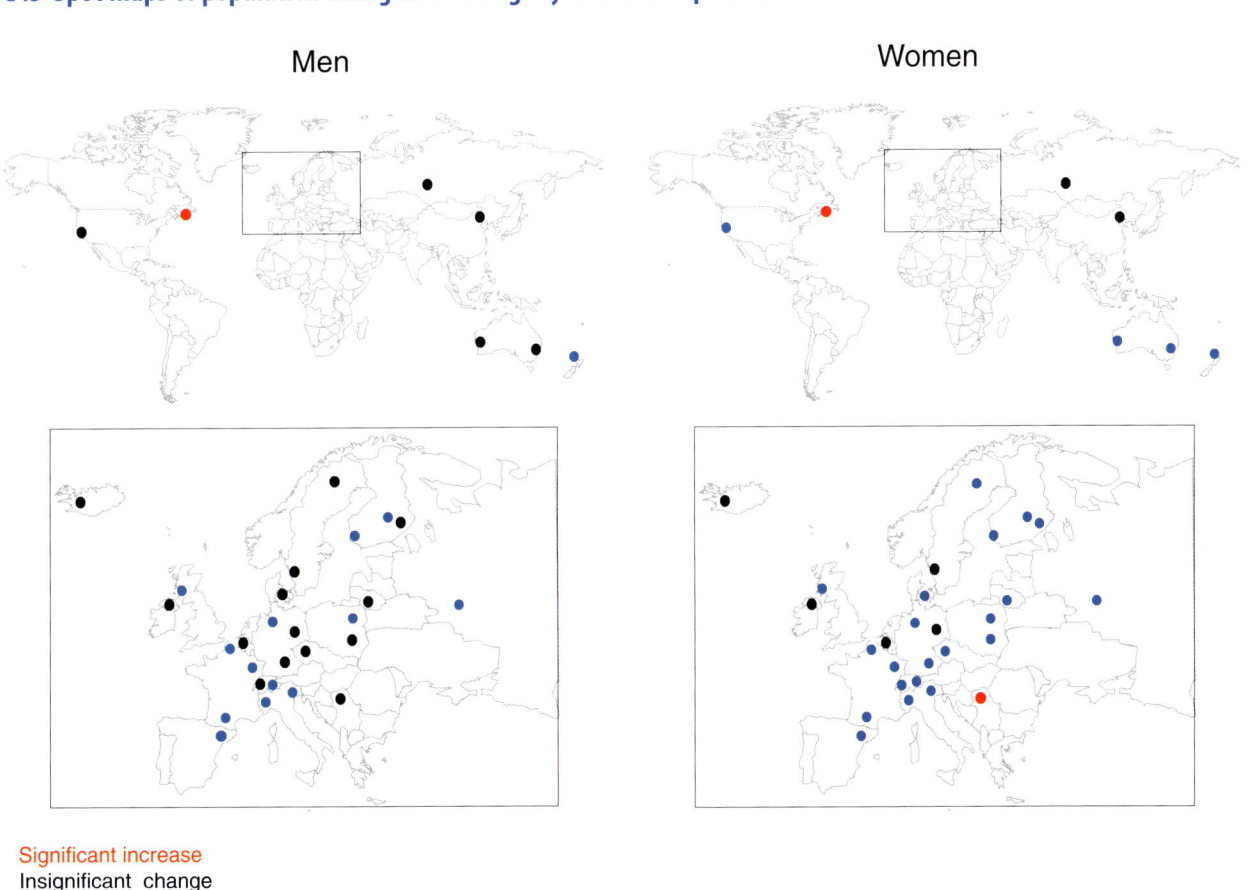

Risk factors: total blood cholesterol

Notes in italics are repeated to help random browsers—systematic readers should ignore them

1. *The timing of the initial and final surveys differed by population. These surveys were usually eight to ten years apart but the interval could be as little as six years. The calendar years and months varied. See G10 and MONICA Quality assessment of age, date of examination and survey periods.*

2. Results are shown as the estimated mean total cholesterol in millimoles per litre (mmol/l) in the 35–64 age group. *The results are age-standardized to minimize any effect of differing age structures on the apparent findings. See #38 Population Prevalence and Trends, #39 Age Standardization.*

3. To convert to and from SI Units: 200 mg/dl = 5.17 mmol/l; 10 mmol/l = 387 mg/dl.

4. *The graphs characterize men and women over a thirty-year age band in each survey for each population with a single value, but levels and trends vary with age.* Age-specific data are published in the MONICA Data Book of population surveys, table 6.2.2 (*1*), and early results in MONICA Publication 11 (*2*).

5. *Survey results could be influenced by failure to participate by some of those selected for the survey. The issue is complex. Different methods of recruitment and sampling were used in different populations. There is more than one definition of response rates. See #28 Sampling, #29 Recruitment and Response rates, MONICA Quality assessment of participation rates, sampling frames and fractions (1).*

6. Cholesterol is one of the classic coronary risk factors, measured in blood as serum or plasma cholesterol. It is otherwise known as total cholesterol because it includes different fractions (such as low, intermediate and high-density lipoprotein, HDL-cholesterol). It is not influenced appreciably by time of day or fasting/non-fasting status, so it can be measured without special preparation.

7. Cholesterol was the only classical risk factor in MONICA dependent on the laboratory. Ensuring and maintaining comparability of different laboratories across ten years and 21 countries was a complex problem. Laboratory readings can drift. MONICA established a quality control centre for lipid measurement in Prague in the Czech Republic, which worked with its equivalent in Atlanta in the USA. See #33 *Cholesterol*, MONICA Manual Part III, Sections 1, 2 (*1*), MONICA Quality assessment of data on cholesterol (*1*), MONICA Quality assessment of data on awareness and treatment of cholesterol (*1*), the MONICA Data Book of population surveys, tables 6.2.1–6.2.7 (*1*), and MONICA Publication 13 (*2*).

8. Participants in the MONICA surveys consented to venepuncture. Blood was taken from an arm vein with minimal or no use of a tourniquet. It was analysed according to a written protocol as plasma or serum, for total and HDL-cholesterol, some being deep-frozen and stored for future reference. See #33 *Cholesterol*, MONICA Manual Part III, Sections 1, 2 (*1*).

9. The scale for men and women is the same. Mean cholesterol levels were similar in the two sexes. Compared with historical population differences there was relatively little variation between most populations, with mean readings ranging between 5.5 and 6.3 mmols/l. The population with the highest readings varied between men and women and the initial and final surveys. China-Beijing, CHN-BEI, see #55 had the lowest mean total cholesterol in all four graphs by a considerable margin.

10. The readings here are age-standardized so they conceal age differences. There is a steeper age gradient in women so that their cholesterol readings are lower than those in men of the same age at 35–44, but they are higher at age 55–64. Age-specific readings are given in the MONICA Data Book of population surveys, table 6.2.2 (*1*), and early results in MONICA Publication 11 (*2*).

11. The Data book contains tables covering a number of other data items concerning cholesterol, such as the percentage of participants above and below certain cut points, HDL-cholesterol, and in later surveys the reported frequency of earlier measurement and treatment. See the MONICA Data Book of population surveys, tables 6.2.1–6.2.7 (*1*). This Monograph discusses only total cholesterol. Despite our efforts, standardization for epidemiological comparison of measurement of HDL-cholesterol in the MONICA decade was unsatisfactory and failed to meet our criteria for formal publication. See MONICA Quality assessment of data on HDL-cholesterol (*1*).

1. **See Monograph CD-ROM or MONICA Website http://www.ktl.fi/monica/.**
2. **Full references and summaries of MONICA Publications appear in #85/86.**

G44 Average blood cholesterol concentration in the initial risk-factor survey

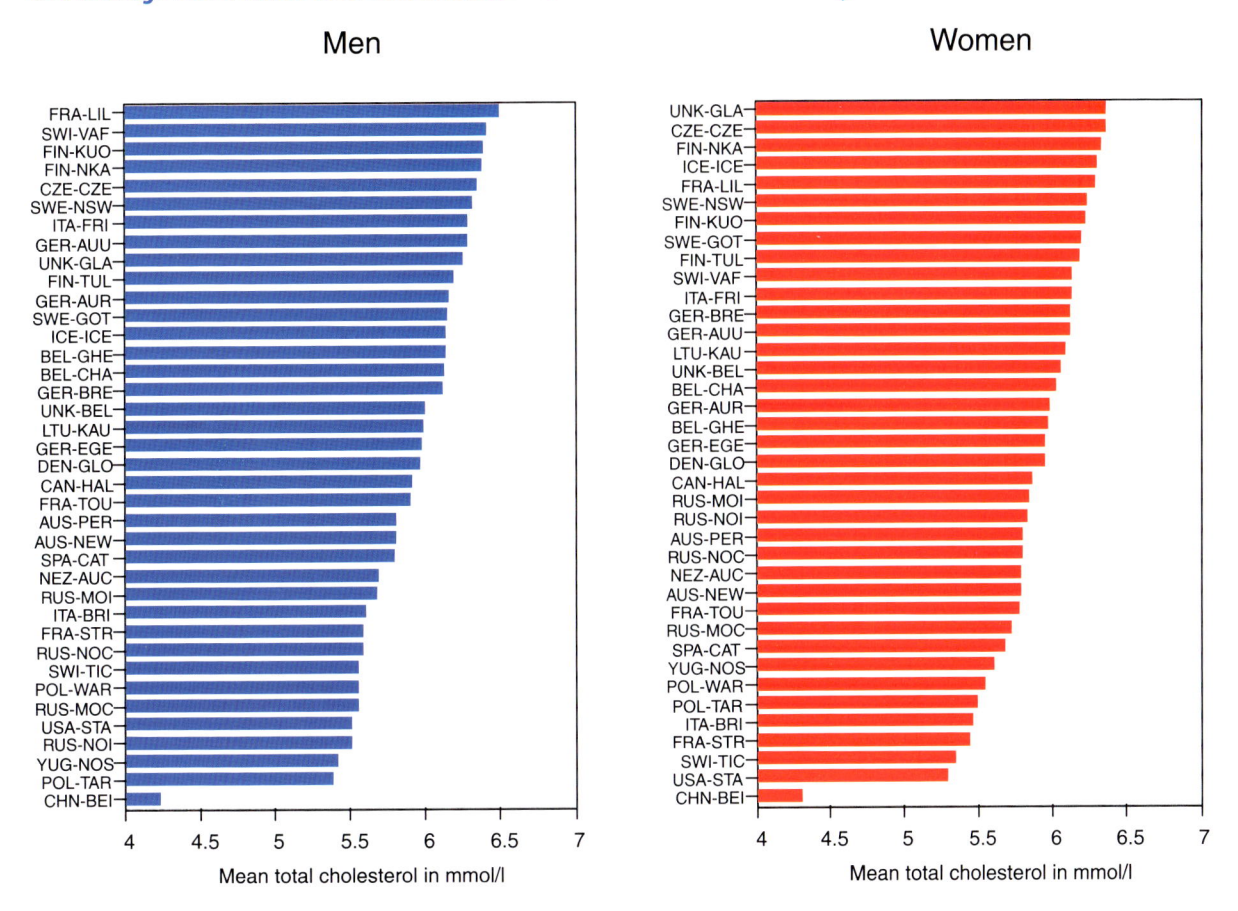

Men / Women
Mean total cholesterol in mmol/l

G45 Average blood cholesterol concentration in the final risk-factor survey

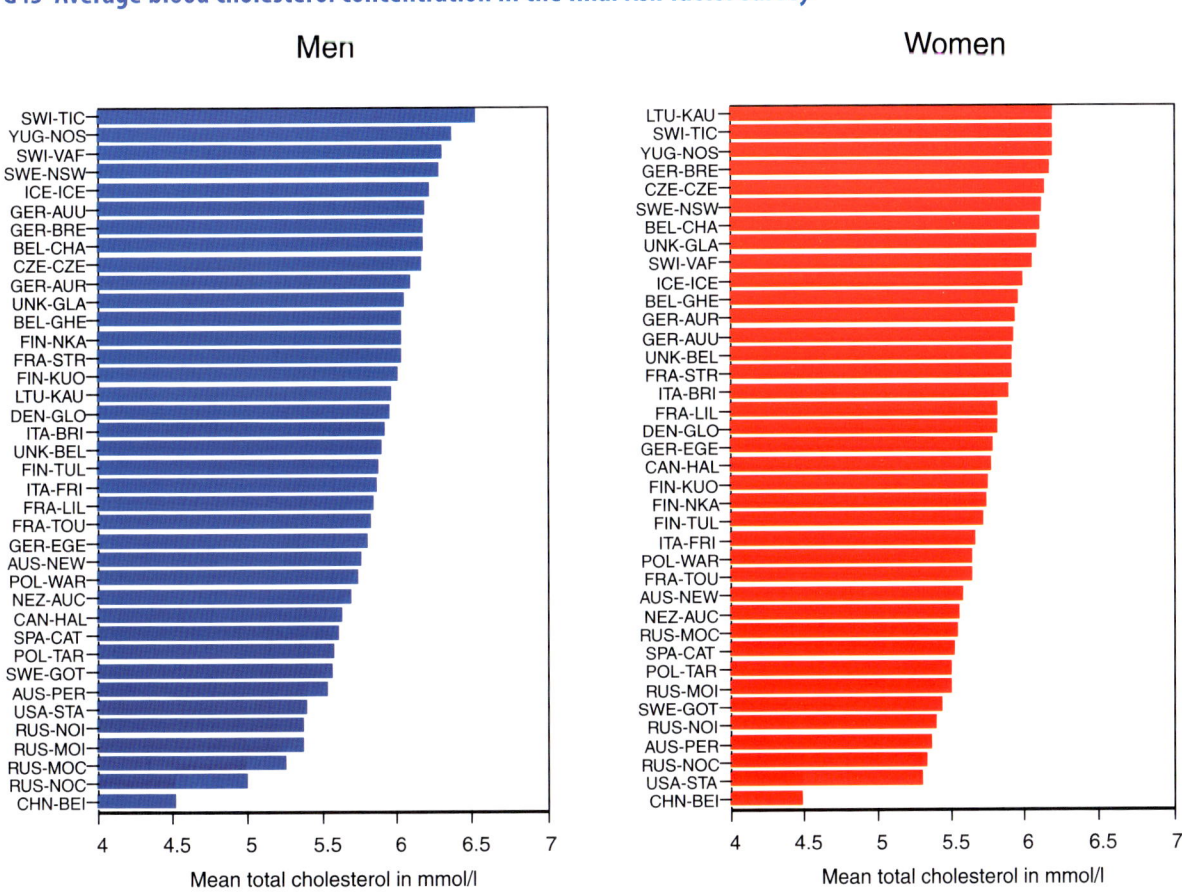

Men / Women
Mean total cholesterol in mmol/l

Notes in italics are repeated to help random browsers—systematic readers should ignore them

G46

1. *Calculation of trends is explained in #38 Population Prevalence and Trends.*

2. *The initial and final surveys did not take place exactly ten years apart. G46 incorporates corrections to standardize the differences, as if they were being measured across ten years.*

3. *Horizontal bars in G46 show the 95% confidence intervals around the estimated annual trend. The smaller the length of the bars, the more precise the trend estimate. If the bars fail to cross the zero line, the estimated trend is considered to deviate significantly from zero. Declining trends are shown to the left of the zero line, increasing trends, to the right.*

4. *To convert to and from SI Units: 200 mg/dl = 5.17 mmol/l; 10 mmol/l = 387 mg/dl.*

5. *Confidence intervals are similar for men and women; the population surveys sampled them in similar numbers.*

6. G46 shows similar trends in total cholesterol in men and women, in the various populations. Two-thirds of the male populations show a decrease, tending to the left of zero. Ten show an increase, right of zero. In women, results are virtually the same, although specific populations vary a little in their ranking. Age-specific data are available in the MONICA Data Book on population surveys table 6.2.2 (*1*).

G47

7. *G47 is a spot map showing the geographical distribution of the results shown in G46. Some of the confidence intervals in G46 include zero. These populations are marked with black spots. Those with a significant decrease in cholesterol levels are shown with blue spots while a significant increase is shown with a red spot. 'Significant' is statistical, meaning that the change is large enough for it to be unlikely to have arisen by chance when random sampling variation is taken into account. Significant changes and differences can occur through undetected bias, such as a drift in laboratory standards over time. These findings have not been adjusted for measurement quality.*

8. Many populations show a significant decline in cholesterol between the initial and final surveys. Seven male and five female populations show an increase. There is some apparent geographical clustering of results.

9. Results shown here should be interpreted in association with the MONICA Quality assessment of data on total cholesterol (*1*), and with G56 (see later). The quality of total cholesterol data, despite intense attempts at standardization in the planning of MONICA, raises more questions than the quality of data on other risk factors. G56 shows that some of the more extreme cholesterol trends arose among population RUAs whose cholesterol quality scores were suboptimal. See notes on G56.

10. The only publication specific to cholesterol is MONICA Publication 13 (*2*) on data quality. MONICA Publication 11 (*2*) contained early cross-sectional and age-specific data. Further publications are in preparation and will be listed on the MONICA Website (*1*) as they appear.

1. **See Monograph CD-ROM or MONICA Website http://www.ktl.fi/monica/.**
2. **Full references and summaries of MONICA Publications appear in #85/86.**

G46 Ten-year change in average blood cholesterol concentration

Men — Ten-year trend in total cholesterol in mmol/l

Women — Ten-year trend in total cholesterol in mmol/l

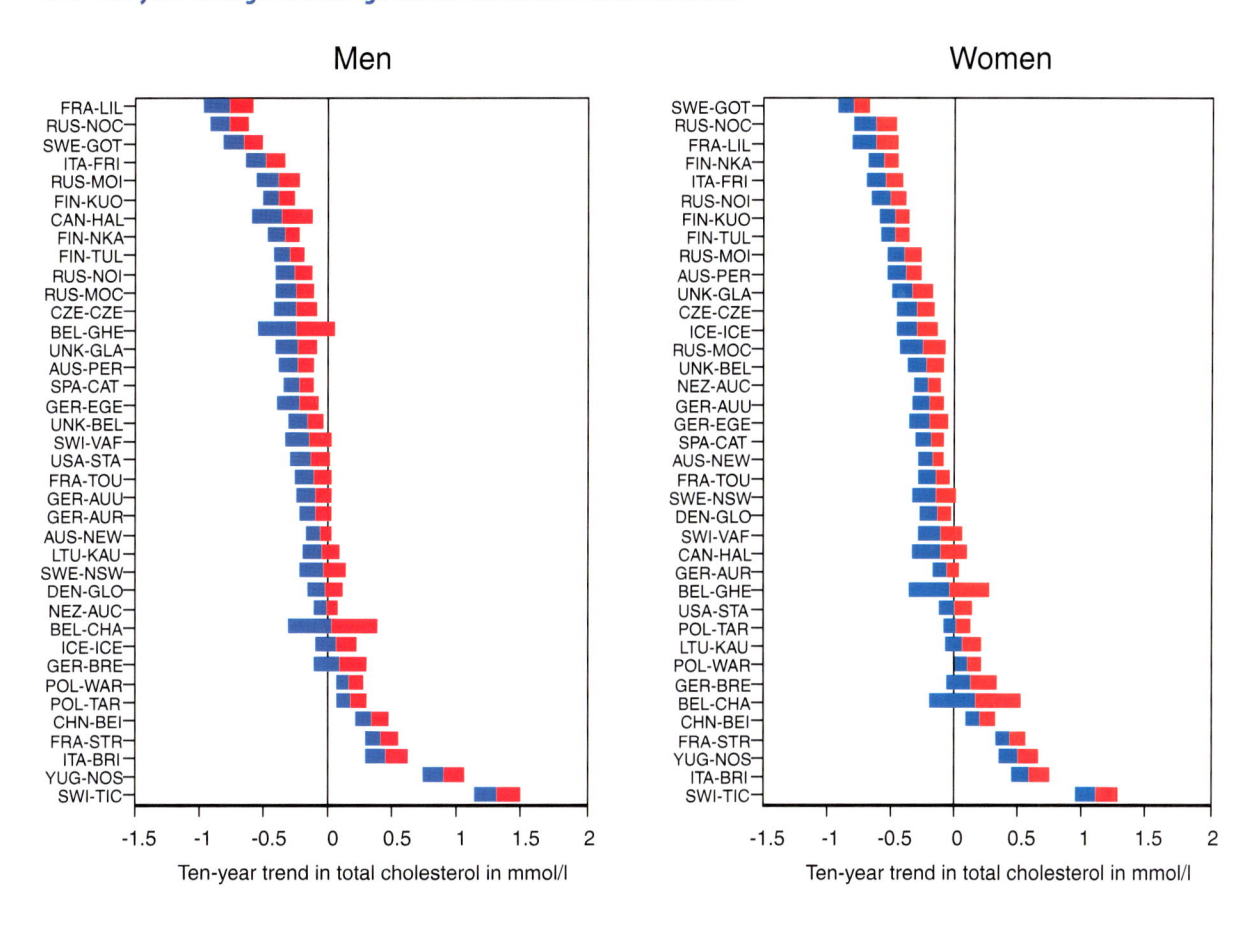

G47 Spot maps of population changes in average blood cholesterol concentration

Men

Women

Significant increase
Insignificant change
Significant decrease

RISK FACTORS: TOTAL BLOOD CHOLESTEROL

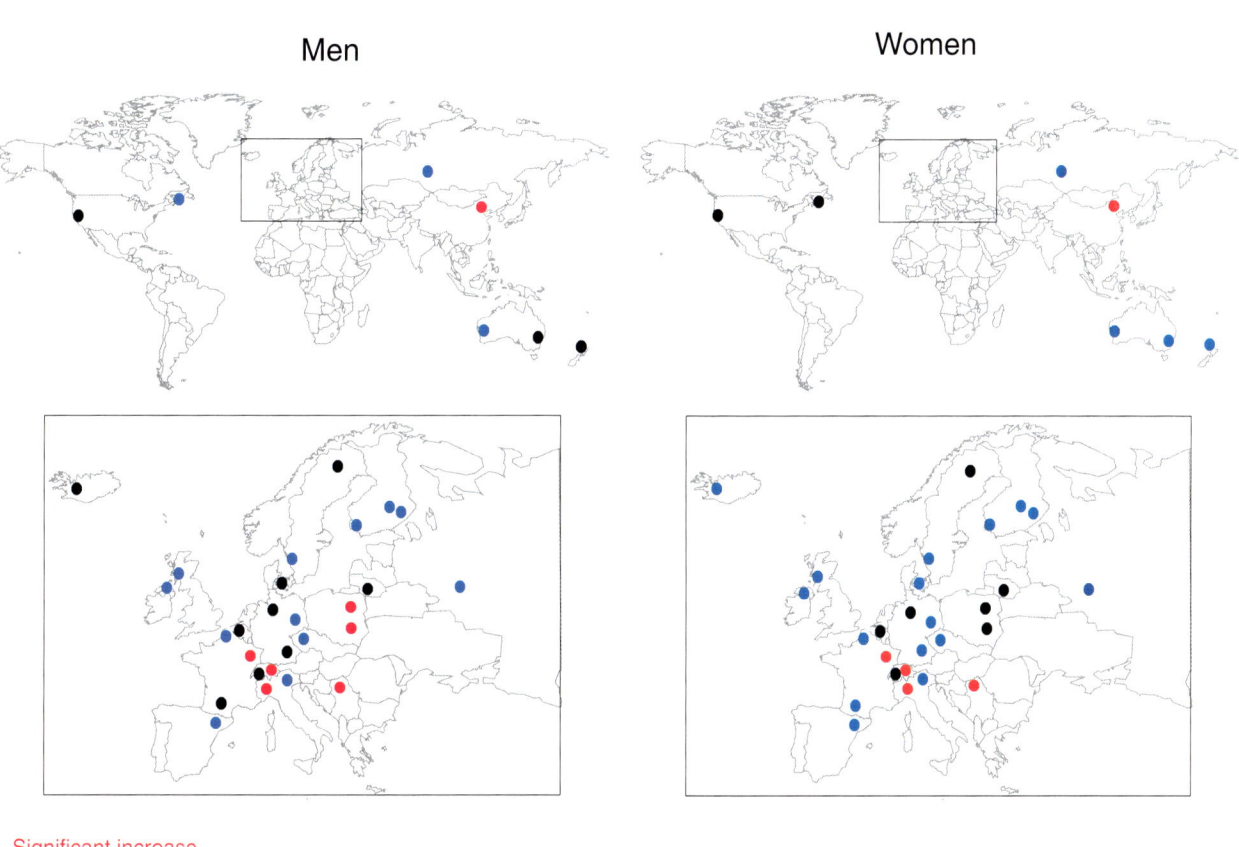

Risk factors: obesity, body mass index

Notes in italics are repeated to help random browsers—systematic readers should ignore them

1. *The timing of the initial and final surveys differed by population. They were usually eight to ten years apart but the interval could be as little as six years. The calendar years and months varied. See G10 and MONICA Quality assessment of age, date of examination and survey periods.*

2. Results are shown as the mean body mass index (BMI) in kilograms per square metre for the 35–64 age group. See #34 *Height, Weight, and Waist Circumference*. The results are age-standardized to minimize any effect of differing age structures on the apparent findings. See #38 *Population Prevalence and Trends*, #39 *Age Standardization*.

3. *The graphs characterize men and women over a thirty-year age band in each survey for each population with a single value, but levels and trends vary with age.* Age-specific data are published in the MONICA Data Book of population surveys, table 6.3.4 (*1*), and early results in MONICA Publication 11 (*2*).

4. *Survey results could be influenced by failure to participate by some of those selected for the survey. The issue is complex. Different methods of recruitment and sampling were used in different populations. There is more than one definition of response rates. See #28 Sampling, #29 Recruitment and Response Rates, MONICA Quality assessment of participation rates, sampling frames and fractions (1).*

5. Body mass index is used as an indicator of obesity or body fat. Weight is corrected by the square of the body height. Although bone and muscle also contribute, the biggest variation between body mass in individuals, particularly in sedentary groups, is in their body fat. Epidemiologists have always been interested in the distribution of body fat, originally using calliper measurement of skin-fold thickness, but this was difficult to standardize. Measurement of abdominal obesity by waist circumference and its ratio with hip circumference became standard just too late for the MONICA protocol for the initial population surveys, although it was introduced into later MONICA surveys. Population surveys need simple techniques. Isotope tests, and weighing under water for body fat estimation can be done in laboratories but not in field surveys. See #34 *Height, Weight, and Waist Circumference*.

6. Participants had their weight and height measured with shoes and outside clothes removed. Measurement, as with blood pressure, appears simple and easy, but there is potential for problems in standardization of measurements, and of equipment, to ensure that population trends are genuine. See #34 *Height, Weight, and Waist Circumference*, MONICA Manual Part III, Section 1 (*1*), MONICA Quality assessment of data on weight and height (*1*), MONICA Quality assessment of data on waist and hip circumference (*1*).

7. The scale for men and women is the same. There was little variation between most population RUAs in the initial survey in men, except for China-Beijing, CHN-BEI, see #55, as previously for cholesterol. There was more variation in women. In the final survey there was again more variation between female populations than in men. Some populations show similar, and some rather different rankings between the two sexes, possibly related to differences in smoking levels by sex. Even a quick glance down the page shows that obesity is increasing between G48 and G49. This is confirmed when you turn the page to G50.

8. The MONICA Data Book of population surveys contains several tables 6.3.2–6.3.7 covering a number of items related to measurements of height, weight, body mass index, obesity cut points, waist and hip circumference and their ratio. Height itself is of epidemiological interest, as a marker of nutritional status in early life.

9. Obesity is not considered a major classical risk factor for coronary disease as are cigarette smoking, blood pressure and cholesterol, but it is of great importance for public health and has generated several papers in MONICA. See #34 *Height, Weight, and Waist Circumference*, MONICA Publications 27, 35, 37, 41 (*2*).

1. **See Monograph CD-ROM or MONICA Website http://www.ktl.fi/monica/.**
2. **Full references and summaries of MONICA Publications appear in #85/86.**

G48 Average body mass index (BMI) in the initial risk-factor survey

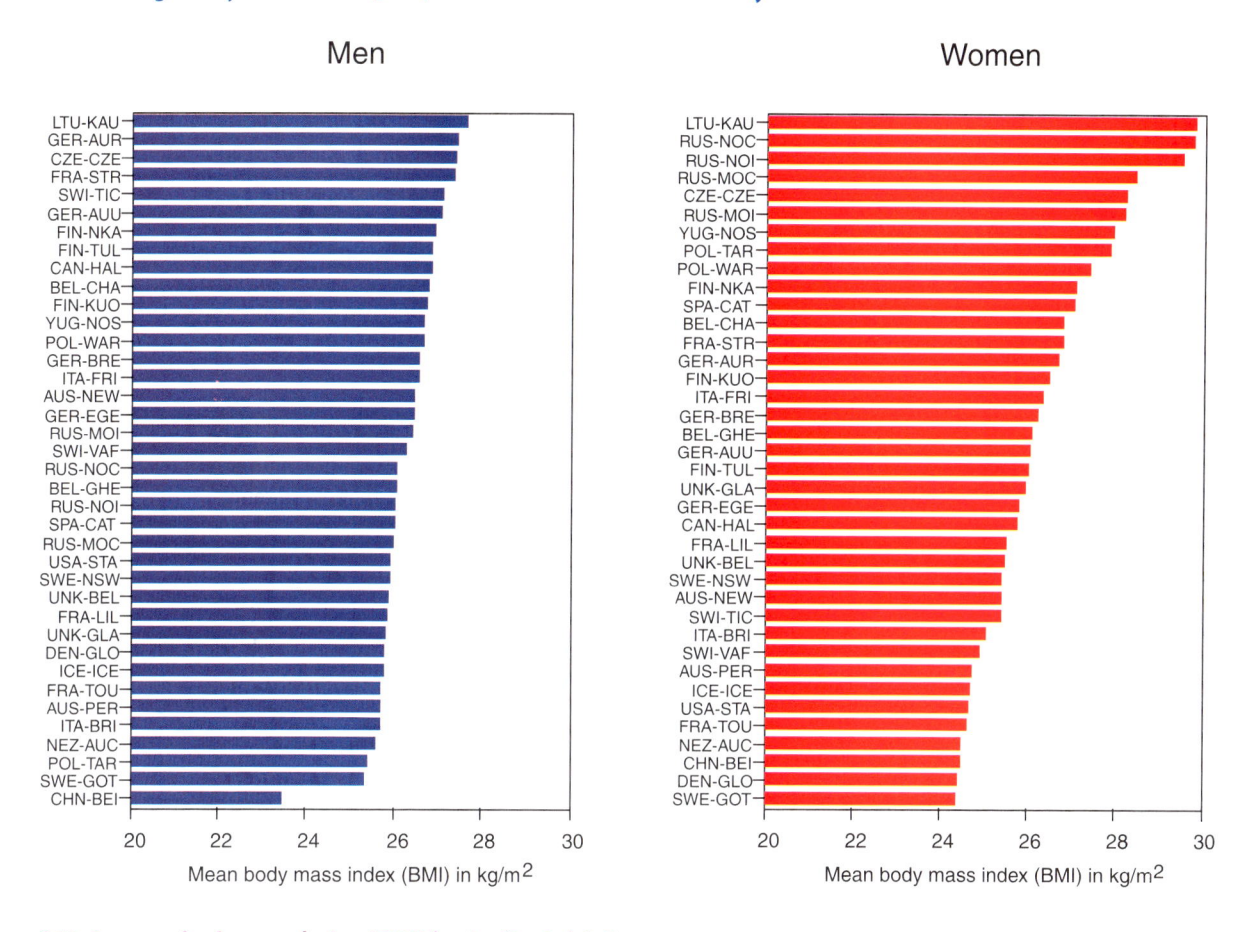

Men — Mean body mass index (BMI) in kg/m^2

Women — Mean body mass index (BMI) in kg/m^2

G49 Average body mass index (BMI) in the final risk-factor survey

Men — Mean body mass index (BMI) in kg/m^2

Women — Mean body mass index (BMI) in kg/m^2

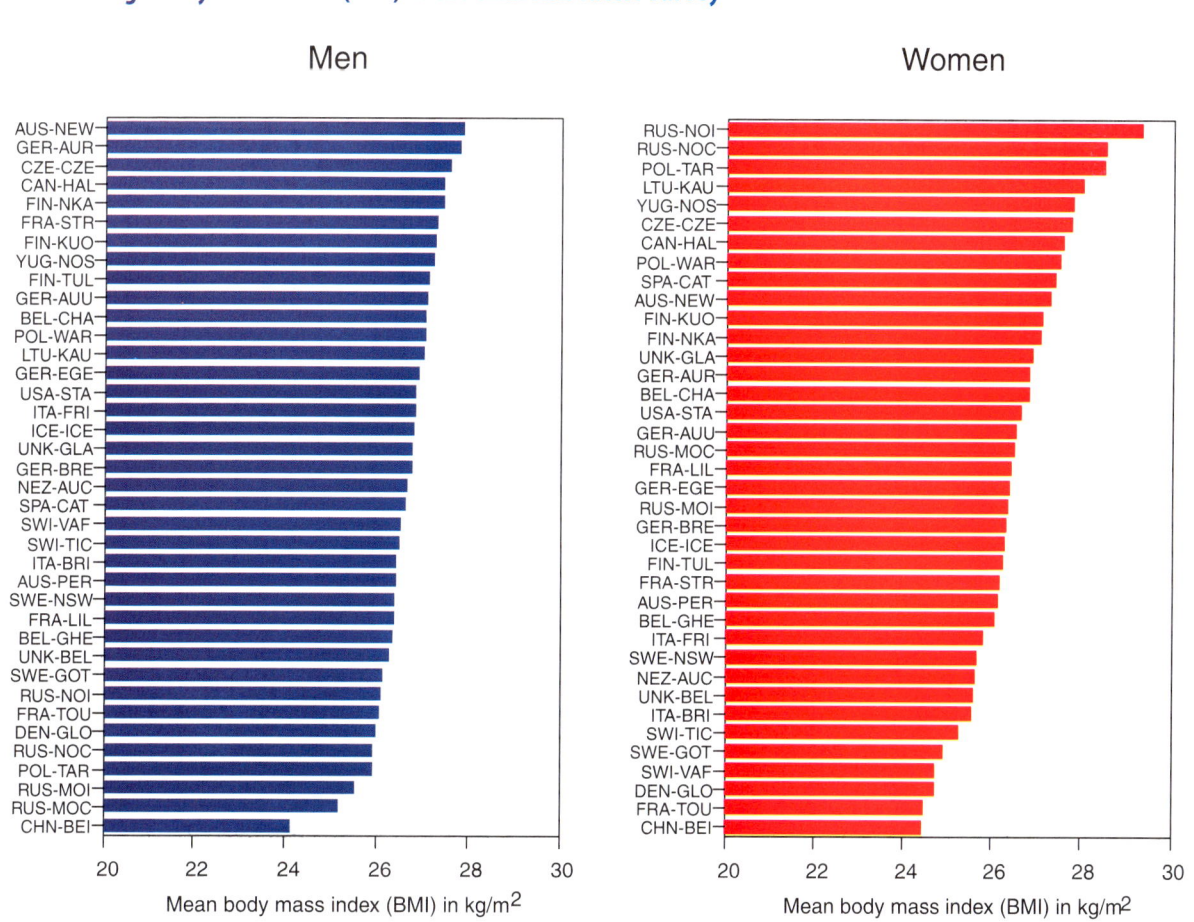

RISK FACTORS: OBESITY, BODY MASS INDEX

Notes in italics are repeated to help random browsers—systematic readers should ignore them

1. *Calculation of trends is explained in #38 Population Prevalence and Trends.*

G50

2. *The initial and final surveys did not take place exactly ten years apart, but this graph incorporates corrections to standardize the differences as if they were being measured across ten years.*

3. *Horizontal bars in G50 show the 95% confidence intervals around the estimated annual trend. The smaller the length of the bars, the more precise the trend estimate. If the bars fail to cross the zero line the estimated trend is considered to deviate significantly from zero. Declining trends are shown to the left of the zero line, increasing trends to the right.*

4. Confidence intervals appear similar for men and women, although possibly a bit wider in more female populations. The population surveys sampled similar numbers of men and women.

5. G50 shows similar trends in body mass index in men and women in the various populations. The majority of male populations show an increase, so that the estimated trend is to the left of zero in only six populations, and to the right in the remainder. In women, there is a similar but less marked pattern with 15 populations showing a decline in body mass index, and the remainder an increase. Changes in women are more extreme at the top and bottom of the graphs than they are in men. Age-specific data are available in the MONICA Data Book of population surveys, table 6.3.4 (*1*).

G51

6. *G51 is a spot map showing the geographical distribution of the results shown in G50. Some of the confidence intervals in G50 include zero. The populations concerned are marked by black spots. Those with a significant decrease in body mass index are shown with blue spots, while a significant increase is shown with a red spot.*

7. Many populations show a significant increase in body mass index between the initial and final surveys. There is some apparent polarization of red and blue across Europe, particularly in women, but this is not consistent.

8. These results should be considered in association with the MONICA Quality assessment of data on weight and height, and with G56 (see later), which plots trends in population RUA results against their quality scores. These suggest that the population increases in body mass index shown here are real.

9. For further information see #34 *Height, Weight, and Waist Circumference*, MONICA Quality assessment of data on weight and height (*1*), MONICA Quality assessment of data on waist and hip circumference (*1*), MONICA Data Book of population surveys, tables 6.3.2–6.3.7 (*1*), MONICA Publications 27, 35, 37, 41 (*2*). Further publications are listed on the MONICA Website as they appear (*1*).

1. **See Monograph CD-ROM or MONICA Website http://www.ktl.fi/monica/.**
2. **Full references and summaries of MONICA Publications appear in #85/86.**

G50 Ten-year change in average body mass index (BMI)

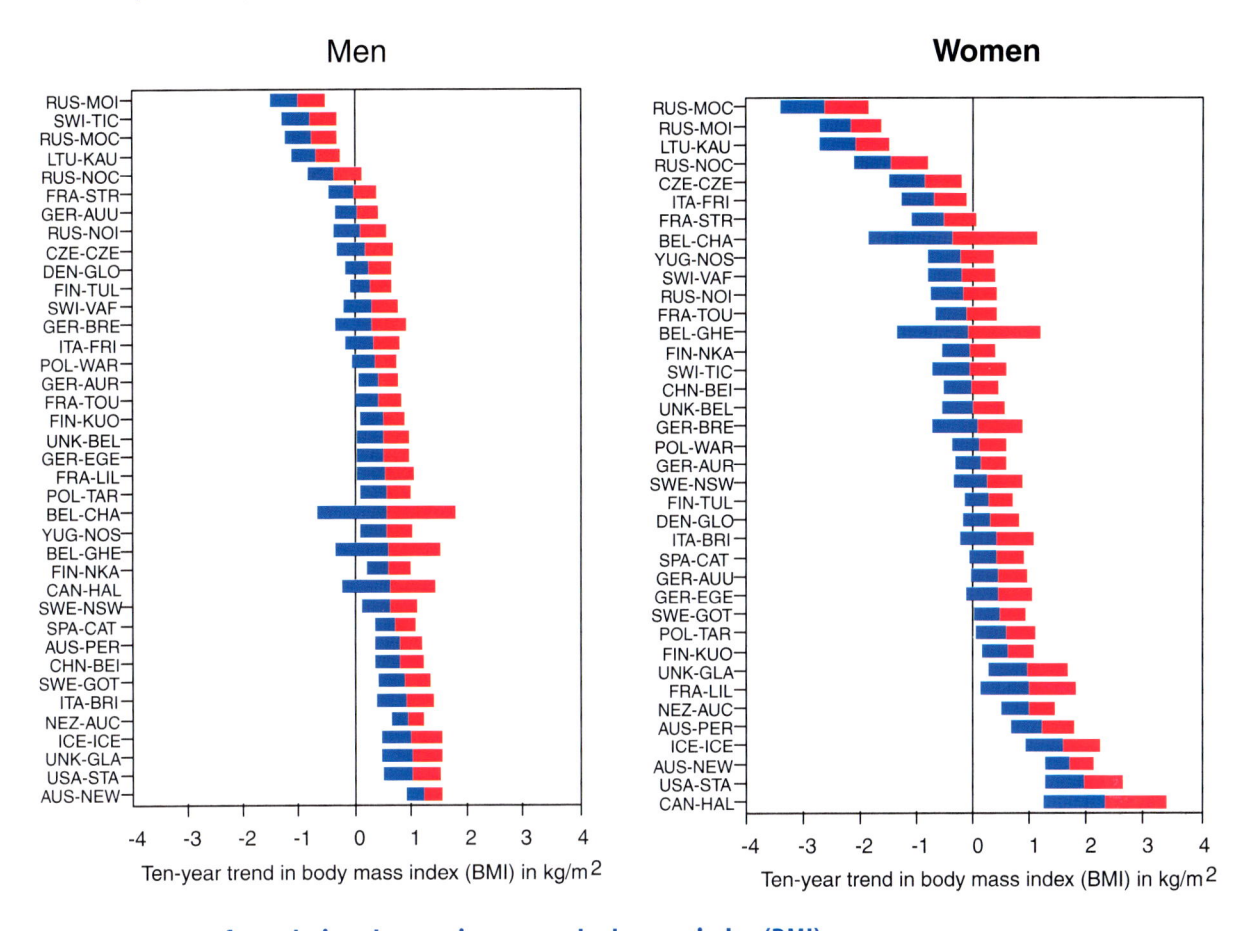

Men

Women

Ten-year trend in body mass index (BMI) in kg/m²

G51 Spot maps of population changes in average body mass index (BMI)

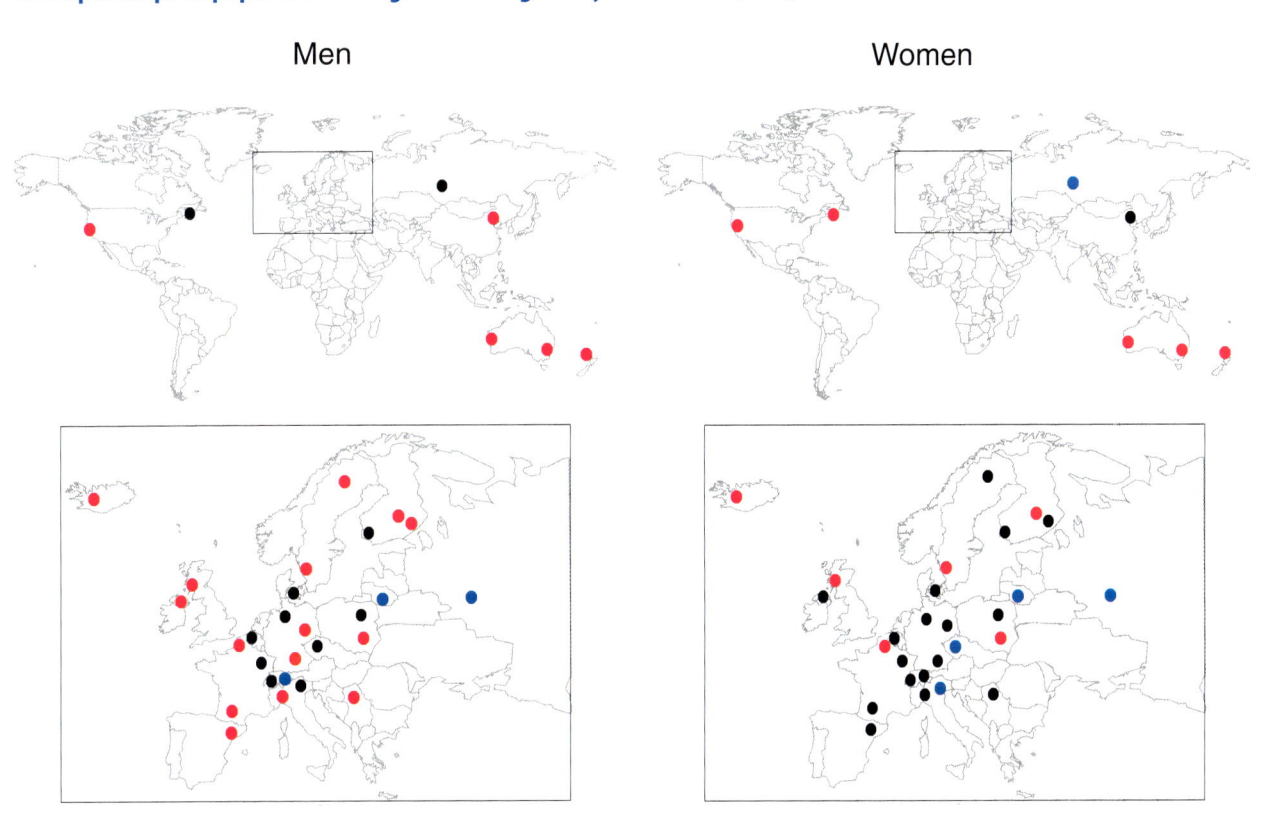

Men

Women

Significant increase
Insignificant change
Significant decrease

RISK FACTORS: OBESITY, BODY MASS INDEX

Risk factors: risk-factor score

Notes in italics are repeated to help random browsers—systematic readers should ignore them

1. *The timing of the initial and final surveys differed by population. They were usually eight to ten years apart but the interval could be as little as six years. The calendar years and months varied. See G10 and MONICA Quality assessment of age, date of examination and survey periods (1).*

2. *Results are shown as the estimated average coronary risk-factor score in the 35–64 age group. The results are age-standardized to minimize any effect of differing age structures on the apparent findings. See #35 Risk-Factor Scores, #38 Population Prevalence and Trends, #39 Age Standardization.*

3. *The graphs characterize men and women over a thirty-year age band in each survey for each population with a single value, but levels and trends vary with age. Age-specific data are not published.* The risk-factor score is derived from risk-factor data published in the MONICA Data Book of population surveys.

4. *Survey results could be influenced by failure to participate by some of those selected for the survey. The issue is complex. Different methods of recruitment and sampling were used in different populations. There is more than one definition of response rates. See #28 Sampling, #29 Recruitment and Response Rates, MONICA Quality assessment of participation rates, sampling frames and fractions (1).*

5. The risk-factor score is used to summarize the presumed contribution of the classical coronary risk factors: cigarette smoking, systolic blood pressure, and total cholesterol, along with body mass index, to coronary risk. The formula is based on follow-up or cohort studies in Europe in which thousands of subjects had such risk-factor measurements and were then followed-up for coronary events. Smoking, blood pressure and cholesterol contribute heavily to the score as classical major risk factors. The contribution of body mass index is smaller, particularly in women. See #35 *Risk-Factor Scores*, MONICA Publications 12, 32, 33, 38 (*2*), and Appendix to 38 published on the MONICA Website (*1*).

6. Although the scale for men and women is similar in G52 and G53, the scores differ on average by about 0.5 units between men and women. Populations rank similarly in men and women, but there are disparities. These may relate to sex differences in smoking rates, which are large in some population RUAs.

7. The risk-factor score is unique among the factors displayed in these charts, in that it is not the same for men and women. Although smoking levels differed in the two sexes, as did blood pressure sometimes, these did not account entirely for the lower score in women in G52 and G53. The statistical coefficients derived for men and women are different. Identical risk-factor values in the two sexes would produce lower scores in women. See #35 *Risk-Factor Scores*. Comparison of the sexes for this item is misleading.

8. The choice of a coronary risk-factor score for testing the MONICA risk-factor hypothesis involved considerable research and planning, some of which is published. See MONICA Publications 12, 32, 33, 38 (*2*) and the Appendix to publication 38 on the MONICA Website and Monograph CD-ROM. (*1*)

9. Coefficients for a stroke risk-factor score are similar but not identical. See #35 *Risk-Factor Scores*.

1. **See Monograph CD-ROM or MONICA Website http://www.ktl.fi/monica/.**
2. **Full references and summaries of MONICA Publications appear in #85/86.**

G52 Average coronary risk-factor score in the initial risk-factor survey

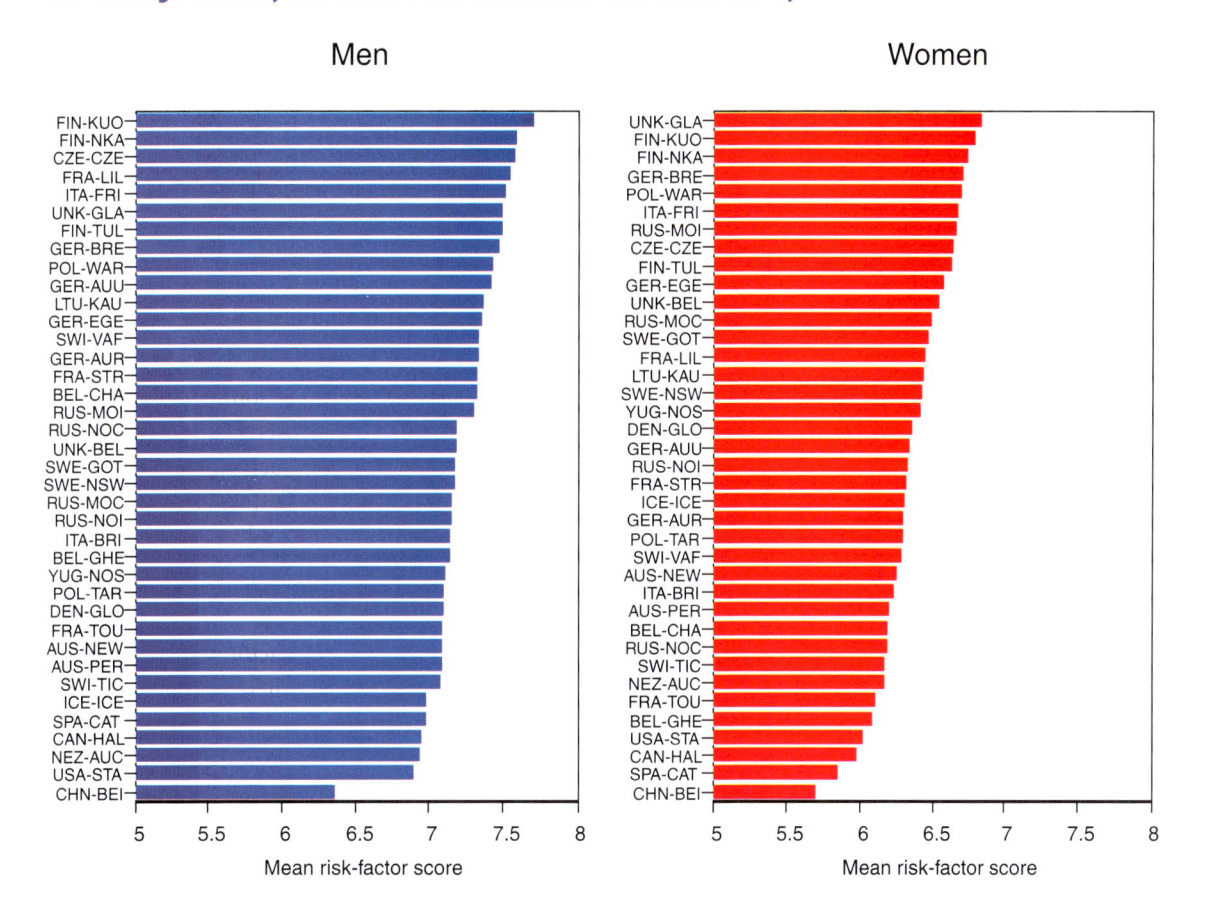

G53 Average coronary risk-factor score in the final risk-factor survey

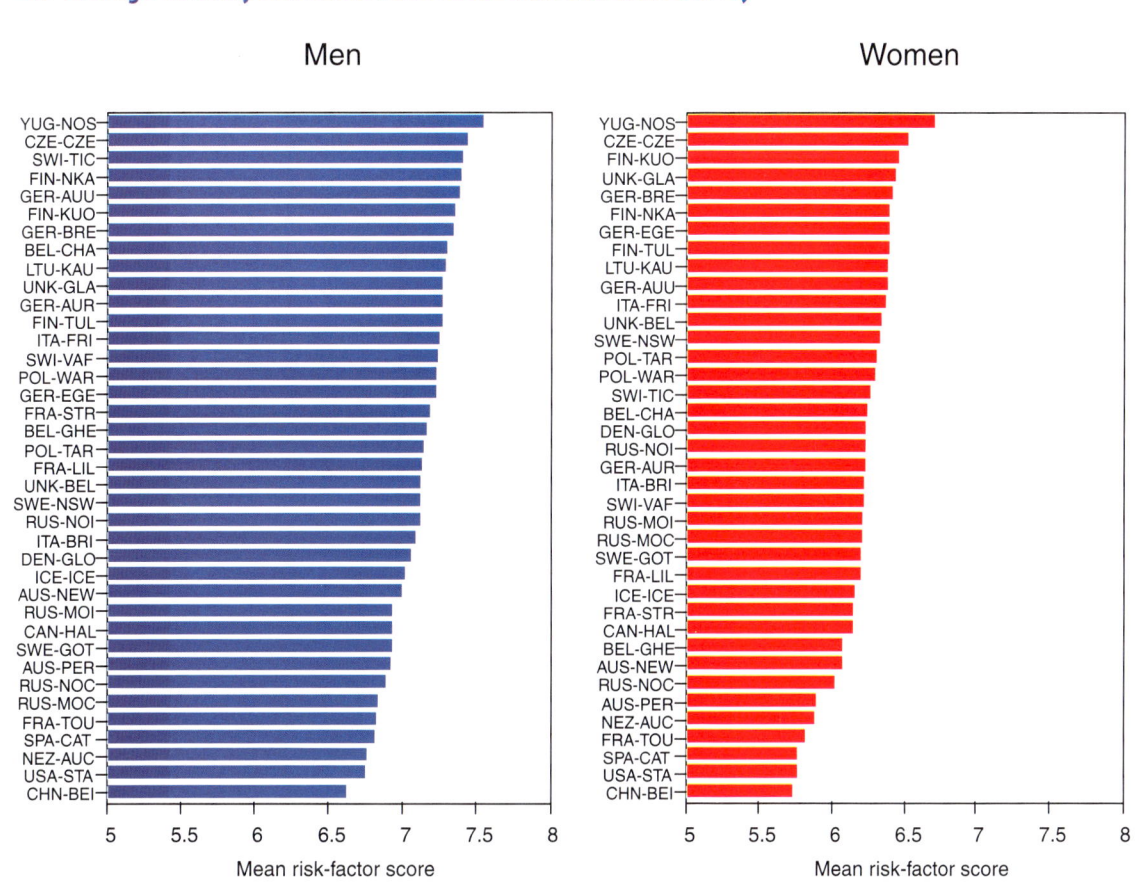

RISK FACTORS: RISK-FACTOR SCORE

Notes in italics are repeated to help random browsers—systematic readers should ignore them

G54

1. *Calculation of trends is explained in #38 Population Prevalence and Trends.*

2. *The initial and final surveys did not take place exactly ten years apart, but this graph incorporates corrections to standardize the differences, as if they were being measured across ten years.*

3. *Horizontal bars in G54 show the 95% confidence intervals around the estimated 10-year trend. The smaller the length of the bars the more precise the estimated trend. If the bars fail to cross the zero line the estimated trend is considered to deviate significantly from zero. Declining trends are shown to the left of the zero line, increasing trends to the right.*

4. *Confidence intervals are similar for men and women; the population surveys sampled them in similar numbers.*

5. G54 shows similar trends in risk-factor scores between men and women in the various populations. The majority of male populations show a decrease, to the left of zero, in all but six populations. In women, there is a similar pattern with all but nine populations showing a decline in risk-factor score. Age-specific data are not published.

G55

6. *G55 is a spot map showing the geographical distribution of the results shown in G54. Some of the confidence intervals in G54 include zero. The populations concerned are marked by black spots. Those with a significant decrease in risk-factor score are marked with blue spots, while a significant increase is shown with a red spot.*

7. Most populations show a significant decrease in risk-factor score between the initial and final surveys. Only three in each sex show a significant increase.

8. The coronary risk-factor score is a derived variable. See MONICA Publications 12, 32 and 33 (*2*). The prime function of the risk-factor score was in testing the coronary risk factor, or First MONICA Hypothesis in MONICA Publication 38 (*2*). The quality scores of the risk factors contributing to the risk-factor score are summarized in the methodological appendix to MONICA Publication 38, published on the MONICA Website and MONICA CD-ROM (*1*).

1. See Monograph CD-ROM or MONICA Website http://www.ktl.fi/monica/.
2. Full references and summaries of MONICA Publications appear in #85/86.

G54 Ten-year change in average coronary risk-factor score

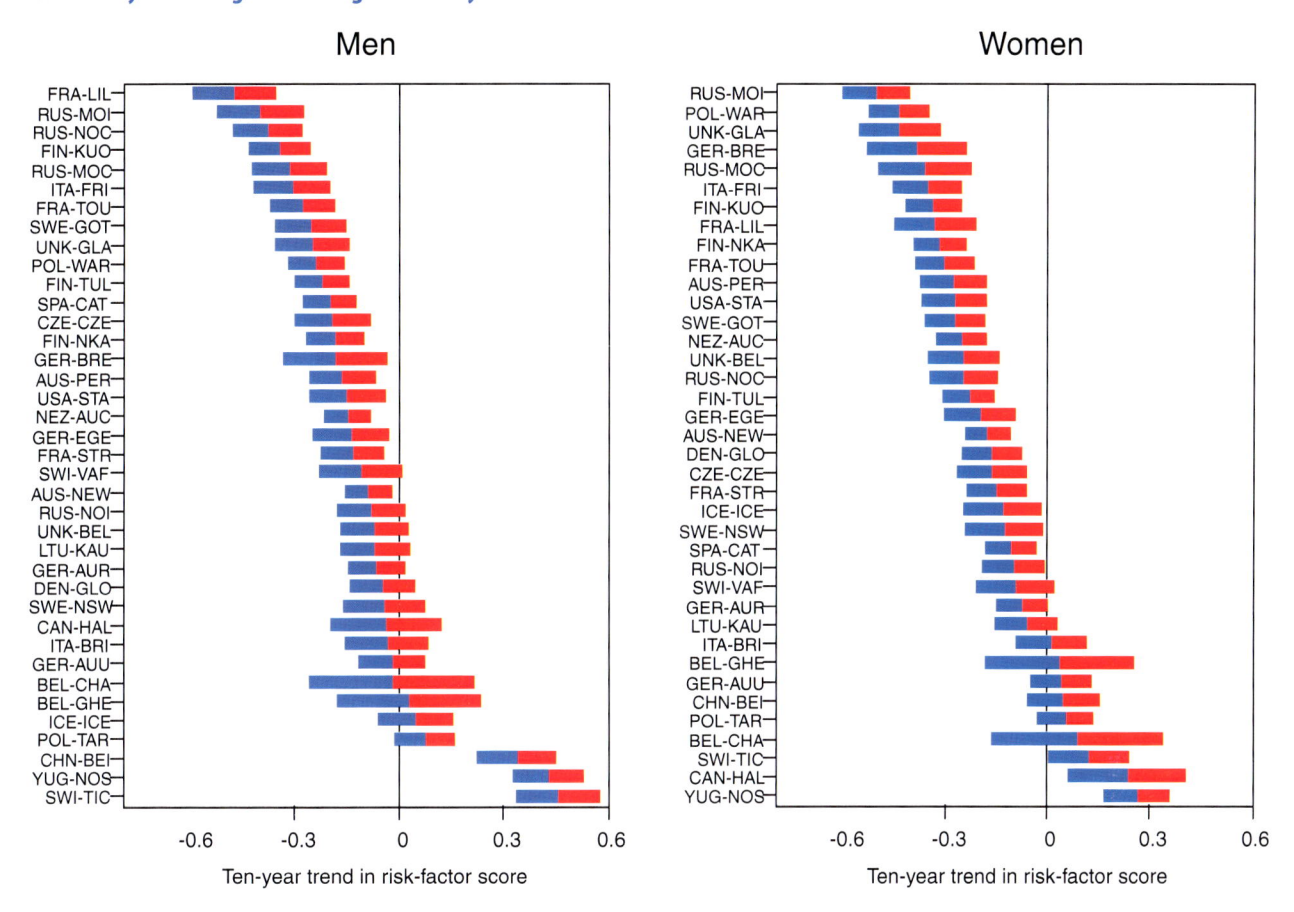

Men

Women

Ten-year trend in risk-factor score

G55 Spot maps of population changes in average coronary risk-factor score

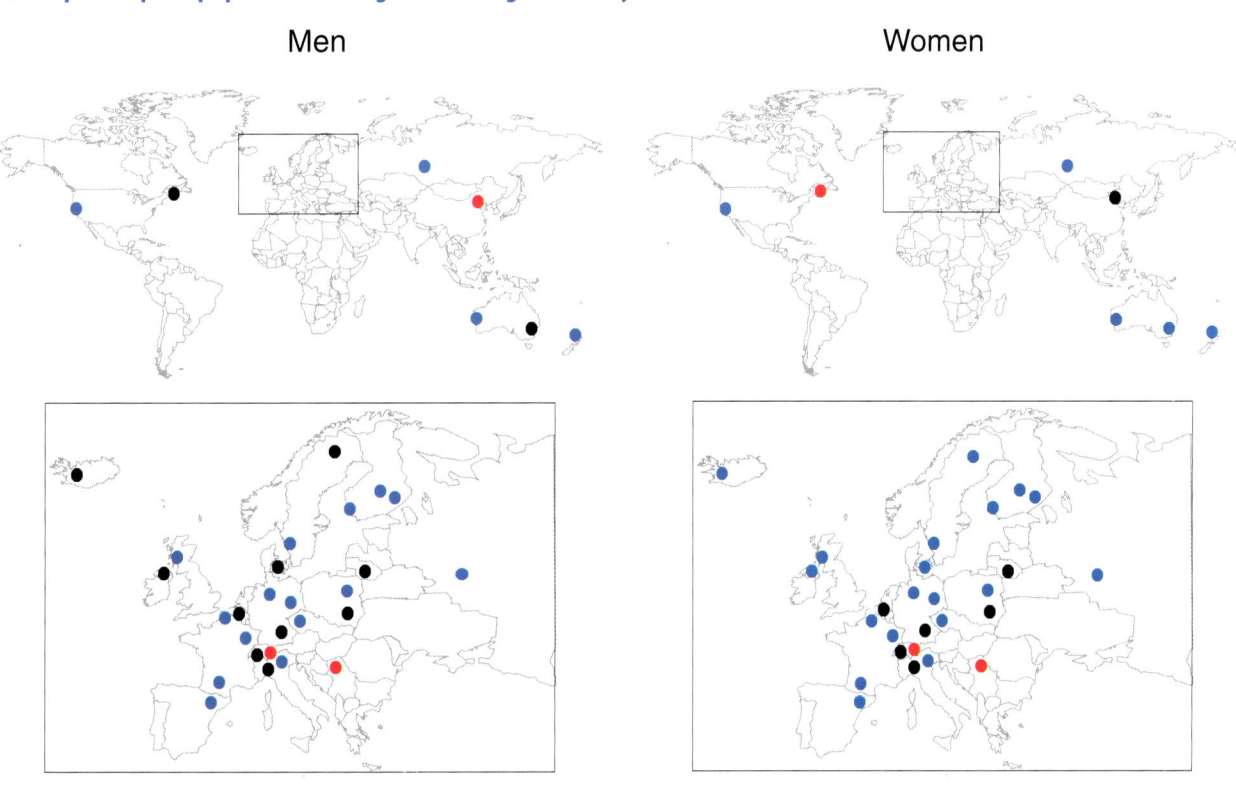

Men

Women

Significant increase
Insignificant change
Significant decrease

RISK FACTORS: RISK-FACTOR SCORE 213

Risk factors: risk-factor quality scores

1. G56 shows scatter plots for the change in each risk factor against the quality score for that factor awarded after assessment of the data in the MONICA Quality assessment reports (1). See #12 Quality Assurance.

2. Quality scores covered items that could be assessed centrally from external quality control, from questionnaires completed by the investigators and from careful analysis of the data. A poor score was not a guarantee that results were unreliable. Conversely, a good score did not guarantee that results were not biased. There could be biases that had not been anticipated or could not be measured and assessed. In MONICA a score of 2.0 was awarded for data of acceptable and consistent quality with no major problems, 1.0 for data with minor problems or inconsistencies and 0.0 where there were significant problems that could not be solved retrospectively. A score of 0.0 is a bad score, but it does not of itself mean that data are unreliable, only that there is major concern about their quality.

3. Scoring was explicit and transparent, and done with the knowledge and cooperation of the investigators concerned. Quality problems are all discussed in the appropriate Quality assessment reports (1). Bias is more important than random error because it is average values that are being compared.

4. Ideally, the great majority of populations would achieve high scores, and the trends being measured would be large in relation to potential measurement errors. Populations with high scores would show the widest variation in risk-factor trends, so there would be no relation between poor scores and extreme results for trends.

5. The manuscript groups decided that MONICA could not exclude populations from hypothesis testing if a few data items were questionable, because almost all centres had some problem with one item or another. Instead it chose to incorporate quality scores into the collaborative analyses. See #12 Quality Assurance, MONICA Publication 38 (2), and its Appendix (1) published on the MONICA Website and CD-ROM.

6. Main results of hypothesis-testing appeared relatively insensitive to whether data quality scores were incorporated or not, and with what weighting. See MONICA Publications 38, 39 (2).

7. In G56 results appear satisfactory for smoking, blood pressure, and body mass index, and less than satisfactory for cholesterol.

8. Two populations with significant increase in total cholesterol between the initial and final surveys had the lowest quality score for this item.

9. Results of quality assessment for total cholesterol were not satisfactory. Those for HDL-cholesterol, not a core risk factor, but of great interest, were worse. This was despite involvement from the start of an external quality control centre, use of standard protocols and preliminary training, and testing with circulation of materials. Methods have advanced since the early 1980s, but standardization and quality control problems never disappear. Anyone denying their existence cannot have looked for them. Investigators in studies such as MONICA need to invest considerably in this area and should assume that they will have problems.

10. The WHO MONICA Project was ahead of its time in the 1980s in placing great emphasis on quality assurance. It also set a precedent by putting all its indicators of performance into the public domain by publishing them on its Website (1).

11. Quality scores aid the interpretation of individual trends. Along with estimates of precision, they were fundamental to the testing of the MONICA hypotheses by providing a means for involving different populations with differing reliability of data. See #40 *Statistical Analysis—relating changes in risk factors and treatments to changes in event rates*, MONICA Publication 38, 39 (2).

1. **See Monograph CD-ROM or MONICA Website http://www.ktl.fi/monica/.**
2. **Full references and summaries of MONICA Publications appear in #85/86.**

G56 Scatter plots by population of change in risk factors against their quality scores

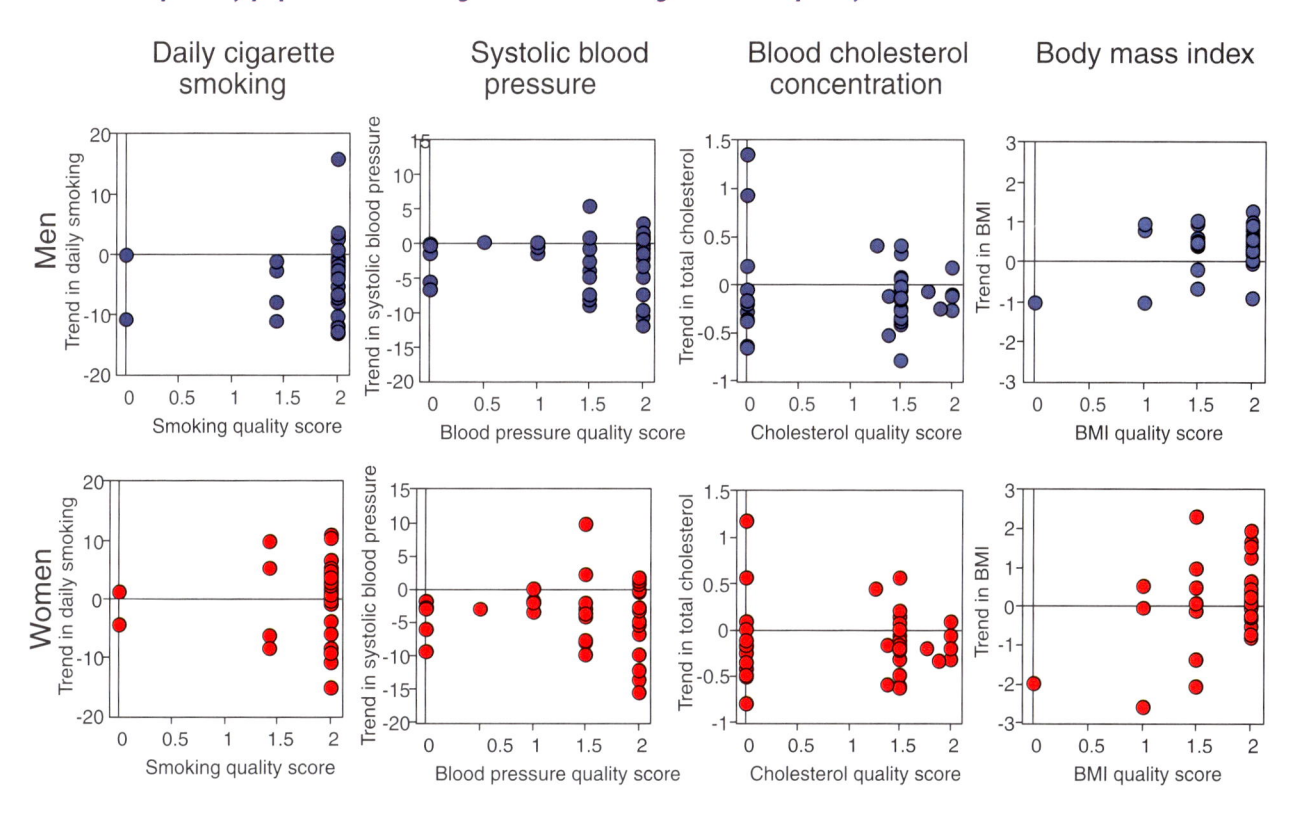

RISK FACTORS: RISK-FACTOR QUALITY SCORES

Eight evidence-based treatments in coronary care

1. Basic coronary-event monitoring did not originally include any treatments or interventions. See G8. When MONICA was planned around 1980, it was not known whether acute coronary care was effective: most coronary deaths were sudden and untreated. The First MONICA, or coronary risk-factor Hypothesis seemed most relevant to disease trends. That acute care influenced survival in coronary events, (or its complement case fatality), was the basis of the Second MONICA or coronary care Hypothesis. The importance of cardiac drugs and treatment in secondary prevention was insufficiently appreciated.

2. For coronary care MONICA investigators were to record all relevant medication and interventions in coronary events for three phases of each coronary event: before the onset, after the onset during the pre-hospital and hospital period, and at discharge from hospital. A minimum of 500 consecutive cases was to be studied in two periods, near the start and at the end of coronary-event registration.

3. The 500 cases included large numbers both of untreated sudden deaths, in which there was difficulty in identifying previous medication, and also of non-fatal possible myocardial infarction, not included in MONICA case definition 1. See #23 *Diagnosing Myocardial Infarction and Coronary Death*. Coronary care data were most complete for non-fatal definite myocardial infarctions, a minority of the 500. Later it was agreed to monitor coronary care continuously, but data remained scanty from the first period.

4. The manuscript group examining the Second MONICA Hypothesis decided to study change in coronary care in non-fatal definite acute myocardial infarction across the two periods against change in major coronary end-points. Event rates, case fatality and mortality could not be measured in non-fatal cases alone, so a contemporaneous or overlapping period of full coronary-event registration was used.

5. The two periods of coronary care in each population, and associated but sometimes longer periods of coronary-event registration were shown in G11. Both coronary care, and coronary-registration periods are a sub-set of the data available. G11 showed that time periods are not the same, and distances between them are unequal, in different populations. Treatment changes are not standardized improvement rates, but simple differences. The manuscript group concentrated on eight evidence-based treatments.

6. G57 and G58 show change in use of beta-blockers, in cases of definite non-fatal myocardial infarction, between two time periods. A blue bar indicates increasing use, the left end is the treatment level per cent in the first period; the right end that in the second. Red bars indicate decreasing use, the right end is the treatment level per cent in the first period; the left end that in the second. The colourless gap to the left is common to both. Beta-blockers were widely used throughout the MONICA period. This explains why the blue and red bars begin a long way from zero

7. G57 shows use of beta-blockers prior to myocardial infarction. Up to one half of new coronary events occur in those with previous angina pectoris, or myocardial infarction, in whom prior treatment might be expected. The other half would have no previous history of coronary heart disease, but some had hypertension. The scale maximum is 50%. G57 shows population RUAs with increasing but also decreasing use before infarction, possibly because of competing drugs for angina and hypertension.

8. G58 shows use during non-fatal definite myocardial infarction. The scale maximum is 100%. Use during infarction increased substantially in many but not all population RUAs as the findings of large randomized controlled trials fed through into practice. There is considerable heterogeneity.

9. Populations, listed alphabetically by country are those described in note 4c for G1 and G2. The asterisk for Swiss women marks missing data.

10. Beta-blockers are only one of numerous treatments and interventions that were recorded. See #24 *Acute Coronary Care*, MONICA Manual Part IV, Section 1, paragraph 4.1.4.3 (*1*), MONICA Quality assessment of acute coronary care data (*1*), the MONICA Data Book of coronary care, tables 11a-p, 12a-p, 13a-p (*1*), MONICA Publication 39 (*2*) the MONICA Second Hypothesis, or coronary care paper. The latter gives the denominators for each of these data points. Its Appendix, published on the MONICA Website (*1*) and Monograph CD-ROM, includes a review of why specific drugs were chosen for this analysis.

1. See Monograph CD-ROM or MONICA Website http://www.ktl.fi/monica/.
2. Full references and summaries of MONICA Publications appear in #85/86.

G57 Change in beta blocker use before myocardial infarction

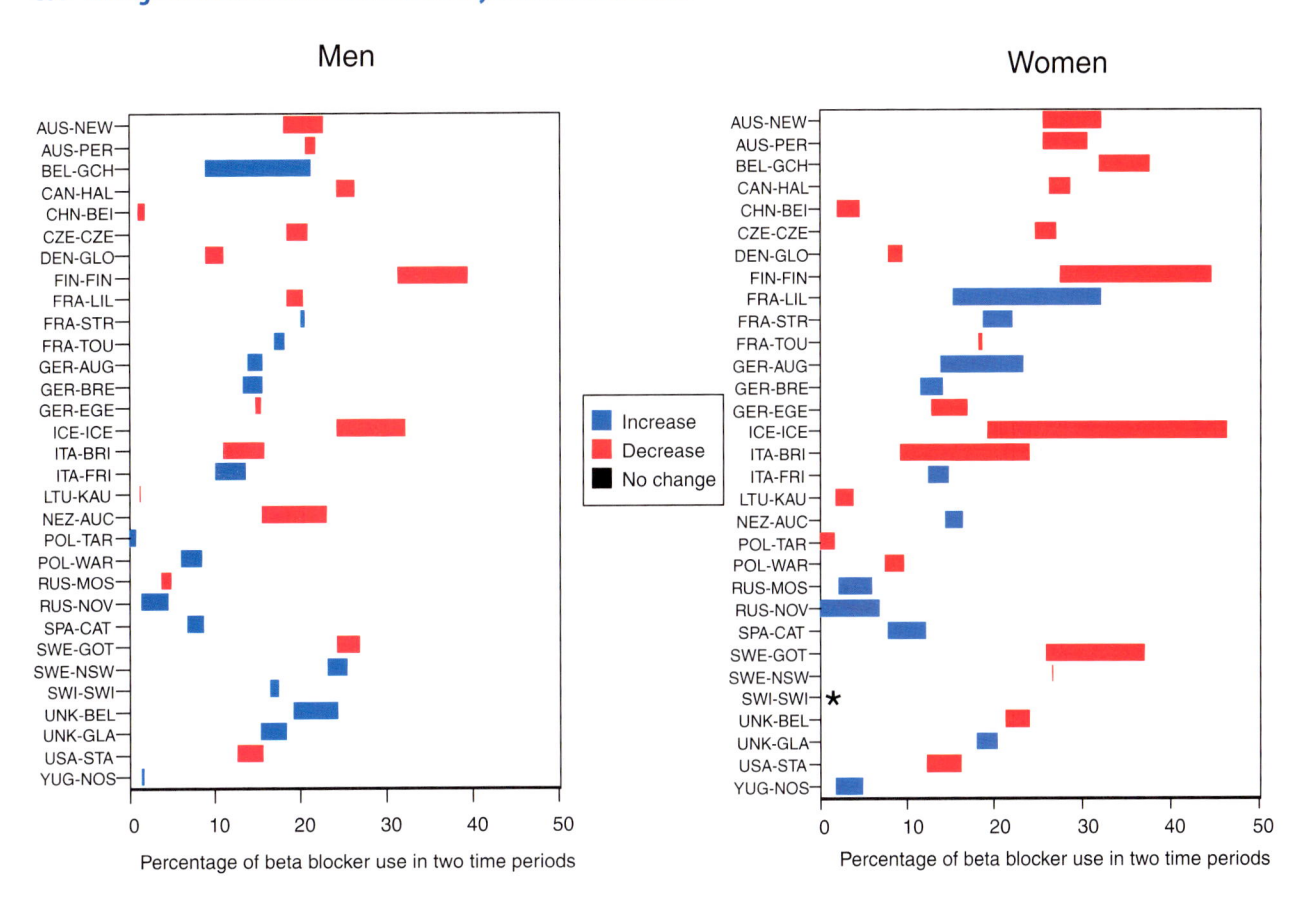

Men

Women

Percentage of beta blocker use in two time periods

- Increase
- Decrease
- No change

G58 Change in beta blocker use during myocardial infarction

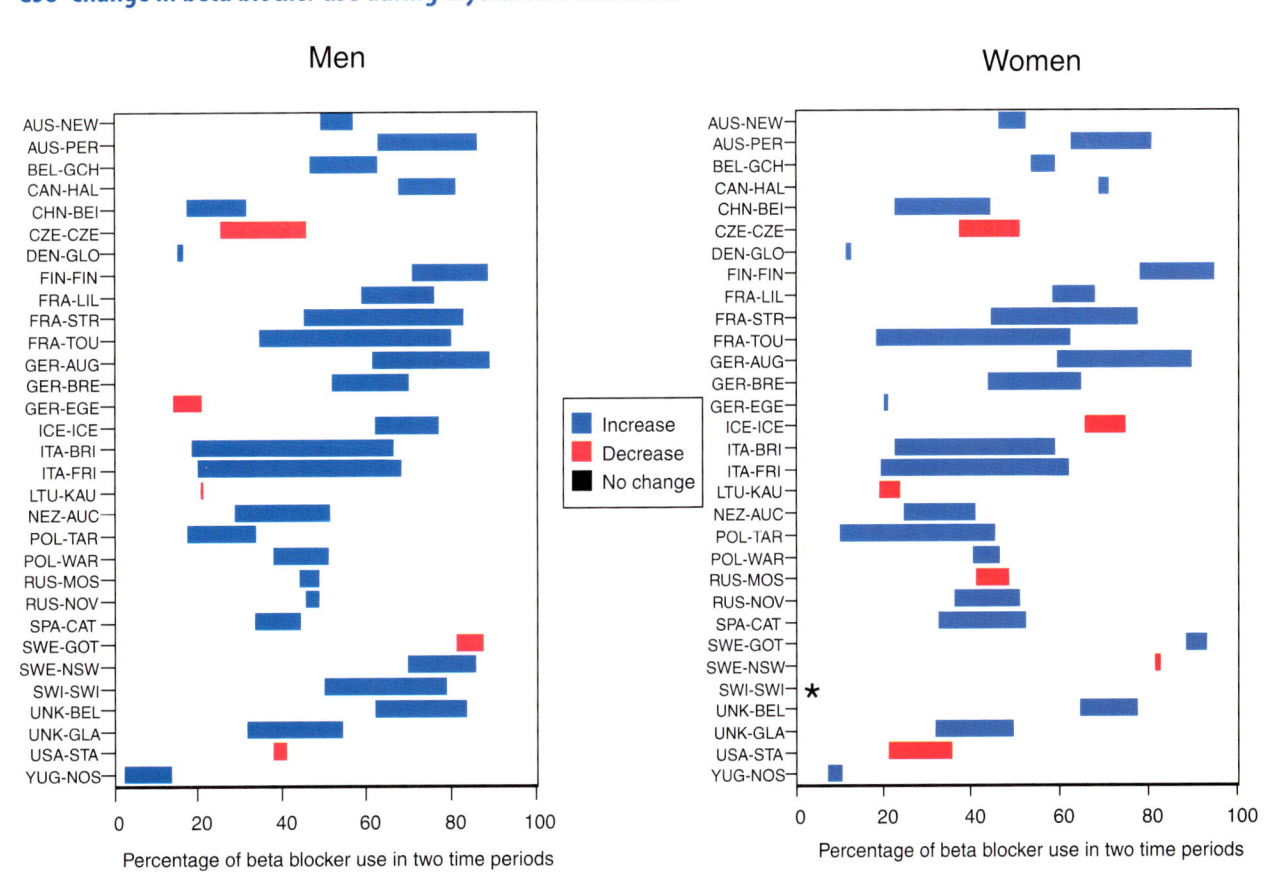

Men

Women

Percentage of beta blocker use in two time periods

- Increase
- Decrease
- No change

EIGHT EVIDENCE-BASED TREATMENTS IN CORONARY CARE

Notes in italics are repeated to help random browsers—systematic readers should ignore them

1. *See background notes at the beginning of this section, for G57 and G58, numbered 1–5.*

2. G59 and G60 show change in use of antiplatelet drugs, (usually aspirin), in the treatment of definite non-fatal myocardial infarction, between two time periods. *A blue bar indicates increasing use, the left end is the treatment level per cent in the first period; the right end that in the second. Red bars indicate decreasing use, the right end is the treatment level per cent in the first period, and the left end that in the second. The colourless gap to the left is common to both.*

3. G59 shows change in use before myocardial infarction. *Up to one half or so of coronary events occur in those with previous angina pectoris, or myocardial infarction, stroke or peripheral vascular disease in which prior treatment might be expected. The other half would have no such history so the scale maximum is 50%.* Antiplatelet drugs were being introduced when MONICA began, both in acute care and in secondary prevention, but the impact on treatment of the major trials came while it was in progress. G59 shows that prior use was found to have increased to up to 30% of cases of non-fatal myocardial infarction coming into care. *Specific changes in particular population RUAs should be cross-referenced with the time periods shown in G1 (1).*

4. G60 shows use during non-fatal definite myocardial infarction. The scale maximum is 100%. Antiplatelet drugs were being introduced when MONICA began, both in acute care and in secondary prevention, but the impact of the major trials came while it was in progress. During MONICA monitoring of coronary care usage of these drugs increased by 70% in some populations making this the largest increase in use of any of the treatments we studied. *Specific changes in particular population RUAs should be cross-referenced with the time periods shown in G1 (1).*

5. *Populations, listed alphabetically by country, are those in note 4c for G1 and G2. The asterisk for Swiss women marks absent data.*

6. Antiplatelet drugs are only one of numerous treatments and interventions that were recorded. See #24 Acute Coronary Care, MONICA Manual Part IV, Section 1, paragraph 4.1.4.3 (1), MONICA Quality assessment of acute coronary care data (1), the MONICA Data Book of coronary care, tables 11a-p, 12a-p, 13a-p (1), MONICA Publication 39 (2) the MONICA Second Hypothesis, or coronary care paper. The latter gives the denominators for each of these data points. Its Appendix, published on the MONICA Website (1) and Monograph CD-ROM, includes a review of why specific drugs were chosen for this analysis.

1. **See Monograph CD-ROM or MONICA Website http://www.ktl.fi/monica/.**
2. **Full references and summaries of MONICA Publications appear in #85/86.**

G59 Change in antiplatelet (aspirin) use before myocardial infarction

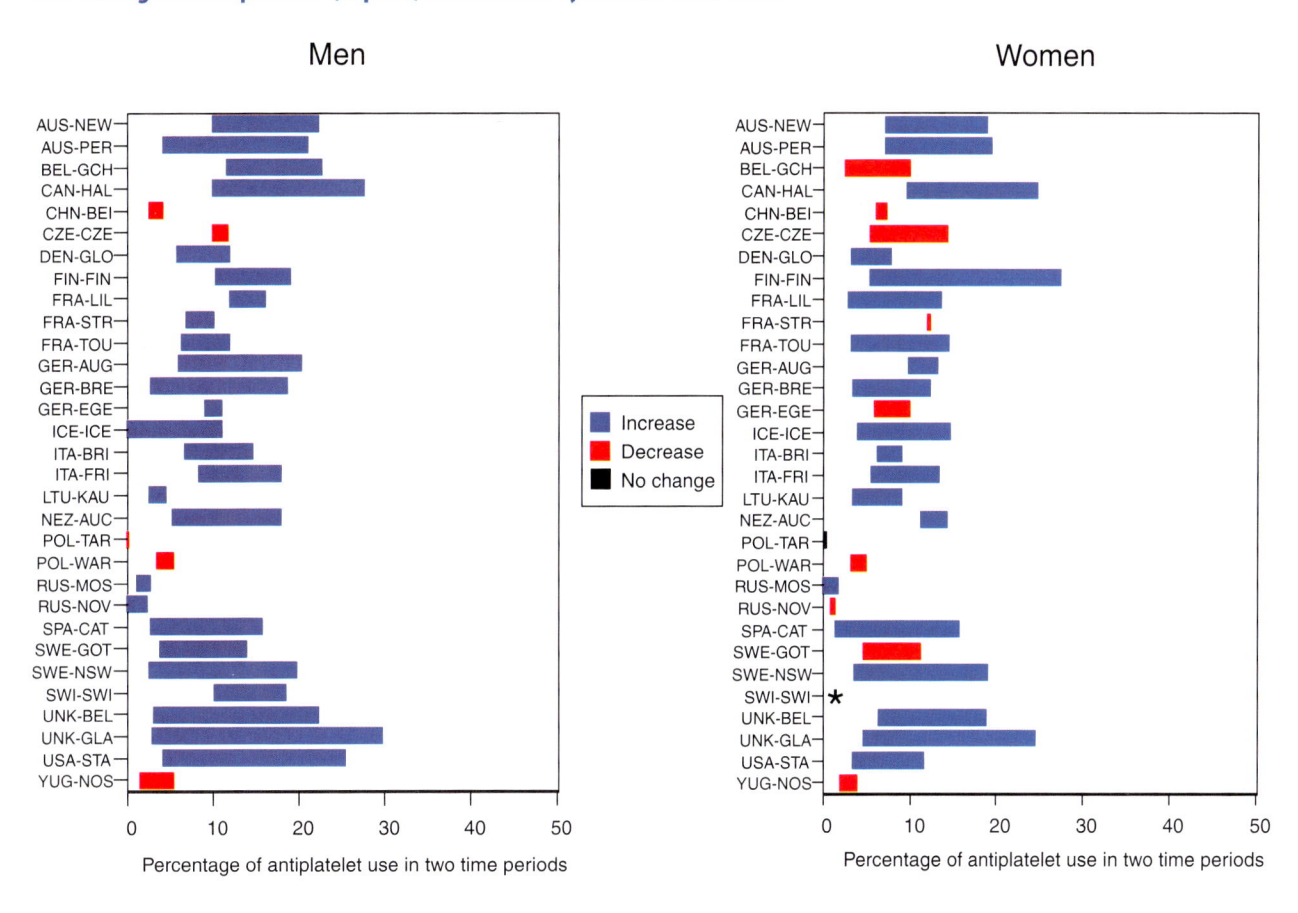

Men

Women

G60 Change in antiplatelet (aspirin) use during myocardial infarction

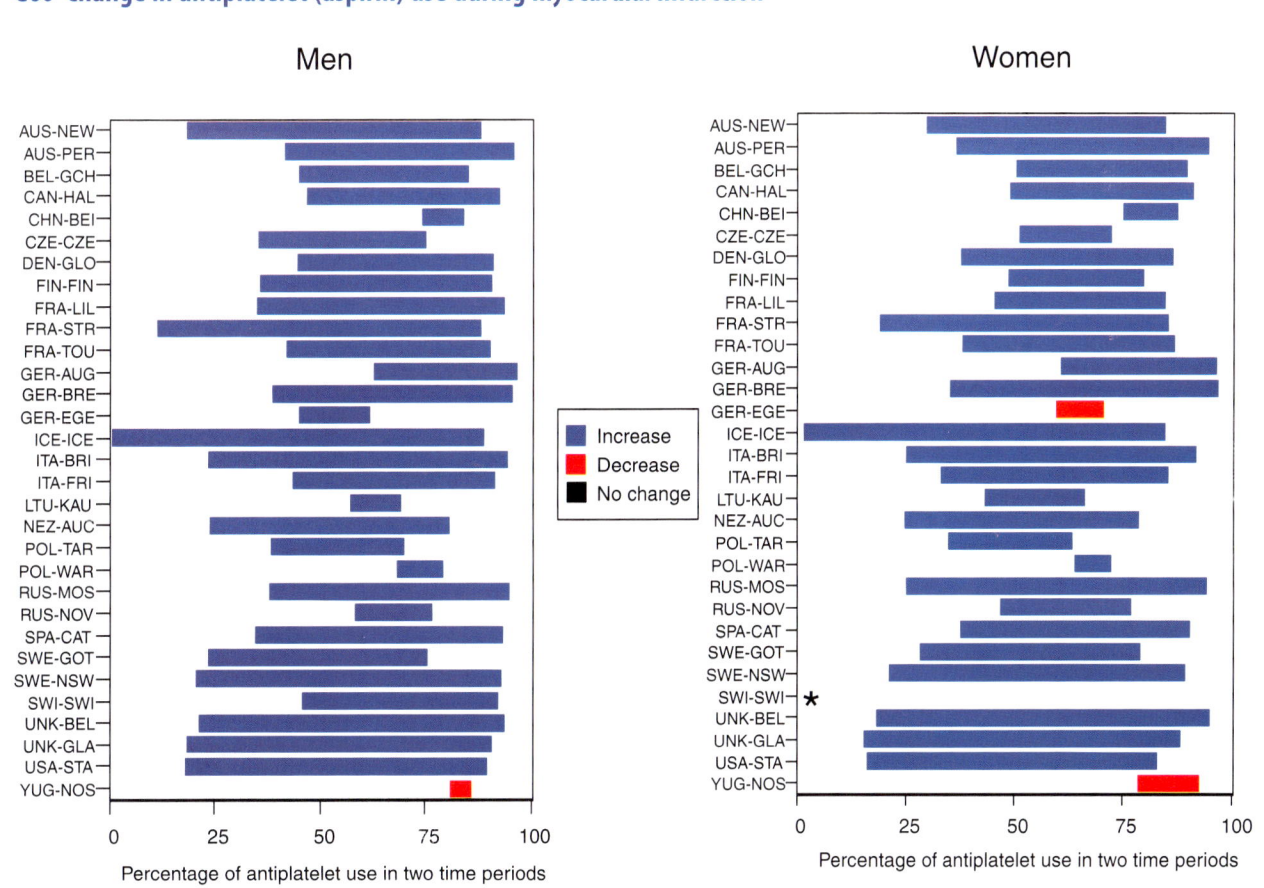

Men

Women

EIGHT EVIDENCE-BASED TREATMENTS IN CORONARY CARE

Notes in italics are repeated to help random browsers—systematic readers should ignore them

1. *See background notes at the beginning of this section, for G57 and G58, numbered 1–5.*

2. G61 and G62 show change in use of ACE inhibitor drugs (angiotensin-converting-enzyme inhibitors), in the treatment of definite non-fatal myocardial infarction, between two time periods. *A blue bar indicates increasing use, the left end is the treatment level per cent in the first period; the right end that in the second. Red bars indicate decreasing use, the right end is the treatment level per cent in the first period, and the left end that in the second. The colourless gap to the left is common to both.*

3. G61 shows change in use before myocardial infarction. *Up to one half or so of coronary events occur in those with previous angina pectoris, or myocardial infarction, or other atheromatous disease, the other half would have no such history although some will have a history of hypertension. The scale maximum here is 50%.* When MONICA began ACE inhibitor drugs were just about to be introduced, both in acute coronary care and in the treatment of hypertension and heart failure. The impact on treatment of the major trials came while it was in progress; recent suggestions of general use for secondary prevention of coronary heart disease post-dated the MONICA study. G61 shows that prior use increased from almost zero to as much as 18% of cases of non-fatal myocardial infarction coming into care, presumably much of it for previously detected hypertension. *Specific changes in particular population RUAs should be cross-referenced with the time periods shown in G11.*

4. G62 shows use during non-fatal definite myocardial infarction. The scale maximum is 100%. ACE inhibitors were just about to be introduced when MONICA began, but the impact of the major trials on their use for left ventricular dysfunction during myocardial infarction came while it was in progress. During MONICA monitoring of coronary care, use of these drugs increased from low levels up to as much as 50% in some populations making this one of the larger increases in the use of the eight treatments we studied. The colourless gaps to the left of the blue bars in G62 suggest that ACE inhibitors were more widely used in men than women for myocardial infarction in the first period. *Specific changes in particular population RUAs should be cross-referenced with the time periods shown in G11.*

5. *Populations, listed alphabetically by country, are those in note 4c for G1 and G2. The asterisk for Swiss women marks absent data.*

6. ACE inhibitors are only one of numerous treatments and interventions that were recorded. *See #24 Acute Coronary Care, MONICA Manual Part IV, Section 1, paragraph 4.1.4.3 (1), MONICA Quality assessment of acute coronary care data (1), the MONICA Data Book of coronary care, tables 11a-p, 12a-p, 13a-p (1), MONICA Publication 39 (2) the MONICA Second Hypothesis, or coronary care paper. The latter gives the denominators for each of these data points. Its Appendix, published on the MONICA Website (1) and Monograph CD-ROM, includes a review of why specific drugs were chosen for this analysis.*

1. **See Monograph CD-ROM or MONICA Website http://www.ktl.fi/monica/.**
2. **Full references and summaries of MONICA Publications appear in #85/86.**

G61 Change in angiotensin converting enzyme (ACE) inhibitor use before myocardial infarction

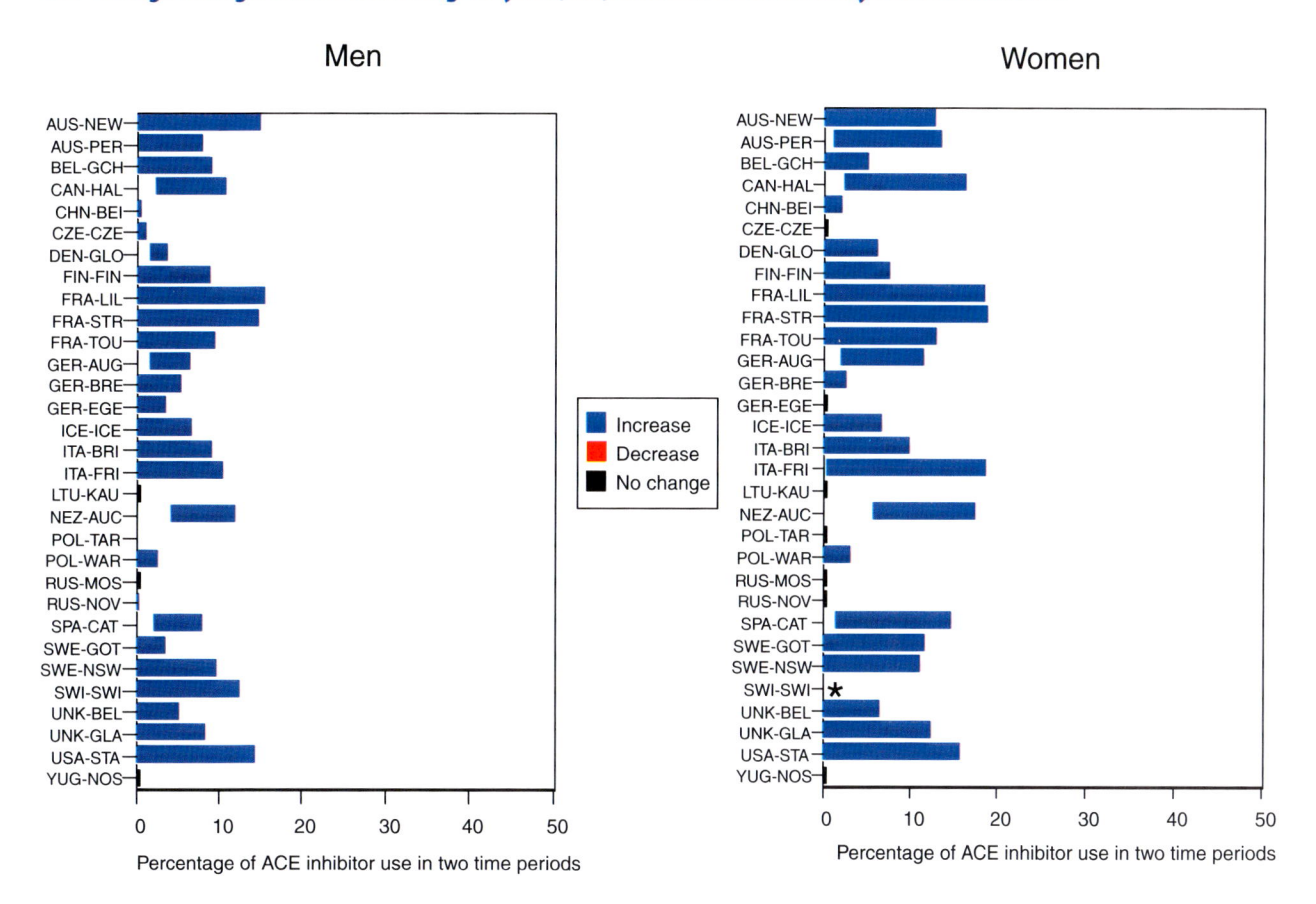

Men

Women

Percentage of ACE inhibitor use in two time periods

Legend: Increase (blue), Decrease (red), No change (black)

G62 Change in angiotensin converting enzyme (ACE) inhibitor use during myocardial infarction

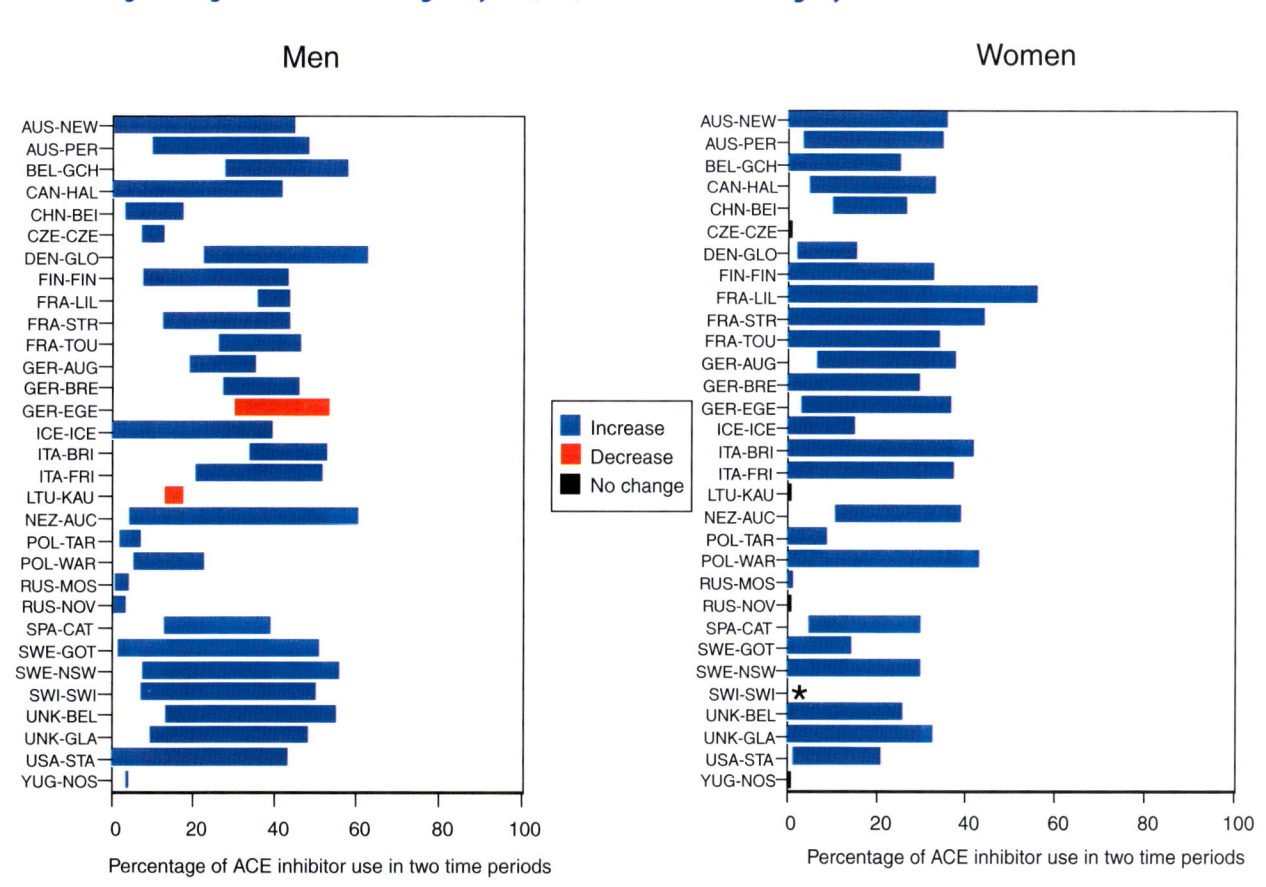

Men

Women

Percentage of ACE inhibitor use in two time periods

Legend: Increase (blue), Decrease (red), No change (black)

Notes in italics are repeated to help random browsers—systematic readers should ignore them

1. *See background notes at the beginning of this section, for G57 and G58, numbered 1–5.*

2. G63 shows change in prior coronary artery revascularization and G64, change in use of thrombolytic therapy in the acute treatment of definite non-fatal myocardial infarction between two time periods. *A blue bar indicates increasing use, the left end is the treatment level per cent in the first period; the right end that in the second. Red bars indicate decreasing use, the right end is the treatment level per cent in the first period; the left end that in the second. The colourless gap to the left is common to both.*

3. G63 shows coronary artery revascularization procedures any time before the myocardial infarction being considered. Up to one half of coronary events occur in those with previous angina pectoris, or myocardial infarction, in which prior procedures might be expected. The other half would have no previous history of coronary heart disease. The scale maximum is 50%. Coronary artery bypass surgery was long established when MONICA began, but not common in most MONICA populations. It was supplemented by coronary angioplasty more recently. Prevalence of prior procedures in victims of heart attack is questionable as a measure of the use of such procedures in the general population, but it was the only measure available in the core data for MONICA. See #18 *Health Services*. G63 shows low prevalence in most populations and considerable disparities, but a net increase over time in the majority. *Specific changes in particular population RUAs should be cross-referenced with the time periods shown in G11.*

4. G64 shows use of thrombolytic drugs during non-fatal myocardial infarction. The scale maximum is 100%. Thrombolytic therapy was part of the coronary care revolution, occurring while MONICA was monitoring change. G64 shows a major increase in usage, not quite as much as for antiplatelet drugs, but from a lower level, in many populations. There is marked heterogeneity between populations, unlike antiplatelet drugs, perhaps reflecting the financial cost, and the complexity of administration, compared with aspirin. *Specific changes in particular population RUAs should be cross-referenced with the time periods shown in G11.*

5. *Populations, listed alphabetically by country, are those in note 4c for G1 and G2. The asterisk for Swiss women marks absent data.*

6. These are only two of numerous treatments and interventions that were recorded. *See #24 Acute Coronary Care, MONICA Manual Part IV, Section 1, paragraph 4.1.4.3 (1), MONICA Quality assessment of acute coronary care data (1), the MONICA Data Book of coronary care, tables 11a-p, 12a-p, 13a-p (1), MONICA Publication 39 (2) the MONICA Second Hypothesis, or coronary care paper. The latter gives the denominators for each of these data points. Its Appendix, published on the MONICA Website (1) and Monograph CD-ROM, includes a review of why specific drugs were chosen for this analysis.*

1. **See Monograph CD-ROM or MONICA Website http://www.ktl.fi/monica/.**
2. **Full references and summaries of MONICA Publications appear in #85/86.**

G63 Change in coronary artery revascularization (bypass graft or angioplasty) before myocardial infarction

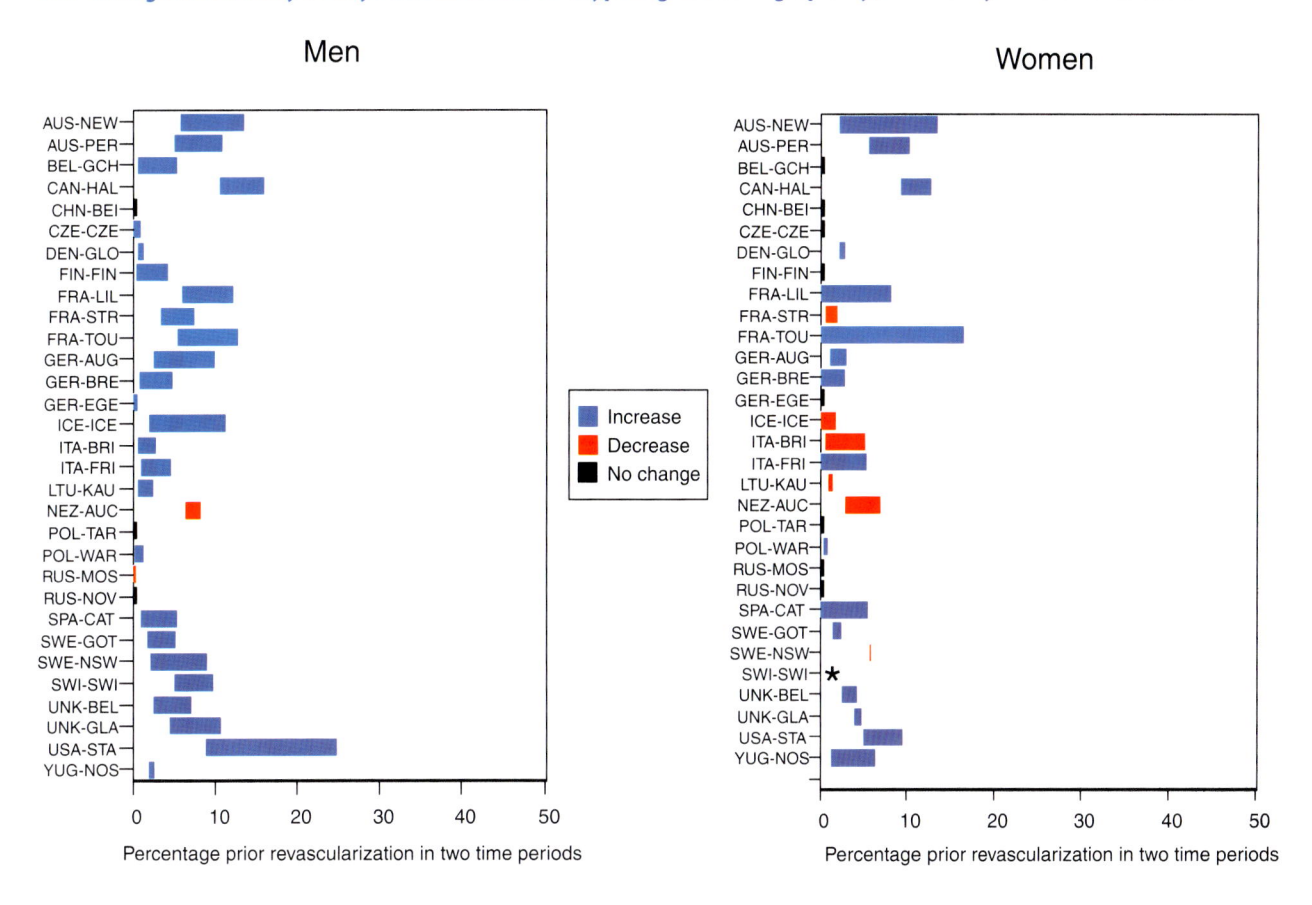

Men

Percentage prior revascularization in two time periods

Women

Percentage prior revascularization in two time periods

G64 Change in thrombolytic drug use during myocardial infarction

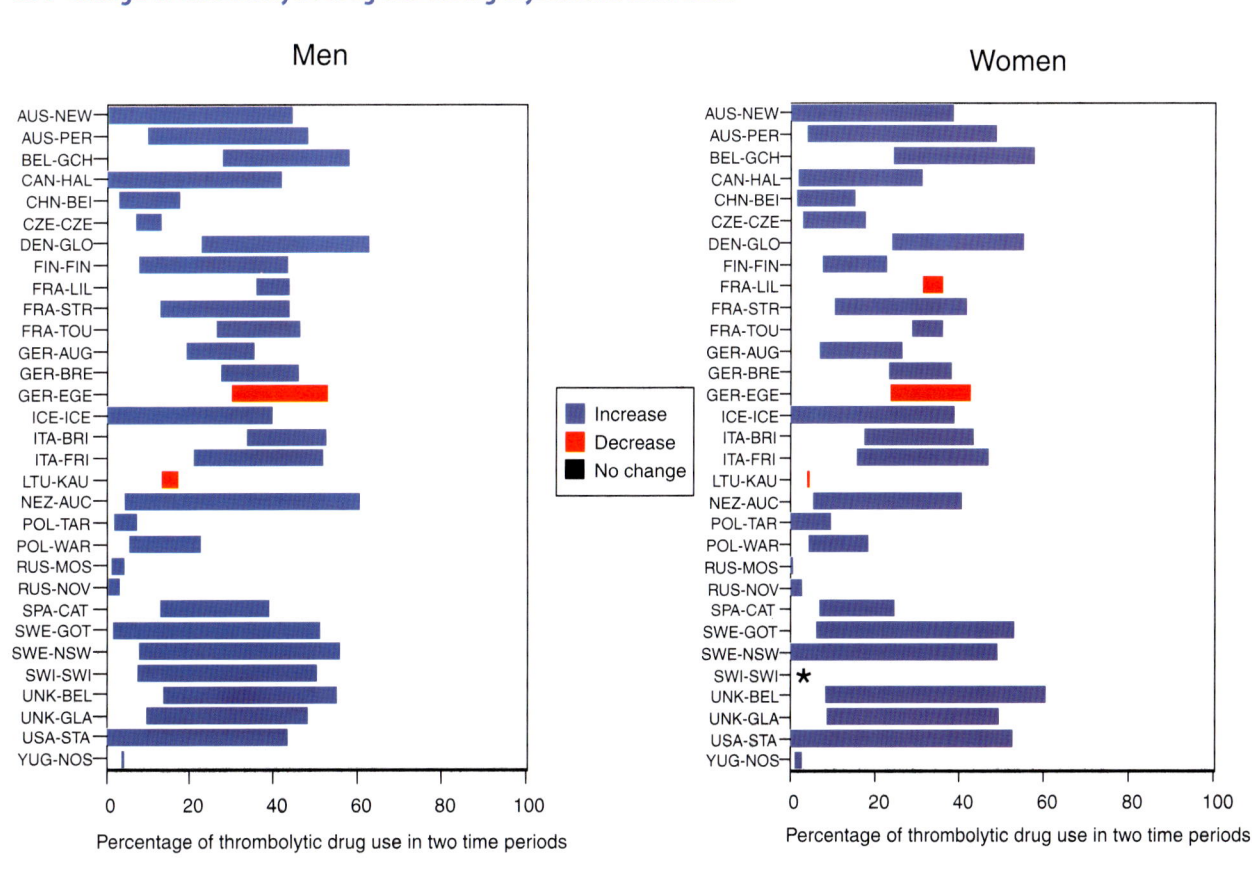

Men

Percentage of thrombolytic drug use in two time periods

Women

Percentage of thrombolytic drug use in two time periods

EIGHT EVIDENCE-BASED TREATMENTS IN CORONARY CARE

1. In order to test the Second or coronary care Hypothesis, MONICA needed an index of coronary care equivalent to the risk-factor score used in the First Hypothesis.

2. The manuscript group was divided between those promoting a sophisticated score, incorporating carefully judged weightings of each component (Weighted Treatment Score), and those who wanted a simple pragmatic score reflecting implementation of evidence-based treatments (Equivalent Treatment Score). See #25 *Treatment scores*, and MONICA Publication 39 (*2*) Appendix. (*1*).

3. Both were tested. A strong correlation was found. The Weighted Treatment Score was strongly affected by one component, because of the heavy weighting given to it, prior coronary artery revascularization procedures (see G63). The simpler score was adopted.

4. The Equivalent Treatment Score, is simply one eighth of the sum of all eight of the treatments per cent, shown in G56 to G64. Three drug groups, beta-blockers, antiplatelet, and ACE-inhibitors, score twice each, once for use before the onset of myocardial infarction, and once for use afterwards. Treatments at hospital discharge were not included in the score but would have been very highly correlated with use in the event.

5. The Equivalent Treatment Score has the greatest contribution from treatments that changed most, in absolute percentage terms, between the two coronary care periods in MONICA. The leader was antiplatelet drugs (aspirin), during the attack (see G60).

6. G65 shows populations listed alphabetically by country, as in previous treatment graphs. The asterisk for Swiss women indicates missing data. G66 shows their ranking by change between the two coronary care periods, as in earlier formats.

7. Note that maximum change in G65, giving a high rank in G66 implies a low start and a high finish point. Populations could rank highly for either or both of these reasons. The actual finishing score was similar in many populations, some of which started with a high score, and therefore ranked only for moderate change. G65 needs to be studied with G11, and with MONICA Publication 39 (*2*), which tabulates numbers and time periods precisely. Differences in population RUAs with high finishing scores from other treatments were often influenced by discrepancies in their use of beta-blockers during infarction in the second period (see G58).

8. Inequality of coronary care periods and the distance between them inhibit simple comparison of the rate of introduction of new therapies. It did not affect the testing of the coronary care hypothesis because end-point changes were compared for similar periods. See later section, G77.

9. The rate of introduction of different therapies can be compared using the MONICA Data Book of coronary care tables 11, 12, 13 (*1*). Treatments tended to be introduced fairly rapidly in a non-linear manner. Only a minority of populations, however, have treatment data for all their years of registration. Years are grouped in the Data Book.

10. Graphs here and the tables in MONICA Data Book on coronary care, tables 11a-p, 12a-p, 13a-p and in MONICA Publication 39 (*2*), show no significant sex bias in the use of evidence-based medication in definite myocardial infarction in the MONICA population RUAs over the decade that was studied. This is despite widespread reporting in the literature of the existence of such a problem. This question is being analysed in a paper being prepared at the same time as this Monograph.

11. Further papers on coronary care are in preparation at the time of writing the Monograph. They will be listed on the MONICA Website as they appear (*1*).

1. **See Monograph CD-ROM or MONICA Website http://www.ktl.fi/monica/.**
2. **Full references and summaries of MONICA Publications appear in #85/86.**

G65 Change in Equivalent Treatment Score

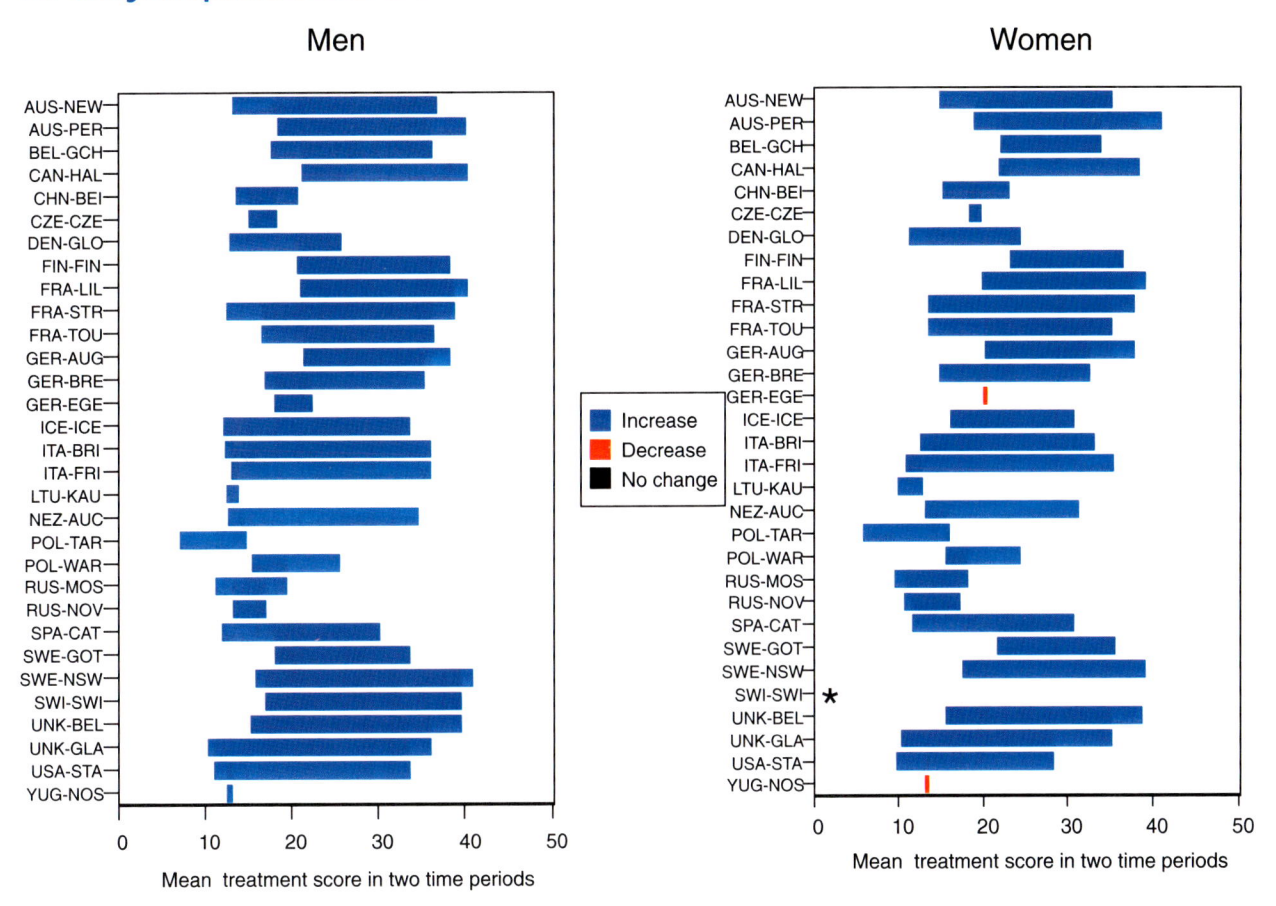

Men

Women

G66 Populations ranked by change in Equivalent Treatment Score

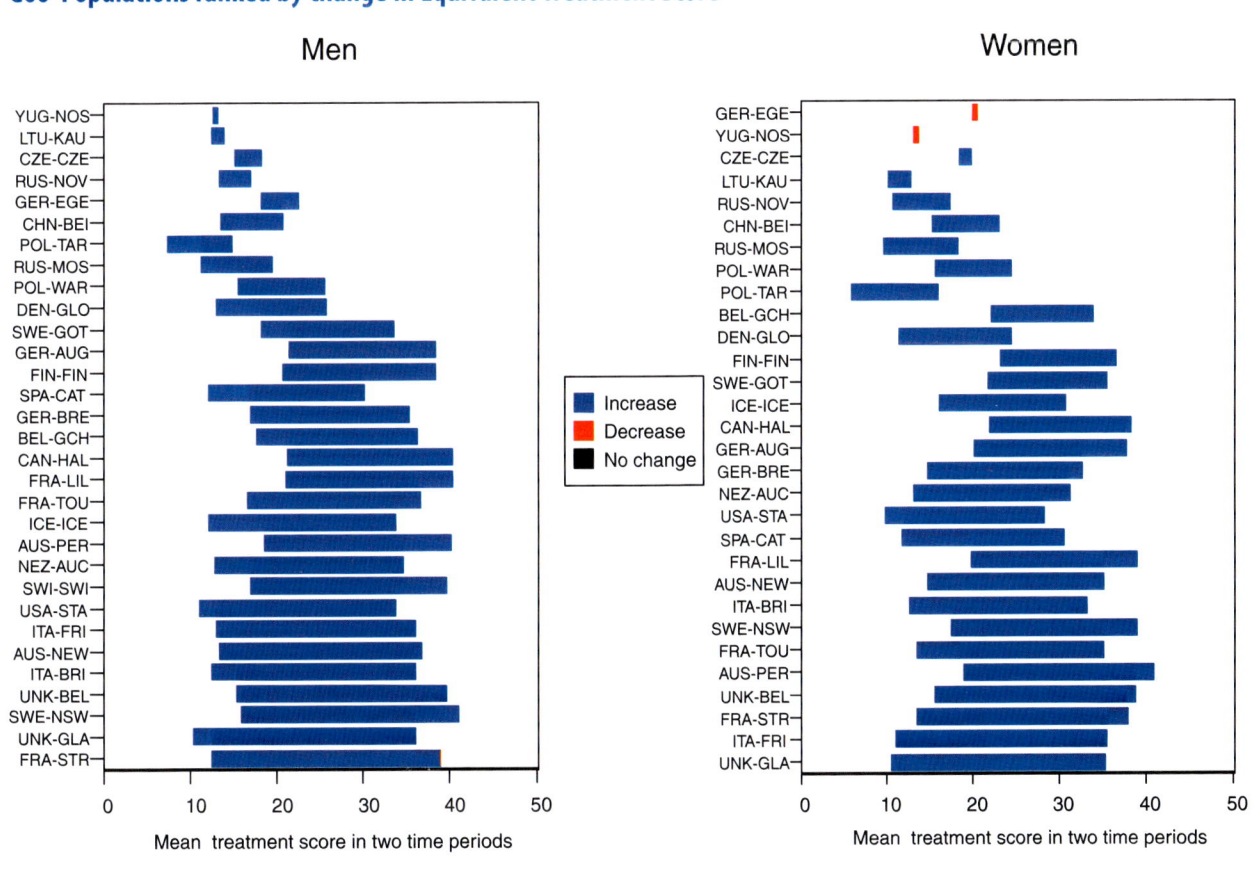

Men

Women

EIGHT EVIDENCE-BASED TREATMENTS IN CORONARY CARE

G67

1. These scatter plots are part of the procedures for testing MONICA findings to see if they are likely to be genuine, or unduly influenced by variations in data quality.

2. A data quality score for coronary care was derived from a number of items. See #12 *Quality Assurance*, MONICA Quality assessment of acute coronary care data, (*1*) MONICA Publication 39 (*2*), Appendix (*1*), (published on MONICA Website and on the Monograph CD-ROM). Such items included the frequency with which coronary care records were missing when they should have been completed, and the frequency with which data were coded as not known, along with other items. The acute coronary care quality score is the same for both sexes in each population RUA.

3. Changes in treatments during the MONICA study period were very large in relation to possible sources of error.

4. Both the greatest and the least changes in Equivalent Treatment Score occurred in populations with high scores for data quality. There were few poor scores for data quality. These were associated with the middle range of treatment changes.

5. It is therefore unlikely that MONICA findings on coronary care are significantly affected by data quality.

G68

6. This shows the geographical distribution of changes in the Equivalent Treatment Score. Large treatment changes are shown in blue while modest ones are shown in red. There is a more striking geographical polarization of results than for any of the previous MONICA spot maps.

7. The previous warning, that unequal periods and different times are being compared, is still true. Examination of G11 however, shows that while a late first coronary care recording period and early second period does apply to some red spot populations (in Germany-East Germany, GER-EGE, #65, they were close together) it does not apply to most. The geographical polarization is therefore real.

8. The polarization of results does raise problems for interpretation of the coronary care hypothesis (see later). If populations are clustered together, can they be considered independent in terms of statistical testing? What else might be happening? See discussion in MONICA Publication 39 (*2*).

1. **See Monograph CD-ROM or MONICA Website http://www.ktl.fi/monica/.**
2. **Full references and summaries of MONICA Publications appear in #85/86.**

G67 Scatter plot of change in Equivalent Treatment Score against the acute coronary care quality score

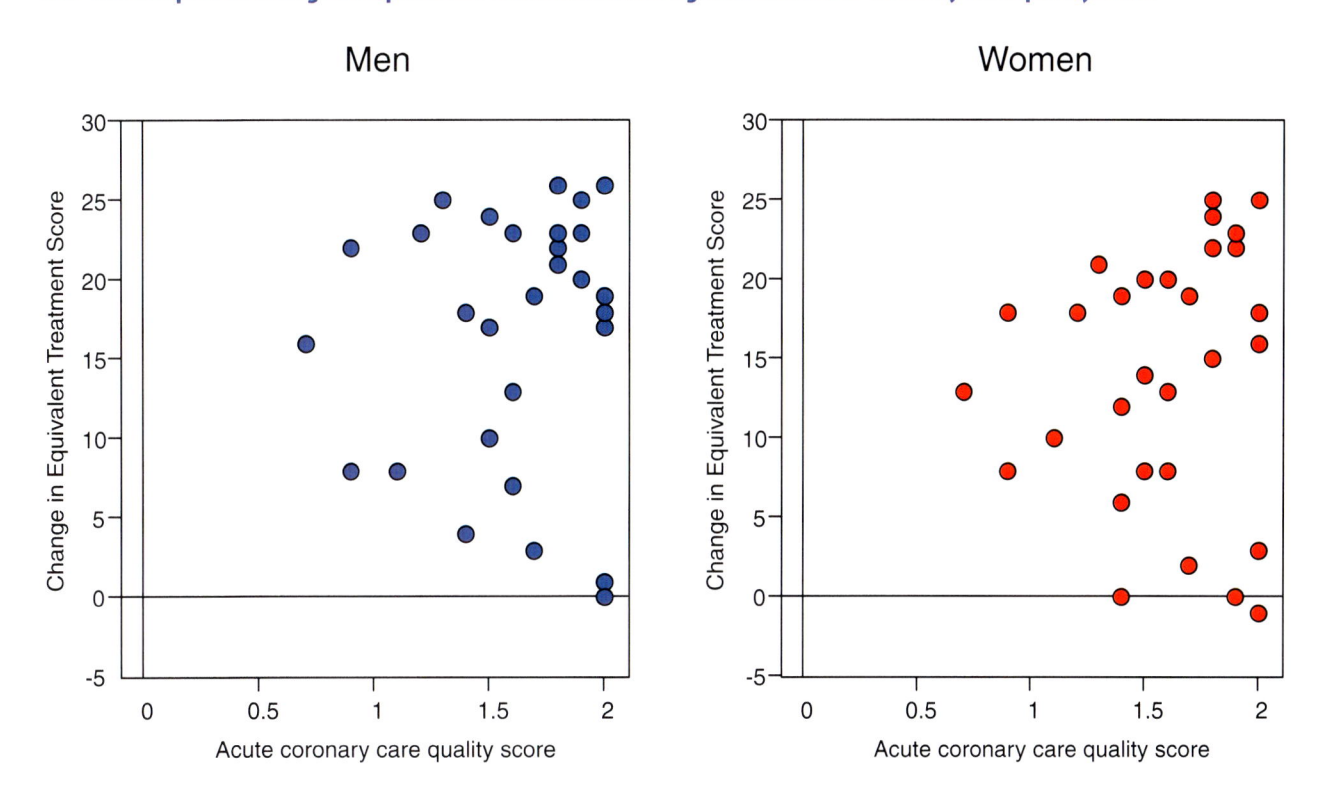

Men

Women

G68 Spot maps of population changes in Equivalent Treatment Score

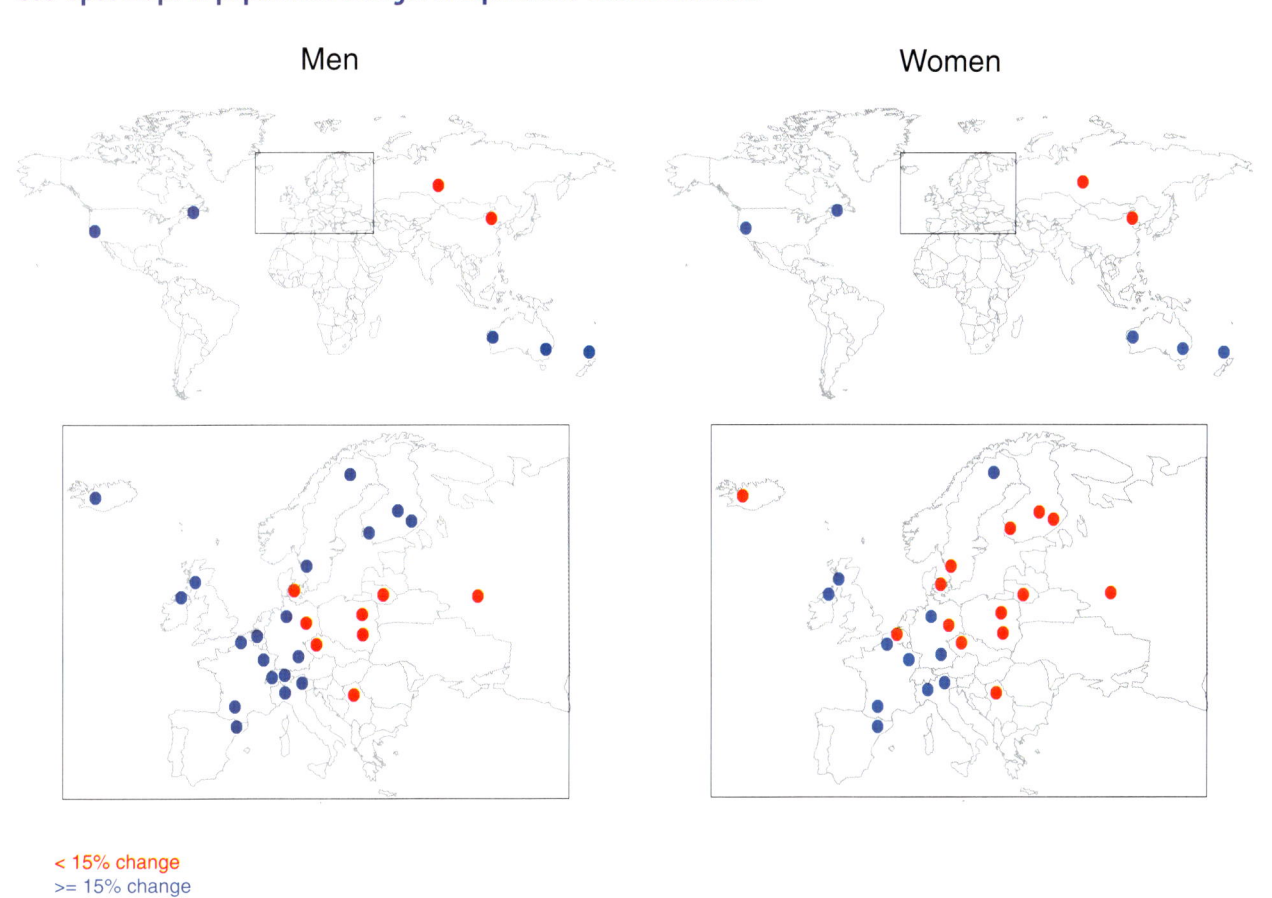

Men

Women

< 15% change
>= 15% change

EIGHT EVIDENCE-BASED TREATMENTS IN CORONARY CARE

Hypotheses: coronary disease and coronary risk factors

1. The following four graphs were plotted during the testing of the First MONICA, or coronary risk-factor Hypothesis, about the association between change in coronary risk factors and change in coronary-event rates. The detailed presentation, along with these graphs, is found in MONICA Publication 38 (*2*). Much of the technical discussion is in its Appendix, published on the MONICA Website and the Monograph CD-ROM (*1*). See also #2 *MONICA Hypotheses and Study Design*, #35 *Risk-Factor Scores*, #40 *Statistical Analysis—relating changes in risk factors and treatments to changes in event rates*.

2. Each coloured point in the plots identifies the location of a MONICA population RUA. It shows how much its risk factors changed in ten years on the x-axis, and how much its event rates changed on the y-axis. Populations are identified in G69 and G70 by their abbreviated 2-letter codes in place of the seven-character identifications, one letter for country, and one for population. See *Appendix* and #51–83.

3. A strong simultaneous association between any change in the coronary-risk score, calculated from changing levels of classical risk factors, and changes in coronary-event rates in the same populations would result in the MONICA populations being arranged along a gradient, or regression line from near the bottom left corner of each plot towards the top right. Calculated regression lines, their equations and 95% confidence limits are added to G69 and G70.

G69

4. The results in G69 come from the whole registration period. They show a modest relation between changes in the risk-factor score and changes in coronary events but also a considerable scatter of populations. At any level of change in the risk-factor score there is considerable variation in the trends in coronary-event rates. Results in men might be considered more precise than in women because of their larger number of coronary events but the gradient of the calculated regression line is small. The variation in the trends in coronary-event rates is badly predicted from the trends in risk factors. In addition a two per cent per year reduction in coronary-event rates is predicted when there is no change in the risk-factor score. The gradient of the regression line in women is more positive, but the MONICA populations are still very scattered about the graph.

G70

5. G70 shows what happens when a lagged (= delayed) registration period is used (see G8). The justification is that change in risk factors must precede a decline in coronary risk, perhaps by a number of years. A time lag was introduced for the beginning of the study period, but not for the end, because most of the final surveys were done at that time or after the end of the event registration periods. Results still show considerable scatter of populations, but the gradients of the regression lines are now considerably steeper. See MONICA Publication 38 (*2*), for a full discussion of the rationale for the lagged registration period.

6. These graphs provoked considerable discussion. Results neither prove nor disprove the coronary risk-factor hypothesis. They can be used to assess the potential contribution of risk-factor change to changing coronary-event rates in whole populations, but there is considerable uncertainty. This leaves potential room for other risk factors or determinants of trends in coronary-event rates, but without actually proving that they exist. One of these is probably drug treatment, see G77.

7. For further information see MONICA Publication 38 (*2*), its appendix on the MONICA Website (*1*) and CD-ROM, the subsequent *Lancet* correspondence and citations of this paper.

1. See Monograph CD-ROM or MONICA Website http://www.ktl.fi/monica/.
2. Full references and summaries of MONICA Publications appear in #85/86.

G69 First MONICA Hypothesis: change in coronary-event rates against change in coronary risk-factor score, full registration period

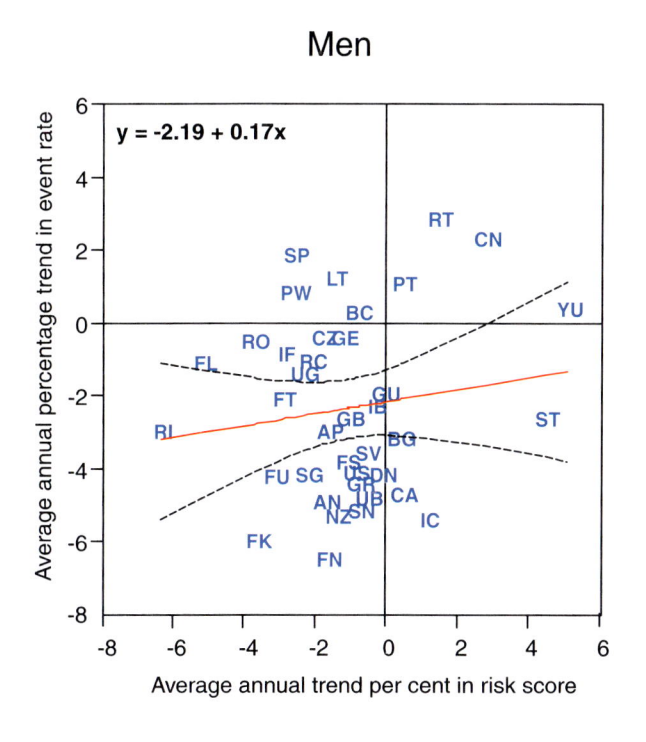

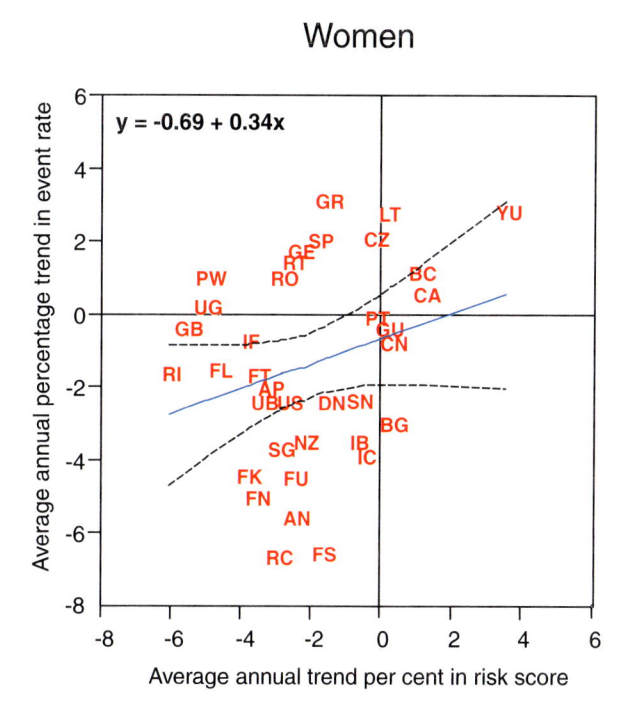

Men

$y = -2.19 + 0.17x$

Women

$y = -0.69 + 0.34x$

G70 First MONICA Hypothesis: change in coronary-event rates against change in coronary risk-factor score, lagged registration period

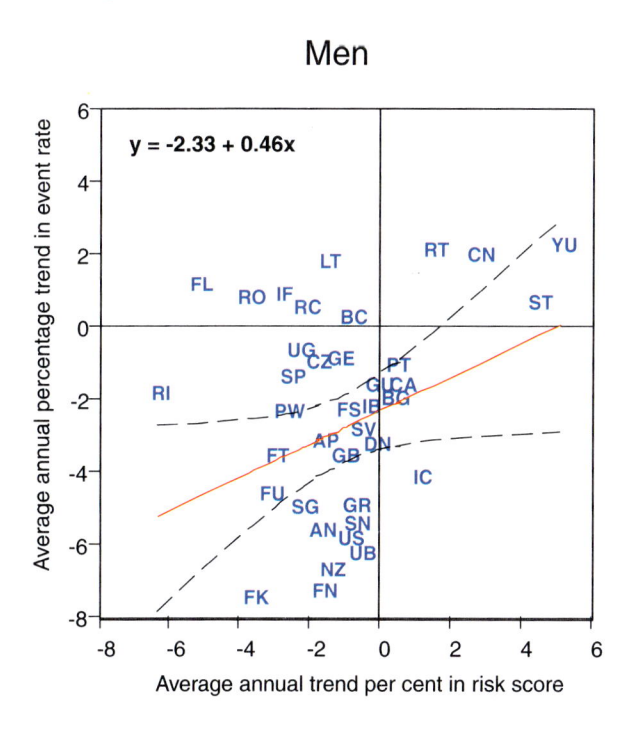

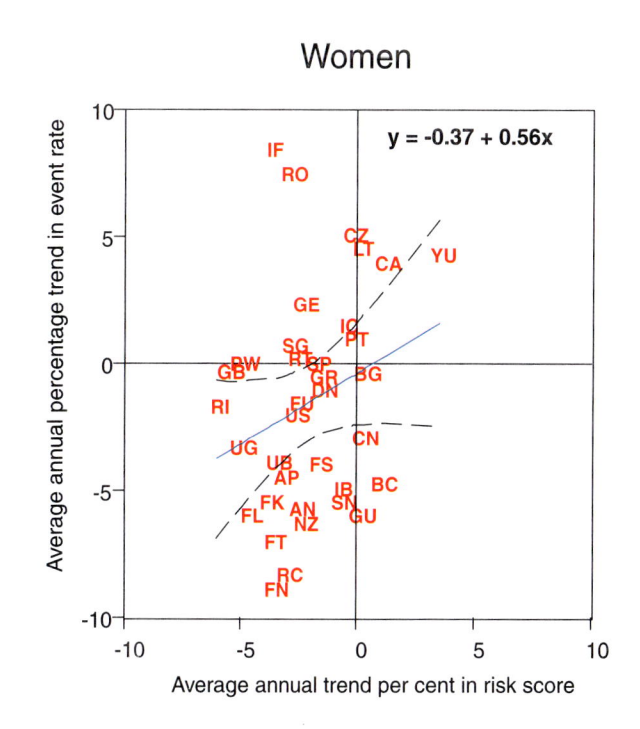

Men

$y = -2.33 + 0.46x$

Women

$y = -0.37 + 0.56x$

1. These graphs should be looked at in association with the notes on G69 and G70.

2. Coronary risk is known to be multi-factorial, so that the effect of one risk factor will be confounded and modified by what is happening to the others. G71 and G72 show changes in coronary-event rates in different populations, in relation to the change in single risk factors, without any correction for the effects of the others. See #35 *Risk-Factor Scores*. Populations are not individually identified, as they were in G69 and G70. Coloured spots are used to mark them. Because the same population results are used in each graph, their positions along the y-axis will be constant for each sex and registration period, but the position on the x-axis will vary with the risk factor concerned. Calculated regression lines have been added but without the accompanying equation or 95% confidence limits.

G71

3. G71 uses the full registration period. Again there is considerable variation in the change in coronary-event rates of populations for any given change in risk factor, without any clear overall pattern. Gradients are rather flat or even negative in the case of body mass index, but five of the eight graphs show a positive gradient for the regression line. In each risk-factor plot the majority of populations show a trend in one direction (usually decreasing). The regression line may be strongly influenced by one or two outlying populations at the other extreme (increasing, but with body mass index, reversed).

G72

4. G72 uses the lagged (= delayed) registration period explained in the notes on G70 and shown in G8. The pattern of the scatter plots and the associated regression lines do change but not in a consistent manner. These graphs should be studied in association with MONICA Publication 38 (*2*) where the contribution of each individual risk factor is estimated in the tables. There is detailed discussion of how the manuscript group interpreted the results in the paper. There were contributions from others in the subsequent correspondence and citations that followed it. Technical information is found in the appendix on the MONICA Website and CD-ROM (*1*). See MONICA Web Publication 20.

1. **See Monograph CD-ROM or MONICA Website http://www.ktl.fi/monica/.**
2. **Full references and summaries of MONICA Publications appear in #85/86.**

G71 First MONICA Hypothesis: change in coronary-event rates against change in individual coronary risk factors, full coronary-event registration period

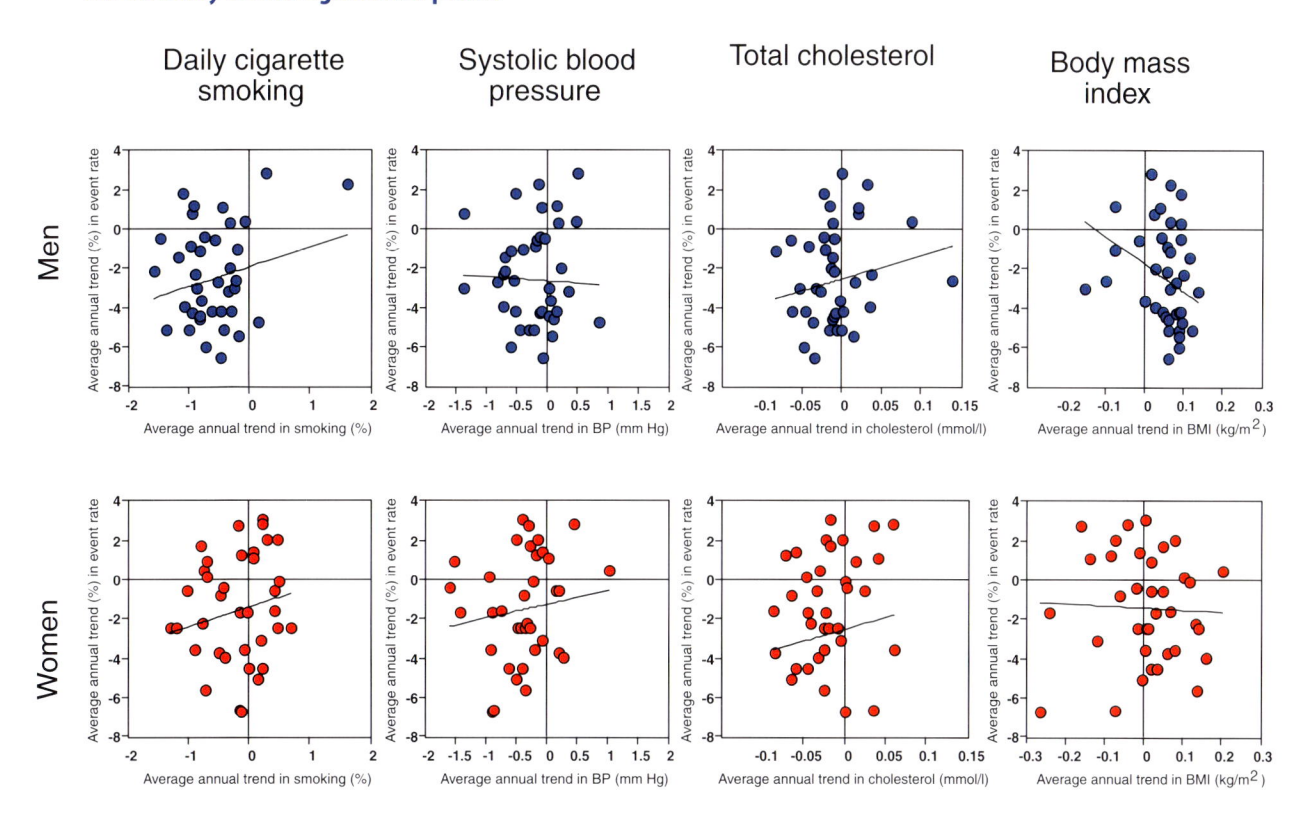

G72 First MONICA Hypothesis: change in coronary-event rates against change in individual coronary risk factors, lagged coronary-event registration period

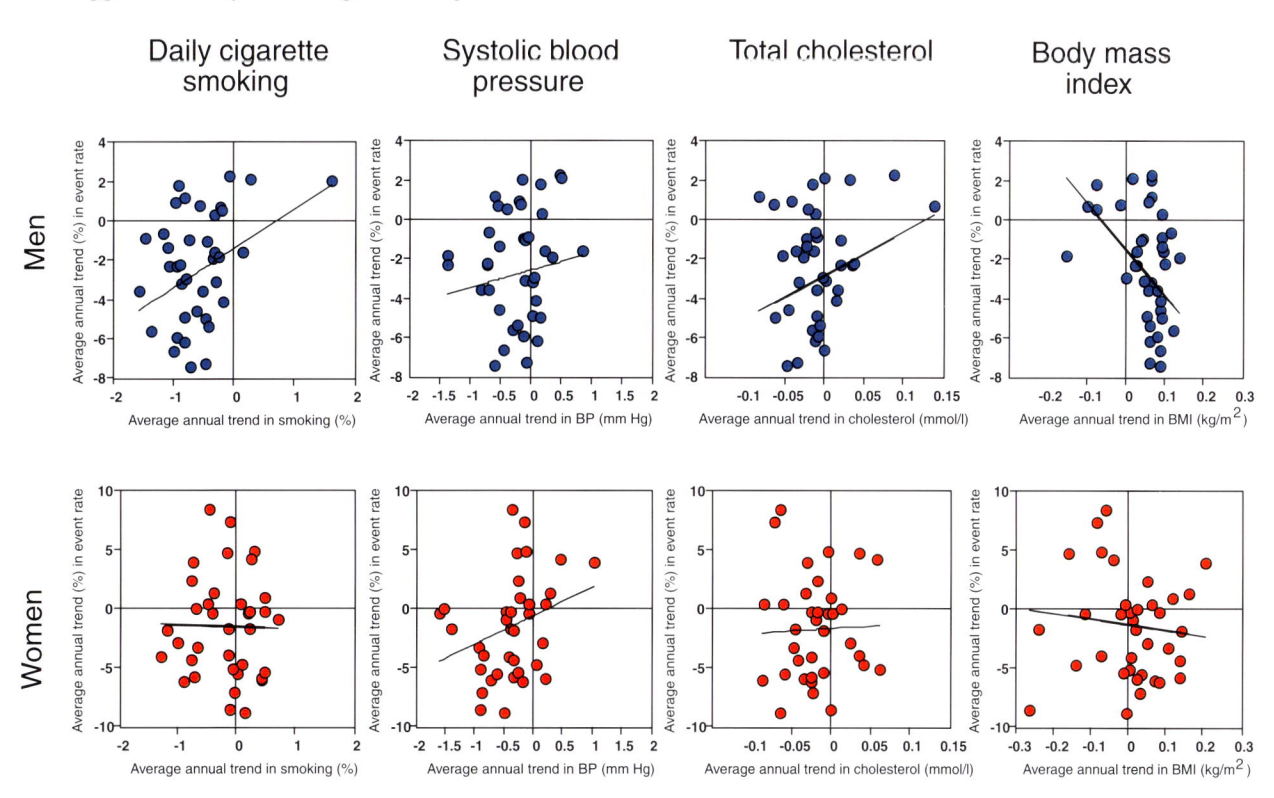

Hypotheses: stroke and stroke risk factors

Notes in italics are repeated to help random browsers—systematic readers should ignore them

1. *The next four graphs were plotted during the testing of the First MONICA stroke, or risk-factor Hypothesis, concerning the association between changes in cardiovascular risk factors and change in stroke-event rates. A manuscript containing these graphs was in preparation for publication at the same time as this Monograph, linked with a technical appendix similar to MONICA Publication 38 (2) for coronary events and its Appendix (1), MONICA Web Publication 20. This analysis is very much in parallel with that for coronary disease. See MONICA Publication 45 and MONICA Web Publication 30, and also #2 MONICA Hypotheses and Study Design, #35 Risk-Factor Scores, #40 Statistical Analysis—relating changes in risk factors and treatments to changes in event rates.*

2. *Each coloured point in the plots identifies the location of a MONICA population RUA, showing how much its risk factors changed in ten years on the x-axis, and how much its event rates changed on the y-axis. Populations are identified in G73 and G74 by their abbreviated 2-letter codes in place of the seven-character identifications, one letter for country, and one for population. See #90 Appendix and #51–83.* The number of stroke population RUAs is only 40% of the number for coronary-event registration. The precision with which trends in stroke-event rates can be estimated within each population is limited by the numbers of strokes in the 35–64 age group.

3. A strong simultaneous relation between any change in the stroke-risk score, calculated from changing levels of classical risk factors, and related changes in stroke-event rates in the same populations would result in the MONICA populations being arranged along a gradient, or regression line from near the bottom left corner of each plot towards the top right. Calculated regression lines, their equations and 95% confidence limits are added to G73 and G74. Note that the scale of the y-axis in the stroke graphs is different from that in the preceding graphs G69–G72 for coronary disease. This distorts simple visual comparison of the gradients of regression lines, but not whether they are positive or negative.

G73

4. The analysis in G73 used the whole registration period. It fails to show any meaningful relation between changes in the risk-factor score and changes in stroke event rates in men as the gradient is virtually flat. At any level of change in the risk-factor score there is considerable variation in the trends in stroke-event rates. Results in women are different in that the calculated regression line shows a positive gradient. Both plots show little change in predicted stroke-event rates when there is no change in the risk-factor score. The number of data points is limited and it is possible to argue that results in both men and women may be being influenced by a small number of outlying populations. However, sensitivity analyses have not shown that re-analysis using different weightings for data quality scores, or omitting certain populations make a significant effect on the results of these findings, so they are comparatively robust.

G74

5. G74 shows what happens when a lagged (= delayed) registration period is used (see G9). The justification is that change in risk factors must precede a decline in stroke risk, perhaps by a number of years. A time lag was introduced for the beginning of the study period, but not for the end, because most of the final surveys were done at that time or after the end of the event registration periods. Results still show considerable scatter of populations. The gradients of the regression lines are now considerably steeper than in G73. That for women shows a more strongly positive or increasing trend with increase in risk-factor score. That for men shows a more strongly negative or decreasing trend with increasing risk-factor score. These results are contradictory and difficult to explain. Comparison shows that certain population RUAs had contrasting stroke-rate trends in men and women although their risk-factor changes were similar.

6. Interpretation of these graphs is a matter for discussion. The MONICA study was designed primarily to investigate and explore trends in coronary-event rates in male populations. For stroke results it was underpowered both in numbers of populations and in its ability to measure trends in event-rates with precision. It appears from these results that stroke risk-factor scores, used for estimating stroke risk in individuals, are less successful in predicting or explaining changes in the risk of stroke in whole populations. See MONICA Publication 45.

1. **See Monograph CD-ROM or MONICA Website http://www.ktl.fi/monica/.**
2. **Full references and summaries of MONICA Publications appear in #85/86.**

G73 First MONICA stroke Hypothesis: change in stroke-event rates against change in stroke risk-factor score, full stroke-event registration period

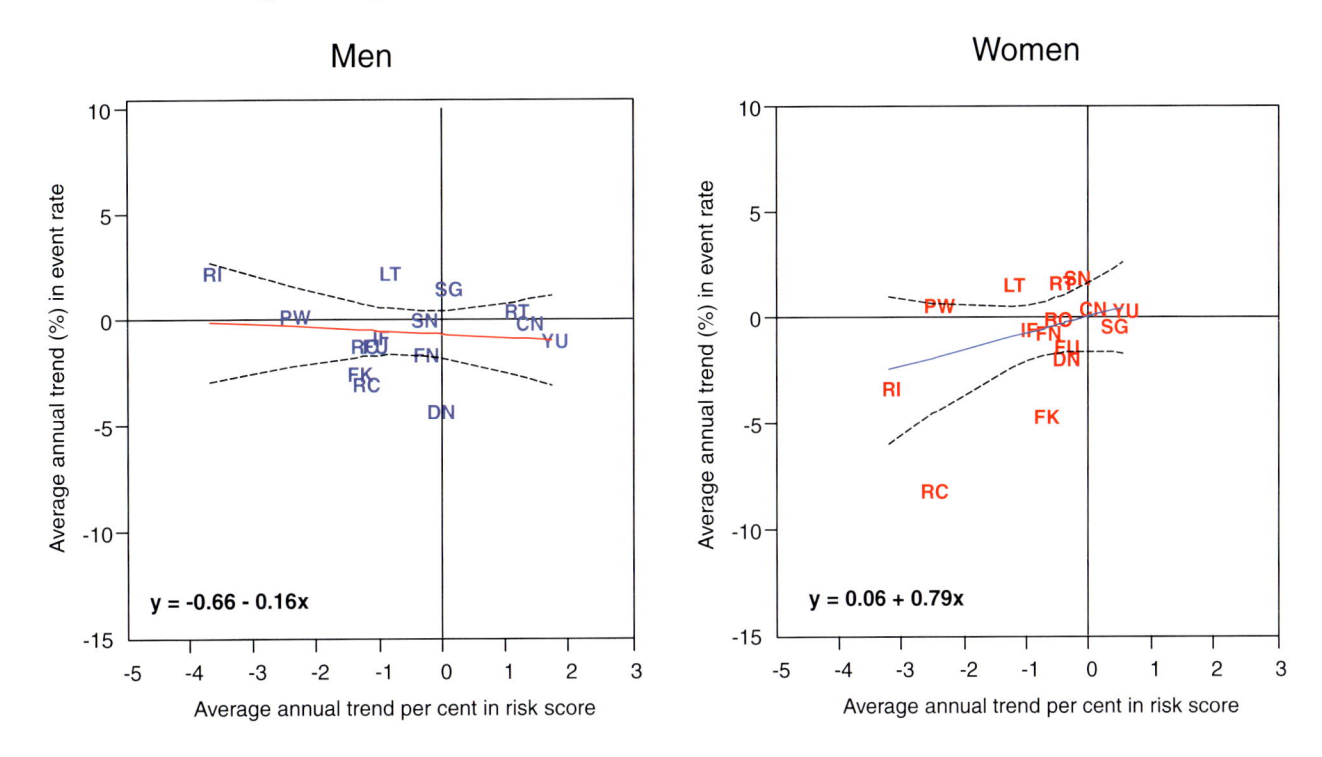

Men

$y = -0.66 - 0.16x$

Women

$y = 0.06 + 0.79x$

G74 First MONICA stroke Hypothesis: change in stroke-event rates against change in stroke risk-factor score, lagged stroke-event registration period

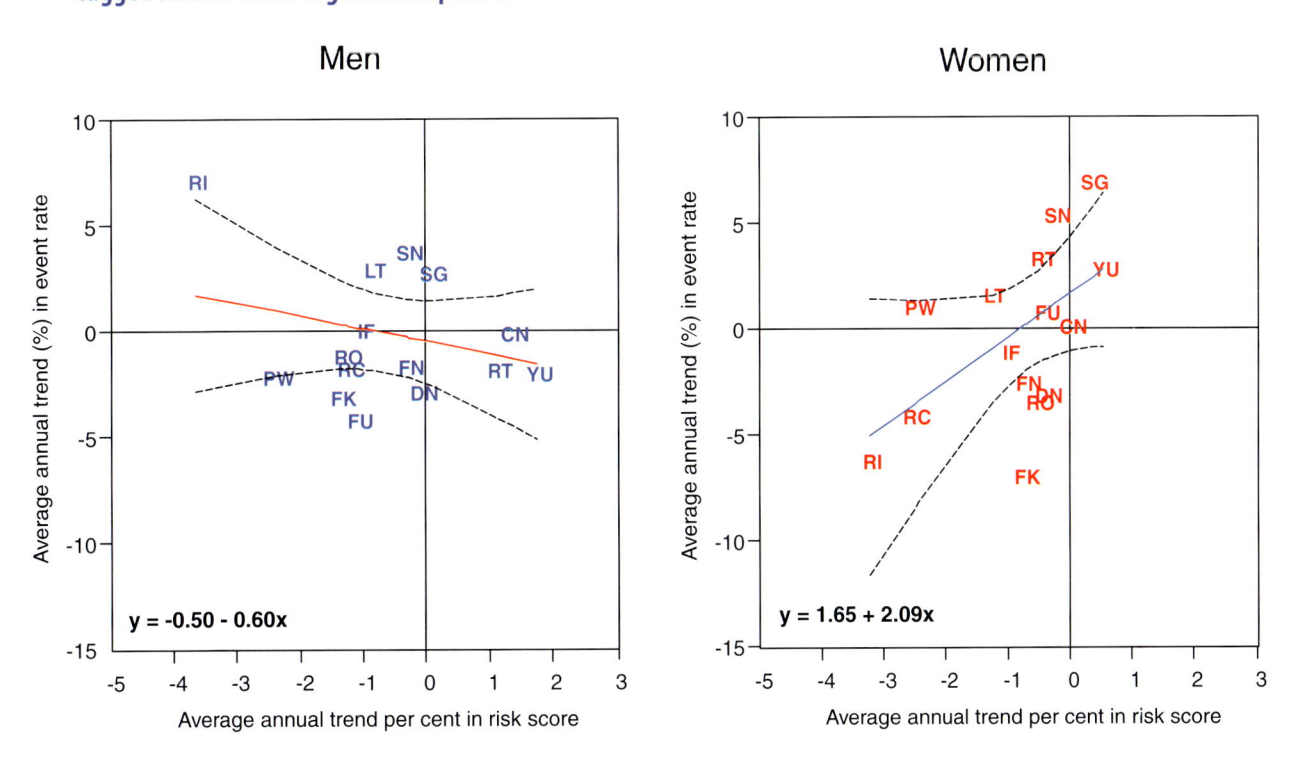

Men

$y = -0.50 - 0.60x$

Women

$y = 1.65 + 2.09x$

Notes in italics are repeated to help random browsers—systematic readers should ignore them

1. *These graphs should be looked at in association with the notes on G73 and G74.*

2. *Although related strongly to blood pressure stroke risk is multi-factorial, so the effect of one risk factor will be confounded and modified by what is happening to the others. The weighting of cardiovascular risk factors for a stroke risk score is different from that for coronary events. See #35 Risk-Factor Scores. G75 and G76 show changes in stroke-event rates in different populations, in relation to the change in single risk factors, without any correction for the effects of the others. Populations are not individually identified as they were in G73 and G74. Coloured spots are used to mark them. Because the same population results are used in each graph, their position along the y-axis will be constant for each sex and registration period, but the position on the x-axis will vary with the risk factor concerned.*

3. G75 uses the full stroke-event registration period. There is considerable variation in the estimated trends in stroke rates, as seen in the previous graphs. Change in individual risk factors does not seem to be an effective method of explaining this variation. The calculated regression line is virtually flat for three of the risk factors in men, and negative for the fourth, body mass index. In women there is a positive gradient for three factors, although weak in relation to the trends that were observed, but a weak negative gradient for cigarette smoking.

4. G76 uses the lagged (= delayed) period, explained in notes on G74 and shown in G9. There is no obvious change in the results in men other than that the negative slope of the calculated regression line in body mass index becomes more negative. In women, as in G73 and G74 the results are again rather contradictory. This is not surprising given the contradictory trends in some population RUAs for men and women for similar risk-factor results. Change in cigarette smoking shows no effect on stroke rates but change in blood pressure, total cholesterol and body mass index all show gradients in the expected positive direction. Of these the most important contribution, and the most predictable from the literature, is for change in systolic blood pressure. It is difficult to explain why there is no similar effect in men.

5. These results are a matter for debate. They are discussed in MONICA Publication 45. One contributory factor may be the geographical origin of the populations concerned. Changes in stroke rates occurred in eastern Europe at a time of severe economic upheaval unaccompanied by major changes in cardiovascular risk factors. These populations accounted for nearly half of those in this study.

6. For further information on the general problem of these analyses with respect to coronary and stroke events see MONICA Publications 38 and 45 (*2*) and the Appendices (*1*), MONICA Web Publications 20 and 30.

1. **See Monograph CD-ROM or MONICA Website http://www.ktl.fi/monica/.**
2. **Full references and summaries of MONICA Publications appear in #85/86.**

G75 Change in stroke-event rates against change in individual stroke risk factors, full stroke-event registration period

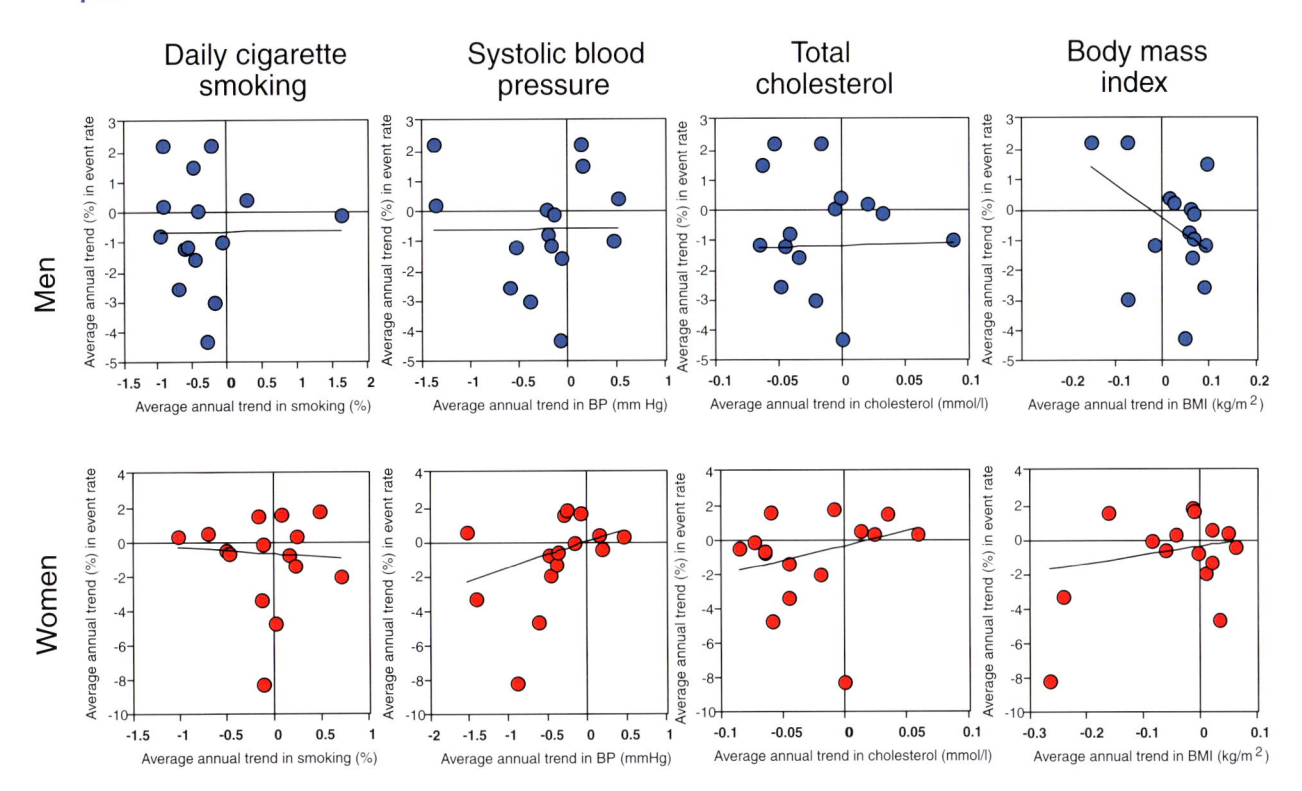

G76 Change in stroke-event rates against change in individual stroke risk factors, lagged stroke-event registration period

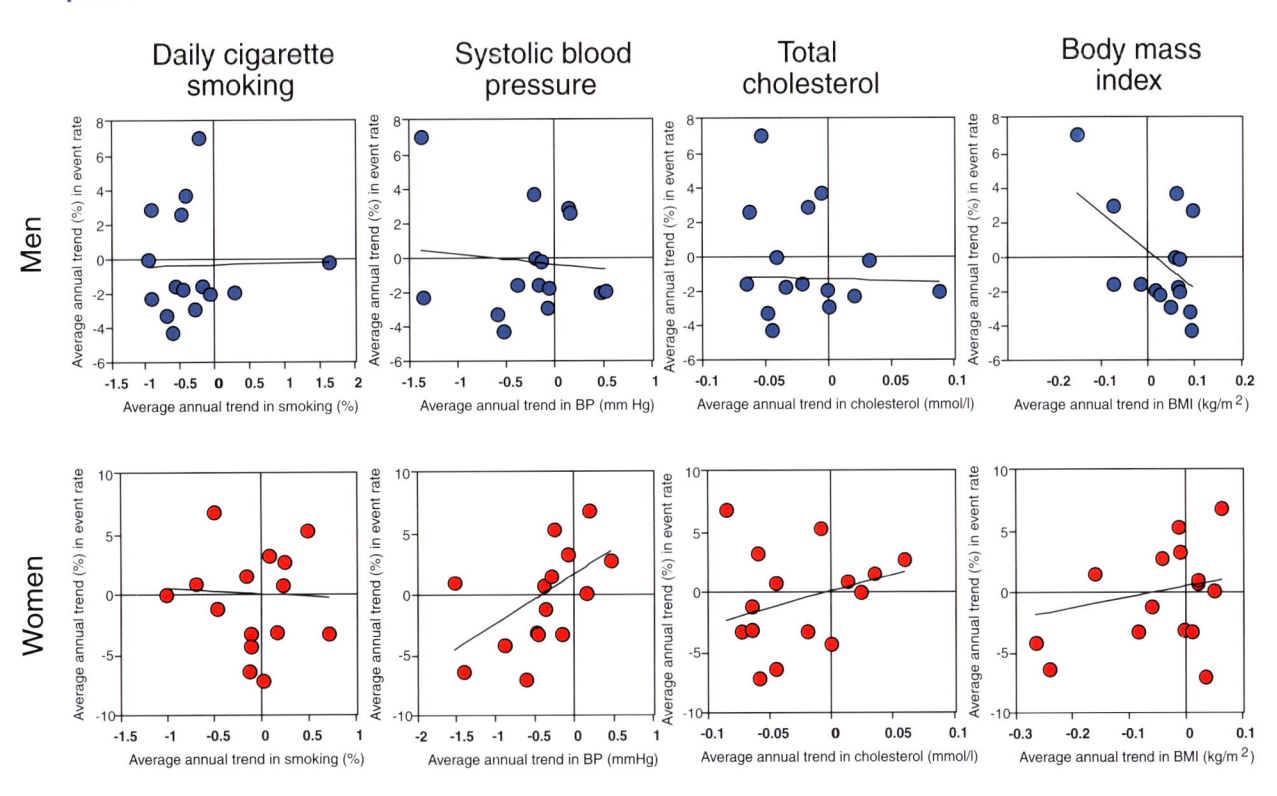

HYPOTHESES: STROKE AND STROKE RISK FACTORS

Hypotheses: coronary care

1. G77 shows the results of the analyses made to test the Second MONICA, or coronary care Hypothesis, relating changes in treatment of coronary events to changes in case fatality, and subsequently to changes in coronary-event rates and mortality rates. They were published and discussed in MONICA Publication 39 (*2*), and its methodological Appendix (*1*). See also the subsequent *Lancet* correspondence.

2. Trends in end-points were in G15, G18 and G22; in treatments and Equivalent Treatment Score in G57–G66. Populations are as for the latter (abbreviations on the following page); time periods as in G11.

3. The MONICA coronary care hypothesis relates increasing treatment with decreasing coronary end-points. If there is an effect, the fitted regression lines and equations (along with the 95% confidence limits) should show decreasing or negative gradients.

4. The original hypothesis was framed in terms of acute coronary care and 28-day case fatality. This is tested in G77a. Most coronary deaths occur out of hospital and are not treated in the attack. Analyses are possible to see whether it is the hospital or pre-hospital component of deaths that are declining—the latter would emphasize secondary prevention rather than acute care.

5. The eight evidence-based treatments we examined were highly correlated so we could not apportion responsibility for the observed benefits. It is even conceivable in this observational study of whole populations (an 'ecological analysis') that extraneous unmeasured factors might have been responsible. See discussion in MONICA Publication 39, and the subsequent correspondence and citations.

6. The manuscript group examined other coronary end-points. There was a significant association between treatment change and change in coronary-event rates, and a stronger one still for change in mortality rates. See G77b and G77c. The results are very strongly positive.

7. There is a relation between change in mortality and associated change in case fatality and coronary-event rates. (See discussion of G22 and G23). The original hypotheses related risk factors to coronary-event rates, and treatments to case fatality. The results of the initial analyses of trends in end-points, see G23, suggested that case fatality had less effect on mortality trends than did event rates. It was a puzzle therefore that new treatments are more strongly related to change in mortality rates than they are to case fatality—and that an effect of change in risk factors has been more difficult to demonstrate.

8. In retrospect it is not surprising that the systematic introduction of powerful drugs on a large scale by sophisticated health-care systems had a more measurable impact on coronary end-points than that of the population changes in risk factors, which were small and difficult to measure. In another decade results could be different. Risk factors are now under pharmacological attack.

9. Some MONICA populations had good information but most were unable to provide data for sudden coronary deaths on previous history and medication. MONICA as a whole could not separate first presentations of coronary disease, susceptible to risk-factor change, from disease progression where drugs for secondary prevention are important. Analyses in individual populations, although worth doing, will lack the power of the MONICA collaboration.

10. MONICA results on change in coronary end-points are polarized between east and west (see G24, G25), as are those for treatment (see G67, G68), complicating interpretation of their association.

11. Analyses for the MONICA First and Second Coronary Hypotheses, MONICA Publications 38 and 39 (*2*), are still to be integrated. It will be necessary to define population RUAs that can be analysed for both studies together, and plan how to cope with a time-lag for risk factors, but not for coronary care. New MONICA publications on this and other subjects will be listed on the MONICA Website as they appear.

1. **See Monograph CD-ROM or MONICA Website http://www.ktl.fi/monica/.**
2. **Full references and summaries of MONICA Publications appear in #85/86.**

G77a Second MONICA Hypothesis: change in case fatality against change in Equivalent Treatment Score

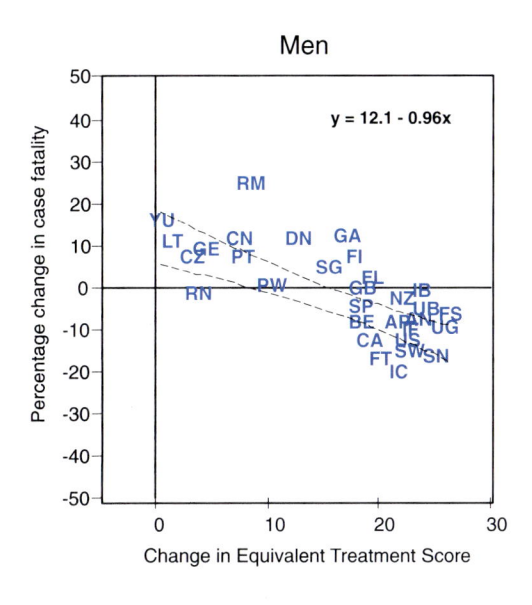

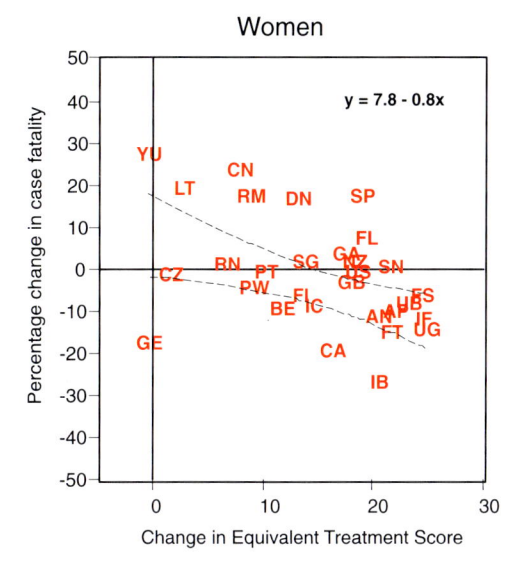

G77b Second MONICA Hypothesis: change in coronary-event rates against change in Equivalent Treatment Score

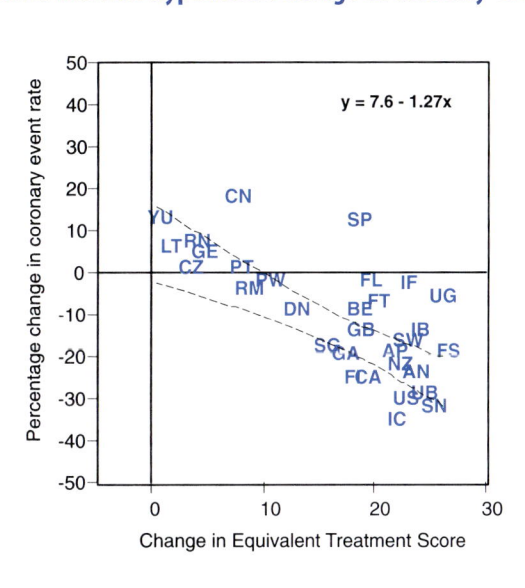

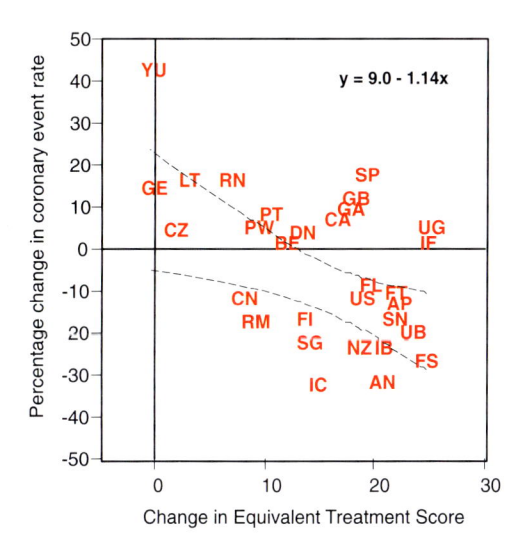

G77c Second MONICA Hypothesis: change in MONICA coronary heart disease (CHD) mortality rates against change in Equivalent Treatment Score

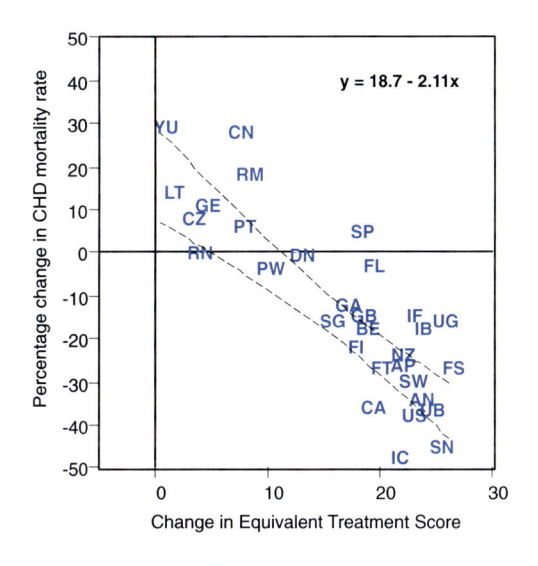

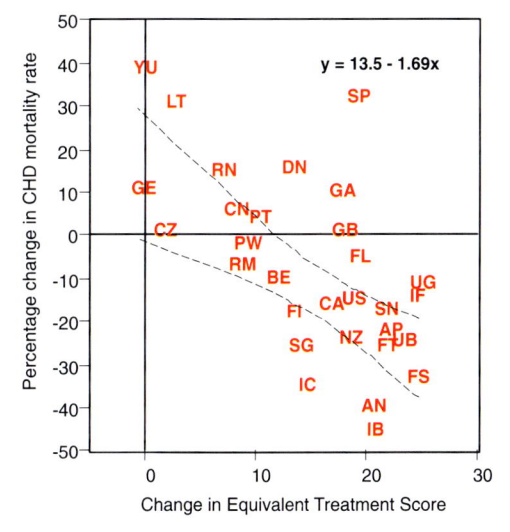

Appendix

Reporting Unit Aggregates (RUAs) used in different MONICA Graphics

Country	Population (RUA)	MCC	Abbreviation	Abb2	RUs	Graphics Numbers
Australia	Newcastle	11	AUS-NEWa	AU	1–5	1–8, 10–25, 36–72, 77
	Perth	10	AUS-PERa	AP	2	10, 36–56, 69–72
		10	AUS-PERb	AP	2–3	1–8, 11–25, 57–68, 77
Belgium	Charleroi	12	BEL-CHAa	BC	2	1–8, 10, 12–25, 36–56, 69–72
	Ghent	12	BEL-GHEa	BG	1	1–8, 10, 12–25, 36–56, 69–72
	Ghent/Charleroi	12	BEL-GCHa	BE	1–2	11, 57–68, 77
Canada	Halifax	15	CAN-HALa	CA	1	1–8, 10–25, 36–72, 77
China	Beijing	17	CHN-BEIa	CN	1	1–77
Czech Republic	Czech Republic	18	CZE-CZEa	CZ	1–6	1–8, 10, 12–25, 36–56, 69–72, 77
		18	CZE-CZEb	CZ	1–5	11, 57–68, 77
Denmark	Glostrup	19	DEN-GLOa	DN	1	1–77
Finland	FINMONICA	20	FIN-FINa	FI	2–3, 6	11, 57–68, 77
	Kuopio Province	20	FIN-KUOa	FK	3	1–10, 12–56, 69–76
	North Karelia	20	FIN-NKAa	FN	2	1–10, 12–56, 69–76
	Turku/Loimaa	20	FIN-TULa	FU	6	1–10, 12–56, 69–76
France	Lille	59	FRA-LILa	FL	1	1–8, 10–25, 36–72, 77
	Strasbourg	54	FRA-STRa	FS	1	1–8, 10–25, 36–72, 77
	Toulouse	55	FRA-TOUa	FT	1	1–8, 10–25, 36–72, 77
Germany	Augsburg	26	GER-AUGa	GA	1–2	1–7, 11, 57–68, 77
	Augsburg rural	26	GER-AURa	GR	2	8, 10, 12–25, 36–56, 69–72
	Augsburg urban	26	GER-AUUa	GU	1	8, 10, 12–25, 36–56, 69–72
	Bremen	24	GER-BREa	GB	1	10, 36–72, 77
		24	GER-BREb	GB	1–2	1–8, 11–25
	East Germany	23	GER-EGEa	GE	4, 17, 19	1–8, 12–25
		23	GER-EGEb	GE	17, 19	10, 36–56, 69–72
		23	GER-EGEd	GE	19	11, 57–68, 77
Iceland	Iceland	28	ICE-ICEb	IC	1–3	1–8, 11–25, 57–68, 77
		28	ICE-ICEc	IC	1	10, 36–56, 69–72
Italy	Brianza	57	ITA-BRIa	IB	1	1–8, 10–25, 36–72, 77
	Friuli	32	ITA-FRIa	IF	1–5	1–77
Lithuania	Kaunas	45	LTU-KAUa	LT	1	1–77
New Zealand	Auckland	33	NEZ-AUCa	NZ	1	1–8, 10–25, 36–72, 77
Poland	Tarnobrzeg Voivodship	35	POL-TARa	PT	1–2	1–8, 10–25, 36–72, 77
	Warsaw	36	POL-WARa	PW	1–2	1–77
Russia	Moscow Control	46	RUS-MOCa	RC	1	3–10, 12–56, 69–76
	Moscow Intervention	46	RUS-MOIa	RI	2	3–10, 26–56, 69–76
		46	RUS-MOIb	RI	2–3	12–25
	Moscow	46	RUS-MOSa	RM	1–3	1–2, 11, 57–68, 77
	Novosibirsk Control	47	RUS-NOCa	RO	3	3–10, 26–34, 36–56, 69–76
		47	RUS-NOCb	RO	3–4	12–25
	Novosibirsk Intervention	47	RUS-NOIa	RT	1	3–10, 12–34, 36–56, 69–76
	Novosibirsk	47	RUS-NOVa	RN	1, 3–4	1–2, 11, 57–68, 77
Spain	Catalonia	39	SPA-CATa	SP	3	1–8, 10–25, 36–72, 77
Sweden	Gothenburg	40	SWE-GOTa	SG	1	1–77
	Northern Sweden	60	SWE-NSWa	SN	1–2	1–77
Switzerland	Switzerland	50	SWI-SWIa	SW	1, 3	11, 57–68, 77
	Ticino	50	SWI-TICa	ST	3	1–8, 10, 12–25, 36–59, 69–72
	Vaud/Fribourg	50	SWI-VAFa	SV	1	1–8, 10, 12–25, 36–59, 69–72
United Kingdom	Belfast	34	UNK-BELa	UB	1	1–8, 10–25, 36–72, 77
	Glasgow	37	UNK-GLAa	UG	1	1–8, 10–25, 36–72, 77
USA	Stanford	43	USA-STAa	US	1–4	1–8, 10–25, 36–72, 77
Yugoslavia	Novi-Sad	49	YUG-NOSa	YU	1	1–77

MCC = MONICA Collaborating Centre, Abb2 = short abbreviation, RU = Reporting Units. Populations are described in #51–#83. See MONICA Manual Part I, Section 1, Paragraph 4 and Part I, Appendix 2 for description of Reporting Units and of MONICA Collaborating Centres.

Index

Numbers without a prefix refer to page numbers. They are in bold type where discussion is substantial and contains cross-references, for example, to relevant sections of the MONICA Manual, MONICA Quality Assessment Reports, or MONICA Data Books and to other sources. Prefix P identifies the subject of a numbered MONICA Publication (see #85, 86). Prefix W identifies a numbered MONICA Web Publication, see #87, also available in the accompanying Monograph CD-ROM Part 1. MONICA Memos are not indexed here but the listing in #88 can be scanned visually; alternatively you may search the listing electronically in the Monograph CD-ROM Part 2. Individual populations are not indexed here (see alphabetic listing on pages iv and v) and the population pages 91–128 are indexed as a group and not individually—their content is standardized (see #50) but varies as to local research interests and continuing activity.

A

ACE (Angiotensin converting enzyme) inhibitors, 50, **220–21**
Acute coronary care, *see* Coronary care
Acute myocardial infarction (AMI), *see* Myocardial infarction
Age standardization, xviii, 73, **75–76**, 81, 170, 174, 184, 186, 194, W6
Ambulance services, 37
Angina pectoris, 5, 42, 48, 216
Anonymity, *see* Confidentiality
Antioxidant vitamins, 19, 85
Antiplatelet drugs, 50, **218–19**, W17
Archiving, 13
ARIC (Atherosclerosis Risk in Communities) Study, xii, 20
Aspirin *see* Antiplatelet drugs
Attack rate, xviii, 4
Authorship, 79
Autopsy, *see* Post-mortem

B

Background, 1
Beta blockers, 50, **216–17**
Bethesda conference, xii, **2**, 30
Bias, 36, 57, 59
BIOMED programme, ix, 14
Blood cholesterol, *see* Cholesterol
Blood pressure, *and see* Risk Factors, 1, 4, **62–64**, 68, **198–201**, 230, 234, P14, P20, P31, W9
Blood pressure control, W15
Blood sugar, *see* Diabetes
Body mass index (BMI), *and see* Risk Factors, xviii, **66–69**, **206–09**, 230, 234, P27, P41

C

CABG, *see* Coronary Artery Bypass Grafts
CAD, *see* Coronary heart disease
Calendar years and dates, 91–128, 164, 166, W6
Carbon monoxide, 61, 194
Cardiovascular disease (CVD) *and see* Cardiovascular mortality, xviii, 3, **28–29**, 85, 160
Cardiovascular Diseases Unit, Geneva, 12
Cardiovascular epidemiology, xii, xiii
Cardiovascular mortality, 4, 35, 85, **160–63**, P1, P11, P17

Cardiovascular Survey Methods, xii, 2, 31, 61
CARPFISH, xviii
Case fatality, xviii, 4, 41, **72–73**, **76**, 174, 186, 193, 236, P16, P19, P29, P36, P39, P40, W24
Cause of death, 35, **160–63**
Centers for Disease Control (CDC) Atlanta, 65, 87
Cerebral haemorrhage, *see* Stroke
Cerebrovascular disease, *see* Stroke
CHD, *see* Coronary heart disease
Cholesterol, *and see* Risk Factors, xviii, 4, **64–66**, 68, **202–05**, 230, 234, P13, W10
Cholesterol awareness and control, W16
Cigarette smoking, *see* Smoking
Coefficients, 5, 67, 69
Cohort studies, 27, 83, 91–128
Cold pursuit, xviii, 26, 39, 164
Communications, 10, 18, 22, 71
Conference on the Decline, *see* Bethesda conference
Confidence intervals (CI), xviii, 77, 172, 196
Confidentiality, **23**, **26–28**
Consultants, 12
Coordinating centre, 9
Core data, 38, 60, 83, 127
CORMORANT, xviii
Coronary artery bypass grafts (CABG), 37, 50, **222–223**
Coronary artery revascularization procedures (CARP), 37, 50, **222–23**
Coronary care, coronary care unit (CCU), mobile coronary care unit (MCCU), xviii, 2, 5, **30–1**, 37, 48, 168, **216–27**, **236–37**, P39, W4, W21–23, W29
Coronary care hypothesis, *see* Hypothesis
Coronary death, *see also* Coronary event, xviii, 46
Coronary event, xviii, 17, 46, 72, **170–83**, **228–231**, 236, P36, P38, P39,
Coronary events: definition, **46–47**, P16
Coronary-event registration, 40, **41–49**, 164, P16, W2, W25
Coronary heart disease *and see* Coronary event, ..mortality xviii, 29
Coronary-heart disease mortality rates, 160, **176–83**, 236, P8, P16, P30, P36, P39
Cotinine, 61, 194

Council of Principal Investigators (CPI), 6, **7–9**
Cross-sectional analyses, 32, 62, 65, 83, 91–128, P1–P31
CVD, *see* Cardiovascular Disease

D

Data Book(s), *see* MONICA Data Book(s)
Data entry, ..format, ..management, ..transfer, 13, 27, 36, **71–81**
Dates, *see* Calendar years
Death certificates, xiv, 20, 35, 43
Death rates, *see* Mortality rates
Decline in mortality, 2
Defibrillator, defibrillation, 2, 37
Demographic data, 5, **36–37**, 72, 170, W3
Developing countries, 10, 20, 28
Diabetes Mellitus, xiv, 67
Diagnostic classification, criteria, 30, **43–47**, **54–55**, P10, P16, P21
Diastolic blood pressure, *see* Blood Pressure
Diet, 4, 19, 85
Drug companies, ix
Drugs, 2, 19, 48–49, 50, 88, **216–227**

E

EARWIG, xviii
Ecological analysis, 48, 77, P17, P26, P30, P38, P39, P45
Educational status, W14
Electrocardiogram (ECG), 16, 25, 30, 39, **44–47**
Enzyme(s), 39, 47
Epstein, Fred, 2, 4, 31
Equivalent Treatment Score, 50, **224–27**, 236
Ethics, **26–28**
European Commission, ix, xv
European Congress of Cardiology, xii, 31
European Convention on Human Rights, 26
European guidelines, xv
European Myocardial Infarction Registers, xiv, 2, 30, 39, 46
European Regional Office of WHO, xiv, 2, 9, 12, 30, 86
Event rate, *and see* Coronary, Stroke xviii, **72**, **75–76**, P36

241

Event registration, *and see* Coronary, Stroke, 17, 25, 40, **43–55**, P16
Evidence-based, 50
Exercise, *see* Physical activity
External quality control, **15–18**, 25, 39, **44–47, 53, 64–66**
Ex-smokers, 61, 194

F

Failed and failing centres, 12, 22, 32, 39, 127
Fatality, *see* Case fatality
Follow-up, *see also* Cohort studies, 27, 68
Framingham, xii, 1, 65
Fruit and vegetables, xiv, 86
Funding, ix, 10, 14, 20, 91–128

G

Genetics, 29, 91–128
Global burden, xiv, 29
Graphics, *see* MONICA graphics

H

Haemostatic factors, 19, 89
Health promotion, xiv, 29
Height, *also see* Body Mass Index, **66–67**, W12
Health services, 5, 17, **37–38**
High density lipoprotein (HDL)-cholesterol, xviii, 65, 83, W11
Hot pursuit, xviii, 26, **42, 164**
Hypertension, *see* Blood pressure
Hypotheses, xviii, **3–5**, 13, 49, 158, **228–37**, P38, P39, P45

I

Incidence, *and see* Event rate, 4, 5
Informed consent, **26–28**, 42
Internal quality control, 15
International Classification of Diseases (ICD), xiv, xviii, 35

K

KTL (National Public Health Institute, Finland), *and see* MONICA Data Centre, ix, xiv, 14

L

Lagged registration period, 164, 166, **228–35**
Lipids, *and see* Cholesterol, 16, 25
Local options, 91–128
Longitudinal studies, *see* Cohort studies

M

Manual, MONICA Manual, xviii, **4–6**, 18, W1, CD-ROM
Manual(s) of operations, 9, 22, 39, 87
Manuscript(s), Manuscript groups, 22, 78
Marital status, W14
Medical care, *and see* Coronary care, 4, 37
Medication, *see* Drugs
Menopausal status, W18
Minnesota code, 16, 31, **44–47**
Minnesota Heart Survey, xii, 31
MONICA Collaborating Centre(s) (MCCs), 6, 7, 13, 25, 38, 91–128, **239**
MONICA Congresses, 8

MONICA Consultants, 10
MONICA Database, xvi, 13, 85, CD-ROM
MONICA Data Books, W25-W29, CD-ROM
MONICA Data Centre (MDC), ix, 6, **13–15**, 79
MONICA family, xvi, 33
MONICA Graphics, xii, xvii, 32, 80, **157–237**, CD-ROM
MONICA hypotheses, *see* Hypotheses
MONICA Management Centre (MMC), 6, **11–13**
MONICA Manual, *see* Manual
MONICA Memos, 7, 23, 32, 38, **148–156**, CD-ROM Part 2
MONICA Monograph, xvi, 8
MONICA naming, 4, 31
MONICA Protocol, 2, 8, 3–5, 32, 158, P2, **W1**, CD-ROM
MONICA Publications, **78–79**, **129–47**
MONICA Quality assessment reports, 15, 26, 37, 57, 60, 63, 77, 164, **W2–W18**
MONICA Quality Control Centre(s) (MQCs), 6, **15–18**, 25
  for Lipid Measurement, 16, 25
  for ECG Coding, 16, 25
  for Event Registration, 17, 25
  for Health Services, 17
MONICA Reference Centre(s) (MRC), 6, 7, **18–19, 83–89**
MONICA Steering Committee (MSC), 6, **9–11**, 12, 23, 32
MONICA Website, 24
Monitoring, 3
Monograph CD-ROM, xvi, **244**, CD-ROM Part 1, Part 2
MORGAM Study, ix, 15, 91–128
Morris, Jerry, 30, xi
Myocardial infarction, *and see* Coronary event v, xviii, 2, 30, 42, **46–51**, P16
Myocardial infarction community registers, *see* European *ibid*
Morbidity, xiv, 3, P8
Mortality, mortality rates, *and see* Coronary, Stroke, xiv, xix, 3, P16, P36

N

National Heart, Lung and Blood and Institutes (NHLBI), ix, xii, 2, 8, 14, 20
National Public Health Institute, *see* KTL
Necropsy, *see* Post-mortem
Noncommunicable diseases, xiv, 12, 29
Non-response, 59
Null hypothesis, *see* hypothesis
Nutrition, 4, 19, 85

O

Obesity, 5, **66–68, 206–9**, P37
Objectives, *see* MONICA Objectives
Observer variation, 45, 63
Official mortality, *see* Routine mortality
Optional studies, 13, **18–19**, 60, **83–89**, 91–128
Organization, **6–19**
Overweight, *see* Obesity

P

Participation rates, *see* Response rates
Passive smoking, 60, 61, 83
Percutaneous transluminal coronary angioplasty (PTCA), *see also* Coronary artery revascularization procedures, 37, 50, **222**
Physical activity, xiv, 4, 19, 87
Pilot studies, 22, 39, 41
Pisa, Zbynek, 2, 10, 11, **30–31**
Polyunsaturated fatty acids (PUFA), 19, 85
Populations, *and see* Reporting Unit Aggregates, 20, 76, **91–128**, 158, **239**
Population demographics, *see* Demographic
Population size, 21
Population surveys, 6, 27, 39, **57–69**, 74, **85–89**, 166, **194–215**
Possible myocardial infarction, **46–47**, P16, P24
Post-mortem, 26, 43, 46, 47, 192
Pre-hospital deaths, 2, 41, 47, 73, 174, 236
Prevalence, **74–76, 194–211**
Prevention, *see also* Secondary Prevention, xix, **28–29**
Primary prevention, *see* Prevention
Progress reports, 38
Proportional mortality, **162–3**
Protocol, *see* MONICA protocol
Psychosocial, 19, 31, **86**
Publication(s), 32, 78, 84, 91–128, **129–47**
Publication rules, 8, 79

Q

Quality assurance, Quality control, xii, xix, 9, 13, **15–18, 25–26**, 30, 32, 36, 45, 47, 62, 64, 67, P4, P5, P13, P14, P20
Quality scores, 25, 39, 45, 63, 77, 178, 192, 214, 226, W23, W28
Questionnaire, **59–61**, 87, 88

R

Randomized controlled trials (RCTs), 48
Random-zero sphygmomanometer, 63
Rapporteur, xix, 4, **30–34**
Record form, **43–44**, 53, 59
Record linkage, 27, 91–128
Recruitment, **20–22, 58–59**, 127–8
Register, registration, registration procedures, xix, 6, 26, 39, 53, 164
Registration period, 91–128, 164, 166, **228–35**
Regression, 21, 69, 77, **228–37**, P44
Regression-dilution, 69
Reporting Unit (RU), Reporting Unit Aggregate, (RUA), xix, 21, 38, 158, **239**
Response rates, **58–59**, W7
Risk factor(s), *and see* Blood pressure, Smoking, Cholesterol, Body Mass Index, xix, 1, 3, 4, 5, 32, **194–215**, 230, 234, P3, P9, P11, P17, P30, P32, P33, P38, P43, P45, W20, W27
Risk-factor hypothesis, *see* Hypothesis
Risk-factor score, 5, **68–69, 210–13**, P12, P45, W30, P32, P33, P38, W20
Risk-factor survey, *see* Population survey
Routine mortality data, xiv, **35**, 72, **160–163, 176–79**

S

Sampling, 39, 57, W7
Sampling frames, 27, **57–59**, W7
Seasonal variation, 64, 166, W6
Secondary prevention, xix, 48, 50

Seven countries study, xii, 1, 31, 65
Sex differences, 69, 170–225, P23, P30
SI units, *see* Système International
Size of study, 21
Smoking, *and see* Risk Factors, 1, 4, **59–62**, 69, **194–97**, 230, 234, P27, P34, P42, W8
Smoking deception, 62, 194
Sphygmomanometer, 63, 198
Sponsors, ix
Spot maps, 165, 182, 190, 196, 200, 204, 208, 212, 227, 226
Stamler, Jeremiah, 5
Statistical analysis, 13, 77, P12, P15, P22, P28, P44, W20, W30
Strasser, Tom, 4, 31
Stroke, xix, 40, **53–56**, **184–93**, P18, P19, P21
Stroke case fatality, *see* Case fatality
Stroke diagnosis, **54–55**
Stroke event rates, **184–93**, **232–235**, P19, P25, P26, P45
Stroke hypotheses, *see* Hypotheses
Stroke mortality rates, 160, **188**, P6, P19
Stroke registration, **53–55**, 166, P5, P18, W5, W26, W28

Stroke sub-types, 54
Subarachnoid haemorrhage, 55, 192, P40
Sudden death, *and see* Coronary death, 5, 26, 35, 174, P16
Survival, *see* Case fatality
Système International (SI) units, xviii, xix, 198, 204

T

Telephone conferences, 23
Ten-day seminars, 2
Test case-histories, 17, 30, 39, 47, 53
Testing, 15, 25, 39, 44, 64
Thiocyanate, 61, 83, 194
Thrombolysis, 43, 50, **222–23**
Tobacco, *see* Smoking
Total cholesterol, *see* Cholesterol
Training, 15, 25, 39, 44, 64, 77
Treatment, 50, **216–27**, **236–37**
Treatment hypothesis, *see* Hypotheses
Treatment scores, **50–51**, **224–27**, **236–7**, P39, W22
Trends, 2, 4, 5, **72–74**, 158–237, P25, P36, P38, P39, P45

U

Unclassifiable deaths, 47, **176–79**

V

Validity, validation, 35, 36, 62
Venepuncture, 65, 202
Vitamins, *see* Antioxidant vitamins
von Willebrand's factor, 89

W

Waist circumference, **66–68**, P35
Waist-hip ratio, **66–68**, P35
Website, *see* MONICA Website
Weight, 4, **66–68**, P27, P41, W12
Weighted Treatment Score, 50, 224
World Health Organization Headquarters, Geneva, ix, xiv, 2, 12
World Health Report, xiv
World Health Statistics Annual(s), xiv, 65, 75
World Standard Population, 75
World War II, xiv, 75
World Wide Web, *see* MONICA Website

Introduction to the CD-ROMs

(This introduction predates completion of the CD-ROMs which should be consulted for later information)

Attached to this book are two CD-ROMs titled 'CD-ROMs for MONICA Monograph and Multimedia Sourcebook Part1 and Part 2'.

Contents of the CD-ROMs

The CD-ROMs include:

1. A copy of the basic MONICA documentation, which has been published in the World Wide Web (WWW):
   - the MONICA Manual;
   - all quality assessment reports of the MONICA data;
   - the MONICA data books, which present aggregate data for each population on:
     — population surveys;
     — coronary events;
     — acute coronary care;
     — stroke events.

2. Copies of other WWW-publications from the MONICA Project. They are appendices to papers published in scientific journals, providing methodological details or additional tables. The WWW-publications published up to December 2002 are included.

3. A screen presentation on "Things to remember when analysing the collaborative MONICA data". It highlights the differences between analyzing data from a single population and that from 30 populations, includes checklists for data analysis, and provides information on the definitions of variables and statistical method used in MONICA.

4. A description of the MONICA Archive which is a long-term store of the Project's data base. The MONICA Archive has been designed to facilitate ease of use of the data for scientific analysis by anyone permitted access to the data.

5. A sample analysis data set. This includes:
   - population demographics and mortality data;
   - Health services data;
   - Population survey data (20% sample for each Reporting Unit and survey);
   - Coronary event and acute coronary care data (20% sample for each Reporting Unit);
   - Stroke event data (20% sample for each Reporting Unit).

   The sample analysis data set was extracted from the 'basic analysis data set' of the MONICA Archive, using systematic sampling of the survey and event registration data.

   Each data component has an introductory text with references to the data collection procedures, the format and specification of the data in the data set, references to the documentation of the quality of the data, and the directory and name of the data file.

6. A slide presentation of the MONICA Graphics with a spoken commentary, taking you through section #89 *MONICA Graphics* of this Monograph, making this a 'Monograph and Multimedia Sourcebook'.

7. Scanned images of other MONICA documents not available as MONICA publications or on the WWW. These include MONICA Memos and similar documents filed in the MONICA Data Centre.

How to use the CD-ROMs

To use the CD-ROMs you will need a personal computer (PC) with a CD-drive and a WWW-browser. Insert the CD-ROM in the CD-drive and open the file "contents.htm" with the WWW-browser. You will get the table of contents of the CD-ROM, which leads you to the various documents and files or to further instructions. Items 1–6 (above) are on the first CD-ROM (Part 1) and item 7 (scanned images) is on the second CD-ROM (Part 2).

Kari Kuulasmaa